Reproductive Medicine for Clinicians

Volume 4

Series Editors

Joseph G. Schenker, Department of Obstetrics and Gynecology, Hebrew University, Jerusalem, Israel

John J. Sciarra, Department of Obstetrics and Gynecology, Northwestern University Department of Obstetrics and Gynecology, Chicago, USA

Liselotte Mettler, Obstetrics and Gynaecology, University Hospital Schleswig-Holst Obstetrics and Gynaecology, Kiel, Germany

Andrea R. Genazzani, Int. Soc. of Gynecological Endocrinology, Pisa, Italy

Martin H. Birkhaeuser, University of Bern, Professor emeritus for Gynaecological Endocrinology and Reproductive Medicine, Gartenstrasse 67, CH-4052, Basel, Switzerland

This series will focuses on and presents developments in knowledge and practice within all aspects of reproductive medicine.

It will help to cover the important gap between the new possibilities offered by the most recent investigations and technical developments and the application in clinical practice.

The series will be a useful tool for professionals and practitioners in the fields of Gynecology, Obstetrics, and Human Reproduction. Trainees interested in the most complete information on the developments of reproductive medicine will benefit as well.

This series is published in partnership with the International Academy of Human Reproduction (IAHR).

Andrea R. Genazzani • Joseph G. Schenker
Jerome Strauss • Domenico Arduini
Giuseppe Benagiano • Martin H. Birkhaeuser
David Vasquez Awad
Editors

Ethical, Efficacy and Safety Issues in Contraception

Springer

Editors
Andrea R. Genazzani
International Academy of Human Reproduction
Locarno, Switzerland

Joseph G. Schenker
Department Obstetrics and Gynecology
Hadassah Medical Center
Jerusalem, Israel

Jerome Strauss
Center for Research on Reproduction and Women's Health, Department of Obstetrics and Gynecology
Perelman School of Medicine, University of Pennsylvania
Philadelphia, PA, USA

Domenico Arduini
Department of Obstetrics and Gynecology
Tor Vergata University
Rome, Italy

Martin H. Birkhaeuser
Division of Gynaecological Endocrinology and Reproductive Medicine
University of Bern
Bern, Switzerland

Giuseppe Benagiano
Faculty of Medicine and Dentistry
Sapienza University of Rome
Rome, Italy

David Vasquez Awad
National Academy of Medicine
Bogotá, Colombia

ISSN 2523-3599 ISSN 2523-3602 (electronic)
Reproductive Medicine for Clinicians
ISBN 978-3-032-07321-1 ISBN 978-3-032-07322-8 (eBook)
https://doi.org/10.1007/978-3-032-07322-8

This Springer imprint is published by the registered company Springer Nature Switzerland AG
The registered company address is: Gewerbestrasse 11, 6330 Cham, Switzerland

Introductory Remarks

In 2022, the Earth's population surpassed 8 billion people, resulting in a call to action for programs to address family planning and women's health to maximize longevity and quality of life.

Contraception refers to methods and devices used to prevent or reduce the likelihood of pregnancy. The use of contraception varies widely among different populations, and it is influenced by various factors including health, cultural, social, economic, and educational factors.

This book offers an update on the importance of contraception and outlines the modalities that can be used to achieve target birth rates based on basic research and clinical studies conducted over the past 60 years.

Furthermore, this book considers the ethical and religious issues related to the control of reproduction and improvements in women's health from the point of view of monotheistic religions originating in the Middle East: Judaism, Christianity, both from the Catholic and Protestant points of view, as well as Islam.

Natural methods of contraception based on fertility awareness are examined and discussed; as well as hormonal contraception, including the molecules employed, their mechanism of action, routes of administration, and specific effects on the genital tract, liver, coagulation, cardiovascular system, bones, and brain.

Particular needs of patients with endometriosis, adenomyosis, fibromatosis are explored in detail, as well as the metabolic effects of combined hormonal contraception in polycystic ovary syndrome. The contraceptive needs of patients with benign breast diseases, breast cancer, and other cancers are reviewed.

Contraception was also analyzed for its benefits to women with menstrual cycle disorders, abnormal uterine bleeding, as well as in women who are postpartum, lactating, or experiencing premature ovarian failure or symptoms of perimenopause.

Progestin only contraception is also considered according to the different methods of administration: oral, intrauterine, subcutaneous implants, and intramuscular injections.

Contraception was analyzed according to its impact on quality of life and sexuality.

The brain as a target of hormonal contraceptives was also examined for the choice of the optimal combination of molecules for symptom management, as well as for their impact on migraine and other pain disorders. Furthermore, specific chapters are dedicated to emergency contraception and reversible male contraception.

This book tends with two important chapters on Sexual and Reproductive Rights for women and "in NO to violence against women" in the world, and on the importance of contraception to preventing women from Sexual Violence.

In introducing this volume, I would like to extend my thanks to the International Federation of Gynecology and Obstetrics (FIGO) for its support, as well as to the Scientific Societies that endorsed it (listed in alphabetical order): Associazione Ginecologi Universitari Italiani (AGUI), Associazione Italiana di Ginecologia Endocrinologica (AIGE), Associazione Ostetrici Ginecologi Ospedalieri Italiani (AOGOI), European Society of Contraception and Reproductive Health (ESC), European Society of Gynecology (ESG), Federación Latinoamericana de Sociedades de Obstetricia y Ginecología (FLASOG), International Society of Gynecological Endocrinology (ISGE), Population Council, Società Italiana di Ginecologia e Ostetricia (SIGO). Last, I would like to express my gratitude to the pharmaceutical companies that supported the organizing of the workshop, "Contraception Today," in Rome in March 2024, which served as the foundation of this Volume.

Declarations

Competing Interests The author(s) has no competing interests to declare that are relevant to the content of this manuscript.

Ethics Approval The author(s) declares that this manuscript does not include primary research with human participants.

The author(s) declares that this manuscript does not include primary studies involving animals.

International Academy of Human Reproduction
Locarno, Switzerland

Andrea R. Genazzani

Reproductive Medicine for Clinicians. Ethical, Efficacy, and Safety Issues in Contraception

Universal health coverage cannot be achieved without ethical access to the full range of family planning commodities as a health right [1]. These commodities are deemed as life-saving and address reproductive health needs that should be integrated in all programs related to women's health [2]. These assess the broader impact of contraceptive use on public health outcomes, including reductions in unintended pregnancies, maternal mortality, and abortion rates. Additionally, they recognize the value of family planning as central to sustainable development which addresses politics, population demographics and dynamics, socio-economics, culture, climate change, and environmental sustainability and partnerships. Health system factors such as the normative environment [3], competent, and motivated HRH address of shortages, supportive supervision, their turn over, and unbiased service provision [4]. Additionally, as family planning commodities are evolving and innovative technologies [5] are advanced, they need to find a total marketing approach [6] for stocking and supply logistics in to assimilate their access and commensurate with the development of necessary infrastructure, dedicated fiscal space [4, 7], capacity building of human resource, and programmatic monitoring cycles. Furthermore, we need to recognize whether demands are met, contraceptive prevalence rates are increased, and both total fertility rate and unmet needs are reduced. Contraception uptake ultimately enhances the resilience and cost-effectiveness to the health system, the individual, and the nation.

Individualized ethics include balanced counseling to make informed decision-making and informed consent, ensuring that individuals have complete and understandable information about the benefits, risks, and alternatives of contraceptive methods, and respecting autonomy and the right to make informed choices about one's sexual and reproductive health. Values and preferences preventing coercive practices in family planning programs, where individuals may be pressured or forced to use certain contraceptive methods, must be abolished and replaced by respecting the voluntary nature of contraceptive choice. Service provision includes medical eligibility and self-care, and regular conduct of monitoring and evaluation, accountability, and learning leveraging the strengthening of ethical contraceptive services.

Regarding access and equity ensuring equitable access (i.e., available, accessible, acceptable, affordable) and equity to contraceptive methods regardless of socioeconomic status, age [8, 9] race, and other inter-sectionalities or geographic location, the unmet need is most notable in LMIC, urban-informal settings, rural populations, and vulnerable populations such as youth, persons living with disability, persons living with HIV, and key populations. This addresses context-specific barriers that prevent marginalized populations from accessing contraception needs interrogation and acted upon. Emergency preparedness and response to contraceptive needs to include in the minimum initial service package (MISP) during humanitarian crisis [10], sexual gender-based violence access to emergency contraception, and post-exposure antiretroviral prophylaxis and commercial sex work include pre-exposure prophylaxis.

In 2019, sexual and reproductive health services fell short of needs in LMICs. Approximately 218 million women of reproductive age in these countries have an unmet need for modern contraception. About half (49%) of pregnancies in LMICs—[11] 1 million annually—are unintended. In 127 million women gave birth each year, and millions of them did not receive adequate pregnancy-related and newborn healthcare. In all, 50 million made fewer than four antenatal care visits, 31 million did not deliver in a health facility, 16 million did not receive the care they need following a major obstetric complication, and 13 million had newborns who did not receive needed care for major complications. Many women whose pregnancies did not end in a live birth also lacked services. In 2 million did not receive the care they need after experiencing a miscarriage, 35 million had abortions in unsafe conditions, and 9 million did not receive the necessary care for complications after an unsafe abortion [12].

Respecting cultural and religious beliefs and practices related to contraception [13–15], balancing respect for cultural norms with the promotion of individual rights and public health, engendering contraception with both the user and their partners meaningfully engaged in the processes promoting contraceptive uptake and sustained utilization, and understanding the effectiveness of different contraceptive methods in preventing pregnancy were typically measured in terms of perfect use and typical use. Methods such as implants, intrauterine devices (IUDs), and sterilization have high effectiveness rates, while methods like condoms and natural family planning have higher failure rates with typical use. Efficacy can be marred by interaction with other drugs, HIV [16], TB medications, gut microbiome, and clinical entities and contraception. Evaluating factors that influence adherence and continuation to contraceptive methods should include ease of use, side effects, and user preferences. Continuation rates vary among methods, with long-acting reversible contraceptives (LARCs) generally having higher continuation rates. More attention to drivers for self-care and service delivery points besides health facilities [17] needs further exploration [18]. Contraceptive efficacy contributes significantly to achieving global health goals.

Medical eligibility criteria is a critical step in eliciting the contraceptive best suited to the individual consumer. Individual comorbidities and identifying of common side effects associated with different contraceptive methods, such as hormonal side effects with oral contraceptives among patients with VTE, diabetes, or insertion-related complications with IUDs, such as translocation, and monitoring for rare but serious complications, such as blood clots with hormonal methods or perforation with IUDs. A thorough history with medical and reproductive clerkship, past performance with contraceptives and physical examination can be performed. This recognizes contraindications for certain contraceptive methods, particularly in individuals with specific health conditions (e.g., smoking and hormonal contraceptives, history of thrombosis). Tailoring of contraceptive choices based on individual health profiles and risk factors [19]. Evaluating the long-term safety of contraceptive methods, including potential impacts on fertility after discontinuation and long-term health outcomes and conducting ongoing research inclusive of longitudinal cohorts and post-market surveillance to monitor safety over time remain an unmet need.

Empowering individuals to make informed decisions by providing comprehensive information about the ethical, efficacy, and safety considerations of contraceptive methods a critical pathway in programmatic success. Ensuring healthcare providers are well-trained and motivated to offer balanced and unbiased information. Additionally, addressing the clients' myths, misconceptions, and misinformation.

Personalized care that tailors contraceptive counseling and options to the individual's needs, preferences, and health status. Respecting individual autonomy while providing guidance based on the best available evidence. Policy and advocacy that promote ethical practices, ensure equitable access, and support safe and effective contraceptive options. Engaging with stakeholders, including communities, healthcare providers, and policymakers, to address ethical, efficacy, and safety issues in contraception. Strengthening of service delivery points, data collection and evidence synthesis further informing the health system challenges, policies, advocacy, and programmatic impact.

Declarations

Competing Interests The author(s) has no competing interests to declare that are relevant to the content of this manuscript.

Ethics Approval The author(s) declares that this manuscript does not include primary research with human participants.

The author(s) declares that this manuscript does not include primary studies involving animals.

Kihara Anne-Beatrice

International Federation
of Gynaecologist and Obstetricians
London, UK

Partnership for Maternal, Neonatal
and Child Health – Health Care
Professional Association Contingency
Geneva, Switzerland

University of Nairobi, Department of Obstetrics
and Gynaecology
Nairobi, Kenya

References

1. Hardee K, Jordan S. Advancing rights-based family planning from 2020 to 2030. Open Access J Contracept. 2021;12:157–71. https://doi.org/10.2147/OAJC.S324678. PMID: 34531690; PMCID: PMC8438348.
2. Nelson AR, Cooper CM, Kamara S, Taylor ND, Zikeh T, Kanneh-Kesselly C, Fields R, Hossain I, Oseni L, Getahun BS, Fiedler A, Schuster A, Tappis H. Operationalizing integrated immunization and family planning services in rural Liberia: lessons learned from evaluating service quality and utilization. Glob Health Sci Pract. 2019;7(3):418–34. https://doi.org/10.9745/GHSP-D-19-00012. PMID: 31558598; PMCID: PMC6816810.
3. Hellwig F, Moreira LR, Silveira MF, Vieira CS, Rios-Quituizaca PB, Masabanda M, Serucaca J, Rudasingwa S, Nyandwi A, Mulu S, Rashad H, Barros AJD. Policies for expanding family planning coverage: lessons from five successful countries. Front Public Health. 2024;12:1339725. https://doi.org/10.3389/fpubh.2024.1339725. PMID: 38808004; PMCID: PMC11131167.
4. Nkhoma L, Sitali DC, Zulu JM. Integration of family planning into HIV services: a systematic review. Ann Med. 2022;54(1):393–403. https://doi.org/10.1080/07853890.2021.2020893. PMID: 35098814; PMCID: PMC8812772.
5. Hemmerling A, Christopher E, Young Holt B. Towards a roadmap to advance non-hormonal contraceptive multipurpose prevention technologies: strategic insights from key stakeholders†. Biol Reprod. 2020;103(2):289–98. https://doi.org/10.1093/biolre/ioaa092. PMID: 32639007; PMCID: PMC7401408.
6. Mozumdar A, Acharya R, Mondal SK, Shah AA, Saggurti N. India's family planning market and opportunities for the private sector: an analysis using the total market approach. Int J Health Plann Manag. 2019;34(4):1078–96. https://doi.org/10.1002/hpm.2753. Epub 2019 Mar 15. PMID: 30874332; PMCID: PMC6919306.
7. Mbachu CO, Agu IC, Ekwueme CN, Ndu A, Onwujekwe O. A narrative review of evidence to support increased domestic resource mobilization for family planning in Nigeria. BMC Womens Health. 2023;23(1):235. https://doi.org/10.1186/s12905-023-02396-y. PMID: 37149568; PMCID: PMC10164324.
8. Africa Gender and Media Initiatives. Robbed of choice: forced and coerced sterilization experiences of women living with HIV in Kenya. 2012.
9. UNFPA. The right to contraceptive information and services for women and adolescents. Briefing paper. Centre for Reproductive Rights; 2010.
10. Habtu Y, Kaba M, Mekonnen H. What do service providers in Southern Ethiopia say about barriers to using youth-friendly sexual and reproductive health services for adolescents?: qualitative study. Reprod Health. 2021;18(1):32. https://doi.org/10.1186/s12978-021-01092-0. PMID: 33563296; PMCID: PMC7871377.
11. IAWG. Minimum initial service package. https://iawg.net/resources/minimum-initial-service-package-misp-resources#:~:text=The%20minimum%2C%20life%2Dsaving%20sexual,within%2048%20hours%20wherever%20possible (cited on 22/7/2024, 10.00 am).
12. Guttmacher adding it up: investing in sexual and reproductive health. 2020. https://www.guttmacher.org/report/adding-it-up-investing-in-sexual-reproductive-health-2019 (cited 22/2/2024, 10.40 am).
13. Alomair N, Alageel S, Davies N, Bailey JV. Factors influencing sexual and reproductive health of Muslim women: a systematic review. Reprod Health. 2020;17(1):33. https://doi.org/10.1186/s12978-020-0888-1. PMID: 32138744; PMCID: PMC7059374.
14. Endler M, Al-Haidari T, Benedetto C, Chowdhury S, Christilaw J, ElKak F, Galimberti D, Gutierrez M, Ibrahim S, Kumari S, McNicholas C, Mostajo Flores D, Muganda J, Ramirez-Negrin A, Senanayake H, Sohail R, Temmerman M, Gemzell Danielsson K. Are sexual and reproductive health and rights taught in medical school? Results from a global survey. Int J Gynaecol Obstet. 2022;159(3):735–42.

15. Dune T, Ayika D, Thepsourinthone J, Mapedzahama V, Mengesha Z. The role of culture and religion on sexual and reproductive health indicators and help-seeking attitudes amongst 1.5 generation migrants in Australia: a quantitative pilot study. Int J Environ Res Public Health. 2021;18(3):1341. https://doi.org/10.3390/ijerph18031341. PMID: 33540735; PMCID: PMC7908584.
16. USAID. Evidence for contraceptive options and HIV outcomes (ECHO) trial. https://www.usaid.gov/sites/default/files/2022-05/USAID_ECHO_Fact_Sheet_Updated_Oct._2019.pdf (cited on 22/7/2024 10.15 am).
17. Juma PA, Mutombo N, Mukiira C. Women's attitudes towards receiving family planning services from community health workers in rural Western Kenya. Afr Health Sci. 2015;15(1):161–70. https://doi.org/10.4314/ahs.v15i1.22. PMID: 25834545; PMCID: PMC4370145.
18. Sigdel A, Bista A, Sapkota H, Teijlingen EV. Barriers in accessing family planning services in Nepal during the COVID-19 pandemic: a qualitative study. PLoS One. 2023;18(5):e0285248. https://doi.org/10.1371/journal.pone.0285248. PMID: 37146025; PMCID: PMC10162517.
19. Altshuler AL, Gaffield ME, Kiarie JN. The WHO's medical eligibility criteria for contraceptive use: 20 years of global guidance. Curr Opin Obstet Gynecol. 2015;27(6):451–9. https://doi.org/10.1097/GCO.0000000000000212. PMID: 26390246; PMCID: PMC5703409.

Contents

Part I
Ethical and Religious Issues Related to Reproduction Control and Women's Health

Chapter 1
Jewish Law (Halakha) and Contraception

Joseph G. Schenker

1.1 Introduction

Support for the regulation of individual fertility can be found in all cultures, and at all times, even in those societies in which social and religious rules have favored the abundant production of children. A variety of mostly primitive and ineffectual methods of contraception were used in many cultures. To this day, some peoples use very primitive methods of contraception. The first known medical application of contraception is found in an Egyptian papyrus from 1850 BCE, which portrays a solution introduced into the vagina. Another papyrus from 1550 BCE describes a cotton cork stopper used as a contraceptive device for many years.

Contraceptive knowledge had a written basis from the works of Aristotle in the fourth-century BC through a variety of Greek and Roman medical writings. The scientific basis for contraception up to the late seventeenth century was spread through Europe by Islamic physicians. Dissemination of birth control methods did not begin until the twentieth century.

Various contraceptive methods have been used for millennia. An extensive secular literature exists concerning the history of contraceptive methods. Equally ancient are the ethical, religious, and legal questions involved. Some methods of antiquity are still in use; others are no longer used; others have been modified and

Joseph Schenker—Presented "Contraception Today" International Academy of Human Reproduction. Rome, 6 March 2024.

J. G. Schenker (✉)
Department Obstetrics Gynecology Hebrew University, Hadassah Medical Center, Jerusalem, Israel
e-mail: joseph.schenker@mail.huji.ac.il

A. R. Genazzani et al. (eds.), *Ethical, Efficacy and Safety Issues in Contraception*, Reproductive Medicine for Clinicians 4,
https://doi.org/10.1007/978-3-032-07322-8_1

modernized; and yet others have been recently developed and continue to undergo change [1, 2].

Early Birth Control Methods from Around the World Included

- Condoms (external and internal) made of animal bladders, linen, silk, or plants.
- Spermicides made of acacia, honey, rock salt, or crocodile dung.
- Sponges made of moss, grass, or bamboo.
- Plant-based oral contraceptives like the Silphium plant growing in North Africa.

1.2 Religion and Medicine

Religion and medicine have been interrelated since the beginning of human history. The partnership of religion and medicine has not always been either holy or healthy. Medicine, for its part, is related to religion in its emphasis on the supreme values of human life and health and through its assistance in the development of medical services.

1.3 The Jewish Law—Halakha

Halakha—the word is derived from the Hebrew root that means "to go or to walk"—is the collective body of Jewish religious law, including the biblical written law (the 613 mitzvot, or commandments), Torah, and the later Talmudic and rabbinic oral law as customs and traditions [3].

Torah—the foundation of the Written Law—the first five books of the Scripture, is the origin of authority. This definition is derived from the ancient tradition and the belief concerning the original revelation on Mount Sinai, when God Gave the Torah to Moses and to the Jewish people, the recipients. The Torah is not an ordinary text of law. It is an expression of God's revelation, teaching, and guidance for man, which includes moral values as well as practical laws.

The Oral Law—interprets, expands, and elucidates the written Torah—establishes new rules and customs. The authority is derived from the written Torah. The dominant parts of the Oral Law are as follows [4]:

1. *The Mishnah*—consists of six major sections (orders) that cover all aspects of human life. The final form was established early in the third century.
2. *The Talmud*—for approximately three centuries after the final compilation of the Mishnah, the great interpreters studied the six orders of the Mishnah and wrote a monumental composition, the Talmud.

   The great interpreters (Amoraim) included within the Talmud commentaries and interpretative studies of the Mishnah and the Midrashim, and established regulations and new customs. The Amoraim in Babylon composed the Babylonian Talmud, while the Amoraim in the Holy Land composed the Jerusalem Talmud.

During the period of Jewish sovereignty in Judea, laws were made by the Sanhedrin, a body of 71 leaders gathered for this purpose, and by local courts with 23 judges. After the fall of the Second Temple, Halakha became primarily the creation of rabbinic literature.

3. *The post-Talmudic codes* were compiled with the intention of assisting access to the laws, regulations, and customs of the Talmudic Halakha. Up to the sixteenth century, different scholars summarized and reviewed the Halakhic conclusions of the Talmud in the post-Talmudic codes. Among the scholars were Rashi (1040–1105), Rabbi Moshe Ben Nachman (1195–1270), and Rabbi Menachen Ben Shlomo Hameiri (1249–1316). The most prominent post-Talmudic codes are the Sheilot, Halakhot, Maimonides, the Piskey Harosh, and the Shulchan Aruch.
4. *The Responsa* is a term usually confined to written replies given to questions on all aspects of Jewish law by qualified authorities from the time of the later Geonim to the present day.

For thousands of years, Halakah has been the main legal and ritual source of the religion and ethical life of Jews. As their circumstances have changed, it has been reinterpreted and made relevant to current science. Although Judaism acknowledges the continuous development of the Halakah, interpretation and discussion are still being pursued by rabbinical studies. On the one hand, Jewish law regards both the study and practice of medicine as a duty and a religious obligation. On the other hand, from a practical point of view, conflicts occasionally arise between Halakah and medicine.

There is no central authority in Judaism. Jews believe that there is a single God who not only created the universe, but with whom every Jew can have an individual and personal relationship. Different communities and individuals pick and choose different rabbinic authority. Rabbinic authority in Judaism relates to the theological and communal authority attributed to rabbis, who serve the Jewish community.

In addition to answering questions about Jewish law and rituals, a congregational rabbi may often be consulted for advice on personal matters. Permission for use of contraception is carefully considered for each individual couple by a Halakhic authority.

1.4 Halakha and Reproduction [5]

The Jewish faith is greatly concerned with reproduction, and the Jewish precepts are found in Talmudic commentaries, law codes, moral tracts, and above all in rabbinical literature.

The duty of procreation—"*Be fertile, multiply, and fill the earth*" (Genesis 1:27) [6]—is a mitzvah. It is the first commandment *given to man*.

In Judaism, sexual relations are a good thing within marriage. In fact, they were prescribed in two separate commandments of God. One was the commandment "*Be fertile, multiply, and fill the earth*" (Genesis 1:27) and the other asserts that a man must not withhold from his wife "her food, her clothing, or her conjugal rights" (Exodus 21:10) [7].

The fact that these were two separate commandments meant that a man's duty to have sexual relations with his wife was independent from his duty to propagate, and consequently, the duty to fulfill the woman's sexual needs continued even after the man had fulfilled the duty to propagate, that is, after he has begotten two children, one male and one female in accordance with the verse in Genesis "*male and female He created them*" (Genesis 1:27) [6].

1.5 Contraception Practice in the Talmud Period

Twisting violent movements by a woman after intercourse were thought to result in the expulsion of semen from her vaginal tract.

- Coitus interruptus. Based on (Genesis 38:8) [8]

  > And Judah said to Onan, go into thy brother's wife, and marry her, and raise up seed to thy brother. And Onan knew that the seed should not be his; and it came to pass, when he went in unto his brother's wife, that he spilled it on the ground, lest that he should give seed to his brother. Onan was killed by God for 'spilling his seed,' which is often taken as divine condemnation of coitus interruptus. (Genesis 38:8)

- Unnatural or anal intercourse is said by some to be the act of Er and Onan to prevent Tamar from becoming pregnant.
- Cup-roots—*cup of ikrim* composed of different herbs may cause sterility.
- Moch—contraceptive tampon. The tampon can be inserted before intercourse and serve *as a* mechanical barrier to sperm. It can be introduced after intercourse to absorb the sperm [9].
- The safe period—time during a woman's menstrual cycle during which conception is least likely to occur (usually immediately before or after menstruation).

The practice of contraception during Talmudic period is written in a passage called "The Beraita of the Three Women" forming the basis for Jewish teaching on contraception. It states that a woman may use a "moch" or "cup of ikrim" in three circumstances—where a pregnancy would seriously harm the woman: the woman is underage (age is not mentioned), pregnant endangers her health, or nursing (Yavamot 12b) [9].

1.6 Halakha Law—Criteria for Contraceptive Practice

The duty "*Be fertile, multiply, and fill the earth*" (Genesis 1:27) rests on the man, any form of male contraception or sterilization is prohibited by Traditional Jewish Law.

In addition, Halakha prohibits masturbation, emitting semen for naught, the destruction of semen (*hashata zera*) and castration.

However, some rabbinical authorities encourage male contraception when the use of contraception is important for the safety and health of the man and his partner. In this regard, these authorities prioritize human health and safety over the male's duty to procreate.

There is essentially no dispute in the Jewish tradition that contraception should be used when the health of the mother may be at risk, based on "The Beraita of the Three Women. It states that a woman may use a 'moch'" (*a contraceptive—tampon, device* as in Yavamot 12b) [9].

Economic difficulties and inconveniences of raising children are not indications for the practice of birth control.

Criteria for Choosing a Contraceptive Method

- It should be without medical side effects.
- It should be effective.
- It should be reversible.
- It should be easy to use.
- It should not interfere with normal sexual relations.

1.7 Natural Contraceptive Methods

- Twisting violent movements by a woman after intercourse—*Permissible*
- Douches—*Prohibited by most orthodox authorities.* Anything that involved wasting seed.
- Abstinence—*Prohibited*
- Abstinence not only is the seed prevented from fulfilling the function of procreation, but also based upon the biblical commandment of *Ona* [8].
- In orthodox Judaism, intercourse and sexual pleasure apart from procreation are considered important in a marriage. A Mitzvah that obliges the husband to be attentive and responsive to his wife's emotional and intimate needs.
- Coitus Interruptus—*Prohibited.* Based upon the biblical commandment of *Onan* (Genesis 38:8). In post-Talmudic Codes, The Shulchan Aruch ("Set Table" is the most widely accepted code of Jewish law ever written. Compiled in the sixteenth century by Rabbi Joseph Karo, state that wasting sperm is considered to be a sin greater than any sin in the Torah).
- Safe period—*May be Permissible.* If it does not interfere with law of NIDAH and abstinence. *NIDAH*, biblically based in the Torah, prevent a menstruating woman

from having sexual relations with her husband both during menstrual period and for a period of seven "white days" following. The Woman takes a bath—*Mikveh* for immersion after the niddah period has ended.

1.8 Acceptable Contraceptives

Condom

Female condom refers to a plastic cup inserted into vagina and anchored by external ring. The first female condom made from a gout bladder was used over 2000 years in Greece.

The male condom was introduced by Dr. Condom in Europe, primarily developed to prevent syphilis in the seventeenth century. The rubber condom was introduced in the eighteenth century.

Accordingly, rabbinical authority's condom use as male contraceptive is *strictly forbidden "Emission of semen for naught."*

Almost all Jewish religious authorities would permit the use of condom to protect against sexually transmitted disease like HIV and syphilis.

1.9 Barrier Methods—Vaginal Diaphragm and Cervical Cap

Barrier methods of contraception are described in the Egyptian medical papyri, but only within the last 150 years, have they undergone improvements in shape, materials, and effectiveness. One of the most important advances of the nineteenth century is the development of the occlusive *pessary*. Two basic types of occlusive pessary are still in use.

The cervical cap, a small high domed device, fits over the cervix, and the vaginal diaphragm, larger, flatter, and disc-shaped. Both were developed by advances in rubber technology.

Rabbinic authorities disagree about the use of the diaphragm—some forbid it because it blocks the passage of semen, while others state that it is not forbidden because the semen enters the woman's body in a normal manner.

The barrier methods diaphragm and cervical cap based on the Talmudic statement is approved on the basis of the Talmudic statement "The BERAITA of three women." The use of "MOCH," an absorbent material inserted into the vagina during intercourse, was allowed for minors, in cases that pregnancy will harm seriously pregnant woman and for lactating woman that may affect the newborn.

1.10 Intrauterine Device (IUD)

In 1909, Richter described a "thread pessary," which rested entirely inside the uterus and was only for contraceptive use.

Years later, in 1928, Ernest Gräfenberg, a Jewish gynecologist in Germany [10] and Ota [11], in Japan 1934 reported their experience with intrauterine rings made of copper and silver. The device caused infection and was condemned by the German medical community.

The use of the IUD was stopped by Nazi—contraception—a threat to the Aryan race. Therefore, the practice of contraception was forbidden in Germany and Axis-allied, Japan.

Dr. Oppenheimer a Jewish gynecologist in Germany settled as a refugee in Jerusalem where he continued to practice contraception by insertion self-made silk-worm gut ring—IUD. In 1959, Oppenheimer published his 28 years of successful clinical results of 1000 insertion of silkworm gut rings in his patients who were mainly Jewish orthodox women.

Oppenheimer's publication [12] stimulated the reintroduction and development of different types of IUDs for contraception practice.

Lippes' plastic loop with a trapezoidal shape was first distributed in 1962 and quickly became the most widely prescribed IUD.

The mode of IUD contraceptive action is not established. According to our study, it prevents implantation [13, 14].

Most rabbinical authorities approve the use of the IUD because it does not destroy semen, does not interfere with normal coitus and sexual pleasure, does not prevent the fulfillment of the wife's conjugal rights, and is a reversible method.

1.11 Contraceptive Pill

The contraceptive pill was developed by Dr. Gregory Pincus with the support of American women's rights campaigner Margaret Sanger. Pincus, Rock, and Garcia tested the hormonal preparation of estrogen and progesterone on women, Puerto Rico study [15]. The first oral contraceptive pill, Enovid, was approved in 1960 by the U.S. Food and Drug Administration (FDA).

In the Talmud, there are several discussions of a so-called cup of roots. "Judith, the wife of Hiyya, having suffered agonizing pains of childbirth, changed her clothes and appeared before a Rabbi to ask a question 'Is a woman commanded to propagate the race?' He replied 'No.' And relying on this decision, she drank a sterilizing potion" (Yavamot 65b) [16].

Rabbinic authorities today seem to prefer the birth control pill as a modern cup of roots. It allows intercourse to proceed naturally ad unimpeded, allowing the fulfillment of the wife's conjugal rights. Also in the case of the pill, there is no "waste of seed."

1.12 Emergency Contraception

The term "postcoital contraception" commonly refers to any drug or device employed after intercourse to prevent pregnancy. The potential methods are insertion of an IUD within 72 hours of intercourse or administration of hormonal agents. The methods may be permissible since the mode of action is prevention of implantation. The method should not be is used as a routine method of contraception, since repeated use may cause medical complications.

1.13 Male Sterilization

Male castration is forbidden based on the Bible "You must not offer to the Lord an animal whose testicles are bruised, crushed, torn, or cut. You must not do this in your own land" (Torah-Vayikra 22:24) [17]. The Sages understand "You must not do this" to be a prohibition on damaging the reproductive organs, and "in your land" to be an extension of the prohibition to any male, animal, or human. The penalty for castrating is lashes. Based on the Torah statement, vasectomy is forbidden.

1.14 Female Sterilization

Female sterilization is the most widely used contraceptive method in the world today mainly practiced in the developing world to prevent population explosion. Tubal ligation, a permanent birth control method (which may be reversible), is available to women who experience difficult pregnancies and do not want any more children [18]. Most rabbinical authorities approve of tubal ligation. Others say that since the surgical procedure damages the reproductive organs (fallopian tubes), it is prohibited. As long as it is possible for a woman to take hormonal preparations or wear an IUD, tubal ligation is prohibited.

1.15 Jewish Religious Movement (Dominations)

Different groups have developed among Jews from ancient times and especially in the modern era. The Orthodox, Reform, and Conservative movements are the three major ones today. Orthodoxy is the only movement formally and legally recognized by the State of Israel. Non-Orthodox movements have remained largely a feature of Judaism in the Diaspora.

1.16 Reform Judaism

Reform Judaism is a religious movement that has modified or abandoned many traditional Jewish beliefs and practices in an effort to adapt Judaism to the modern world.

Originating in Germany in 1809, it spread to the United States in the 1840s under the leadership of Rabbi Mayer Wise. Reform Judaism gained ground with the children and grandchildren of these immigrants, especially in the 1930s among refugees from Nazi Europe. Reform Judaism responds to a growing desire among non-Orthodox Jews for some traditional practices; responding to this, they introduced ritual into synagogue services and home observances.

Many of the changes in Reform Judaism have to do with women's participation in public worship and in religious affairs. First, women are permitted to become rabbis. Second Reform synagogues have mixed seating, as distinct from segregation during Orthodox worship. In Orthodox congregations' women are located behind a mechitza, or curtain. Third, women in Reform Judaism can be honored in the synagogue and called up to read from the Torah. Girls have bat mitzvah and women may wear a tallit, or prayer shawl, and be included on synagogue boards of management.

Reform Judaism does not observe daily public worship, strict dietary laws, or the restriction of normal activities on the Sabbath. The Reform movement first considered questions of the new treatment of infertility, IVF.

Reform Judaism has generally been the most liberal with regard to birth control, allowing individual followers to use their own judgment in what, if any, birth control methods they might wish to employ.

1.17 Conservative Judaism

The Conservative movement developed in Europe and the United States in the 1800 as Jews reacted to the changes brought about by the Jewish emancipation and as a reaction not to Orthodox Judaism but to Reform Judaism, which was increasingly felt to be abandoning too many of the tenets of traditional Judaism. The time of Conservative Judaism's greatest expansion was during and after the horrors of World War II, which led many Jews to reidentify with some form of religion.

From its earliest day, the Conservative movement showed a willingness to respond to contemporary issues, which attracted increasing numbers followers the majority of whom were not committed to rigid observance of Halakha.

Conservative Judaism has generally been liberal with regard to contraceptive practice allowing individual followers to use their own judgment s to what, if any, birth control method they might wish to employ. Individuals may address the Rabi for consultation.

Declarations

Competing Interests The author(s) has no competing interests to declare that are relevant to the content of this manuscript.

Ethics Approval The author(s) declares that this manuscript does not include primary research with human participants.

The author(s) declares that this manuscript does not include primary studies involving animals.

References

1. Encyclopedia Britanica. History of birth control. https://www.britannica.com/science/birth-control/History-of-birth-control
2. Schenker JG, Rabenou V. Contraception: traditional and religious attitudes. Eur J Obstet Gynecol Reprod Biol. 1993;49:15–8.
3. Schenker JG, Halperin M. Jewish family practice and their evolution. Glob Bioeth. 1995;8(1–3):35.
4. Schenker JG. Women's reproductive health: monotheistic religions perspectives. Int J Gynaecol Obstet. 2000;70(1):77–86.
5. Schenker JG. Assisted reproductive technology: perspectives in Halakha (Jewish religious law). Reprod Biomed Online. 2008;17(Suppl 3):17–24.
6. Bible – Genesis 1:27.
7. Bible – Exodus 21:10.
8. Bible – Genesis 38:8.
9. Babylon Talmud – Yavamot 12b.
10. Grafenberg E. Silk als Antikoncipiens Geburen. Berlin: Kurt Bebedix; 1928. p. 50.
11. Ota R. A study on birth control with an intrauterine instrument. Jap J Obstet Gynecol. 1934;17:210.
12. Oppenheimer N. Prevention of pregnancy by Gräfenberg ring method. Am J Obstet Gynecol. 1959;78:446.
13. Yarkoni S, Zer T, Schenker JG. Chorionic gonadotropin in women fitted with intrauterine device. Infertility. 1980;3(1):23–7.
14. Rozin S, Schwartz A, Schenker JG. Studies of the mode of action of intrauterine contraceptive device. Obstet Gynecol. 1967;30(6):855–61.
15. Rock J, Pincus G, Garcia C-R. Effects of certain 19-nor steroids on the human menstrual cycle. Science. 1956;124:891–3.
16. Talmud – Yavamot 65b.
17. Bible – Vayikra 22:24.
18. Fasouliotis JS, Schenker JG. Voluntary and involuntary sterilization: medical, ethical, legal and religious aspects. Ginekol Pol. 1999;70(8):558–72.

Chapter 2
Global Population Growth and Family Planning: A Catholic Theological-Ethical Approach to Responsible Parenthood and Socio-ecological Sustainability

Martin M. Lintner

2.1 Clarification of the Terminology

Before we go more deeply into the topic, I would like to clarify some terminology. I have already used different terms in the title and introduction, such as birth control, birth regulation, contraception, conception regulation, responsible parenthood, and family planning.

Terms commonly used in the 1960s and 1970s, particularly birth control or birth regulation, are now considered outdated and are no longer used in current discourse. In contrast to contraception, birth control or birth regulation not only includes the prevention of unplanned pregnancy, but also measures such as abortion with the intention of reducing the number of births. The term contraception, on the other hand, which continues to be used frequently, places a priori a negative linguistic emphasis on the prevention of conception, in contrast to conception regulation. However, the term contraception remains justified with regard to the methods used specifically in order to prevent pregnancy. This usually refers to the use of condoms, vaginal rings, barrier methods, or oral contraceptive pills, which make the sexual act infertile. Contraception also includes methods to bring about infertility by sterilization, such as tubal ligation in women or vasectomy in men. With regard to the so-called natural methods, which restrict sexual intercourse to the infertile period in a woman's cycle and which help to determine this period as precisely and safely as possible, it is more appropriate to speak of conception regulation or of family planning. Since the regulation of conception and of births as a whole is part of a parent's responsible family planning, the two terms "responsible parenthood" and "family

M. M. Lintner (✉)
PTH Brixen, Brixen, Italy
e-mail: martin.lintner@pthsta.it

A. R. Genazzani et al. (eds.), *Ethical, Efficacy and Safety Issues in Contraception*, Reproductive Medicine for Clinicians 4,
https://doi.org/10.1007/978-3-032-07322-8_2

planning" are those that will be generally used in what follows, although the majority of the ecclesiastical documents to which I will refer use a different terminology.

2.2 The Development of Catholic Teaching on Responsible Parenthood and Family Planning

The connection between global population growth and family planning has preoccupied the Catholic Church since the early 1960s. Indeed, a Papal Commission on this issue was created by John XXIII in March, 1963. The original task of the Commission was to prepare a Papal message to the leaders of the United Nations on demographic problems.[1]

However, it turned out that the work of the Commission, which after John's death was confirmed by his successor Paul VI, focused more and more on the question of the moral evaluation of hormonal contraceptives, which were being marketed for the first time in the United States in those years. After Paul VI withdrew this question from the Second Vatican Council, the Council Fathers did not comment on it. However, they took a stand on the question of which aspects parents should take into account when passing on life. They interpreted the task of transmitting and educating human life as participation of spouses in God's creative love.[2] Finally, they affirm that parents should form an appropriate judgment:

> Let them thoughtfully take into account both their own welfare and that of their children, those already born and those which the future may bring. For this accounting they need to reckon with both the material and the spiritual conditions of the times as well as of their state in life. Finally, they should consult the interests of the family group, of temporal society, and of the Church herself. The parents themselves and no one else should ultimately make this judgment in the sight of God. (*Gaudium et spes*, no. 50)

In the Encyclical *Humanae vitae* (1968),[3] Paul VI explicitly speaks of responsible parenthood. By this he means that spouses must consider various interrelated aspects. He mentions inter alia the biological and psychological processes, as well as the knowledge and consideration of the functions associated with them. Finally,

---

[1] See Marengo, Gilfredo: *La nascita di un'enciclica. Humanae Vitae alla luce degli Archivi Vaticani*, Vatican City 2018; Lintner, Martin M.: *Cinquant'anni di Humanae vitae. Fine di un conflitto – riscoperta di un messaggio*, Brescia 2018; id.: "From *Humanae Vitae* to *Amoris Laetitia*: 50 years of controversy over the Church's doctrine on Birth Control," in: *Marriage, Families & Spirituality* 24 (2018), 3–27.

[2] Cf. Second Vatican Council: *Gaudium et spes*. Pastoral Constitution on the Church in the Modern World (1965), no. 50–51; online: https://www.vatican.va/archive/hist_councils/ii_vatican_council/documents/vat-ii_const_19651207_gaudium-et-spes_en.html (01.04.2024).

[3] Paul VI: *Humanae vitae*. Encyclical Letter on the Regulation of Birth (1968); online: https://www.vatican.va/content/paul-vi/en/encyclicals/documents/hf_p-vi_enc_25071968_humanae-vitae.html (01.04.2024).

with regard to the health, economic, emotional and social situation, responsible parenthood means, according to Paul VI, that either, after careful consideration, a couple decides generously to have more children, or, for serious reasons and in accordance with the moral law, they decide to temporarily or permanently refrain from having more children (cf. *Humanae vitae*, no. 10). Finally, he appeals to the state authorities to solve the problem of population growth through a wise and forward-looking family and education policy that safeguards the moral law and the freedom of citizens (cf. ibid., no. 23).

Already the year before, in *Populorum progessio* (1967),[4] Paul VI had emphasized the right of the political authorities to take measures that decelerate the rate of population growth:

> There is no doubt that public authorities can intervene in this matter, within the bounds of their competence. They can instruct citizens on this subject and adopt appropriate measures, so long as these are in conformity with the dictates of the moral law and the rightful freedom of married couples is preserved completely intact. (ibid., no. 37)

Unfortunately, these statements from *Populorum progressio* were not subsequently taken to a deeper level and further reflected upon, because the controversial reactions to *Humanae vitae* overshadowed and dominated the debate. The history of the impact of *Humanae vitae* has largely been limited to the controversial discussions about the moral rejection of the so-called "artificial" contraception—including all methods and actions either before, at the moment of, or after sexual intercourse which specifically intend to prevent procreation (cf. *Humanae vitae*, no. 14). It is well known that many theologians and also bishops wanted to elaborate a more differentiated criteriology with regard to the moral judgment of the methods of family planning. This involves, for example, recognizing the fertility of the marriage as a whole, not just of the individual sexual act, taking into account also the intentions of a married couple, and respecting the health and the physical and mental well-being of the spouses. As an example, I quote the Joint Synod of the dioceses in the Federal Republic of Germany, the so-called Synod of Würzburg (1971–1975), which stated in this regard:

> The judgement on the method of regulating conception, which in the sense of responsible parenthood belongs to the decision of the spouses, must not be made arbitrarily, but should be made in a fundamental mentality of willingness to transmit life and must include in the conscientious examination the objective norms presented by the Magisterium of the Church. The method used must not coerce, endanger the health of either partner, emotionally harm or impair their capacity for love.[5]

The Roman Magisterium of the Church rejected such considerations, which ultimately would not have condemned unconditionally the morality of the use of

[4] Paul VI: *Populorum progressio*. Encyclical on the Development of Peoples (1967); online: https://www.vatican.va/content/paul-vi/en/encyclicals/documents/hf_p-vi_enc_26031967_populorum.html (01.04.2024).

[5] Gemeinsame Synode der Bistümer in der Bundesrepublik Deutschland in Würzburg (1971–1975): "Beschluss Ehe und Familie," in: *Offizielle Gesamtausgabe*, vol. 1, Freiburg/Basel/Wien 1976, 423–457 (my translation).

"artificial" methods. One consequence was that the impression that the Church was against any form of regulation of procreation and family planning became more and more entrenched. This false impression has also been reinforced by the fact that John Paul II, during his long pontificate (1978–2005), focused very much on inculcating the normative teaching of the moral condemnation of "artificial" contraception. From a theological standpoint, it is important to acknowledge that the non-reception of *Humane vitae* has ramifications that extend beyond the Church's teachings on sexuality, family, and family planning. From a theological perspective, it is important to acknowledge that the non-reception of *Humane vitae* has ramifications that extend beyond the Church's teachings on sexuality, family, and family planning. It also impacts the authority of the Church's Magisterium, the infallibility of its teachings, and the role of the *sensus fidelium*, that is, the faithful's collective sense of faith, as well as the role of experience and dialogue in shaping the Church's moral teachings.[6]

Nevertheless, it must be noted that the Church not only did not forbid conception regulation and family planning, but in fact emphasized it as part of parental responsibility. This can be demonstrated with the aid of some passages in the *Catechism of the Catholic Church*,[7] which declares that "a particular aspect of this responsibility [i.e. to transmit human life and to educate the children] concerns the *regulation of procreation*. For just reasons, spouses may wish to space the births of their children" (no. 2368). According to the *Catechism*, various aspects are decisive for an ethical judgment. These include, on the one hand, the intentions and motivations of the spouses—"It is their duty to make certain that their desire is not motivated by selfishness but is in conformity with the generosity appropriate to responsible parenthood" (ibid.)—and, on the other, the methods chosen, which should not contradict the dignity of the person and must comply with the objective criteria of morality:

> When it is a question of harmonizing married love with the responsible transmission of life, the morality of the behavior does not depend on sincere intention and evaluation of motives alone; but it must be determined by objective criteria, criteria drawn from the nature of the person and his acts, criteria that respect the total meaning of mutual self-giving and human procreation in the context of true love. (ibid.)

As I have already mentioned, the Church's Magisterium considers that these objective criteria are to be met exclusively in the choice of the so-called "natural" method of conception regulation:

---

[6]As this issue is not subject matter of this essay, please see, e.g., Curran, Charles E., *"Humanae Vitae" and the sensus fidelium. On moral issues, the church must learn from the experiences of baptized people*, in: National Catholic Reporter, June 25, 2018; online: https://www.ncronline.org/news/humanae-vitae-and-sensus-fidelium (01.04.2024); Schockenhoff, Eberhard, *Die Nicht-Rezeption einer Lehre durch die Gläubigen als Chance: "Humanae vitae" als ungewollter Anstoß zu einem theologischen Paradigmenwechsel*, in: Birgit Aschmann/Wilhelm Damberg (edd.), *Liebe und tu, was du willst? Die "Pillenenzyklika" Humanae vitae von 1968 und ihre Folgen*, Leiden NL 2020, 349–375; https://doi.org/10.30965/9783657760220_014; Thiel, Marie-Jo, *Réformer l'éthique sexuelle catholique*, in: Études, Février 2024, n°4312, 79–91.

[7]*Catechism of the Catholic Church*, second edition, Vatican City 2019; online: https://www.usccb.org/sites/default/files/flipbooks/catechism/II/ (01.04.2024).

> Periodic continence, that is, the methods of birth regulation based on self-observation and the use of infertile periods, is in conformity with the objective criteria of morality. These methods respect the bodies of the spouses, encourage tenderness between them, and favor the education of an authentic freedom. (ibid., no. 2370)

Under the pontificates of Benedict XVI and Francis, the emphasis has shifted from the normative evaluation of methods of conception regulation to their existential significance for spouses.

Benedict XVI, for example, said that it is very significant for a couple to know each other, especially the female body and its rhythms, and that a couple's relationship is characterized by this mutual knowledge. For him, the question of how a couple practices conception regulation is not primarily a question of the method used, but rather of a lifestyle and relationship style. With regard to the use of contraceptives, he said, without revising the teaching of Paul VI, that mutual responsibility is also a decisive criterion with regard to health.[8]

Pope Francis speaks of the "need to return to the message of the Encyclical *Humanae vitae* […], which highlights the need to respect the dignity of the person in morally assessing methods of regulating birth" (*Amoris laetitia*, no. 82).[9] However, he does not primarily address the normative evaluation of conception regulation methods, but emphasizes, on the one hand, that parents must form and examine their conscience in order to make a responsible decision and, on the other hand, that a social climate must be promoted that is life- and child-friendly in order to counter a mentality that is often hostile to life (cf. ibid., no. 222).

It should be borne in mind, however, that this doctrine of contraception has always been understood by the Church as referring to marital relations. The discourse on non-marital relations, according to the Church's teaching, must be approached differently.

Furthermore, in a recent document, members of the *Pontifical Academy for Life* in the light of a broader and humanizing overall approach argue for a rethinking of the permissibility of hormonal contraception and for overcoming the alternative between "natural" and "artificial" methods:

> As in the case of the methods, which already make use of specific techniques and scientific knowledge, there are situations in which two spouses who have decided or will decide to have children can make a wise choice in a specific case which, without contradicting their openness to life, does not provide for it at that moment. The wise choice will be made by an appropriate evaluation of all the possible techniques in relation to the specific situation, obviously excluding abortion. These choices are far from the 'contraceptive mentality' and anti-natalism rightly criticised by *Humanae vitae* and *Familiaris consortio*. In the perspec-

---

[8] See Benedict XVI: Address to Participants in the International Congress on the 40th Anniversary of the Encyclical "Humanae Vitae" (10.05.2008); online: https://www.vatican.va/content/benedict-xvi/en/speeches/2008/may/documents/hf_ben-xvi_spe_20080510_humanae-vitae.html (01.04.2024).

[9] Francis: *Amoris laetitia*. Post-Synodal Apostolic Exhortation on Love in the Family (2016); online: https://www.vatican.va/content/francesco/en/apost_exhortations/documents/papa-francesco_esortazione-ap_20160319_amoris-laetitia.html (01.04.2024).

tive we have outlined, the alternative between 'natural' and 'artificial' methods should be transcended: the radical question is played out in the concretely possible forms of a generous and no less demanding responsibility for the gift of procreation.[10]

2.3 Moral Criteria for Methods of Family Planning

We can, therefore, state that the Church is in favor of responsible family planning through conception regulation and also in favor of appropriate measures to decelerate the global population growth. The Church defends the principle of responsible parenthood, which means that the parents themselves should ultimately decide in their conscience how many children to have and when to have them, taking into account various aspects such as the protection of the spouses' health and psychological well-being, especially that of the woman, as well as social and financial circumstances. Whether the magisterial position that "artificial" methods of contraception fundamentally contradict the dignity of the person and the objective criteria of morality can be justified in an ethically stringent argument, and plausible manner, is still controversial. Apart from this issue, the following fundamental aspects for moral evaluation of family planning should be mentioned.

The basic principle is respect for the dignity of the person, that is, not only her freedom and moral self-determination, her private and family life, but also her physical and psychological integrity, as well as her health. How many children a couple wants to have is their free (not arbitrary) decision and must not be prescribed by state authorities.[11]

Family planning is also a question of the well-being of the spouses and the success of their relationship, as well as of the well-being and flourishing of the already born and of the future children.

With regard to the psychological well-being of a couple, the effectiveness and safety of the contraceptive method has a major impact, especially for the woman, on how a partnership is experienced and how sexual intimacy can be lived, whether it can be freely and unconditionally enjoyed or is associated rather with the fear of an unplanned pregnancy.

An important postulate that should be emphasized at this point, however, is that family planning and the prevention of an unplanned pregnancy is the joint responsibility of both partners, of man and woman, and that the burden of this responsibility should not be shifted unilaterally onto the woman.

In order to protect the freedom and moral self-determination of a couple, and in particular of the woman, it is necessary that the spouses are comprehensively

---

[10] Casalone, Carlo et al.: *La gioia della vita. Un percorso di etica teologica: Scrittura, tradizione, sfide pratiche*, Vatican City 2024, 129–130 (no. 172) (my translation).

[11] See, e.g.: Schockenhoff, Eberhard: *Genug Platz für alle? Bevölkerungswachstum, Welternährung und Familienplanung,* Schwabenverlag, Ostfildern 1992; Leisinger, Klaus M.: *Hoffnung als Prinzip. Bevölkerungswachstum: Einblicke und Ausblicke*, Basel et al. 1993.

informed and educated, both medically and ethically, about the various methods. The aim must be to protect the health and the psychological well-being, to guarantee individual freedom and moral self-determination in the field of sexual behavior, and to prevent unplanned pregnancies. The crucial difference between contraception, that is, the prevention of fertilization, and the destruction of already fertilized eggs (e.g., by preventing them from implanting in the uterus) must also be emphasized, so that the mode of action of drugs and the mechanism of the so-called "emergency contraception" such as the "Plan B morning-after pill" after unprotected sex must be examined carefully. It should only be mentioned at this point that this argument is based on the assumption that a new human being has been created with the completion of the fertilization process and that this being already has undivided human dignity, including the right to life.[12]

In order to guarantee freedom of choice, comprehensive and non-ideological counseling on the various forms of hormonal and non-hormonal contraceptive methods, not only for women but also for men, is necessary. Improving contraceptive methods for men—in addition to the condom and as alternatives to sterilization by vasectomy—remain an unmet need, and there is still a lot of medical research to be done in this area.[13]

In this regard, it is interesting to note that in Germany, for example, there is a clear trend reversal in the choice of contraceptive methods in recent years. The number of women using hormonal contraception has continued to fall since 2020. This prompted the German Society of Gynaecology and Obstetrics (DGGG), together with specialist societies from Austria and Switzerland, to draw up for the very first time and present detailed S2k guidelines on non-hormonal contraception in January, 2024.[14] The guidelines for doctors on non-hormonal contraception is an interesting novelty. It covers natural family planning (NFP) and fertility awareness-based (FAB) methods as well as barrier methods that do not require the use of hormones. The use and effectiveness of non-hormonal contraceptive methods is discussed in detail, in order to provide couples with the best possible counseling. The guidelines contain recommendations that are based on current developments in society—for example, as mentioned before, the fact that condoms are now used more frequently than hormonal pills for contraception—and that respond to new sensitivities among couples, especially among women. Younger women in

[12] On the debate about the moral status of the Pre-Embryo, see e.g.: Shannon, Thomas A., Wolter, Allan B.: "Reflections on the Moral Status of the Pre-Embryo," in: *Theological Studies* 51 (1990), 603–626; Vorster, Jakobus M.: "A Christian Ethical Perspective on the Moral Status of the Human Embryo," in: *Acta Theologica* 31 (2011), 189–204.

[13] See e.g. Sitruk-Ware, Regine-Wang, Christina: "Contraceptive methods for men: an unmet need," in: *GREM Gynecological and Reproductive Endocrinology & Metabolism* (2024), 2–3/2023, 92–96; https://doi.org/10.53260/grem.234027.

[14] The document is available online: https://register.awmf.org/de/leitlinien/detail/015-095 (01.04.2024).

particular, between 18 and 29 years old, believe that contraception with hormones has "negative effects on body and soul".[15]

Education about the safe and effective use of natural family planning is also particularly important in regions where access to medical or contraceptive products, whether hormonal or non-hormonal, may be limited. Methods of conception control must be affordable, accessible and manageable in real life situations. Naturally, the efficiency and safety of the method play a significant role.

It is to be welcomed that the different forms of contraception are studied under various aspects without ideology, and especially with regard to women's health and the possible effects on the quality of a couple's relationship in a broader perspective. Family planning cannot be viewed in isolation; it is always integrated into the overall context of the organization of a relationship and family life.

2.4 Global Population Growth and Family Planning in the Context of the Eco-social Crisis

In the last section, I would like to briefly address the question of responsible parenthood in the context of the global eco-social crisis that we are experiencing today. I find it worrying, for example, when female representatives of the "last generation," as they call themselves, take the decision to be sterilized and speak of a "birth strike" because they consider it irresponsible to bring children into the world today.[16] At a recent meeting, Pope Francis addressed the topic and formulated a decisive message:

> The problem is not *how many of us there are in the world*, but *the world that we are building*—this is the problem; not children, but selfishness, which creates injustice and structures of sin, to the point of weaving unhealthy interdependencies between social, economic and political systems.[17]

I find it plausible that there are ecological limits to the growth of the world's population. At the same time, it is important to warn against reductionist measures

---

[15] Cf. Bundeszentrale für gesundheitliche Aufklärung (BZgA): Studie "Verhütungsverhalten Erwachsener 2023" (16.11.2023); online: https://www.bzga.de/fileadmin/user_upload/PDF/pressemitteilungen/daten_und_fakten/Infoblatt_BZgA-Studiendaten_Verh%C3%BCtungsverhalten_2023.pdf (01.04.2024); Ärzteblatt.de: "S2k-Leitlinie zur nicht hormonellen Empfängnisverhütung erschienen" (05.02.2024); online: https://www.aerzteblatt.de/nachrichten/149093/S2k-Leitlinie-zur-nicht-hormonellen-Empfaengnisverhuetung-erschienen (01.04.2024).

[16] See e.g. McGroarty, Beth: "Some Millennials Going on "Birth Strike" Because of Climate Change" (07.05.2019); online: https://globalwellnessinstitute.org/global-wellness-institute-blog/2019/05/07/some-millennials-going-on-birth-strike-because-of-climate-change/ (01.04.2024).

[17] Francis: *Address at the Fourth Edition of General States on Natality* (10.05.2024); online: https://www.vatican.va/content/francesco/en/speeches/2024/may/documents/20240510-statigenerali-natalita.html (01.06.2024).

of limiting population growth. Furthermore, the problem of population development is complex and is linked not only to the number of people.[18]

It is also essentially a question of the fair distribution of available resources, the utilization of land for the production of plant-based foods, and the reduction of global meat consumption in order to be able to use more land for the production of plant-based foods for humans instead for livestock. It is also crucial to significantly reduce carbon dioxide emissions, especially in industrialized countries.

In addition, the connection between the common good and a country's birth rate must be taken into account, insofar as a low or even negative birth rate also has a negative impact on a country's social welfare and pension systems. For Pope Francis, for instance, "the birth rate is the first indicator of the hope of a people. Without children and young people, a country loses its desire for the future",[19] he said.

Couples' decisions on the number of children also depend on various factors such as prosperity, health care, reduced mortality rate of children, social and financial security in old age, education, especially for women, strengthening women's rights in patriarchal societies, and social protection of women against sexual violence and exploitation. This is particularly relevant because in many regions the rate of unplanned pregnancies is very high: between 30% and 40%.[20]

It should also be borne in mind that in many cultures, a high number of children represents a kind of status symbol and that a great deal of cultural sensitivity and education is needed, in order to reduce the number of children.

The aim of family planning, however, must not simply be to reduce the birthrate, but rather to promote the common good and to achieve eco-social justice. Moreover, birth control must not be an expression of a pessimistic attitude toward humanity, but must rather be based on a fundamental attitude of love for humanity and for people, so that it can truly protect human dignity and promote people's freedom and self-determination.

The issue of birth control and contraception, therefore, must be placed in a broader context: from measures to ensure social justice to protecting the freedom of family planning, from promoting women's education and strengthening the social role of women to a functioning healthcare and social welfare system, from education about birth control methods to the acceptance of measures to control population growth. Acceptance is a necessary prerequisite for protecting the freedom of couples, so that the control of population growth is not imposed on them.

---

[18] Cf. e.g. Müller, Johannes: "Bevölkerungswachstum und Armut. Sozialwissenschaftliche Fakten und sozialethische Überlegungen," in: *Amos international* 7 (2013) 1, 3–12; id.: "Entwicklung der Weltbevölkerung," in: Schaupp, Walter (ed.): *Ethik und Empirie. Gegenwärtige Herausforderungen für Moraltheologie und Sozialethik* (SthE142), Fribourg et al. 2014, 155–170; Vogt, Markus: *Christliche Umweltethik. Grundlagen und zentrale Herausforderungen*, Freiburg i. Br. et al. 2022, 616–638.

[19] Francis: *Address at the Fourth Edition of General States on Natality* (10.05.2024).

[20] Cf. Vogt: *Christliche Umweltethik*, 628.

2.5 Final Statements and Summary Theses

1. Recalling the teachings of the Catholic Church:

   (a) It upholds the principle of responsible parenthood, which means that a married couple has the responsibility to decide on the number and timing of the children they wish to give birth to. This decision should take into account the well-being of the spouses, the children, the family, and society, as well as social, ecological, and financial conditions.
   (b) It is recognized that the public authorities have the right to adopt appropriate measures, so long as these are in conformity with the moral law and the rightful freedom of couples is preserved intact.
   (c) In terms of moral law, the Magisterium of the Catholic Church takes the position that for a married couple only consideration of the woman's fertility cycle is permissible, that is, NFP (natural family planning) and FABMs (fertility awareness-based methods) such as various symptothermal methods, while many theologians, ethicists, and believers argue in favor of overcoming the alternative between "natural" and "artificial" methods and consider the use of contraceptives to be morally legitimate as long as the method used does not coerce, endanger the health of either partner, especially of the woman, or emotionally harm or impair their capacity for love.
   (d) Pope Benedict XVI and Pope Francis emphasize that conception regulation is not just a question of a method, but of a lifestyle and of how a marital relationship is lived, especially including sensitivity towards the woman's body. At the same time, at the social level, they advocate overcoming antinatalism and promoting a child-friendly climate.

2. In order to protect the freedom and self-determination of a couple and in particular of the woman, it is necessary that the spouses are comprehensively informed and educated about the various methods, both medically and ethically. Besides knowledge, acceptance too is a necessary prerequisite for protecting the freedom of couples, so that the measures of family planning are not imposed on them.
3. Family planning and the prevention of unwanted pregnancies must not be left unilaterally to the woman, but is a profound ethical responsibility of the couple, that is, also of the man. It is particularly important to emphasize this, because in many regions of the world, the proportion of unwanted pregnancies is very high, presumably 30–40% of all pregnancies.
4. Couples' decisions on the number of children depend on various factors such as prosperity, health care, reduced mortality rate of children, social and financial security in old age, education, especially for women, strengthening women's rights in patriarchal societies and social protection of women against sexual exploitation, and so on.
5. In the context of today's global eco-social developments, measures for family planning and for decelerating the global population growth must also take account of global justice issues with regard to distribution of available resources.

The aim of family planning must not simply be to reduce the birthrate, but rather to promote the common good and to achieve eco-social justice.

6. The issue, therefore, must be placed in a broader context: from measures to ensure social justice to protecting the freedom of family planning, from promoting women's education and strengthening the social role of women to a functioning healthcare and social welfare system, and from education about birth control methods to the acceptance of measures to control population growth.

Declarations

Competing Interests The author(s) has no competing interests to declare that are relevant to the content of this manuscript.

Ethics Approval The author(s) declares that this manuscript does not include primary research with human participants.

The author(s) declares that this manuscript does not include primary studies involving animals.

Chapter 3
"Be Fruitful, and Multiply"? Contraception from the Perspective of Protestant Theology

Georg Pfleiderer

3.1 Introduction

The subject of the ethical problems of contraception has almost disappeared from recent Protestant sexual ethics. The problems connected to it have largely been transferred from the field of normative ethical theory to the realm of the individual practice and responsibility of each couple. This is at least the case for present-day academic and church theology in the German-speaking world (but not only there). Regarding this liberalization, academic Protestant ethics differs from "fundamentalist" evangelical theologies mainly in the United States, from the most of the fast-growing Pentecostal churches in the Global South, and from official Greek and Russian Orthodox theologies. Such conservative theologies assert that the Bible contains a concept of the Christian family that entails different roles for the father as the head of the family and the mother as the care-taker of a great number of children, if possible. In this context, fertility is understood as God's gift and even more as God's demand; and contraception, particularly with technical (e.g., chemical) tools, is mostly perceived as an intervention in the course of God's creation.

For centuries, such a restrictive understanding of family life and procreation was in fact widespread among Christian churches, including Protestant churches. It is probably true that it changed largely due to the influence of modern societies, of their individualism, egalitarianism, and their criticism of patriarchal family structures. It is not true, however, that these modern developments and ideas are hostile to original Christian ethics as conceived in the New Testament. On the contrary, modern theology can show that a reasonable and self-determined approach to fertility fits fundamental Christian ethical values much better than more or less

G. Pfleiderer (✉)
University of Basel, Basel, Switzerland
e-mail: Georg.Pfleiderer@unibas.ch

A. R. Genazzani et al. (eds.), *Ethical, Efficacy and Safety Issues in Contraception*, Reproductive Medicine for Clinicians 4,
https://doi.org/10.1007/978-3-032-07322-8_3

uncontrolled fertility. There is also no evidence that the Bible sweepingly condemns technical instruments of birth control.[1]

Supporting this claim is the subject of Sect. 3.2 of this chapter. Section 3.3 examines the development of ethical views on contraception in German-speaking Protestantism in the twentieth and twenty-first centuries as an example of the destiny of conservative sexual ethics in anti-modern theology under the conditions of modernization and the success of the rediscovery of original Christian liberalism. Section 3.4 provides a short summary.

3.2 Sexual Ethics and Procreation in the New Testament

To understand the ethics of partnership and procreation in the New Testament, one has to understand the basic conditions and fundamental ideas of early Christianity. To beg with, the Jesus movement depicted in the Christian Bible was a first-century eschatological (or apocalyptic) Jewish movement. This means that its founder, Jesus of Nazareth, his immediate followers, and also early Christians after his death believed in resurrection and lived expecting the immanent arrival of the "kingdom of God" (Mk 1:15). This "kingdom" was conceived as a "new world," transcendent yet still immanent and real. It would completely change the social and even natural conditions of human and creaturely life. As the prophets in the Old Testament had promised: "The wolves shall dwell with the lambs, and the leopards shall lie down with the goats" (Is 11:6). As all evildoers would be excluded from this kingdom, all enmity among human beings would end, and only love would remain. It would represent an eternal life with perfect justice and equality and with no poverty or social differences. Since God or his eternal son, Jesus Christ, would serve an immediate government, all political and social institutions separate from God were expected to come to an end. It was likewise expected that the institution of marriage would end: "When the dead rise from the dead, they will no longer marry as they do here on earth. It will be completely different: they will be like the angels of God in heaven" (Mt 22:30).

This eschatology was theoretical (a concept of interpreting reality) but also practical: already in Jesus's preaching, it was addressed to every single individual. It demanded a completely new self-understanding: Would you be willing to participate in the anticipation of God's kingdom by loving your enemy and by renouncing all your obstructive property and possessions and any advantages you have due to a prominent social position? This is what following Jesus originally entailed. In exchange, it offered participation in a community of followers, in the church, understood as the "body of Christ." In this transcendent community, all social differences had ended. "Here is neither Jew nor Greek, here is neither slave nor free, here is

[1] This was the position of the Roman Catholic Church since the *Encyclica Casti Connubii* by Pope Pius XI (1930).

neither male nor female; for you are all one in Christ Jesus" (Gal 3:28). The Christian community thus conceived itself as the new egalitarian "family of God." All creaturely relationships and all social differences were excluded from it. This means that the fundamental social order—the biological family and descent, and with them sexuality and procreation—were no longer a decisive part of religious identity. These subjects were simply ignored.

As the preaching and the practice of Jesus demonstrate in many ways, Christian ethics is an ethics of a loving, self-determined, and responsible humanism. It is an attitude of a general acceptance of all creatures and their right to live and develop as beloved children of God, whom Jesus called "Abba," the familial (Aramaic) term for "dad." It also required a strong self-consciousness, spontaneity, and self-determination. Although Jesus did not set aside the Jewish Law of Moses, he did take the liberty to interpret every command according to the fundamental general meaning of creaturely self-understanding and love.

It should be evident that under the conditions of the world as it is, and even more so as it was for early Christians—patriarchal, unfair, brutal, with hunger, deprivations of all kinds, violence, and suppression and persecution by a rough and hostile Roman state—living according to such an idealistic, utopic religious concept not only entailed high demands on the individual's willingness to renounce many worldly things; it also required individuals to mediate theoretically between the expectation of the kingdom of God as the "eon to come" and the perpetual "present eon." This ontological and chronological mediation was particularly prepared by Paul with his understanding of the crucifixion and resurrection of Jesus Christ as the apocalyptic event marking the beginning of the coming of the new eon. In that understanding, the relationship between the "eon to come" and "the present eon" can be conceived in a dialectic of "already and not yet." This dialectic served as a general key to the system of mediations initiated in the preaching and practice of Jesus.

Strictly understood, such a radical ethics of messianic existence was only practiced by Jesus himself and an inner circle of his followers who had abandoned their civil existence and walked with him through Galilee and Palestine. But as the Gospels show, there were also other "friends" of Jesus who remained sedentary and employed in their ordinary professions. The family of Maria, Martha, and Lazarus is the most prominent example. Jesus did not criticize them but acknowledged their lifestyle by visiting them frequently in their houses. An existence as an "itinerant charismatic" (Gerd Theissen) was thus not the only and obligatory form of being a follower of Jesus or of being a Christian after his death. And regarding the (Roman) state, Jesus himself coined a formula of mediation and adaptation: "Render unto Ceasar the things that are Ceasar's" (Lk 20:25). Without such a distinction, Jesus's preaching of the divine kingdom to come could have been confused with a program of political protest, which actually happened despite such statements when Jesus was crucified as the supposedly self-declared "king of the Jews."

Mediating between the eschatological concept of the divine kingdom and the conditions of this world has thus accompanied Christian ethics from its very beginnings. Despite its utopic radicalism, it always had aspects of a "compromise," as the famous liberal Protestant theologian Ernst Troeltsch put it. On the other hand, that readiness for compromise also intensified in the generations after the first Christians. In the so-called pastoral Epistles of the New Testament, which are attributed to Paul but were composed by theologians (to some extent in his spirit) several decades later, one can note manifest signs of a far-reaching "civilization" (Adolf von Harnack) of the early Christian communities. Instead of "love," "piety" in the sense of loyalty to God, but also to a given social order, became the leading cardinal virtue. The so-called house rules in the pastoral Epistles presuppose a Christian ethics that more or less follows the social and gender relationships of the ancient pagan or Jewish patriarchal family. This change was concomitant with the fact that instead of single unmarried or widowed women, married men and their whole families (who were probably not consulted) were increasingly the dominant group converting to the Christian faith.

Nevertheless, this development should not be understood as a simple decline in the original ethical and religious radicalism to a later culture of uninspired if not cowardly compromise. Certain compromises were necessary from the beginning to maintain the truly transcendent—today we would say the truly religious—character of the idea of the coming kingdom of God. This transcendence was not esoteric. It had significant ethical (and political) implications for living under the conditions of this eon, implications that can be detected in the house rules of the pastoral Epistles. While they presuppose given social and gender differences—such as the superordination of the husband over his wife and of parents over their children and also the presence of slaves—the Epistles demand a loving attitude and, at least to some extent, reciprocity.

In addition, adherence to the truly transcendent character of the kingdom to come did not entail a strict structural differentiation between religion and politics, as implied by the modern concepts. From a normative theological perspective, the temporal aspect of the "kingdom to come" always involved a willingness to overcome the conservative structures of given social orders and to contribute to a social order that came closer to the ideals of justice, love, and peace, which will be perfectly realized in the kingdom of God.

If we apply these general insights to the ethical subjects of marriage, procreation, and contraception, we can say that from the perspective of a Christian ethics (based on the New Testament), there is no reason to take the responsibility for procreation and contraception away from the individual couple. Sexuality is not a separate sphere of human communication that should follow a separate command of God or a normative image of "the Christian family." It is part of the free self-determination and loving interaction of the free and equal "children of God." "*[P]ost Christum natum*," after the birth of Jesus Christ as the unique son of God, the famous Swiss theologian Karl Barth argues, "the procreation of the human race ('Be fruitful and multiply!,' Gn 1:28) has ceased to be an unconditional commandment" (p. 301) [1]. Christianity takes up God's promise to Abraham to have "descendants as numerous as the stars in the sky and as the sand on the seashore" (Gn 22:17), but the preferred method of multiplication is by mission and individual decision, not by sexual procreation. The main purpose of marriage is thus not the production of children but the loving partnership of the couple. Giving birth to children is the free gift of God to free creatures. Giving birth to children entails great responsibility, and nobody should be able to force the burden of this responsibility on somebody else. There are, however, many people who can help parents so as to make them able and willing to bear such a responsibility.

Because having children is a free responsibility, there also cannot be any ethical condemnation of specific technical instruments of contraception, as long as they are instruments of contraception, not of abortion.[2]

3.3 Discourses on Procreation and Contraception in (German-Speaking) Protestant Ethics from the Twentieth and Twenty-First Centuries

3.3.1 1930s–1960s: Toward the Sexual Self-Determination of Married Couples

As in every religious tradition and every society, sexual ethics and family ethics have always been a major ethical field for regulating the behavior of ordinary people in Christianity. Nevertheless, the Protestant Reformation particularly concentrated with even greater intensity on the family as a religious unit in its own right. The rediscovery of the individual and their immediacy to God, which was Luther’s revolutionary theological insight, led to a strong relativization of the official church and the clergy. Such strengthening of the individual and individual belief strengthened the importance of religious and general education. In his “Sermon on Keeping Children in School” [2], Luther published on this pedagogical interest. For centuries, the Protestant pastoral family—starting with Luther and his wife Katharina’s own household—was a role model for family life in general.

In modernity, as theology and the church struggle with an increasingly secular society, this vital social function of the Christian, or Protestant, family has served as something like an ideological icon. The more individualism, pluralism, and secularism have taken hold of society, the more theologians and churches have stressed *the* Christian family as a core value of Christian ethics. Interestingly enough, even the Catholic Church—despite its very different understanding of the church—has adopted this strategy. While enforcing Christian dogma had been the central field of interest of both the Roman Catholic and Protestant churches, in modernity, starting with the age of Enlightenment and its separation of rational and religious truth, ethics and especially sexual and family ethics became the preferred field in the churches’ public struggles for a Christian identity. The price of this development was that theology and the churches had difficulties accepting that modern

[2] There are, to be sure, instruments where this distinction might be unclear, depending on the understanding of pregnancy, but this discussion cannot be pursued here.

individualism and pluralism were actually not hostile, anti-Christian values but ideas and creatures of themselves. The result of this misjudgment was a permanent belated reaction in Protestantism to the development of modern sexual ethics. Such effects and tendencies can be particularly observed in the history of Protestant theological discourses on contraception in the twentieth and twenty-first centuries.

In the 1930s, conservative Protestant theologians' resistance to modernization in the field of sexual ethics was motivated by their sympathy for ethnonationalist ideologies. In his *Christian Ethics*, published in 1936, the conservative Lutheran theologian Reinhold Seeberg argues: "[I]t must not be forgotten that *a nation's survival depends on the fertility of marriages*. Once the rationalization or artificial infertility of married life has taken root in a nation, it is difficult to remove. This is the road to national suicide" (p. 252) [3]. Liberal discourses on sexuality and birth control were treated as an element of secularization, of the dechristianization of society and the dissolution of traditional Christian family values: "Social conditions and excessive individualism and demands for a high standard of living are to blame for the fact that celibacy has become much more common in modern life, but also for the fact that marital fertility is artificially restricted. People want to enjoy nature and at the same time despise the order instilled in it by the Creator. … Various artificial means of preventing conception and abortion are not only used in families without any compelling reason but are also widespread among unmarried people, thus paving the way for an immoral and undisciplined life. And both celibacy and the deliberate restriction of births entail grave socioethical dangers" (p. 249) [3].

However, even such conservative positions like Seeberg's did not deny that procreation and birth control must be considered as subjects of individual and matrimonial responsibility. In the middle of twentieth century, Protestant theologians usually acknowledged that modern living conditions, the development of medicine, and the rapid decline of infant mortality formed the basis for the use of birth control and decreasing fertility rates. Since the high phase of industrialization around 1900, Protestant theologians commonly argued that a restrictive prohibition of contraceptives would lead to more illegal abortions, particularly among working-class people. Similarly, even if theologians were quite critical of typical modern developments—like extended adolescence due to longer education, the emancipation of women, the effects of individualization and of the anonymization of modern urbanity—they usually accepted that such processes had resulted in a new social reality that could not simply be controlled by moral appeals. Nevertheless, this did not prevent them from trying to shape women's sexual self-determination in particular.[3]

Despite such restrictions, Barth summarizes the contemporary theological discourses on birth control in his family ethics from 1951 by stating that the "freedom of the disposition" of the woman and the couple is affirmed by virtually all theologians. Barth even maintains: "Today there are no longer any fundamental

[3]In 1964, Helmut Thielicke still argued that there was a moral difference in avoiding pregnancy between a woman who did so because of work that was an economic need or a true profession and a woman for whom an occupation was just a hobby or who selfishly renounced having children for the purpose of self-realization (p. 732) [4].

differences within Christianity either. ... The question is in fact fundamentally affirmed today in almost universal agreement" (p. 301) [1]. And this applied not only to German-speaking Protestant theologians but also to the Lambeth Conference of Anglican Bishops and "partly to the Catholic Magisterium."[4]

As stated, it cannot be overlooked that the development of Protestant sexual ethics in modernity is deeply intertwined with the development of modern societies. Protestant theologians analyzed how the distinction between "natural" and "non-natural," or "artificial," methods of contraception made in Pope Pius XI's influential *Encyclical Casti Connubii* from 1930[5] was itself a reaction to developments in medicine and technology in the nineteenth and twentieth centuries. Protestant theologians, be they Lutheran or Reformed, always argued that such a difference is itself artificial. And using a notebook and calculator to register "infertile days" would be no less "artificial" than "artificial" contraceptives.

According to Barth, the general tendency to liberalize the ethics of contraception did not mean, however, that theologians would abstain from any ethical reflections on this subject. Virtually all Protestant theologians agreed that the most radical intervention, sterilization, is the most problematic. Regarding the ethical differentiation between other available methods of contraception, Barth's argumentation in his ethics from 1951 may be quite representative of a general attitude among Protestant theologians of that time. On a scale that seemed to combine criteria of intensity of sexual abstention and intervention, he distinguished between complete abstinence, temporary abstinence, coitus interruptus, and mechanical contraceptives [1]. The first he considered difficult and as threatening the love and loyalty of partners. Temporary sexual abstinence, on the other hand, would deprive sexual intercourse of its spontaneity and "festive" character [1]. The practice of coitus interruptus was associated with—to quote the then very influential Swiss physician Theodor Bovet [4]—"psychological and physiological dangers" (p. 308) [1]. And of the technical contraceptives, it had to be noted that none of them were completely reliable.

Barth drew a methodological conclusion from this negative result of normative ethical judgment on the different means of contraception. As each of these methods had its specific pros and cons, theological advice should restrict itself to the recommendation that each couple should deal with this problem with a free consciousness, not in fear or doubt, and through shared reflection and decision by both the man and the woman.[6]

---

[4] However, Barth could not ignore one difference between the official Roman Catholic position and the average contemporary Protestant. Protestant theologians accepted the personal responsibility of the married couple for its procreation because they believed that churches should not react with any kind of punishment to a violation of what they conceived of as responsible Christian behavior [1].

[5] This distinction and doctrine were maintained in the *Encyclica Humanae Vitae* by Pope Pius XI (1968) as well as by Pope Benedict XVI (p. 124–128) [5].

[6] He added: "the embarrassment [connected to all of these methods] should go as far as possible to the expense of the man" (p. 310) [1].

A perhaps rather unintended consequence of the slow process of the liberalization and individualization of sexual ethics was that social and political aspects of birth control—namely, problems of population planning and the ongoing practices of the forced sterilization of mentally retarded girls and women—were not much discussed in Protestant sexual ethics. Only in 1960s did German theologians become aware of the problems of the fast-growing populations in developing countries, the "explosion of the population" (p. 740) [4]. And even when it did so, conservative theologians like Helmut Thielicke argued: "The general approval of contraception or even its elevation to a legal requirement … would turn the exception into the rule, pervert the order of creation and take the responsible decision away from the individual. This would enthrone the unrestrained rule of libido in (and outside) marriage. Not the libido but only its consequences would be limited" (p. 743) [4].

3.3.2 *After the Sexual Revolution of the 1960s: The Struggle for Defending Marriage*

Despite such conservative judgments, which demonstrate a persistent tendency to shape women's individual sexual self-determination, the majority of German Protestant theologians in the 1960s put family planning into the hands of couples. The individualization of sexual morality had more or less won. However, it must be said that this was only true within a specific frame: the frame of marriage. Among unmarried couples, not only contraception but also sexual encounters in general were more or less morally banned.

The struggle to defend this restriction became formative for the theological debates on sexuality and contraception in the period after the mid-1960s. Initially, conservative and liberal theologians agreed that marriage was the basis for legitimate sexual intercourse, but they argued differently. While conservative theologians referred to a divine "order of creation," liberal theologians referred to a theory of individual subjectivity (many conservative theologians did so as well, in addition to referring to a divine order). True individual subjectivity (and true individual freedom) could only be realized and rightly understood as a holistic entity of the mind, soul, and body from a life-long perspective. The "wholeness" and integrity of an individual person was spiritually and intellectually based on their religious beliefs. The decisive and fundamental practice of such individuality, intimacy, and privacy was sexuality. Thus, only within the frame and borders of a personally and, after intense consideration, voluntarily started marriage—only within this life-long binding decision—could individual personality and individual freedom be perfectly realized. In theory, this was true for both sexes, according to their complementary gifts and conditions.[7]

[7] For this theory in nineteenth-century liberal (and conservative) theologians, see, e.g., Christian Palmer (p. 382) [6] or Christoph Ernst Luthardt (p. 57) [7], who refers to the German idealist

Although considered worldly, marriage has almost been treated as a holy sacrament in modern Protestant theology and in many Protestants' lives. It was not a sacrament in the formal Roman Catholic sense but in a moral and religious sense. It was considered the core and basis of Christian life. It is obvious that despite its affinity to modern individualism and self-determination, this sanctification of marriage made Protestant theology quite unfit for the sexual revolution of the 1960s.

At the turn to the 1970s, the federation of the (West) German churches, the Evangelical Church in Germany, formed a committee to formulate a new sexual ethics. In the committee, the liberals and conservatives had a hard time agreeing on a common text. In the end, the 1971 "Memorandum Regarding Questions of Sexual Ethics" [8] was a paper of compromise. The fault lines are easy to see and run mostly between the different chapters. The first chapter recalls the fundamental convictions regarding sexuality of traditional (modern) Protestantism and dresses them in contemporary, sociological language: "The coexistence of people ... requires a constant shaping of sexual life, as it has been found in institutions, customs, and traditions, because a mere ego-related living out of drives, which makes the partner the mere object of one's own needs, threatens both the life of the individual and the coexistence of the community" (p. 147) [8]. The moral condemnation of contemporary sexual practices is quite harsh: "Partner exchange and group sexuality show how little the participants have succeeded in integrating their genitality into their overall human sexuality and thus into a personal partnership" (p. 152). Nevertheless, in the chapter on the "sexual practices of the youth" (p. 153), the text has a tone that was a bit more sympathetic to the social changes in sexual behavior: "However, the need to take a differentiated view of processes of sexual development is also recognized. Therefore, sexual intercourse between engaged or committed couples in a holistic, personal relationship, which is linked to the intention of permanence, is viewed fundamentally differently than 'trying it out' with changing partners" (p. 154). For such unmarried couples, contraceptives could be tolerated (p. 155–56).[8]

In contrast to this ambiguity and underlying conservatism of West German theological ethics, a contemporary paper by an East German theological committee

J. G. Fichte: "The unmarried person is only half human." With this ideal of marriage, modern (liberal) Protestantism was confident it could overcome the compromise Christianity had always made between eschatological, transcendent ideals and the demands of reality.

[8] For such unmarried couples, "all procedures that affect life that has already begun or lead to the termination of pregnancy must be excluded as methods of birth control" [8] (p. 157). It is not entirely clear what this concretely means, as the next chapter on abortion declares that "according to current scientific knowledge, life begins with fertilization, the fusion of germ cells." However, the text goes on: "The beginning of pregnancy is now scientifically defined as the implantation of the living germ in the uterus. Any intervention that destroys the incipient life is the killing of nascent life" (p. 158). Does this mean that contraceptives that inhibit nidation are acceptable or not? It is not clear; it is a compromise, readable in two ways. On the background of its fundamental heterosexual convictions, it is not surprising that the memorandum clearly labels homosexuality a "sexual abnormality" (p. 164) that should not be condemned but medically and psychologically treated. Despite such dominate conservatism, the Synod of the Evangelical Church of Germany (ECG) did not acknowledge the memorandum as an official church document.

from 1969 is much more sensitive and tolerant. Even if the sexual practices of young people are treated in a chapter titled "Education Toward Marriage," there are sentences like the following: "The helplessness of most parents in the face of their children's premature sexual intercourse is a particular problem" (p. 205) [9]. The paper also unfolds the influential concept of "responsible parenthood": "We prefer the term responsible parenthood because other terms, such as family planning, birth control or regulation, or conception regulation only describe the problem technically or, like contraception, only negatively. … The intention of responsible parenthood can be expressed in one thesis: every child has the right to love, joy, and security from the moment of its conception" (p. 206).[9]

It took the West German churches at least two more decades to reach this standard of a modern sexual ethics. A short paper by the Conference of the German Lutheran Bishops from 1981 only lists changes in sexual behavior and public morality, including the widespread use of contraceptives, in the introduction, culminating in the statement that all these developments could arouse "doubts and reservations about marriage as a public institution" (p. 58) [10]. In the 1970s and 1980s, many official papers of West German churches were directed against this diagnosed "crisis of marriage" (p. 7) [11] in the form of the acceptance "nonmarital cohabitation" [11]. To broaden the front, after the visit of Pope John Paul II to Germany in 1980, the Evangelical Church in Germany formed an ecumenical committee together with the Roman Catholic Bishops and Dicastery for Promoting Christian Unity. Together they warned: "Without the institutional constitution of marriage …, the desired cohabitation remains exposed to destructive insecurity; this leads to a constant threat to trust, even where this is not initially recognized or admitted" [12]. Four years later (1985), the Evangelical Church in Germany had come to the insight that "the increase of nonmarital cohabitation" does not necessarily mean that "loyalty, love, and reliability have lost their esteem" (p. 6) [12]. Nevertheless, the paper concludes: "Marriage is the basic form of cohabitation between a man and a woman, and the church opposes its devaluation or relativization. Nonmarital cohabitation should not be equated with marriage and should not be legalized. Those who live in such unions retain their place in the Christian community. Marriage as a comprehensive and reliable life partnership of a man and a woman is God's gift and task for us" (p. 17) [12]. Even though it was losing ground in society and even among the

[9]The text contains many sensitive and self-critical insights: "It is decisive for a true understanding of marriage that in sexual intercourse the partners turn their full love to each other. … The work of clearing up the unfortunate constriction that we have known since the early church tradition, according to which the only 'decent' thing left in sexual intercourse was the production of children, has not yet been completed. This one-sided understanding has also found its way into Protestantism and has continued to have an effect into our century. Despite all the changes that have taken place in the meantime, more people are probably still more biased than we think, especially those influenced by this Christian tradition" (p. 206–7) [9]. Or: "Responsible parenthood includes the experimental and mutually considerate use of methods and means to regulate conception. The reluctance to consult a specialist or marriage counselor about the questions that arise here must be reduced so that married couples do not allow themselves to be driven into mutual incomprehension out of uncertainty and ignorance" (p. 207).

majority of its members, the Evangelical Church in Germany concentrated on its core staff: pastors. Despite the concession that "marriage-like partnerships (are) valued differently by social ethicists" (p. 130) [13], "partnerships without a marriage certificate" (p. 23) were prohibited for pastors or vicars. Even students of theology were not to practice it.

In none of these official church documents from the 1980s were contraceptives as such explicitly discussed. They were tacitly accepted.

3.3.3 *Around the Millennium (1990–2015): The Debate on the Status of Human Embryos*

In the 1990s, the debates on sexual ethics in German Protestant churches shifted again. They begin to be dominated by ethical debates about the implications and consequences of in vitro fertilization. These were debates on the ontological and ethical status of embryos and thus the question of the beginning of human life. The subject of contraceptives came only indirectly into these debates, namely, regarding contraceptives that inhibited nidation.

In 1989, a significant ecumenical paper was published by the Evangelical Church in Germany, the German Roman-Catholic Bishops, and all the other churches of the Working Group of Christian Churches in the Federal Republic of Germany: "God is a Friend of Life" [14]. The paper declares that human life definitively begins with "the fusion of the egg cell and the sperm cell .... This human being is individual life from the beginning and the case of subsequent cell division, which leads to the creation of identical twins, does not cancel out this fundamental fact—the further process of development is a continuous process and does not have any obvious junctures at which something new is added" (p. 43) [14]. The consequences of this maximalist position for nidation-inhibiting contraceptives were not discussed.

This was at least slightly different in another significant paper by the Evangelical Church in Germany published in 2002 entitled "Dealing with Life in the Spirit of Love" [15]. The committee that worked on this paper, the Chamber for Public Responsibility, declared that it had difficulties finding a common position on the problem of when human life begins. Some members argued for the moment of the fusion of the egg and the sperm cell; others for the moment of nidation. The paper ends by recommending a "tuistic" ethics, which means "an attitude that, in view of existing uncertainties and disagreements, advocates low-risk and cautious options for action (particularly in legal terms)" (p. 35). This result seems to support the position of the first group. The committee admits that the supporters of this position must be asked "whether [they are] prepared to follow the practical consequences that seem to result from this view: reluctance to use contraceptive methods that inhibit nidation as well as in vitro fertilization because of its consequential problems; life protection for embryos from the moment of fertilization" (p. 20). The question remained open in the paper and in the further discussions on sexual ethics in German Protestant churches. In recent years, they have turned to very different subjects, namely, the acknowledgment of homosexual marriages. German Protestant churches have done so one after another since 2016; Swiss churches have also acknowledged marriage for everyone.

3.4 Zeitgeist or Holy Ghost? Contraception, Protestant Sexual Ethics, and the Divine Truth: A Conclusion

As I have shown, over about the last hundred years, Protestant sexual ethics in German-speaking countries, particularly as observed in Germany, have developed more or less in one direction: from a paternalist, conservative ethics guided by an image of the normative, heterosexual, patriarchal Christian family, preferably with many children and very little birth control, to the acknowledgment of a variety of sexual orientations and relationships guided by an ideal of mutual love and care between the partners and also for the children, if there are any and be they the offspring of those two partners or of an earlier partner. Regarding contraception, the guiding principle of "responsible parenthood" has remained, but all concrete questions are left to couples, except that abortion must not be a regular instrument of Christian family planning.

How are we to judge this development? It is evident that academic and church theology followed the zeitgeist, though with longer or shorter delays. Recently, the delay seems to have become even shorter. Is this willingness to adapt to blame for any of the church's problems? From an ecumenical perspective, many Christians argue that it is. The Western Protestant mainline churches went in a direction in which the Roman Catholic Church, the Greek and Russian Orthodox Churches, and many fundamentalist churches in the worldwide family of Protestant churches do not want to follow them.

This is definitely a problem. But the question is: for whom? What should have become clear is that a modern theological interpretation of the Bible and a modern academic interpretation of Christian life in modern societies probably cannot come to a different result. Individual freedom, love, care, and mutual understanding are the foundations of personal, individual life and of social and family life as well—rightly understood already in the New Testament in the preaching and life of Jesus of Nazareth. "The Christian family" is not a certain sociobiological entity but an assembly of all people of good will; in the New Testament: the followers of Jesus. Family planning and contraception are not a question of Christian or non-Christian identity but a practical problem for all sexually active people. "Let him who is without fault cast the first stone" (Jn 8:7).

Declarations

Competing Interests The author(s) has no competing interests to declare that are relevant to the content of this manuscript.

Ethics Approval The author(s) declares that this manuscript does not include primary research with human participants.

The author(s) declares that this manuscript does not include primary studies involving animals.

Bibliography

1. Barth K. Church dogmatics. Vol. 3, the doctrine of creation. Part 4. 3rd ed. Zurich: Theologian Verlag; 1969.
2. Luther M. A sermon or sermon that children should be kept in school (1530). In: Dr. Martin Luther's works: critical complete edition. Vol. 30. Part 2. Weimar: Böhlau; 1909. p. 526–88.
3. Seeberg R. Christian ethics. Stuttgart: Kohlhammer; 1936.
4. Thielicke H. Theological ethics. Vol. 3, unfolding. Part 3, ethics of society, law, sexuality and art. Tübingen: J.C.B. Mohr; 1964.
5. Benedict XVI life and love: about marriage and family. Augsburg: Saint Ulrich; 2008.
6. Palmer C. The morality of Christianity. Stuttgart: A. Liesching; 1864.
7. Luthardt CE. Compendium of theological ethics. 2nd rev. ed. Leipzig: Dörffling & Franke; 1898.
8. Evangelical Church in Germany. Memorandum on questions of sexual ethics (1971). In: The memoranda of the Evangelical Church in Germany. Vol. 3, marriage, family, sexuality, youth. Gütersloh: H.G. Mohn; 1981. p. 139–73.
9. Sexual Ethical Commission from the Protestant Regional Churches of the GDR. Opportunities for marriage today (1969). In: The memoranda of the Evangelical Church in Germany. Vol. 3, marriage, family, sexuality, youth. Gütersloh: H.G. Mohn; 1981. p. 186–209.
10. Bishops' Conference of the VELKD Declaration on Marriage (1978). The memoranda of the Evangelical Church in Germany. Vol. 3, marriage, family, sexuality, youth. Gütersloh: H. G. Mohn; 1981. p. 57–61.
11. Evangelical Church in Germany. Non-marital partnerships. In: Marriage and non-marital partnerships: Positions and considerations of the Evangelical Church in Germany. EKD Texts 12. Hanover: Evangelical Church in Germany; 1985. p. 2–17.
12. Evangelical Church in Germany and thc German Bishops' Conference. Yes to marriage (1981). In: Marriage and non-marital partnerships: positions and considerations of the Evangelical Church in Germany. EKD Texts 12. Hanover: Evangelical Church in Germany; 1985. p. 24–7.
13. Evangelical Church in Germany. The marriage of the pastor and the pastor: reflections of the church conference of the Evangelical Church in Germany (1981). In: Marriage and non-marital partnerships: positions and considerations of the Evangelical Church in Germany. EKD Texts 12. Hanover: Evangelical Church in Germany; 1985. p. 18–23.
14. Evangelical Church in Germany and the German Bishops' Conference. God is a friend of life: challenges and tasks in protecting life (1989). Special representative ed. Trier: Paulinus; 2000.
15. Chamber for Public Responsibility of the Evangelical Church in Germany. Dealing with life in the spirit of love: argumentation aid for current medical and bioethical questions. EKD Texts 71. Hanover: Evangelical Church in Germany; 2002.

Chapter 4
Islamic Law and Reproduction

Gamal I. Serour and Ahmed G. Serour

In Islamic society the family, formed through marriage, is the basic social unit. Marriage and family formation are great responsibilities and are subject to specific regulations. The relationship in marriage is described in the Qur'an as two major qualities: love (passion, friendship, companionship), and mercy (understanding, reconciliation, tolerance, forgiveness).

The Holy Qur'ān says, "And one of [Allah's] signs is, that He has created for you mates from yourselves that you may dwell in tranquility with them, and has ordained between you Love and Mercy" Holy Quraan (21:30).

"وَمِنْ آيَاتِهِ أَنْ خَلَقَ لَكُم مِّنْ أَنفُسِكُمْ أَزْوَاجًا لِّتَسْكُنُوا إِلَيْهَا وَجَعَلَ بَيْنَكُم مَّوَدَّةً وَرَحْمَةً ۚ إِنَّ فِي ذَٰلِكَ لَآيَاتٍ لِّقَوْمٍ يَتَفَكَّرُونَ"
(قرآن كريم سورة الروم 21:30)

In Islam, children are the adornment of life and one of its two joys. The Holy Qur'an says "Wealth and children are the adornment of this present life" (Qu'ran 18:46).

" الْمَالُ وَالْبَنُونَ زِينَةُ الْحَيَاةِ الدُّنْيَا ۖ وَالْبَاقِيَاتُ الصَّالِحَاتُ خَيْرٌ عِندَ رَبِّكَ ثَوَابًا وَخَيْرٌ أَمَلًا "
(قرآن كريم سورة الكهف 18:46)

As children are gifts in the hands of their parents, they must be cared for physically, mentally, and educationally and be provided with all support they need. Such care cannot be achieved without family planning and contraception.

G. I. Serour (✉)
the Egyptian IVF Center, Cairo, Egypt

International Islamic Center for Population Studies and Research, Al Azhar University, Maadi, Egypt
e-mail: giserour1@link.net

A. G. Serour
the Egyptian IVF Center, Cairo, Egypt

A. R. Genazzani et al. (eds.), *Ethical, Efficacy and Safety Issues in Contraception*, Reproductive Medicine for Clinicians 4,
https://doi.org/10.1007/978-3-032-07322-8_4

The Prophet (PBUH) says, “You are all responsible for your subjects” (Sahih El Bokhary 853).

The leadership of Al-Azhar believes that family planning and the inability to conceive are two sides of the same coin. Thus, attention and guidance should be outlined in Islamic society on both family planning and the management of infertility. Availability and access to infertility management would promote the use of contraception. Couples would be encouraged to practice family planning if they know that should they decide to have a baby they will be helped to do so [7].

4.1 Sources of Islamic Law

It is important to understand the terminology of the ruling principles in Islam. Sharia means the right way or the right path of religion. Its sources in chronological order are the holy Qur’an followed by the authenticated hadith (saying or deeds) of Prophet Mohamed (PBUH), Igmaa, and analogy. Thus, Sharia is a total divine Islamic discourse that includes guidance on spiritual, moral, legal, economic, social, and political issues. Sharia requires deciphering, discovery, and interpretation of its primary sources by individuals, knowledgeable in religion, to be applicable in everyday life. This human source of information is called Fiqh. Fiqh is not divine though it is often conflated with God’s law.

Islamic law is the product of the efforts of jurists in their theoretical jurisprudence to outline the legal aspects of Sharia. Islamic law applied in courts is sometimes different though interrelated with Islamic law outlined by Sharia. The Broad Principles of Islamic Jurisprudence are the basic nature of actions is their permissibility unless prohibited by a text (*IBAHA*), no harm and no harassment, necessity overrides prohibition and choice of the lesser harm.

4.2 Deriving Rulings on Contemporary Issued in Islam

To derive Islamic rulings on a contemporary issue, one turns first to the primary sources of Sharia’a. The primary sources of Sharia in chronological order are the Qur’an, the Sunna, and Hadith, which are the authentic traditions and sayings of Prophet Mohammed (PBUH) as collected by specialists in Hadith, the unanimous opinions of Islamic Scholars or (*Igmaa*), and analogy (*Kias*), which is the intelligent reasoning used to rule on events not mentioned by the Quran and Sunna by matching against similar or equivalent events previously ruled on. In matters not discussed by primary sources of Shari’a. Muslims refer to secondary sources of Sharia, which include the choice of one of several lawful options *Istihsan*, the views of the Prophet’s companions, current lawful customs, public welfare, and the rulings of previous divine religions if not contradicting the primary sources of Sharia’a.

Sharia'a can accommodate different honest opinions as long as they do not conflict with the spirit of its primary sources and are directed to the benefit of humanity.

Differences in the opinion of Islamic scholars on matters that need (*ijtihad*), as it is not mentioned in the primary sources of Sharia, are acceptable. The Prophet—PBUH—has venerated this Ijtihad and said, "When a ruler judges with Ijtihad and succeeds, he is rewarded twice; but if he fails (in his trial), he is rewarded only once" (Sahih El Bukhari 7352).

4.3 Human Reproduction in Islamic Societies

The duty of the family and the society at large is to provide their children with the best possible health care, education, justice, equality, and upbringing, which is almost impossible without family planning. However, large families had been the norm in most Muslim countries. With the recent increase in the cost of living, education, housing, and increased participation of mothers in the labor force, it became almost impossible for large families to maintain these ideal standards for their children in most of the Muslim world.

Furthermore, too early, too many, and too close pregnancies are associated with increased maternal and child mortality and morbidity and unsafe abortion [13, 14]. Consequently, to ensure that marriage fulfills tranquility, love, and mercy among parents and physical, mental, and educational care for the children, family planning is indispensable at the family level and a must at the country level based on the available services and resources [13, 14].

Increased population growth due to the high fertility rate and low contraceptive prevalence in most Muslim countries has had a negative impact on development and achieving sustainable development goals (SDGs) by 2030 as projected by United Nations.

Family planning (FP) is planning for a family and not merely contraception. It involves when, how often, how many children to have, and when to stop childbearing.

The use of contraceptives to space births has been met with some cultural resistance in the Islamic world based on the false belief that it is against Islamic Shari'aa (Haram) due to misinterpretation of some verses in the Holy Qur'an and sayings of Prophet Mohamed (PBUH). This resulted in low contraceptive prevalence and high unmet needs for modern contraceptives which led to high fertility rates and increased population growth rates in many countries in the Muslim world. In a recent cross-sectional study of 663 Muslim women (age 15–49 years) in two countries in Kenya (Wajir and Lamu) by Abdi et al., the leading reason for the non-use of contraception was the false belief that FP is not allowed in Islam [2, 3].

Contrary to the belief that Islam calls for unlimited reproduction and forbids family planning (*tanzim al-nasl*), Islam has encouraged procreation. Islamic Shariah provides guidance to promote, protect, and care for women's and children's health.

Though the Islamic Law has affirmed the importance of marriage, family formation, and procreation, it has also emphasized the healthcare of the woman and her children and the preservation and protection of the environment and future generations. Family planning seeks to achieve these objectives, especially in overpopulated and low resource countries [10, 21, 22].

In planning for a family, practices vary from family to family and from one country to another, according to their circumstances, available healthcare services, and resources. Some countries suffer from rapid population growth, limited resources, and poor healthcare and educational systems. In such countries, proper planning of families is urgently needed together with other means of development. This is in concordance with the principle of avoidance of possible harm (*daf al darar al-muhtamal*) and the secular principles of beneficence, non-maleficence, justice [4], protection of the environment, responsibility toward future generations, and human solidarity [27]. With the current fertility rate, the projected global Muslim population will increase from 1.6 billion in 2011 to 2.2 billion in 2030 [32]. Furthermore, unplanned births have implications for population dynamics and women and newborn mortality and morbidity rates. Because of a low rate of contraceptive use, most Muslim countries suffer from high maternal and child mortality rates, high adolescent pregnancy rates, and unsafe abortion [28, 29]. Improving access to family planning reduces poverty and hunger and averts 32% of all maternal deaths and nearly 10% of childhood deaths [5]. Thus, family planning as it contributes to the preservation of the life of the mother and the child to be born fulfils two of the five objectives of Shari'aa, namely, preservation of self and progeny.

4.4 Islamic Law and Human Reproduction

4.4.1 Islamic Law and Contraception

Shari'aa has called for child spacing and family planning. A thorough review of the Qur'ān reveals no text (*nass*) prohibiting contraception or planning of pregnancy. On the contrary, planning of families seems to be permitted by several verses in the Qur'an, and traditions of the Prophet (PBUH) [10].

The Qur'ān encourages breastfeeding for 2 years, which is in itself a natural method of Family Planning.

The Holy Qur'ān says, "Mothers may breastfeed their children two complete years for whoever wishes to complete the nursing [period]" Holy Qur'an (2:233).

" ۞ وَالْوَالِدَاتُ يُرْضِعْنَ أَوْلَادَهُنَّ حَوْلَيْنِ كَامِلَيْنِ ۖ لِمَنْ أَرَادَ أَن يُتِمَّ الرَّضَاعَةَ "
(سورة البقرة 2:233)

The Holy Qur'an also says, "And We have commended unto man kindness toward parents. – His mother beareth him in weakness upon weakness, and his weaning is in two years – Give thanks unto Me and unto thy parents. Unto Me is the journeying" (Lokman: 14).

(وَوَصَّيْنَا الْإِنسَانَ بِوَالِدَيْهِ حَمَلَتْهُ أُمُّهُ ، وَهْنًا عَلَىٰ وَهْنٍ وَفِصَالُهُ ، فِي عَامَيْنِ أَنِ اشْكُرْ لِي وَلِوَالِدَيْكَ إِلَيَّ الْمَصِيرُ (14))

While the Qur'ān was being revealed, the Prophet Mohamed (PBUH) learned that his Companions (*sahābah*) were practicing coitus interruptus (*al-azl*) and he did not prohibit it. Thus *al-'azl* for reversible contraception is permissible (*jāiz*), lawful, and the majority of jurists agree that it is permitted [10].

Imam al-Ghazālī (d. 505/1111) also allowed *al-'azl*, with the wife's consent, for health and economic reasons and even to preserve a woman's figure and beauty for the continued enjoyment of her life with her husband [11, p. 491]. Modern reversible methods of contraception such as contraceptive pills, implants, injectables, intrauterine contraceptive devices, or condoms by analogy are similar to coitus interruptus (Al-Azl).

Most scholars have endorsed reversible contraceptive methods available today [17].

There are Prophetic reports which stress the idea that Muslims must search for lawful provision and sustenance for their families to provide a good quality of life for their children. Such provisions cannot be achieved without family planning.

An authenticated Hadith says, "A multitude of children is one of two cases of poverty, while a few children is one of two cases of ease" (Narrated by Qudaei).

(كثرة العيال أحد الفقرين وقلة العيال أحد اليسارين". (حديث شريف رواه القضاعى "

The Prophet (PBUH) said, "The most grueling trial (Juhd al balaa) is to have plenty of children with no adequate means" (authenticated Hadith by al Seyuti and al-Hakim).

(جهد البلاء كثرة العيال مع قلة الشيء ". (رواه السيوطى والحاكم "

Despite these clear instructions in Islamic law on permissibility of FP, in many Muslim societies, contraception is not widely accepted or practiced because of misinterpretation of some verses in the Holy Qur'an and some Hadiths of the Prophet Mohamed (PBUH). These misinterpretations have unfortunately been passed from one generation to another as a cultural norm with the misconception that it is supported by Islam.

The Holy Qur'an says, "Don't kill your children for fear of want, we provide sustenance for them and for you, the killing of them is a great sin" Al-Isra sura (17:31).

" وَلَا تَقْتُلُوا أَوْلَادَكُمْ خَشْيَةَ إِمْلَاقٍ ۖ نَحْنُ نَرْزُقُهُمْ وَإِيَّاكُمْ ۚ إِنَّ قَتْلَهُمْ كَانَ خِطْئًا كَبِيرًا "
(سورة الإسراء 17:31)

The prevention of pregnancy by contraceptives is not killing children. Contraception prevents the sperm of the husband from meeting and fertilizing the egg of the wife and does not involve the killing of a fetus. These Holy verses in the Qur'an are referring to the pre-Islamic Arabic custom of burying children in fear of poverty.

One of the Qur'anic verses which is often quoted in support of a ban on contraceptive use is "No creature is there crawling on the earth, but its sustenance is on Allah" Holy Qur'an (11:6).

" وَمَا مِن دَابَّةٍ فِي الْأَرْضِ إِلَّا عَلَى اللَّهِ رِزْقُهَا "

6:11) سورة هود)

The Holy Qur'an emphasizes that Allah ensured that every creature existing on earth shall be provided with sustenance, but it does not call for uncontrolled population growth without resources for its sustenance. It also calls for strong nations which are not necessarily large in number. The Holy Qur'an says,

> How oft, by Allah's will. Has a small host vanquished (defeated) a large host. Al-Baqrah sura (2:249)

"كَم مِّن فِئَةٍ قَلِيلَةٍ غَلَبَتْ فِئَةً كَثِيرَةً بِإِذْنِ اللَّهِ ۗ"
2:249) سورة البقرة)

Also, some argue that FP contradicts the Prophet's Hadīth which states, "Marry and beget many children and I will pride myself in you before other nations on the Day of Judgment" (Authenticated by Abu Dawod).

"تناكحوا تناسلوا تكاثروا فإني مُباهٍ بكم الأمم يوم القيامة"
(حديث شريف رواه أبو داود)

The Hadith does not mean the large size and weak and non-productive nation. The Prophet's companions asked him (PBUH) are we few then? He (PBUH) replied you are then many, but like rain bubbles and GOD will make your enemies not afraid from you.

". قالوا أو مِن قلَّةٍ نحن يومئذ يا رسول الله ؟ قال: بل أنتم يومئذٍ كثير، ولكنكم غثاء كغثاء السَّيل، ولينزعنَّ الله من قلوب أعدائكم المهابة منكم "

4.5 Contraception and Old and Contemporary Islamic Jurists

Imam Shawkānī says in his book *Nayl Al-Awtār*: "There is no dispute [or] disagreement among scholars in permitting '*Azl*, provided that the free wife's consent is obtained, for she is a companion in sexual intercourse" [24, vol. 6, p. 233].

Several jurists and institutions have expressed support for reversible family planning. The al-Azhar Committee of Fatwa on 10 March 1953 indicated that using a medicine to prevent pregnancy for a short duration is not forbidden according to the Shāfi'īs. The committee acknowledged this point of view because it beneficial for people and avoids harm. According to the *fatwā*, the fear of too many pregnancies, which are likely to weaken the mother without having time to rest and regain her health, is considered lawful.

The *fatwā* cites this verse of the Holy Qur'an: "God intends every facility for you; He does not want to put you to difficulties" Holy Qur'an (2:185).

"....يُرِيدُ اللَّهُ بِكُمُ الْيُسْرَ وَلَا يُرِيدُ بِكُمُ الْعُسْرَ .... "
2:185) سورة البقرة)

The *fatwā*, however, indicates that permanent prevention of pregnancy forever is considered prohibited.

The late Sheikh of al-Azhar and former mufti of Egypt sheikh Sayyid Tantāwī noted in 1988: "There is no harm to stop pregnancy for a term to bring the child up well. This conduct of employing means permitted by Allah is an honest behavior" [26].

In general, the four schools of Islamic law allowed family planning: The opinion in the Mālikī and Hanbalī schools is permission with the wife's consent, as it is in the Zaydī Shīī School. The Imāmi Shafi preferred to obtain the wife's permission at the time of the marriage contract.

The late Egyptian scholar Sayyid Sābiq (1915–2000) noted that Islam is willing to increase progeny (children), for this is a sign of the power of nations and countries. However, Islam in certain conditions does not forbid planning for having children by using a contraceptive or by applying any other means to prevent pregnancy. He observed that planning is allowed if the family has many children and cannot afford to bring up more children in a decent way, or when the wife is weak, or if the man is poor, or if there is a contagious disease in any of them. In such conditions, contraception is permitted. Some scholars see that planning in such cases is not only permissible, but is also recommendable [13].

The late Saudi scholar Sheikh Abd al-Azīz Ibn Bāz recommended family planning in cases where pregnancy would harm the mother's health or when repeated pregnancies would affect the mother's care of her children [12].

The late Grand Imam of al-Azhar, Sheikh Mahmūd Shaltūt, noted that Muslim jurists have agreed that abortion after a baby is given life—that is, after 4 months of pregnancy—is a forbidden crime. No Muslim is allowed to do it, for it is a crime against a living human being. If continuation of pregnancy means the death of the mother, Islamic law in its general rules recommends the lesser of the two harms, that is, abortion. But abortion before life is given to it, before 4 months, is a matter of dispute. Some say it is permitted and not prohibited and others say it is forbidden or undesirable" [23, pp. 249–255].

Several formal statements (*fatwās*) have been issued over the years from different parts of the Muslim world, which includes a *fatwā* from the mufti of Egypt in 1937, by Sheikh Abd al-Majīd Salīm permitting FP according to the Hanafīs; a *fatwā* from Singapore by Tuan Haji Ali in 1955; a *fatwā* from Turkey by the Advisory Council on Religion in 1960); a *fatwā* from Iran by Ayatollah Baha'eddin Mahallati in 1964; a *fatwā* from Malaysia by Haji Abdel Jalil Hassan in 1964; a *fatwā* from Yemen by the president of the High Court of Appeals in 1968; and a *fatwā* from Lebanon by Sheikh Shamsuddin on Sterilization in 1971 [17].

One of the issues which is often discussed by legislators in many Muslim countries suffering from increased population growth and high fertility rates is it lawful for the State to enact laws on family planning which compel parents to limit family size particularly if such laws are in the national interest? Islam ensures that family size is to be decided by agreement between the husband and wife. No one imposes his or her will on married couples. How can the State then support coercive laws which ignore the needs and circumstances of individual families?

However, the state can help people to make responsible decisions by providing them with all the necessary information to avoid too many pregnancies and too close pregnancies. This can be done through several channels, including sexual and reproductive health (SRH) education at schools and universities, provision of quality family planning services, mass media information, faith-based organizations, and informed religious Imams [17]. The state has to abolish incentives to have large families through the criminalization of child labor and improving the standard of living of the people. The state has to provide contraceptives or make them available and affordable, and to provide quality healthcare services in the primary healthcare units and family planning clinics [17].

In Muslim countries, the State must advocate that the provision of contraceptives is a human right and is consistent with the ethical principles of autonomy, beneficence, nonmaleficence, and justice which are deeply rooted in Islam [20].

4.6 Obstacles to the Use of Contraceptives in the Muslim Societies

(a) Does the use of contraceptives impair fertility?

- It is often quoted that contraceptives impair fertility. However, none of the modern methods of contraception impairs fertility. Fertility is restored shortly after stopping the method used.

(b) Is the use of contraceptives associated with harmful side effects on the health of women?

- On the contrary, when properly used contraceptives save the lives of women and children, and improve the quality of their lives.

The benefits of the use of contraceptives to prevent adolescent pregnancy, too-close pregnancies, too many pregnancies, and unwanted pregnancies far outweigh any associated risks. Risks associated with the use of contraceptives are few and mild, and can be minimized by the proper choice of method for each couple as recommended by WHO eligibility criteria [30, 31].

Some contraceptives protect women from contracting STIs, protect women from the development of malignant diseases of the reproductive system, and improve menstrual symptoms such as heavy bleeding and painful menstruation.

4.6.1 Islamic Law and Infertility Treatment

Infertility treatment is encouraged in Islam. Soon most countries will have population growth below the replacement level including some Muslim countries. While this may have a beneficial impact on the environment, underpopulation and family building are of growing concern in many countries with very low fertility [8].

There is no dispute in the Muslim world on the use of conventional methods of treatment of infertility. However, when assisted reproductive technology (ART) was introduced for the treatment of infertility in 1978 by Steptoe and Edwards [25], it was met with great resistance, denial, and rejection in the Muslim world [18]. The society and infertile couples thought by seeking ART for the treatment of infertility that they are challenging God's will by trying to render barren women fertile [18].

The primary sources of Sharia encouraged marriage, family formation, and procreation.

The Holy Quran Says: (49). ……….. He creates what He wills. He bestows female (offspring) upon whom He wills, and bestows male (offspring) upon whom He wills (50) Or He bestows both males and females, and He renders barren whom He wills. El Shoura: 49–50.

يَخْلُقُ مَا يَشَاءُ ۚ يَهَبُ لِمَن يَشَاءُ إِنَاثًا وَيَهَبُ لِمَن يَشَاءُ الذُّكُورَ (………… (49)) (الشورى 49–50) أَوْ يُزَوِّجُهُمْ ذُكْرَانًا وَإِنَاثًا ۖ وَيَجْعَلُ مَن يَشَاءُ عَقِيمًا ۚ
إِنَّهُ عَلِيمٌ قَدِيرٌ

ART was not mentioned in the primary sources of Sharia. However, procreation within the framework of marriage was encouraged as it preserves humankind, which is one of the five objectives of Sharia'a.

The attitude of patients changed from rejection, doubt, feelings of shame, guilt, and secrecy to seeking ART for the treatment of their infertility when Fatwas were issued by Al Azhar in 1980 (Gad El Hak 1980). The Fatwa emphasized that: If ART is indicated for a couple (Husband and Wife) as a necessary line of treatment it is permitted and even encouraged as it preserves humankind. In the Muslim world, there are two sects: the Sunni (90%) and the Shiaa (10%). The Sunni Fatwa agreed to the permissibility of ART between husband and wife, with fertilization of the egg from the wife with the sperm of the husband, and the transfer of the fertilized egg to the wife, the owner of the egg during the validity of marriage contract. The Fatwa does not approve of egg donation, sperm donation, embryo donation, or surrogacy.

However, the Shariaa Fatwa opened the way to third-party donation of egg, sperm, embryo, and surrogacy via fatwa from Ayatollah Ali Hussein Khameini in 1999. However, sperm donation was prohibited later on. For the Shiaa, the Preservation of marriage was prioritized over preservation of lineage. Preservation of both is required for Sunni [18, 19]. The Islamic Republic of Iran has had legislation on Embryo Donation since 2003 [1].

Sex selection technologies for non-medical reasons have been condemned on the grounds that their application discriminates against female embryos and fetuses, so perpetuating prejudice against the girl child and social devaluation of women [6]. To avoid discrimination against the female child, sex selection should not be performed for selection of sex of the first child in the family or in families who have children of both sexes or for selection of one sex only whether male or female [9].

In Muslim societies, reproductive medicine physician should properly counsel their patients, in societies where sex selection is allowed, before agreeing to it, to ensure that the procedure does not contribute to discrimination on the basis of sex or gender and is performed for the protection of the interest of the mother and the family in some societies [16].

Respect for embryos advances step by step with their morphological development and growth [15].

God says, "The embryo grows from a clot to a lump of flesh then boned flesh and finally a fully grown infant" (23–14).

قال تعالى: ....ثُمَّ خَلَقْنَا النُّطْفَةَ عَلَقَةً فَخَلَقْنَا الْعَلَقَةَ مُضْغَةً فَخَلَقْنَا الْمُضْغَةَ عِظَامًا فَكَسَوْنَا الْعِظَامَ لَحْمًا ثُمَّ أَنشَأْنَاهُ خَلْقًا آخَرَ ۚ فَتَبَارَكَ اللَّهُ أَحْسَنُ الْخَالِقِينَ *
((المؤمنون – 14

قال تعالى: "... فَإِنَّا خَلَقْنَاكُم مِّن تُرَابٍ ثُمَّ مِن نُّطْفَةٍ ثُمَّ مِنْ عَلَقَةٍ ثُمَّ مِن مُّضْغَةٍ مُّخَلَّقَةٍ وَغَيْرِ مُخَلَّقَةٍ لِّنُبَيِّنَ لَكُمْ ۚ وَنُقِرُّ فِي الْأَرْحَامِ مَا نَشَاءُ إِلَىٰ أَجَلٍ مُّسَمًّى......."*
((الحج – 5

Organ differentiation occurs 42 days after fertilization. Ensoulment of the fetus occurs after 120 days. However, some authorities consider it to occur as early as 42 days post-fertilization.

" إذا مر بالنطفة ثنتان وأربعون ليلة بعث الله إليها ملكاً فصورها وخلق سمعها وبصرها وجلدها ولحمها وعظامها "
(رواه مسلم عن ابن أسيد الغثارى)
" إن أحدكم يجمع خلقه فى بطن أمه اربعين يوماً "نطفة" ثم يكون "علقة" مثل ذلك ثم يكون "مضغة" مثل ذلك ثم يرسل إليه الملك فينفخ فيه الروح"
(رواه البخاري ومسلم عن ابن مسعود)

This old threshold of 40 days and upward from conception has been brought to as early as 14 days by researchers as recent progress in embryology has established that the individuality of the "new being" begins at this date [15].

This concept has been affirmed by scholars and researchers from various Muslim countries during the International Seminar on Dilemma of Stem Cell Research held in Cairo Nov. 2007 and organized by IOMS, WHO/EMRO, and Al Azhar [18].

Embryo testing and research for prevention and treatment of diseases, and for the advancement of scientific knowledge and benefit of humanity, is therefore allowed before 14 days post fertilization and on surplus embryos donated for research with the free informed consent of the couple.

Declarations

Competing Interests The author(s) have no competing interests to declare that are relevant to the content of this manuscript.

Ethics Approval The author(s) declares that this manuscript does not include primary research with human participants.

The author(s) declares that this manuscript does not include primary studies involving animals.

References

1. Afshar L, Bahgari A. Embryo donation in Iran: an ethical review. Dev World Bioeth. 2013;13(3):119–24.
2. Abdi B, Okal J, Serour G, Temmerman M. Children are a blessing from God – a qualitative study exploring the socio-cultural factors influencing contraceptive use in two Muslim communities in Kenya. Reprod Health. 2020;17:44.
3. Abdi B, Okal J, Serour G, Were V, Temmerman M, Gichangi P. Pattern and determinants of contraceptive use among the Muslim women in Wajir and Lamu counties in Kenya: a cross-sectional study. BMC Womens Health. 2024;24:53. https://doi.org/10.1186/s12905-024-02892-9.
4. Beauchamp TL, Childress JF. Principles of biomedical ethics. 7th ed. New York: Oxford University Press; 2013.
5. Cleland J, Conde-Agudelo A, Peterson H, Ross J, Tsui A. Contraception and health. Lancet. 2012;380(9837):149–56. https://doi.org/10.1016/S0140-6736(12)60609-6.
6. Fathalla MF. The girl child. Int J Gynecol Obstet. 2000;70:7–12.
7. Fathalla MF. Introductory remarks. In: Vayena E, Rowe PJ, Griffin PD, editors. Current practices and controversies in assisted reproduction. Geneva: WHO; 2002. p. 41–9.
8. Fauser BCJM, Adamson DG, Boivin J, Chembers GM, de Geyter C, Dyer S, Inhorn MC, Schmidt L, Serour GI, Tarlatzis B, Zegers-Hochschild F. Declining global fertility rates and the implications for family planning and family building: an IFFS consensus document based on a narrative review of the literature. Hum Reprod Update. 2024;30(2):153–73.
9. FIGO Ethics Committee and FIGO WSRR. FIGO 34 Committees Int. JGO. 2006.
10. Gad El Hak AGE, Serour GI, editors. Some gynecological problems in the context of Islam. Cairo: The International Islamic Center for Population Studies and Research, al-Azhar University; 2000.
11. al-Ghazālī MAH. Ihyā' 'Ulūm al-Dīn. Beirut: Dār ibn Hazm; 2005.
12. Ibn Bāz. 'Abd al-'Azīz. "al-Qawl al-Fasl fī hukm al-'azl." https://binbaz.org.sa/fatwas/1906./القول-الفصل-في-حكم-العزل.
13. Omran AR. Family planning in the legacy of Islam. New York: Routledge; 1992.
14. Serour GI, Omran A. Ethical guidelines for human reproduction research in the Muslim world. Cairo: International Islamic Center for Population Studies and Research, al-Azhar University; 1992. https://alazhar-iicpsr.org/.
15. Serour GI. Ethical implications of human embryo research. Publications of the Islamic Educational, Scientific and Cultural Organization (ISESCO) 1421 A.H./2000 A.D.; 2000.
16. Serour GI, Dickens B. Assisted reproduction developments in the Islamic world. Int J Gyn Obst. 2001;74:178–93.
17. Serour GI, Hod Hod. Family planning and the opinions of contemporary imams of jurisprudence manual. International Islamic Center for Population Studies and Research (IICPSR); 2021. p. 103.
18. Serour GI, Serour AG. The impact of religion and culture on medically assisted reproduction in the Middle East and Europe. RBM Online. 2021;43(3):421–33.
19. Serour GI. Reproductive BioMedicine on line. RBM Online. 2008;17, Suppl 3(4):34–8.
20. Serour GI. Islam and the four principles. In: Gillon R, editor. Principles of health care ethics. London: Wiley; 1994. p. 75–91.
21. Serour GI. Attitudes and cultural perspectives on infertility and its alleviation in the Middle East area. In: Vayena E, Rowe PJ, Griffin PD, editors. Current practices and controversies in assisted reproduction. Geneva: WHO; 2002. p. 41–9.
22. Serour GI. What is it to practice good medical ethics? A Muslim perspective. J Med Ethics. 2015;41:121–4.
23. Shaltūt M. al-Fatāwā. Cairo: Dār al-Shurūq; 1988.
24. Shawkānī M i A. Nayl al-Awtār. Cairo: Dār al-Hadīth; 1998.

25. Steptoe PC, Edwards RG. Birth after the reimplantation of a human embryo. Lancet. 1978;2:366.
26. Tantāwī, Muhammad Sayyid (1988). Birth planning and the religious point of view. Cairo: IICPSR, al-Azhar University.
27. UNESCO. The universal declaration on bioethics and human rights. Paris: UNESCO; 2005.
28. UNFPA State of the World Population Report. My body is my own. 2021.
29. UNFPA State of the World Population Report. The power of choice. 2018.
30. WHO. Medical eligibility criteria for contraceptive use. 5th ed.; 2015. http://apps.who.int.
31. WHO. New approach for WHO's medical eligibility criteria for contraceptive use. WHO; 2019.
32. UNFPA State of the orld Population Report. 2014.https://www.un.org.

Part II
Natural Methods of Contraception and Family Planning

Chapter 5
Ovulation, the Intersection in Hormonal Contraception

Mettler Liselotte

5.1 Understanding of Ovulation

Ovulation can best be understood by looking at the historical background of its first descriptions. If a couple cannot conceive and deliver a baby, we speak of "infertility" as an unwanted condition that has been well known since ancient times. However, the first known gynecologic medical text, the Kahoun papyrus (2200–1950 B.C), describes infertility as a disruption in the continuity between the reproductive organs and the digestive tract.

Infertility throughout the millennia started to be better understood when Hippocrates [1] described several causes of infertility and potential therapies. He prescribed "when, a cervix is closed too tightly the inner orifice must be opened using a special mixture of red nitre, cumin, resin and honey…or it could be dilated by inserting a hollow leaden probe into the uterus enabling emollient substances to be poured in." Vesale in the time of Renaissance, much later, published an anatomic atlas, *Humani Corporis Fabrica* in 1543, in which he included anatomic cross sections of female genital organs. Early developments of understanding ovulation and follicular function were slow and went over centuries. Table 5.1 lists some early discoveries relevant to ovulation and follicular function as well as their use to avoid fertilization.

Since the early successful days of ART after the birth of Louise Brown in 1978 [1] still in a spontaneous cycle at that time, controlled ovarian hyperstimulation became the advised concept for a successful outcome of any ART treatment. This concept may change, once optimal ways of single embryo development and transfer

M. Liselotte (✉)
Department of Obstetrics and Gynecology, University Hospitals of Schleswig-Holstein
Campus Kiel, Kiel, Germany

A. R. Genazzani et al. (eds.), *Ethical, Efficacy and Safety Issues in Contraception*, Reproductive Medicine for Clinicians 4,
https://doi.org/10.1007/978-3-032-07322-8_5

Table 5.1 Chronology in understanding ovulation, fertilization, and avoiding pregnancies

1672: De Graaf. *De Mullerium Organis* (follicular functions in the female ovary -thinking that the follicle was the egg) [2]
1707: Martin Naboth *De Sterilitate* (ovarian sclerosis and tubal blockage provoked infertility) [3]
1796: Morgani (the reason of infertility is follicular absence or agenesis) In 1905 Theodoor Hendrik van de Velde (women only ovulate once per menstrual cycle) [4]
1920s: Kyusaku Ogino and Hermann Knaus (ovulation occurs about 14 days before the next menstruation). Ogino used his discovery to develop a formula aiding infertile women to time intercourse to achieve pregnancy [5]
1930: John Smulders used Herman Knaus discovery to create a method for *avoiding* pregnancy. His work called the rhythm method was published with the Dutch Roman Catholic medical association, being the first published system for periodic abstinence. Scientist [6]
1950: Gregory Pincus developed the first oral contraceptives in 1950 [7].

in consecutive cycles to the ovum pick-up cycle, will prove the same safe outcome with healthy children and mothers in spontaneous ovulatory cycles.

It is the aim of the present paper to specify the understanding of ovulation and controlled ovarian hyperstimulation, also referred to as controlled ovarian superovulation.

De Graaf [2] described in De Mullerium Organis already in the year 1672 the ovarian and follicular function, although he mistakenly interpreted the follicle to be the egg. Martin Naboth, in 1707, published De Sterilitate, in which he claimed that ovarian sclerosis and tubal blockage caused infertility. In 1769, Morgani added follicular absence or agenesis as a cause for infertility. While a greater understanding of the etiology of infertility was gained during this time, Renaissance physicians continued to struggle to find an effective treatment to offer their patients [2–4]. Later Ogino and Knaus described independently in Japan and Germany the first female menstrual cycle [5, 6]. John Smulders and Hermann Knaus [6] initiated the groundwork for hormonal contraception by creating a method to avoid pregnancy.

The nineteenth and twentieth centuries were marked by numerous advances which now define what is known as modern medicine today. Reproductive endocrinology was born with the discovery of gonadotropins and their regulation of the menstrual cycle. In 1927, Ascheim and Zondek [10] isolated human chorionic gonadotropin (hCG) from the urine of pregnant women. Soon thereafter in 1930, Cole and Hart discovered equine chorionic gonadotropin, which became known as pregnant mare serum gonadotropin (PMSG) [11]. From these discoveries, the technique of superovulation was born. Methods were developed to superovulate immature mice using PMSG followed by hCG to induce estrus and ovulation. Foreseeing the ethical and medical complications of ovarian stimulation, Edwards and Fowler described an increase in liter size and fetal mortality during superovulation of mice

[12]. Despite already discovered in the late 1920s to early 1930s, it took over 40 years for the technique to be adviced used as a treatment for anovulation in infertility. In his description of the hormones, Gregory Pincus [7] described ovulation. At ovulation, a mature follicle ruptures and releases a mature egg that can be fertilized by sperm. Understanding ovulation is crucial for hormonal contraception. Ovulation is regulated by hormones and ovarian dynamics; by understanding the hypothalamo-ovarian axis (see Chap. 2), possible mechanisms to hinder ovulation were developed for contraception.

5.2 Ovulation Inhibition for Contraception

5.2.1 Introduction

Ovulation stands in the center of hormonal contraception. Since the early input of Gregory Pincus [7], internationally this method of hormonal contraception has been accepted worldwide and led to numerous publications [8, 9]. Congratulations to all the authors and pharmaceutical companies who have worked and will work on it.

5.2.2 Injectable Birth Control

It stops ovulation. It also thickens and decreases the amount of cervical mucus. This makes it difficult for sperm to enter the uterus and tubes to fertilize an egg in the fimbrial parts of the tubes or in the pouch of Douglas. It also decreases the size of the endometrium to a thickness of only 2–4 mm, which does then not allow implantation.

DMPA is injected deep into the muscle, such as in the buttock or upper arm, or injected subcutaneously (under the skin). With either type of injection, this contraceptive is given once every 3 months.

The most common side effects of DMPA are irregular or prolonged bleeding and spotting, particularly during the first few months of use. Only 50% of patients become "amenorrheic" after 1 year of DMPA use. Monthly periods generally return within 6 months of the last DMPA injection. Weight gain is observed sometimes under DMPA injections. Additional benefits of DMPA include a decreased risk of uterine cancer and pelvic inflammatory disease. Because DMPA is long-acting, it should not be used if the patient wants to get pregnant shortly after stopping the medication. Most people are able to conceive within 10 months.

5.2.3 Birth Control Implants

The implant (Nexplanon or Implanon) is a small rod that contains the hormone progestin. It is inserted under the skin into the upper inner arm and is effective for at least 3 years, but can be removed earlier. Insertion and removal can be done on an outpatient basis with local anesthesia.

The contraceptive effect of IMPLANON etonogestrel 68 mg is achieved by several mechanisms that include *suppression of ovulation*, increased viscosity of cervical mucus, and alterations in endometrial thickness.

The implant is one of the most effective methods of birth control. It provides at least 3 years of protection from pregnancy as progestin is slowly released into the surrounding tissues. Depending on when during the menstrual cycle, the implant is placed, backup birth control (for instance, condoms) may be recommended for 1 week following placement. Irregular bleeding is the most bothersome side effect. Fertility returns rapidly after the rod is removed. The most common side effects of the implant are irregular and unpredictable bleedings.

5.2.4 Intrauterine Devices (IUD) with Progestin

There are several intrauterine devices (IUDs) that release a hormone called levonorgestrel (a type of progestin). The two types of levonorgestrel IUDs (Mirena, Liletta) can be left in place for more than 5 years. The other options (Kyleena, Skyla) are somewhat smaller and can be left in place for up to 4 years (Kyleena) or 3 years (Skyla). All of the levonorgestrel IUDs are highly effective in preventing pregnancy. The major mechanism of action of the progesterone receptor agonist, levonorgestrel, is to prevent fertilization. The intrauterine systems, however, thicken the cervical mucus and slightly act on ovulation. Side effects—Although irregular bleeding is common initially after progestin IUD placement, bleeding tends to diminish over time. With ongoing use, people using Mirena or Liletta often experience little or no bleeding. Those who use Kyleena or Skyla are more likely to continue having monthly periods.

5.2.5 Birth Control Pills

Most oral contraceptives contain a combination of *estrogen and progestin*. The combination pill reduces the risk of pregnancy by *Preventing ovulation*, keeping the mucus in the cervix thick and impenetrable to sperm and thinning the lining of the uterus.

The pill makes bleeding more regular, with fewer days of flow and overall lighter flow. Additional benefits of the pill include a reduction in menstrual cramps or pain, risk of ovarian cancer or cancer of the endometrium (uterine lining), acne, and iron-deficiency anemia. One potential downside of the pill is that, in order to maximize efficacy, it must be taken every day, ideally at the same time of day. When taken properly, birth control pills are an effective form of contraception; however, skipping pills or forgetting to restart the pill after the week of period will increase risk of pregnancy. Missed pills are a common cause of pregnancy. In general, if a patient forgets to take a pill (containing hormones), she should take it as soon as possible and take the next one at the usual time. If someone misses more than two pills, a backup method of birth control (condoms) has to be used for 7 days.

The main contraceptive efficacy of combined oral contraceptives (COCs) is *suppression of ovulation* by inhibition of gonadotropin-releasing hormone (GnRH) from the hypothalamus, as well as inhibition of both luteinizing hormone (LH) and follicle-stimulating hormone (FSH), and disruption of the mid-cycle LH surge (Table 5.1). These effects are mediated by both the progestin and estrogen component of the COC working synergistically, but it is estrogen's ability to suppress FSH and thus prevent folliculogenesis that is likely the most important mechanism. The additional estrogen exposure in pills with a shorter pill-free interval, pills with an additional 10 mcg ethinyl estradiol in the placebo week, or continuous-use pills results in a more complete suppression of FSH and less folliculogenesis. However, a substantial number of women can still develop follicles while taking a low-dose COC. Additionally, the estrogen component stabilizes sufficient endometrium growth to maintain a regular withdrawal bleeding pattern (cycle control).

Side effects—Possible side effects of the pill include nausea, breast tenderness, bloating, and mood changes. These typically improve within 2–3 months without treatment (while continuing the pill). Side effects are also Irregular bleeding. Irregular bleeding, also called "breakthrough bleeding" or "spotting," is particularly common during the first few months of taking the pill. It almost always resolves without any treatment within 2–3 months. Forgetting a pill can also cause breakthrough bleeding. Taking birth control pills does not cause weight gain.

When the pill was first introduced in the 1960s, the doses of both hormones (estrogen and progestin) were quite high. Because of this, cardiovascular complications occurred, such as high blood pressure, heart attacks, strokes, and blood clots in the legs and lungs. The pills prescribed today have much lower doses of progestin and estrogen, which has decreased the risk of these complications. As a result, birth control pills are now considered a reliable and safe option for most healthy, nonsmoking people. While today's lower-dose pills do elevate the risk of blood clots, this risk is actually lower than the risk during pregnancy or soon after giving birth.

Experts have studied the possible association between taking the pill and the risk of breast cancer. While these studies have had mixed results, there is some evidence that people who take the pill do have a slightly higher risk of getting breast cancer later in life than those who do not. However, if there is an increase in risk, it is very small, especially in younger people. It is important to balance this against the benefits of the pill, which include not only pregnancy prevention but also a sizable reduction in the risk of ovarian and endometrial (uterine) cancer.

Women are advised not to use estrogen/progestin contraception under the following circumstances: If a patient is over 35 years of age and smokes cigarettes, if a patient could be pregnant or has had blood clots or a stroke in the past (as this increases her risk of blood clots while taking the pill) the pill should not be given. Also we should exclude patients, who have a history of an "estrogen-dependent" tumor (breast or uterine cancer), who have abnormal or unexplained menstrual bleeding (in which case the cause of the bleeding should be investigated before starting the pill). Patients who have active liver disease or who have migraine, headaches associated with certain visual or other neurologic symptoms (aura), which increases their risk of stroke are not advised to take estrogens and/or progestins.

Over time, using continuous-dosing regimens results in fewer bleeding episodes per year (or no bleeding at all); however, many people experience unpredictable breakthrough bleeding when starting a continuous-dosing regimen.

Progestin-only pills—Some pills contain only progestin (sometimes called the "mini pill"); these may be an option for people who cannot or should not take estrogen. This includes those who are breastfeeding or who have worsened migraines or high blood pressure with combination contraceptive pills. Progestin-only pills appear to be as effective as combination pills when taken at the same time every day, but they have a slightly higher failure rate if the patient is more than 3 hours late in taking them. A backup method of birth control should be used for 7 days if one forgets a pill or is more than 3 hours late in taking it. Breakthrough bleeding or spotting is common with both types of progestin-only pills.

Progestin-only pills are available in 28-day packs. Two types of progestin-only pills are available. For one type (containing norethindrone), all 28 pills contain the hormone. For the second type (containing drospirenone), each pack includes 24 hormone pills and 4 placebo pills. The drospirenone pill may be more effective than the norethindrone pill. A disadvantage of the drospirenone pill is that no generic is available, which makes it more expensive.

5.2.6 Vaginal Rings

These are flexible plastic rings that contain *estrogen and a progestin*. The ring is inserted into the vagina, and the hormones are slowly absorbed into the body. This prevents pregnancy, similar to the pill. The ring is kept in the vagina for 3 weeks then is taken out for 1 week, during which the patient will experience bleeding. The following week, it has to be reinserted (Annovera: this type of ring is reusable for approximately 1 year). Other rings (NuvaRing, EluRyng) need to be discarded and to be replaced each month.

As long as the ring remains in the vagina and is not uncomfortable, the ring's position inside the vagina is not important. In any case, rings have to be inserted within the first week of the menstrual period.

Most people cannot feel the ring while it is in place, and in most cases, it is easy to insert and remove. It may be removed for a short time if desired, as discussed below, but should be left in during intercourse. The partner most likely will not be able to feel the ring.

As with the pill, in addition to being an effective method of preventing pregnancy, the vaginal ring also has other potential benefits. These include a reduction in menstrual cramps, iron-deficiency anemia, and the risk of certain cancers.

Risks and side effects are also similar to those of oral contraceptives.

5.2.7 *Birth Control Skin Patches*

Birth control skin patches (Xulane, Twirla) contain *estrogen and progestin*, similar to oral contraceptives. Both patches are similar to the pill in terms of efficacy in preventing pregnancy and *ovulation*. Some people prefer patches because they do not require remembering to take a pill each day; on the other hand, some people do not like having a visible patch on their skin. Neither patch type should be used by people with a body mass index (BMI) of 30 kg/m^2 or higher.

The patch is worn for 1 week on the shoulder, upper back, abdomen, or buttock; one type (Twirla) can also be worn on the upper arm. After 1 week, it is removed and a new one applied. This is done for 3 weeks. During the fourth week, no new patch is applied and withdrawal bleeding will come.

The patch is ideally started on the first day of the period. This approach provides protection from pregnancy immediately.

As with the pill, in addition to being an effective method of preventing pregnancy, the patch also likely has other potential benefits, although studies are limited. These include a reduction in menstrual cramps, iron-deficiency anemia, and the risk for certain cancers.

While efficacy is similar to the pill, the Xulane patch may deliver a higher overall dose of estrogen. Some studies found that this was associated with an approximate doubling of the risk of blood clots compared with use of oral contraceptives. However, other studies found no increase in risk compared with people using the pill. Further study is needed to define this risk.

5.2.8 *Cardiovascular Risks and Infection*

All mentioned methods of hormonal contraception *with ovulation inhibition* carry a slight risk of cardiovascular disease.

One meta-analysis, which included 23 studies, reported that COCs increased the risk of venous thrombosis fourfold. The relative risk of VTE compared with non-use in norethindrone COC users was 3.2 (95% CI, 2.0–5.1), levonorgestrel COC users 2.8 (2.0–4.1), and desogestrel COC users 3.8 (2.7–5.4).

Medically, the key issues relate to reliability and the thrombosis *and infection risk* of each possible method. The most reliable methods are those that are the most straight forward to use, the implant, and the intrauterine device (IUD). The thrombotic risk is greatest with estrogen-containing compounds and the copper IUD which is a non-hormonal, just mechanical IUD that has the greatest risk of pelvic infection, while all non-barrier contraceptives at best have a limited benefit through thickening of the cervical mucus or no protective benefit at all in preventing infection. A good approach is the use of a long-acting reversible form of contraception combined with a male condom for prevention of sexually transmitted diseases.

5.3 Controlled Ovarian Hyperstimulation (COH) for Infertility Treatment and Assisted Reproductive Technologies (ART)

As hormonal contraception, meaning a barrier of fertilization, is equally important as ovulation induction and controlled ovarian hyperstimulation for any infertility treatment we deal in this chapter of our book of contraception also with it.

Only in the twentieth century, medical research brought up an understanding of the pituitary gonadal axis and the role of gonadotropins in the control of ovulation and reproduction (Fig. 5.1). After testing these hormones in different animal species, the use of these hormones for ovulation induction in humans followed. A real achievement in the history of ovulation induction was the isolation and purification of human gonadotropins.

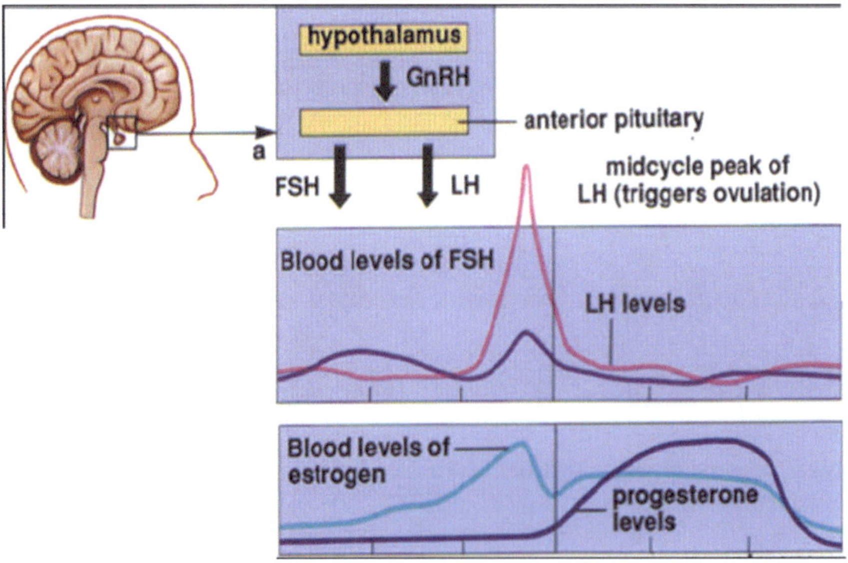

Fig. 5.1 Hypothalamic-pituitary-gonadal (ovary) axis

At the beginning, the amount of urine required and the extraction procedure for human gonadotropins were too complex to serve as a stimulation procedure. It was thought to better derive gonadotropins from the pituitary gland. Table 5.2 specifies the consecutive chronology in understanding details in ovulation induction. Despite intense work in the first half of the twentieth century, ovulation induction started only with GEMZELL in 1958 to be effective in the human [13].

In the 1980s, following the introduction of GnRH analogues (agonists and antagonists) for medical use in various fields, in human reproduction, they are till today a basic entity in every ovulation induction program. Their names usually end in -relin. The most well-known and widely used GnRH analogues are the GnRh agonist leuprorelin (brand name Lupron) and triptorelin (brand name Decepeptyl or in the USA Trelstar) and the GnRh antagonist, cetrorelix (brand name Cetrotide.) The application is performed intramuscularly, subcutaneously daily, and as depot preparations once a month or every 3 months. It is also available as daily application in form of a nasal spray, and recently also orally.

Gemzell's theory was confirmed by Buxton and his colleagues in the United States. This initiated the United States Public Health Service and the Veterans Administration to recruit a large number of hospitals for the extraction and purification of the pituitary tissue. In different centers, induction of ovulation was performed using pituitary extracts, which had primarily FSH activity and hCG as a

Table 5.2 Chronology in understanding ovulation induction

1927: Ascheim and Zondek isolated human chorionic gonadotropin (hCG) from the urine of pregnant women [10].
1930: Cole and Hart discovered equine chorionic gonadotropin, which became known as pregnant mare serum gonadotropin (PMSG). From these discoveries, the technique of superovulation was born [11].
1953: Watson and Crick description of the double helical structure of DNA.
1959: Edwards and Fowler: Superovulation was first described by an increase in liter size and fetal mortality during superovulation of mice. It took 40 years from 1920s till 1959 for the technique to be described as a treatment of anovulation in humans [12].
1958: Gemzell was the first to report induction of ovulation with pituitary-derived gonadotropins [13].
1960: Buxton and his colleagues at Yale University confirmed Gemzell's work in the United States in 1960.
1964: Donini extraction of human gonadotropins (HMG) from human menopausal urine in sufficient quantities; he stated to use of HMG for ovarian stimulation as a treatment for amenorrhea [14].
1972: Walter Fiers: first complete gene sequence of a nucleotide was obtained and published by Walter Fiers.
1974: Shome and Parlow proposed the amino acid sequence of FSH. This was soon followed by the cloning and DNA sequencing of the common alpha subunit then the hormone-specific B subunit. These early studies led the way to the expression of human FSH in Chinese hamster ovary cells, providing a source of bioactive FSH not only for experimental use but also for clinical application.
1971: GnRH was synthesized by Schally et al. [15].

substitute for LH. Although successful in stimulating follicular development, the technique was very expensive and had problems. Pituitary glands from 10 individuals were needed to yield sufficient quantities of gonadotopin to stimulate one patient for one cycle.

In 1970, as a young gynecologist, interested in endocrinology and infertility, I wrote to Andrew Schally, who was at that time in Houston, Texas that I want to buy a few grams of Human pituitary extracts with FSH activity for ovulation stimulation for my patients in Kiel, Germany. The answer was: "dear young doctor, fine, but how many million dollars you have available for this purchase?" Well, the concept of using GnRH, after its synthesis as decapeptide, and after understanding its rhythmical release from the pituitary led to the treatment of hypothalamic amenorrhea with the GnRh pump as normally GnRH is released in pulses at intervals of about 90 to 120 minutes from the hypothalamus. The releasing hormone must be administered in pulses by a pump to increase serum gonadotropin concentrations in patients with GnRH deficiency.

The "extraction of human gonadotropins" (HMG) from human menopausal urine in sufficient quantities was described by Donini in 1964; and later introduced as HMG for ovarian stimulation as a treatment for amenorrhea. In these studies, he identified forms of hyperstimulation and described the untoward side effect of multiple pregnancies as a result of the use of HMG and hCG for ovulation induction. The development of the technique to extract urinary derived gonadotropins provided a safer and more easily available source of FSH and LH, compared to the pituitary extracts, but the purity of the product was still low.

The high levels of co-purified contaminant proteins resulted in hypersensitivity and injection site reactions. While comparable to purified pituitary, many problems appeared with batch-to-batch variations and standardization of the dose from one batch to the next.

The desire to develop a monotherapy with FSH alone was driven by the hopes to provide a more consistent and better-defined dose. This led to the development of urinary FSH with minimal LH activity by Serono. They marketed the product under the name Metrodin. This formulation was used successfully in patients with PCOS and later for superovulation in IVF. Reproductive endocrinologists continued to isolate, purify, and study the regulation and function of hormones and the field of molecular and genetic science exploded. In 1953, Watson and Crick published their classic paper that first described the double-helical structure of DNA [16]. The central dogma: A gene is transcribed to mRNA and mRNA is translated into protein was proposed by Crick in 1958. These two monumental theories ushered in the age of molecular biology. In 1972, the first complete gene sequence was obtained and published by Walter Fiers. Shome and Parlow described the amino acid sequence of FSH in 1974. The cloning and DNA sequencing of the common alpha subunit was possible before the hormone-specific B subunit. The expression of human FSH by Chinese hamster ovary cells provides a source of bioactive FSH not only for experimental use but also for clinical use followed these studies. I very well remember our trials in the late 1980s. Using recombinant human FSH for ovarian stimulation in in vitro fertilization was only possible after 1992 [17, 18].

After immune affinity purification and high-performance liquid chromatography, urinary-derived gonadotropins could be obtained with low levels (<1%) of co-purified non-gonadotropin proteins. A repeatable standard dose of combined human gonadotropins is today giving us multiple gonadotropin formulations for ovulation induction with recombinant FSH and LH in addition to combined gonadotropins purified from urine.

As similar results are today achieved with all these stimulation patterns, the choice is not easy, depending on financial issues and knowledge of the physician. Although downregulation with and without flare-up protocols for GnRh agonists and antagonists are available, a stimulation with purified FSH appears to be the leading strategy. Let us not forget oral agents to introduce ovulation. In 1967, clomiphene was already approved by the FDA for ovulation induction. Today Tamoxifen and Letrozol are used as effective medications and show some benefits.

This brings us to ovulation induction or stimulation, to controlled ovarian hyper-stimulation or superovulation within the field *of assisted reproductive technologies* (Table 5.3). With all the progress in genetics, it is still not possible to decide upon an ovarian hyper-stimulation formula according to the human genome of the individual "mother to be."

In September 1981, at our first Bourne Hall meeting, Patrick STEPTOE, Robert EDWARDS, and Jean Purdy invited their friends, clinicians, and researchers from around the world to Bourne HALL/CAMBRIDGE and we established five contents that are still valuable today. These consents are still guiding all IVF protocols even today:

Table 5.3 Chronology of IVF and ICSI development

1890: Heape isolated and briefly cultured embryos from an Angora female rabbit, transferred the embryos into the reproductive tract of a Belgian hare recipient, and obtained offspring from the transfer.
1944: John Rock published the first report claiming successful in vitro fertilization and cleavage of a human oocyte [20].
1955: Shettles repeated Rocks work and reported successful culture to the morula stage in vitro of a human embryo.
1976: Steptoe and Edwards achieved their first pregnancy with IVF and ET; however, it was an ectopic pregnancy. By this time they had performed well over 100 stimulated cycles and were able to transfer embryos into approximately 70 women without success [21].
1978: Steptoe and Edwards were concerned that their failure in achieving pregnancies was related to the hormonal stimulation and the resulting luteal phase defect. This made them to return to use the natural cycle and then they published the delivery of the first IVF baby, Louise Brown [22].
1981: Bourne Hall meeting: In September 1981, Patrique Steptoe, Robert Edwards, and Jean Purdy invited some 25 clinicians and scientists from around the world to build up basic guidelines for IVF and ET.
1992: The first pregnancy using recombinant human FSH during ovarian stimulation for in vitro fertilization [18].
2023: ESHRE—Copenhagen, Denmark—At least 12 million babies since the first IVF birth in 1978.

1. Stimulated cycles are better than natural cycle for better number of oocytes and better prediction of ovulation and pregnancies
2. Ultrasound to monitor growth of follicles
3. Focus on embryo transfer (ET)/progesterone for luteal phase support—start on the day of follicular puncture
4. Control of culture media and laboratory procedures is essential
5. Effect of CO_2 on oocyte quality with laparoscopy. The first oocyte retrievals were done for years by laparoscopy.

Only between 1982 and 1988 transvaginal ultrasound-guided follicular puncture was developed. Many publications followed this meeting [19].

Since diminished ovarian reserve is diagnosed by blood tests measuring hormone levels, and not by counting eggs, it is difficult to determine the average number of oocytes of someone who has this condition. Stimulation protocols have to be adjusted to poor, normal, moderate, low, and high ovarian responders. Nowadays, the use of IVF has improved the prospects of infertility treatment. The expected outcome of IVF depends greatly on the effectiveness of controlled ovarian hyperstimulation (COH), where exogenous gonadotropins are used to induce folliculogenesis.

The response to stimulation varies substantially among women and is difficult to predict. Several predictive markers of COH outcome are available (e.g., maternal age and ovarian reserve) but no genetic markers have as yet been well established for routine use.

Nowadays, the use of IVF has improved the prospects of infertility treatment. The expected outcome of IVF depends greatly on the effectiveness of controlled ovarian hyperstimulation (COH), where exogenous gonadotropins are used to induce folliculogenesis (Table 5.3).

The response to stimulation varies substantially among women and is difficult to predict. Several polymorphisms in genes involved in FSH signaling, estrogen biosynthesis, folliculogenesis, folate metabolism, and other aspects influence the response to exogenous gonadotropin administration, resulting in differences in COH and IVF outcomes.

Nevertheless, the most studied polymorphism FSHRAsn680Ser is practically the only genetic marker, together with ESR1 PvuII T/C, that could be applied in clinical tests. Although data are accumulating with evidence suggesting that the ovarian response to COH is mediated by various polymorphisms, the optimal biomarkers and the efficacy of the tests still remain to be evaluated. Some results obtained by different research groups are promising; research involving useful predictive panels of genetic markers in COH is still in its infancy.

In addition to the large sample size, these genetic association studies should focus on optimal selection of study samples, which are controlled for ethnicity and geographic origin in order to minimize phenotype heterogeneity. A well-designed study requires also power calculations for the sample size optimization and optimal marker selection. The relatively slow uptake of pharmacogenetics in clinical practice is a result of several factors, including the additional cost of genetic tests, the need for specific laboratory equipment, the lack of proof of the utility of pharmacogenetic tests, difficulty in interpretation of test results, and a lack of knowledge amongst health professionals and also patients regarding pharmacogenetics. However, here is the easy way [24].

Basic parameters for monitoring controlled ovarian hyperstimulation in 2024 are still:

1. *Follicular size, vascularization, and numbers observed by vaginal ultrasound*
2. *Serum estradiol measurements (LH, FSH, and progesterone occasionally)*
3. *Endometrial thickness.*

5.4 Conclusion

Any type of hormonal contraception goes hand in hand with advances in other domains of the medical field as well as the understanding of ovulation, ovulation induction, and controlled ovarian hyperstimulation [23, 24]. Luckily, over the last 60, there have been many advances in relevant technologies: the development of ART and contraception went hand in hand with infection prophylaxis and treatment as well as with modern medical production in many fields. Even with Covid as an example of infectious disease, we are getting closer to irradication with the various vaccines on the market. New medical and medical technical advances in micro invasive surgery (MIS) in gynecology as well as in all medical fields, including robotics, new imaging techniques, inter-operative MRI, and inter operative navigation, lead to success. We advanced in prenatal medicine and also getting ahead in cancer diagnosis and therapy. Particularly *in contraception* new ethical and medical challenges come up daily to take care of situations. A comparison of ART centering on ovulation induction and contraception seems up to date. Artificial Intelligence (AI), ethics, and methods of contraception as well as selected systems for embryo selection in ART are more widely used to guarantee a healthy and successful life and have to be considered in healthcare in 2024.

Acknowledgment Thanks to my Kiel Germany Team of Obstetrics and Gynecology and to my co-worker Barbara Bonin-Mettler.

Declarations

Competing Interests The author(s) has no competing interests to declare that are relevant to the content of this manuscript.

Ethics Approval The author(s) declares that this manuscript does not include primary research with human participants.

The author(s) declares that this manuscript does not include primary studies involving animals.

References

1. Steptoe PC, Edwards RG. Birth after the reimplantation of a human embryo. Lancet. 1978;2(8085):366. Whiteley K. Hippocrates' diseases of women book 1 – Greek text with English translation and footnotes. 2009.
2. De Graaf R. De Mullerium Organis; 1672.
3. Martin N. De Sterilitate; 1707.
4. Morgagni 1769.
5. Kyusaku Ogino (1882–1975) and Herman Knaus (1892–1975) and the Oginus-Knaus method.
6. John Smulders, in the 1930s, the rhythm method.
7. Gregory P. The hormones (5 editions 1948–1964); 1950.
8. Skouby SO. Contraceptive use and behavior in the 21st century: a comprehensive study across five European countries. Eur J Contracept Reprod Health Care. 2010;15:S42–53. https://doi.org/10.3109/13625187.2010.533002. [PubMed] [CrossRef] [Google Scholar].
9. Hall KS, Trussell J. Types of combined oral contraceptives used by US women. Contraception. 2012;86:659–65. https://doi.org/10.1016/j.contraception.2012.05.017. [PMC free article] [PubMed] [CrossRef] [Google Scholar].
10. Kelley K. The Aschheim-Zondek test for pregnancy. Embryo Project Encyclopedia; 2010.
11. Cole HH, Hart GH. The potency of blood serum of mares in progressive stages of pregnancy in effecting sexual maturity of the immature rat. Am J Phys. 1930;83:57–68. [Google Scholar].
12. Edwards RG, Fowler RE. Fetal mortality in adult mice after superovulation with gonadotropins. J Exp Zool. 1959;141:299–322. [PubMed] [Google Scholar].
13. Gemzell CA, Diczfalusy E, Tillinger G. Clinical effect of human pituitary follicle-stimulating hormone (FSH). J Clin Endocrinol Metab. 1958;18(12):1333–48. [PubMed] [Google Scholar].
14. Donini P, Puzzuoli D, Alessio DI. Purification of gonadotrophin from menopausal urine by gel filtration on sephadex. Acta Endocrinol (Copenh). 1964;45:329–34. [PubMed] [Google Scholar].
15. Schally A, Arimura K, Kastin H, Matsuo Y, Baba TW, Nair RMG, Debeljuk L. Gonadotropin-releasing hormone: one polypeptide regulates secretion of luteiinizing and follicle-stimulating hormones. Science. 1971;173:1036–8.
16. Watson JD, Crick FH. Molecular structure of nucleic acids; a structure for deoxyribose nucleic acid. Nature. 1953;171(4356):737–8. [PubMed] [Google Scholar].
17. Devroey P, Van Steirteghem A, Mannaerts B, Coelingh Bennink H. First singleton term birth after ovarian superovulation with rhFSH. Lancet. 1992;340(8827):1108–9. [PubMed] [Google Scholar].
18. Germond M, Dessole S, Senn A, Loumaye E, Howles C, Beltrami V. Successful in-vitro fertilization and embryo transfer after treatment with recombinant human FSH. Lancet. 1992;339(8802):1170.
19. Wikland, et al. Collection of human oocytes by the use of sonography. Fertil Steril. 1983;39:603–8. and many other publications GIFT, ZIFT.
20. Rock J, Menkin MF. In vitro fertilization and cleavage of human ovarian eggs. Science. 1944;100(2588):105–7.
21. Steptoe PC, Edwards RG. Reimplantation of a human embryo with subsequent tubal pregnancy. Lancet. 1976;1(7965):880–2.
22. Steptoe PC, Edwards RG. Birth after the reimplantation of a human embryo. Lancet. 1978;2(8085):366.
23. Mettler L, Dasari-Mettler A, von Otte S. Artificial Reproductive Technologies (ART) and controlled ovarian hyperstimulation. Int J Med Sci Clin Res Stud. 2024;04(03).
24. Agarwal M, Mettler L, Marikinti K. Handbook of ovulation induction. Knowledge Bridge; 2024.

Chapter 6
History and Use of Fertility Awareness-Based Methods

Rachel Peragallo Urrutia

6.1 Background

Fertility awareness-based methods (FABMs) are a group of family planning methods that allow users to track one or more biomarkers to determine the days during each menstrual cycle when the chances of conception would be highest and lowest [1]. FABMs can be used to avoid pregnancy, try to conceive, and/or monitor ovulation and gynecological health.

As a group, FABMs are one of the least commonly used methods of contraception. Nevertheless, they are used by millions of people worldwide. Data from the United States National Survey of Family Growth, 2013–2017 estimate that 3–4% of current female US contraceptive users use FABMs [2]. A similar proportion of the use was described among contraceptive users in the 43 countries that participated in the 2014 Demographic Health Survey [3]. However, these proportions appear to be increasing over the last decade (from 1% of contraceptive users in the 2008 NSFG) [4]. Moreover, an additional proportion of contraceptive users use FABMs along with other methods such as barrier methods [5]. The majority of FABM users in national surveys use a calendar-based method [6]. In addition, the majority of individuals who are actively trying to conceive track ovulation using an FABM [7].

Unfortunately, relative to other methods of family planning, significant misinformation about FABMs persists among contraceptive providers and the public [5, 8]. This may be partly due to the fact that many FABMs are provided directly to users without going through a medical provider unlike for contraceptive drugs or devices. It may also be due to the fact that many health care workers do not believe FABMs

R. P. Urrutia (✉)
Department of Obstetrics and Gynecology, University of North Carolina School of Medicine, Chapel Hill, NC, USA
e-mail: rachel_peragallo@med.unc.edu

A. R. Genazzani et al. (eds.), *Ethical, Efficacy and Safety Issues in Contraception*, Reproductive Medicine for Clinicians 4,
https://doi.org/10.1007/978-3-032-07322-8_6

are a viable option for most contraceptive users and are unable to provide information about these methods [9]. This leaves potential users to seek information in the popular press. Heath care workers who provide contraceptive counseling and education should understand the effectiveness and use considerations of FABMs so that they can provide up to date and transparent information to potential users. The purpose of this chapter will be to review the biological and historical underpinnings of modern FABMs, discuss effectiveness of FABMs for avoiding pregnancy, and provide a summary of key ethical considerations for users and health care providers who are counseling potential users.

6.2 Biological Underpinnings of Modern FABMs

The ability to use FABMs to avoid pregnancy is based on the biological fact that penile-vaginal intercourse can only lead to pregnancy on some, but not all, days of the female menstrual cycle [10]. First, human females are not in a constant state of fecundity but only ovulate at a specific time each cycle. Second, human spermatozoo can survive in the female genital tract for about 5 days. Third, the oocyte has a lifespan of only 12–24 h without fertilization. Therefore, there are only about 5–6 days of potential fecundity in each female cycle. Finally, several bodily signs or biomarkers can be observed to help users predict fecundity at various time points in the menstrual cycle. The period of time during the cycle with high fecundity is known as "The Fertile Window."

The biological Fertile Window is the time during the menstrual cycle when acts of penile-vaginal intercourse could lead to pregnancy. Given the biological facts previously discussed, these acts of intercourse would need to occur in the days leading up to ovulation when sperm can survive in the female genital tract and the day of ovulation where sperm could directly fertilize the oocyte. The existence of the biological Fertile Window has been demonstrated multiple prospective studies (see Fig. 6.1) [10]. In cohorts of couples tracking days of unprotected intercourse and female ovulation through basal body temperature shifts [11–14], cervical mucus [12, 15], and daily multiple urinary hormone monitoring analyzed in a research lab [16, 17], Bayesian methods were used to calculate day-specific probabilities of conception. The probability of conception approached zero at 5–7 days prior to ovulation and 1–4 days after ovulation, depending on the method use to predict ovulation. In the studies using the gold standard measure of ovulation, multiple urinary hormone markers analyzed in a research lab, the Fertile Window began 5 days before ovulation and ended abruptly the day after ovulation: "In every cycle in which conception occurred, there was intercourse at least once during the six consecutive days that ended with the day of ovulation. There was no shorter span of days that included intercourse in every cycle. Conversely, there were 31 cycles in which there was no intercourse during this six-day interval, and none resulted in conception."[17] However, this method of monitoring the Fertile Window is retrospective and cannot be accessed by the typical user.

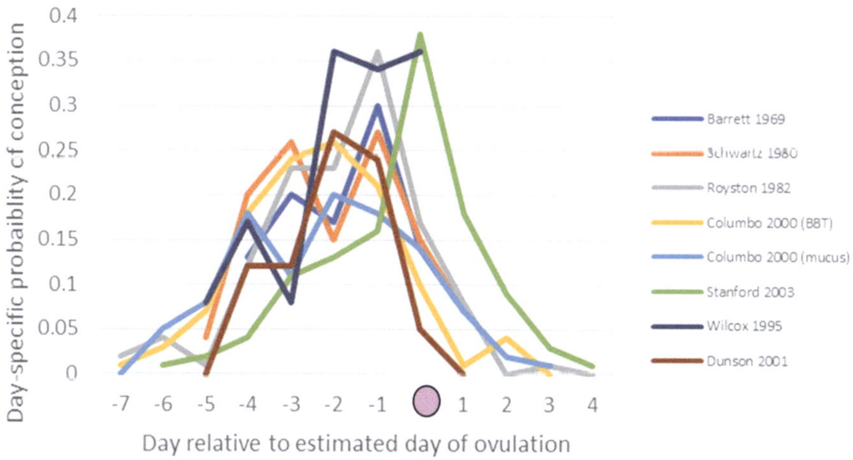

Fig. 6.1 Estimates of day-specific probabilities of conception from prospective studies. Pink circle denotes the day of ovulation. (Graphic generated by and shared with permission from Chelsea Polis, using data from Lynch et al. 2006)

Therefore, for users of FABMs, the biological Fertile Window needs to be prospectively predicted using one or more biomarkers that can be monitored at home by potential users. If everyone experienced 28-day cycles and ovulated on day 14, prediction of the Fertile Window would be relatively simple. However, despite the norms described in textbooks, less than 15% of cycles are 28 days in length, and, of those that are, <25% ovulate on day 14 [18–20]. Figure 6.2 demonstrates how people with different cycle lengths can experience vastly different timing of the Fertile Window relative to menses. Typically, the post-ovulatory or luteal phase of the cycle is the most stable in each individual and between individuals. The larger variation is in the pre-ovulatory or follicular portion of the cycle. As depicted in Fig. 6.2, individuals with early ovulation and 21-day cycles may begin their Fertile Window while they are still menstruating. For individuals with a 28-day cycle, the Fertile Window begins days to a week after the menstrual bleeding ends. For people with longer cycles, the Fertile Window may begin on day 20 or after. Individual users who have predictable cycles will be able to more accurately predict the fertile window in future cycles. Individuals who have a great deal of variation of cycle length and day of ovulation will, by necessity, need to have a wider fertile window to encompass more uncertainty in the prediction [21].

Modern FABMs have been developed to help users predict the timing of the Fertile Window and use this information to determine whether to have unprotected intercourse on a given day of the cycle. Users who want to avoid pregnancy need to avoid intercourse (periodic abstinence) or use an alternate contraceptive method (e.g., barrier methods) during the Fertile Window. Users who desire to conceive could time intercourse during the Fertile Window.

Each FABM uses one or more biomarkers along with a set of rules or a predictive algorithm to determine the Fertile Window. These include menstrual cycle dates,

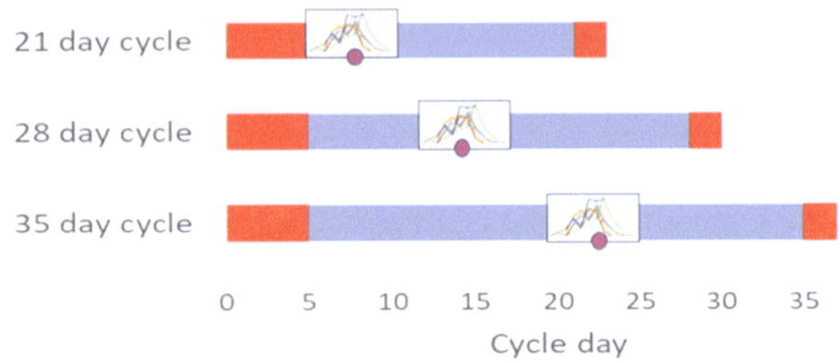

Fig. 6.2 Variability in the timing of the fertile window. (Graphic generated together with and shared with permission from Chelsea Polis)

cervical mucus, basal body temperature, urinary hormones, and cervical consistency and position. Previous **menstrual cycle dates** are correlated with the day of ovulation in future cycles, especially cycles with predictable lengths [21]. **Cervical mucus** consistency changes based on the hormonal milieu in the body. When estrogen dominates prior to ovulation, cervical mucus is more copious, watery, and clear allowing for better motility and survival for sperm. Users can appreciate this type of mucus at the vulva or even through sensation while doing normal daily activities. When ovulation occurs, the abrupt drop in estrogen and rise in progesterone leads to a sudden change in production of mucus; it becomes thicker, stickier, and less clear. This type of mucus can sometimes be appreciated at the vulva but frequently users perceive the absence of mucus at the vulva [22, 23]. Users can be taught to identify this "point of change" in cervical mucus which occurs ±4 days of ovulation [24]. Therefore, changes in cervical mucus can herald the start of the Fertile Window and its end. Basal body temperature (BBT) refers to resting body temperature, typically taken first thing in the morning. BBT typically increases by at least 0.5 °F ±4 days of ovulation. This temperature shift can be used to confirm that ovulation has occurred and predict the end of the Fertile Window but cannot be used prospectively to identify ovulation and the beginning of the Fertile Window [25]. **Urinary hormones**, most commonly estrogen metabolites and luteinizing hormones, can be assessed with home monitors. Rising levels of estrogen prior to ovulation denote days of high fertility (beginning of the Fertile Window), and a Luteinizing Hormone surge occurs within ±1 day of ovulation and predicts the end of the Fertile Window [26]. **Cervical consistency** is a marker that is less commonly used; similar to mucus, when estrogen levels predominate prior to ovulation, the cervix is softer, more open and higher in the vagina. When progesterone predominates after ovulation, the cervix becomes more firm, more closed and drops lower in the vagina [25].

6.3 Historical Underpinnings of FABMs

Historically and traditionally, there has been documented awareness of changing patterns of fertility, referenced in early Hebrew Scriptures from 1500 B.C. In Leviticus, the best timing for sexual intercourse, presumably to promote procreation was starting 8 days after the menstrual period ended, typically the days of peak fertility for those with regular cycles (Leviticus 15). References detailing fairly accurate optimal times of conception, at least for individuals with regular cycles, are present in Hindu, Tao, and Jewish writings from before 1000 A.D. [27–29]. However, other writings from early Greek philosophers shared less biologically correct ideas about timing of fertility [30].

Despite the correct understanding of changing fertility in some cultures, it was not until much later that scientific findings confirmed and clarified these traditional understandings. In 1678, Leeuwenhoek discovered spermatozoa, and, more than 100 years later, in 1827, von Baer discovered the mammalian ovum [31] [32]. Shortly thereafter, in the late 1800s, researchers first began describing biomarkers of changing fecundity that could be observed, such as cervical mucus changes and basal body temperature [33].

The Rhythm method was the first modern FABM to be described by Ogino in the 1920s. This method relied on specific calculations to predict the Fertile Window (using 12 previous cycle lengths, subtract 18 days from your shortest cycle length to determine the first day of your Fertile Window; subtract 11 from your longest cycle length to determine the last day of your Fertile window) [34]. Though the name of the method is frequently used to describe contemporary FABM users, it is the experience of this author that the Rhythm method, as described in the 1920s and 1930s, is very rarely used today.

BBT-based methods were then described beginning in the 1960s by Doerring in Germany and Marshall in the United Kingdom [35, 36]. Users document BBT shift around the time of ovulation and consider themselves unlikely to conceive if intercourse starts on or after the third day of a higher temperature reading. Users of these methods frequently pair it with a calendar calculation (i.e., subtract 19 days from previous shortest cycle length to determine the day of the cycle when the Fertile Window begins). Users who avoided intercourse until after the Fertile Window ended with a BBT shift had lower unintended pregnancy rates than those who had intercourse both prior to the Fertile Window (as determined by calendar calculation) and also after the Fertile Window ended (determined by BBT), but they also had fewer days available for intercourse if they wanted to avoid pregnancy [37].

In the 1970s, an FABM based primarily on changes in the cervical mucus patterns was first described by John and Evelyn Billings (Australia) [38]. This method, eventually called the Billings Ovulation Method, was based upon the rules that conception was more likely once cervical mucus began to change prior to ovulation and was less likely 4 days after the peak mucus day. The peak mucus day was described as the last day of any clear, stretchy or lubricative mucus. This method was further modified to include standardized evaluation of the cervical mucus by Hilgers and was called the Creighton Model FertilityCare™ System [39].

Symptothermal methods were first described in the 1980s by Doring [40]. These methods incorporated cervical mucus changes and basal body temperature changes into one method. Calendar rules such as previous cycle lengths and previous temperature shifts were also incorporated. Some users also substituted observations of cervical opening and consistency instead of cervical mucus. Though many examples of use of symptothermal methods exist, the method most studied regarding effectiveness is the German method called Sensiplan [25].

Symptohormonal methods were first described in the 1990s when home monitoring of luteinizing hormone and estrogen metabolites was first possible [41]. This type of FABM was further refined at Marquette University in the 2000s and is currently used with the Clearblue Fertility Monitor as the Marquette Model [42]. A randomized controlled trial evaluated the effectiveness of use of the urinary hormone monitor only versus use of the monitor plus other symptom changes (e.g., cervical mucus) and found no difference in effectiveness. Therefore, in practice, most users of the Marquette Model focus on use of the hormone monitor.

The Institute of Reproductive Health at Georgetown was interested in developing FABMs that were simple to use and teach among a variety of populations with varying education, literacy, and ability levels. Their research resulted in the development of a simple calendar method called the Standard Days Method, a method for individuals with regular cycles (26–32 days). The Standard Days Method defines the Fertile Window as day 8–19 for all users [43]. The group produced a variety of tools including an Internet application and "Cycle Beads" that can be used to keep track of days of the cycle. The Institute also developed a simple cervical mucus method called the Two-Day Method in which users ask themselves whether they noticed any cervical secretions on that day or the day before [44]. If the answer to either question is yes, they should avoid unprotected intercourse if they do not wish to conceive.

More recent advances include the use of Internet-based predictive algorithms. Natural Cycles was the first and still the only available United States Food and Drug Administration (FDA)-cleared contraceptive app [45, 46]. It allows users to inputs of menstrual cycle dates, basal body temperature, and (optional) luteinizing hormone peak day. Users do not make any decisions about which days are of higher fecundity. The app predicts those days based upon inputs received. More recently, Natural Cycles has been approved for use with Fem Tech devices worn overnight to measure mean resting temperature. These devices (e.g., Oura Ring and Apple Watch) sync automatically with the app each day [47]. This requires less input from users, but they must still check the predictive algorithm in order to make decisions about how likely they would be to conceive with intercourse on that day. An Internet application called Dynamic Optimal Timing was developed and subsequently approved by the FDA [21]. This a calendar-based method with predicted Fertile Window timing based on previous cycle lengths. It learns individual cycle parameters and can be used by people with more varying cycle lengths than the Standard Days Method. It was approved by US FDA as a contraceptive method but is not currently available to consumers. Another advance that may be coming in the future is the incorporation of quantitative urinary hormone measurements into an FABM [48].

6.4 Use and Effectiveness of FABMs

People choose to use contraceptive methods for a variety of reasons. Effectiveness is not the only or most important factor for all individuals who are choosing a contraceptive. Other important factors include cost, side effects, and patient autonomy in starting and stopping [49]. Effectiveness will be improved by good contraceptive fit for the user, which leads to more correct and consistent use [50]. Considerations unique to FABMs should be shared with users so they can select whether and/or which FABM may be the best fit for them. See Table 6.1 for considerations about FABM use. Each specific FABM has additional user considerations such as which biomarkers are tracked, when instruction with an experienced teacher is needed, etc., and these are more fully discussed in an infographic developed by the British Medical Journal [1].

Effectiveness for most contraceptives can be triangulated from prospective trials which are more selective and population-based retrospective studies which are more generalizable. With FABMs, retrospective surveys of contraceptive effectiveness such as the United States National Survey of Family Growth are unable to calculate individual effectiveness estimates for each specific FABM due to low numbers of users. The most recent effectiveness estimate for FABMs from the National Survey of Family Growth was 15 per 100 women years and lumps all FABM users together, probably mostly reflecting calendar-based method users [1]. In 2012, a Cochrane review investigated comparative effectiveness of FABMS but only included randomized controlled trials (RCTs) [51]. This review identified two poor quality trials and concluded that evidence about effectiveness was lacking.

However, it is logistically difficult to randomize participants to very different contraceptive methods; therefore, most contraceptive effectiveness studies are not randomized trials. Therefore, more recent effectiveness reviews for FABMs have included non-randomized prospective studies. Manhart et al. in 2013 identified 29 studies from a search of one database (Medline) published since 1980. Correct use pregnancy rates ranged from 0.4 to 5 pregnancies per 100 woman years and typical use ranging from 1 to 22 pregnancies per 100 woman years [52]. A larger systematic

Table 6.1 User considerations for FABMs

Advantages	No side effects May appeal to those preferring no hormones/devices Encourages body literacy Can be used to try to conceive Compatible with teachings of major religions
Disadvantages	Requires abstinence or use of a second method during fertile window Very unforgiving of incorrect use Long/irregular cycles may complicate use No protection against sexually transmitted infections
Advantage/disadvantage depends on user	Requires partner communication and cooperation Requires careful daily tracking of biomarkers

review was published in 2018 [53]; the search included four scientific databases from inception through June 2017 and identified 74 published articles representing 53 studies. No studies were ranked high quality, 21 ranked moderate quality, and 32 were ranked low quality. The moderate quality effectiveness estimates for each FABM are detailed in Table 6.2. The correct use rates ranged <1 to 12 per 100 women years with most being <5. The typical use rates ranged from 2 to 33 per 100 women years. One limitation of this study is that effectiveness rates for specific FABMs cannot be directly compared given the small number of studies of each method and the heterogeneity of the study designs and populations. However, it appears that methods with multiple markers like the Sensiplan double check method and the Marquette monitor-based methods are most effective. Typical use pregnancy rates for these methods are similar to those for combined hormonal contraceptives. Correct use pregnancy rates for most FABMs are quite low, suggesting that these methods can be used effectively with correct and consistent use. Obviously, potential users should understand the sensitivity of these methods to incorrect use.

FABM effectiveness data is limited for populations with long and/or irregular cycles. A review published in 2022 evaluated effectiveness of FABMs among users

Table 6.2 Effectiveness of specific fertility awareness-based methods for avoiding pregnancy from moderate quality prospective studies

FABM category	Specific FABM method	Typical use pregnancies per 100 woman years	Correct use pregnancies per 100 woman years
Calendar-based methods	Standard Days Method	11–14	5
	Clue Birth Control[a]	(8)	(3)
Mucus-based methods	Two-Day Method	14	4
	Billings	11–34	1–3
	Marquette mucus-only	4–19	3
Basal body temperature-based methods	Bioself	9	–
	Natural Cycles[a]	10 (7)	– (3)
Symptothermal methods	Single-check symptothermal	13	–
	Thyma	11–33	–
	Sensiplan double check	2	<1
Urinary hormone-based methods	Persona	26	12
	Marquette monitor-only	2–7	<1
Symptohormonal methods	Marquette monitor plus mucus	6–7	–

From Peragallo Urrutia et al., Effectiveness of Fertility Awareness-Based Methods for Pregnancy Prevention. Obstetrics & Gynecology 2018 and several newer studies

[a]Estimates in parenthesis were published after June 2017 and were not included in the systematic review

who were amenorrheic and breastfeeding [54]. Only four studies were identified and three were of low quality. Among the included studies, effectiveness estimates for the first year of use after delivery were similar to those of users with regular cycles. No studies evaluated effectiveness among individuals with polycystic ovarian syndrome or other syndromes of abnormal ovulation. One study has evaluated effectiveness in the perimenopausal age among users of the symptohormonal Marquette Model [55]. Effectiveness estimates from that study were similar to those of younger users; however, most users in this study were in their early 40s and not in the late menopause transition when ovulation is more unpredictable.

6.5 Key Ethical Considerations for FABM Users and Their Providers

There are several ethical considerations for potential users of FABMs and the providers who are working with them. The first relates to reduced access to these methods compared with other contraceptive methods. Because most FABMs are not drugs and devices, costs associated with FABM use such as working with experienced instructors, thermometers, hormone monitors, and internet applications are not consistently covered by insurers in some countries like the United States. Furthermore, many providers lack knowledge about FABMs and are less likely to offer these methods as "a viable option" for most contraceptive users due to their perception that clients do not desire these methods, cannot afford supplies, and would want more effective methods [9].

Unfortunately, wherever there are perceived barriers in which providers subjectively offer certain methods to some patients and not to others, existing inequities can be worsened. Whether it is Roma people or North African people in Europe or Black people in the United States, our societies have a habit of forceful reproductive practices on certain populations [56–58]. In the United States, this began with enslavement and complete control of people's reproductive function and has continued with forced sterilization in the early twentieth century and forced LARCs or refusal to remove LARCs in recent years. As one recent Black research participant told us, "They don't want us to have babies" [59]. If providers think that certain methods are appropriate only for some patients due to effectiveness concerns, this introduces an opportunity for the implicit bias of the provider about who should be able to reproduce to impact which patients they discuss use of FABMs with. In the National Survey of Family Growth 2013–2017, Black FABM users were underrepresented compared to all contraceptive users [2].

A common provider level ethical concern is about effectiveness of FABMs and the ability of users to achieve periodic abstinence. FABMs cannot be used to avoid pregnancy in the context of a relationship where the user cannot negotiate the timing of intercourse and/or barrier method use, and potential users should be counseled about this. However, for people in safe relationships, FABM instructors from multiple methods help train users to nurture intimacy in other ways than sexual intercourse. Many users of FABMs have satisfying sexual relationships. In a Sensiplan study, 1/3 of users only used abstinence during the Fertile Window, 1/3 used occasional barrier methods during the Fertile Window, and the remainder used regular barrier methods during Fertile Window intercourse. Frequency of intercourse was similar between groups and was consistent with frequency of intercourse in similarly aged populations. Pregnancy rates were very similar between periodic abstinence users and barrier method users (2.3 vs. 2.1 per 100 women years) [60]. In a large multi-national survey of FABM users encouraged to practice periodic abstinence, most felt that FABM use improved their relationship and their sex life with ¾ of men and women "satisfied" or "very satisfied" with their sex life [61].

Some providers are significantly concerned when they encounter a user of FABMs who has a serious medical risk from pregnancy such as history of placental accreta spectrum disorder, kidney disease, or cardiac disorder. In some of these cases, users may be morally opposed to use of other contraceptive methods. Regardless of the reason someone has chosen to use an FABM, shared decision making is essential. Contraceptive decision-making must be patient-centered regardless of the opinion of the provider and the perceived risks of a particular decision [62]. Patients who desire to use FABMs for whatever reason deserve transparent information and support to help them use that method as successfully as possible despite any provider discomfort about effectiveness. Furthermore, providers knowledgeable about FABMs may be able to help users improve the correctness and consistency of their use or refer to experienced instructors who can help.

A final group of ethical consideration for FABM users relates to the existence of hundreds of fertility applications being marketed directly to consumers. Among hundreds, only one available app has undergone government clearance as a contraceptive (Natural Cycles). However, many consumers may not realize that an app has not undergone effectiveness testing for avoiding pregnancy. Some devices have overstated effectiveness to consumers [63]. Many apps have a proprietary algorithm for calculating the Fertile Window which is not transparently shared with consumers or experts, and in many cases, the determination of the Fertile Window has not been found to be accurate [64, 65]. Furthermore, apps gather lots of intimate data about patients that is sometimes shared with third parties without appropriate transparency about how and with whom this may be shared [66].

For providers who desire additional training about FABMs, Table 6.3 contains a list of resources.

Table 6.3 FABM educational resources for health care providers

FABM information, general	Interactive infographic: https://www.bmj.com/content/366/bmj.l4245/infographic Effectiveness systematic review: https://irp.cdn-website.com/49b279e6/files/uploaded/ACOG_Urrutia-Systematic-Review (1).pdf Self-paced e-learning course: https://ctcsrh.org/ctcsrh-training/fertility-awareness-based-methods-of-contraception/ (1.25 continuing education credit hours) FABM effectiveness webinar: https://rhntc.org/resources/effectiveness-fabms-pregnancy-prevention-webinar FABM counseling webinar: https://rhntc.org/resources/understanding-and-counseling-potential-users-fertility-awareness-based-methods-pregnancy Fertility apps webinar: https://rhntc.org/resources/fertility-apps-new-approach-fabms-webinar Fertility awareness-based methods: Fertility indicator concepts and counseling points job aid: https://rhntc.org/resources/fertility-awareness-based-methods-fertility-indicator-concepts-and-counseling-points-job
FABM information, specific methods	Standard Days Method online module (2 h) https://www.globalhealthlearning.org/course/standard-days-method Two-Day Method resource repository: https://www.irh.org/twoday-method-resource-repository/ Sensiplan materials in English: https://www.replyfertility.com/store/ Sensiplan teacher training: https://www.sensiplan.de/en/professionals/teacher-training Billings ovulation method teacher training: https://woombinternational.org/global-outreach/ Marquette Model teacher training: https://www.marquette.edu/nursing/institute-natural-family-planning/teacher.php Natural Cycles application: https://www.naturalcycles.com/?irclickid=1-vxUvwiHxyKWzy0d1TrVVp4UkCQ2dQZs0Mq3E0&utm_source=affiliate&utm_medium=2003851&utm_campaign=EdgeBingFlow&irgwc=1
FABM instructors	Billings ovulation method: https://billings.life/en/contactbillingslife/billings-ovulation-method-teaching-centres-worldwide-2.html Sensiplan: https://www.sensiplan.de/en/how-do-i-start/sensiplan-counsellor?country=DE Marquette Model: https://www.marquettemethod.com/ Association of fertility awareness professionals: https://www.fertilityawarenessprofessionals.org/find-a-fertility-awareness-educator/ Couple to couple league: https://ccli.powerappsportals.com/en-US/ Read your body educators directory: https://readyourbody.com/educators-directory/

6.6 Conclusion

All methods of pregnancy prevention, including FABMs, have advantages and disadvantages. Offering a wide mix of acceptable and accessible methods is essential to help people achieve their reproductive goals. Users have the right to transparent information and support to use whatever method they choose correctly and consistently. Providing clear information about all contraceptive options is key and requires high-quality scientific evidence. Providers should familiarize themselves with FABMs. Clients seeking FABM information deserve respect and support.

Declarations

Competing Interests The author(s) has no competing interests to declare that are relevant to the content of this manuscript.

Ethics Approval The author(s) declares that this manuscript does not include primary research with human participants.

The author(s) declares that this manuscript does not include primary studies involving animals.

References

1. Urrutia RP, Polis CB. Fertility awareness based methods for pregnancy prevention. BMJ. 2019;366:l4245.
2. Brewer M, Stevens L. Use of fertility awareness-based methods of contraception: evidence from the National Survey of Family Growth, 2013–2017. Contraception. 2021;104:183–7.
3. Polis CB, Bradley SEK, Bankole A, Onda T, Croft T, Singh S. Typical-use contraceptive failure rates in 43 countries with Demographic and Health Survey data: summary of a detailed report. Contraception. 2016;94:11–7.
4. Kavanaugh ML, Jerman J. Contraceptive method use in the United States: trends and characteristics between 2008, 2012 and 2014. Contraception. 2018;97:14–21.
5. Polis CB, Jones RK. Multiple contraceptive method use and prevalence of fertility awareness based method use in the United States, 2013–2015. Contraception. 2018;98:188–92.
6. Frohwirth L, Moore AM, Maniaci R. Perceptions of susceptibility to pregnancy among U.S. women obtaining abortions. Soc Sci Med. 2013;99:18–26.
7. Pérez Capotosto M, Lee CS, Jurgens CY, Wang S, Mitsunami M, Charlton BM, Chavarro JE. Predictors of fertility-awareness-based method use among women trying to conceive and women contemplating pregnancy. Nurs Res. 2023;72:355–62.
8. Turner JV. Misrepresentation of contraceptive effectiveness rates for fertility awareness methods of family planning. J Obstet Gynaecol Res. 2021;47:2271–7.
9. Webb S, Cheng A-L, Simmons R, Peragallo Urrutia R, Jennings V, Witt J. A mixed-methods assessment of health care providers' knowledge, attitudes, and practices around fertility awareness-based methods in Title X Clinics in the United States. Womens Health Rep (New Rochelle). 2020;1:354–65.
10. Lynch CD, Jackson LW, Buck Louis GM. Estimation of the day-specific probabilities of conception: current state of the knowledge and the relevance for epidemiological research. Paediatr Perinat Epidemiol. 2006;20(Suppl 1):3–12.

11. Barrett JC, Marshall J. The risk of conception on different days of the menstrual cycle. Popul Stud (Camb). 1969;23:455–61.
12. Colombo B, Masarotto G. Daily fecundability: first results from a new data base. Demogr Res. 2000;3:39.
13. Royston JP. Basal body temperature, ovulation and the risk of conception, with special reference to the lifetimes of sperm and egg. Biometrics. 1982;38:397–406.
14. Schwartz D, Macdonald PD, Heuchel V. Fecundability, coital frequency and the viability of Ova. Popul Stud (Camb). 1980;34:397–400.
15. Stanford JB, Smith KR, Dunson DB. Vulvar mucus observations and the probability of pregnancy. Obstet Gynecol. 2003;101:1285–93.
16. Dunson DB. Bayesian modeling of the level and duration of fertility in the menstrual cycle. Biometrics. 2001;57:1067–73.
17. Wilcox AJ, Weinberg CR, Baird DD. Timing of sexual intercourse in relation to ovulation. Effects on the probability of conception, survival of the pregnancy, and sex of the baby. N Engl J Med. 1995;333:1517–21.
18. Najmabadi S, Schliep KC, Simonsen SE, Porucznik CA, Egger MJ, Stanford JB. Menstrual bleeding, cycle length, and follicular and luteal phase lengths in women without known subfertility: a pooled analysis of three cohorts. Paediatr Perinat Epidemiol. 2020;34:318–27.
19. Bull JR, Rowland SP, Scherwitzl EB, Scherwitzl R, Danielsson KG, Harper J. Real-world menstrual cycle characteristics of more than 600,000 menstrual cycles. NPJ Digit Med. 2019;2:83.
20. Soumpasis I, Grace B, Johnson S. Real-life insights on menstrual cycles and ovulation using big data. Hum Reprod Open. 2020;2020:hoaa011.
21. Simmons RG, Shattuck DC, Jennings VH. Assessing the efficacy of an app-based method of family planning: the dot study protocol. JMIR Res Protoc. 2017;6:e5.
22. Brown JB. Types of ovarian activity in women and their significance: the continuum (a reinterpretation of early findings). Hum Reprod Update. 2011;17:141–58.
23. Billings EL, Brown JB, Billings JJ, Burger HG. Symptoms and hormonal changes accompanying ovulation. Lancet. 1972;1:282–4.
24. Fehring RJ. Accuracy of the peak day of cervical mucus as a biological marker of fertility. Contraception. 2002;66:231–5.
25. Frank-Herrmann P, Heil J, Gnoth C, Toledo E, Baur S, Pyper C, Jenetzky E, Strowitzki T, Freundl G. The effectiveness of a fertility awareness based method to avoid pregnancy in relation to a couple's sexual behaviour during the fertile time: a prospective longitudinal study. Hum Reprod. 2007;22:1310–9.
26. Tanabe K, Susumu N, Hand K, Nishii K, Ishikawa I, Nozawa S. Prediction of the potentially fertile period by urinary hormone measurements using a new home-use monitor: comparison with laboratory hormone analyses. Hum Reprod. 2001;16:1619–24.
27. Chaturvedi BK. Agni Purana; 2002. books.google.com
28. Niddah 31a ~ When is a woman most fertile? – Talmudology. https://www.talmudology.com/jeremybrownmdgmailcom/2015/11/15/sotah-27a-when-is-a-woman-most-fertile. Accessed 11 Nov 2024.
29. Huang Y, Geng Q. Women become immortal through the use of procreation ability: a study on the fertility concept of female alchemy. Religions (Basel). 2023;14:727.
30. Flemming R. The invention of infertility in the classical Greek world: medicine, divinity, and gender. Bull Hist Med. 2013;87:565–90.
31. Colonna FT. De ovi mammalium et hominis genesi (1827), by Karl Ernst von Baer. 2017.
32. Birkhead TR, Montgomerie R. Three centuries of sperm research. In: Sperm biology. Elsevier; 2009. p. 1–42.
33. Vollman RF. The menstrual cycle. Major Probl Obstet Gynecol. 1977;7:1–193.
34. Tietze C, Potter RG. Statistical evaluation of the rhythm method. Am J Obstet Gynecol. 1962;84:692–8.
35. Marshall J, Rowe B. Psychologic aspects of the basal body temperature method of regulating births. Fertil Steril. 1970;21:14–9.

36. Döring GK. On the reliability of temperature method for contraception. Dtsch Med Wochenschr. 1967;92:1055–61.
37. Marshall J. A field trial of the basal-body-temperature method of regulating births. Lancet. 1968;2:8–10.
38. Weissmann MC, Foliaki L, Billings EL, Billings JJ. A trial of the ovulation method of family planning in Tonga. Lancet. 1972;2:813–6.
39. Hilgers TW, Stanford JB. Creighton model NaProEducation technology for avoiding pregnancy. Use effectiveness. J Reprod Med. 1998;43:495–502.
40. Döring GK, Socher K. Experiences with the sympto-thermal method of family planning. Geburtshilfe Frauenheilkd. 1988;48:106–8.
41. Freundl G, Bonnar J, Flynn A, Frank-Herrmann P, Kirkmann R, Snowden R. Contraception per computer. Hormone system persona – results of studies in Germany. Fortschr Med. 1998;116:47–8.
42. Fehring RJ, Schneider M, Raviele K, Rodriguez D, Pruszynski J. Randomized comparison of two Internet-supported fertility-awareness-based methods of family planning. Contraception. 2013;88:24–30.
43. Arévalo M, Jennings V, Sinai I. Efficacy of a new method of family planning: the standard days method. Contraception. 2002;65:333–8.
44. Arévalo M, Jennings V, Nikula M, Sinai I. Efficacy of the new TwoDay method of family planning. Fertil Steril. 2004;82:885–92.
45. Berglund Scherwitzl E, Gemzell Danielsson K, Sellberg JA, Scherwitzl R. Fertility awareness-based mobile application for contraception. Eur J Contracept Reprod Health Care. 2016;21:234–41.
46. Pearson JT, Chelstowska M, Rowland SP, Benhar E, Kopp-Kallner H, Berglund Scherwitzl E, Acuna J, Gemzell Danielsson K, Scherwitzl R. Contraceptive effectiveness of an FDA-cleared birth control app: results from the natural cycles U.S. Cohort. J Womens Health (Larchmt). 2021;30:782–8.
47. Alzueta E, de Zambotti M, Javitz H, et al. Tracking Sleep, temperature, heart rate, and daily symptoms across the menstrual cycle with the oura ring in healthy women. Int J Womens Health. 2022;14:491–503.
48. Bouchard TP, Fehring RJ, Mu Q. Quantitative versus qualitative estrogen and luteinizing hormone testing for personal fertility monitoring. Expert Rev Mol Diagn. 2021;21:1349–60.
49. Wyatt KD, Anderson RT, Creedon D, Montori VM, Bachman J, Erwin P, LeBlanc A. Women's values in contraceptive choice: a systematic review of relevant attributes included in decision aids. BMC Womens Health. 2014;14:28.
50. Dehlendorf C, Fox E, Sobel L, Borrero S. Patient-centered contraceptive counseling: evidence to inform practice. Curr Obstet Gynecol Rep. 2016;5:55–63.
51. Grimes DA, Gallo MF, Grigorieva V, Nanda K, Schulz KF. Fertility awareness-based methods for contraception. Cochrane Database Syst Rev. 2004;2004:CD004860.
52. Manhart MD, Duane M, Lind A, Sinai I, Golden-Tevald J. Fertility awareness-based methods of family planning: a review of effectiveness for avoiding pregnancy using SORT. Osteopath Fam Physician. 2013;5:2–8.
53. Peragallo Urrutia R, Polis CB, Jensen ET, Greene ME, Kennedy E, Stanford JB. Effectiveness of fertility awareness-based methods for pregnancy prevention: a systematic review. Obstet Gynecol. 2018;132:591–604.
54. Redmond JJ, Jensen ET, Stanford JB, Greene ME, Kennedy E, Urrutia RP. Effectiveness of fertility awareness-based methods for pregnancy prevention during the postpartum period. Contraception. 2022;114:32–40.
55. Fehring RJ, Mu Q. Cohort efficacy study of natural family planning among perimenopause age women. J Obstet Gynecol Neonatal Nurs. 2014;43:351–8.
56. Cronin M. Anarcha, Betsey, Lucy, and the women whose names were not recorded: the legacy of J Marion Sims. Anaesth Intensive Care. 2020;48:6–13.

57. Zampas C, Lamačková A. Forced and coerced sterilization of women in Europe. Int J Gynaecol Obstet. 2011;114:163–6.
58. Powerful Contraception, Complicated Programs: Preventing Coercive Promotion of Long-Acting Reversible Contraceptives | Guttmacher Institute. https://www.guttmacher.org/gpr/2021/05/powerful-contraception-complicated-programs-preventing-coercive-promotion-long-acting. Accessed 15 Nov 2024.
59. Verbiest S, Cene C, Chambers E, Pearsall M, Tully K, Peragallo Urrutia R. Listening to patients opportunities to improve reproductive wellness for women with chronic conditions. Health Services Research; 2022.
60. Frank-Herrmann P, Freundl G, Baur S, Bremme M, Döring GK, Godehardt EA, Sottong U. Effectiveness and acceptibility of the symptothermal method of natural family planning in Germany. Am J Obstet Gynecol. 1991;165:2052–4.
61. Unseld M, Rötzer E, Weigl R, Masel EK, Manhart MD. Use of Natural Family Planning (NFP) and its effect on couple relationships and sexual satisfaction: a multi-country survey of NFP users from US and Europe. Front Public Health. 2017;5:42.
62. American College of Obstetricians and Gynecologists' Committee on Health Care for Underserved Women, Contraceptive Equity Expert Work Group, and Committee on Ethics. Patient-centered contraceptive counseling: ACOG Committee Statement Number 1. Obstet Gynecol. 2022;139:350–3.
63. Polis CB. Published analysis of contraceptive effectiveness of Daysy and DaysyView app is fatally flawed. Reprod Health. 2018;15:113.
64. Duane M, Contreras A, Jensen ET, White A. The performance of fertility awareness-based method apps marketed to avoid pregnancy. J Am Board Fam Med. 2016;29:508–11.
65. Johnson S, Marriott L, Zinaman M. Can apps and calendar methods predict ovulation with accuracy? Curr Med Res Opin. 2018;34:1587–94.
66. Fowler LR, Gillard C, Morain SR. Readability and accessibility of terms of service and privacy policies for menstruation-tracking smartphone applications. Health Promot Pract. 2020;21:679–83.

Chapter 7
Fertility Awareness-Based Methods: New Technologies and Acceptability in Twenty-First Century

Valeria Versace and Domenico Arduini

7.1 The FABMs Ensemble

Fertility awareness-based methods (FABMs) are methods that allow women to recognize the fertile and non-fertile periods of their cycle in order to implement a conscious regulation of fertility. They are based on various biological indicators related to the phases of the menstrual cycle.

We can recognize four groups of indicators used in different FABMs: the rhythm of the menstrual cycle—the "calendar" (most women of childbearing age achieve a regularity of menstrual cycles), the cervical mucus (variations respond to the distinct hormonal stimulations of estrogen and progesterone), the basal body temperature (that rises in the post-ovulatory phase), and urinary hormones (dosage allows us to directly evaluate the hormonal state). Although they are all valid and proven indicators, FABMs obviously differ in the reading and interpretation that are made starting from them; furthermore, diverse FABMs can use only one or combinations of these indicators [1].

For instance, some methods utilize hormonal dosages, of which currently available for personal use are LH and estrogen metabolites; these hormonal tests are generally performed in a defined time window, so that other indicator is needed to combine informations: menstrual cycle data (Persona® contraception monitor) or even cervical mucus (Marquette monitor-based methods). Also cervical mucus is recognized, described, and intepreted differently depending on the method used [2].

V. Versace
Study and Research Center for the Natural Regulation of Fertility, Catholic University of the Sacred Heart, Rome, Italy

D. Arduini (✉)
Department of Obstetrics and Gynecology, Tor Vergata University, Rome, Italy

A. R. Genazzani et al. (eds.), *Ethical, Efficacy and Safety Issues in Contraception*, Reproductive Medicine for Clinicians 4,
https://doi.org/10.1007/978-3-032-07322-8_7

Hence an important first concept emerges, about distinguishing between the validity of the biological marker (e.g., cervical mucus, temperature) and evaluating a method that provides certain rules, calculations, interpretations, and methods of use through that given marker. Therefore, the last and final evaluation of the effectiveness of FABMs must be strictly referred to the single method.

Another important distinction concerns the reading method of the indicator, which can be performed by the woman in person (enabled to reading and interpreting the "body data"), or be delegated to an algorithm in which she gives an informative input and receives an interpretative response and an indication of use. Moreover, a deeper understanding of the physiological changings in the menstrual cycle will explain why only some methods allow the recognition of the pre-ovulatory infertility phase.

7.2 Current Awareness on FABMs

In this paragraph, we would like to consider the current knowledge in the medical cultural panorama about FABMs from a critical point of view.

Starting from latest UN documents regarding contraceptive use [3, 4], where the prevalence of contraceptive use divided by method is reported, we find, under the "traditional" section, the "Rythm" category, in which FABMs are included. Unlike lactactional amenorrhea method (LAM) is reported in the "modern contraceptives" section. We know that the prevalence of the use of FABM is considerably lower than contraceptives methods and studies on large numbers do not allow us to differentiate on the specific use between the different FABMs. But beyond the data, the choice to use the term "Rhythm" to include them denotes at least a lack of knowledge of the methods they are referring to.

Continuing with a critical analysis of the provided scientific information regarding FABMs, we mention guidelines specifically drafted to provide information on FABMs as an emblematic example [5].

Here we find a targeted, extensive, and quite complete discussion where the different methods are described, their basic rationale and how they work. Although some efficacy data are then reported in the text in relation to some methods, the initial data provided "The use of single fertility indicators is not recommended because the typical use pregnancy rate at 1 year is approximately 24%" is taken from the citation of a summary table showing a cumulative efficacy in typical use of FABMs [6]. Without entering into the merits of the study on the efficacy of FABMs, for which we refer to the previous chapter, we would just like to highlight about this same table, also reported in other studies [7]: there are many FABMs and each one displays its own specificities, offers various applications with distinct purposes and related efficacy, therefore it is not sustainable to provide cumulative data because it would be inaccurate in any case. Not respecting the specificity of the single method would be comparable, for example, to lumping together under a single heading short- and long-acting hormonal contraception, reporting the highest Pearl index, in this case of the pill, while we know that LARCs have a far superior efficacy. Conversely, providing a general information expressed "in range" would mean offering a summarizing but still respectful view of the evidence on the different methods, which therefore have different efficacy.

The culture regarding FABMs is enormously burdened by the lacking interest of in-depth comprehension of the topic. In fact, studies that have evaluated clinicians' knowledge about FABMs report poor results, as in a Canadian study in which less than 6% of the doctors involved had adequate knowledge regarding the perfect use of FABMs [8]. Another interesting finding in this study comes from the significant differences in preparation and attitudes toward FABMs among family physicians, gynecologists, and the respective categories of residents: gynaecologists, and in particular, the younger ones were the least informed and least inclined to include FABMs in their counseling of patients.

Unfortunately, the whole of misleading, inaccurate, or lacking information in the cultural, medical, and institutional sources on contraceptive methods effectively excludes FABMs from the scenario of available options in counseling about fertility regulation [9]. An extreme consequence thereof emerges, for example, in this Dutch study: "Professionals considered FABMs as 'not a medical issue', therefore falling outside the scope of their responsibilities" [10].

On the other hand, we have evidence that training doctors and providing tools to support counseling have resulted in a greater appreciation of FABMs both by doctors, who have therefore acquired adequate knowledge to include them in their counseling, and consequently also by patients who seek appropriate information and are able to consciously choose the best option for them [11, 12].

7.3 Which New Technology

The achievement of a more accurate tool in predicting the central event of female fertility, which is ovulation, has always aroused and continues to remain of great interest in research field, as highlighted by the study on "Prediction of ovulation: new insight into an old challenge" [13], published on Nature.

The indicators of female fertility are just those already known and "old but gold": to unite/combine the "old scientific rationale" with "new tools" is necessary in order to rediscover their meaning and improve their applicability also through new technologies.

Hence the complex new chapter of the theme of digitalization and how this compares with FABMs.

In recent years, we have witnessed a burst of applications (apps) development for mobile phones relating to menstrual cycles. Most of them are proposed as a simple monitoring tool, useful for noting and keeping track of events during the menstrual cycle. However, some intend to act as a method of regulation of fertility, both in the contraceptive sense and pregnancy research. At the moment, the two applications FDA approved as "Software Application for Contraception" are Natural Cycles®

(also CE certified as a contraceptive in Europe) and Clue Birth Control [14, 15]. The two differs in many aspects, first in the reported different indication of use and the analyzed variables: the first uses temperature measures and menstrual cycle data through proprietary algorithm, the second one based solely on menstrual cycle data uses the dynamic optimal timing (DOT) algorithm. Both software have been evaluated in efficacy and effectiveness studies [16, 17], even if some critics were raised against, in particular for the study design and interpretation of data [18, 19]. An in-depth review of Duane (2016) [20] offers an analysis of the apps available at that time, distinguishing them by purpose of use, rating the performance with established criteria, and evaluating outcomes deriving from their application, compared to FABMs. Results show a different performance in predicting fertile and non-fertile days, with an acceptable correspondence in only six apps, while in the remaining apps, the information on fertility periods has a high rate of false negatives and positives.

If, on the one hand, digitalization offers women many advantages, such as the simplification of data recording and sharing, on the other hand, it is important to maintain the distinction between evidence- and non-evidence-based applications in fertility regulation.

7.4 Acceptability of FABMs

When dealing with the issue of FABMs acceptability, it is clear that effectiveness is a central theme closely related; for this reason, we refer to the appropriate discussion in the previous chapter. In fact, we are aware that we remain today with the need for more high-quality effectiveness studies for FABMs to prevent pregnancy, especially in specific populations [21].

We therefore take into consideration other important factors that influence the use and acceptability of FABMs. By their very nature, the effectiveness of FABMs is closely related to the motivation that led the woman or couple to choose their use. In fact, when used for the purpose of postponing a pregnancy, approximately 80% of failure rates are reported in literature in groups defined as "low motivation," precisely because the final piece of the process remains patient-centered, based on woman's will [22].

On the other hand, when consciously embraced, the woman or couple keep satisfaction of their use and therefore have a low rate of discontinuation, as reported in this study by Moreau "Contraceptive discontinuation attributed to method dissatisfaction in the United States" in the comparison between pills and FABMS (29.2% vs. 14.6% discontinuation due to dissatisfaction) [23].

This data is obviously connected to the user profile. In fact, many studies that have evaluated populations using different contraceptive methods show significant differences in FABMs users compared to other contraceptive users. In particular, a survey on 6195 women between 2013 and 2017 in the United States reports particular characteristics in the relationship status, education, parity, health insurance status, and religious affiliation among FABMs users, and in reference to them a lower probability of previous use of pills, higher rate of suspension of pills due to side effects, and a greater propensity to have other pregnancies [24].

A crucial point in the choice of a contraceptive method is in fact the presence of side effects, present in most contraceptive methods and absent in the use of FABMs. According to a global systematic review, the issue of side effects and safety of a method is the primary concern of women when faced with the contraceptive choice and even surpasses the efficacy issue [25].

This data makes us reflect on how the topic of contraception is commonly addressed in medical-scientific culture, that is, with a purely quantitative approach. Notwithstanding, this rigor must absolutely not be abandoned, to avoid leaving room for non-scientifically sustainable drifts on this topic. Yet, it needs to be explored also from other points of view: the phenomenon of contraceptive choice involves the person entirely, in many aspects, and therefore cannot be reduced to a mere mechanistic process. Intimate issues such as fertility and procreation deeply affect personal identity, in the biological, relational, psychological, and spiritual dimensions. And so choices inherent in these areas are influenced by multiple social, economic, and psychological factors.

The idea that reproductive choices can derive from a rational calculation process is not realistic. Therefore, the qualitative research strand aims precisely to fill this gap in knowledge of reality, and it is more important than ever to have a deeper and more careful look at this topic.

An example of this approach appears is the interesting study by Dudouet in which the authors address the issue of the use of "fertility apps" through semistructured qualitative interviews. This sheds light on the thoughts, desires, and expectations of women when faced with reproductive choices [26]. The use of fertility apps is motivated in this study in particular by the search for "nonhormonal alternatives, to understand one's body better, particular life-stage and the ability to involve one's partner in contraceptive decisions."

The first motivation captures a particularly mainstream topic, as we can learn looking at social media platforms. Many studies have found a social movement that tends towards a "non-hormonal" contraception, highlighting and often overemphasizing the side effects of hormonal contraception, almost to outline a picture of "hormonophobia" [27].

Data collected by Kolher et al. from an analysis of the contents of the Pinterest platform, defined "pins," show how the OC pills receive the highest number of barriers to use (52.94%) mainly due to side effects, while FABMs resulted well-liked, with the lowest reported barriers rate (25.5%) [28]. Notably, only 5.45% of pins analyzed have a "formal medical institution" origin.

Also, the widespread used social platform TikTok is a lens through which to study this social phenomenon and the informational environment about contraception. Pfender et al. reported a popular use of hastags as #nonhormonalbirthcontrol and #birthcontrolsideeffects [29]. Yet, the negative depiction of hormonal contraception and the citation in favour of FABMs in these videos are far from being evidence based, while most are driven by personal experience and only 26% of videos analyzed were created by clinicians.

As these, other examples could be presented about the perception of contraception in general population, so much that clinicians may be alarmed and concerned about the rampant disorientation in this field and the feeling is of an insourmontable gulf in between the two realities, "medical academic" and social [27]. In a such situation, FABMs represent a symbol of this distance, laying just in the middle between the two sides: the more scientific supports exclude FAMBs from the fertility regulation options, the more the users seek elsewhere informations and alternatives, for example, on social platforms, where the ground can be fertile for the growth of conspiracy theories and hostility to the scientific community. The result on the other side is that clinicians and health providers distance themselves from FABMs even more, relegating them to "non-medical issues" and perpetuating the vicious circle.

Nevertheless, there is a great opportunity to fill this gap, returning to listen to users fears, preferences and desires. On the other hand, we have evidence of the interest of many women in learning a method of knowledge that enables them to manage their fertility and, when asked, they report a high degree of satisfaction in their use [30–32]. Such expectations and women's boost require a response from the scientific community, whose responsibility remains to provide valid scientific evidence to support them.

The application of FABMs, however, goes well beyond the contraceptive field. The fertility self-knowledge tool brings with it many benefits for the person: on a personal level (of identity), it builds a more aware self-image, improves self-esteem and women empowerment, on a relational level it improves dialogue with the partner, as a shared responsibility in reproductive choices is required [33]. Last but not least, by promoting education and fertility awareness, FABMs can become a valid aid in clinical practice, in diagnostic suspicion and monitoring of many endocrinological, gynecological, and metabolic diseases [34].

These final considerations about FABMs applications could easily let us state that "modern contraceptives and FABMs are not equal tools," as they can serve in other ways.

The citation instead comes from the paper "Fertility Awareness Methods Are Not Modern Contraceptives: Defining Contraception to Reflect Our Priorities" [35], quite a vigorous offensive to FABMs, particularly against the suggestion written by Malarcher et al. in "Fertility Awareness Methods: Distinctive Modern Contraceptives" [36]. In particular, the authors move reflection on the fact that FABMs—actually considering only three methods—do not get attention because they are confined by the definition of "traditional" method; according to the authors, this misperception can lead up countries to not prioritize investments on FABMs, moreover, FABMs use is less monitored and counseled, and "we as a community are failing to recognize a valid and important choice to meet client needs" [36].

In fact, the very core of the discussion is whether to include or not FABMs in the category of contraception. It is not a matter of deciding about if they are "modern": in the common sense of modern, they clearly are, since have been recently created and currently studied.

But what about the concept of contraception? Following the definition of modern contraceptive drawn by Hubacher and Trussell as "a product or medical procedure that interferes with reproduction from acts of sexual intercourse" [37], FABMs definitely don't fit in this category.

Understanding FAMBs in their multifaceted essence would result in addressing their pertinence outside the sphere contraception, but in the wider area of family planning, where FABMs and contraceptive methods are equally placed as valid options of choice. Plain language help us to assign and recognize the specificities, peculiarities, and nature of things, while giving the wrong name would lead to erroneous considerations and trickle-down effects on information and counseling.

7.5 Conclusions

7.5.1 More Evidences, More Awareness

In conclusion, strengthened by the solid scientific rationale of FABMs, we expect more evidences to provide robust data on efficacy and effectiveness in the various applications of these methods: avoid pregnancy, search for pregnancy, knowledge, and protection of reproductive health.

In order to achieve this, the whole scientific community should be aware of the nature of FAMBs. To implement course on FABMs in medical education would be highly recommended to fill this knowledge gap among clinicians.

7.5.2 PROs in the Twenty-first Century

In the current social context, non-negligible benefits could derive from the use of FABMs.

Unlocking the potential of FABMs would favor the "participatory" dimension of medicine [38] through patient—women empowerment. The advantages of self-body consciousness can go far beyond management of fertility or medical conditions, but can heal the person, from a psychological frailty, low self-esteem, in a challenging relationship.

Moreover, digitalization offers great potential in this field, as already noticed by the widespread use of fertility apps: this surge of interest would be better enhanced, making it an opportunity for knowledge, education, and prevention.

7.5.3 Personalized Counseling

The goal of reproductive and fertility management can be reached through many different paths, depending on a plethora of influencing factors, bringing to the personal right choice.

Clinicians should accompany users in this tangled travel, with appropriate, comprehensive, and patient-centered reproductive counseling.

Declarations

Competing Interests The author(s) has no competing interests to declare that are relevant to the content of this manuscript.

Ethics Approval The author(s) declares that this manuscript does not include primary research with human participants.

The author(s) declares that this manuscript does not include primary studies involving animals.

References

1. Manhart MD, Duane M, Lind A, Sinai I, Golden TJ. Fertility awareness-based methods of family planning: a review of effectiveness for avoiding pregnancy using SORT. Osteopath Fam Physician. 2013;5:2–8. https://doi.org/10.1016/j.osfp.2012.09.002.
2. Urrutia RP, Polis CB. Fertility awareness based methods for pregnancy prevention. BMJ. 2019;366:l4245. https://doi.org/10.1136/bmj.l4245. PMID: 31296535
3. United Nations Department of Economic and Social Affairs, Population Division. World Contraceptive Use 2022.
4. United Nations, Department of Economic and Social Affairs, Population Division. Contraceptive Use by Method 2019: Data Booklet (ST/ESA/SER.A/435). 2019.
5. FSRH Clinical Guideline: Fertility Awareness Methods. 2015. ISSN 1755-103X. https://www.fsrh.org/Public/Public/Documents/ceu-guidance-fertility-awareness-methods.aspx
6. Trussell J. Contraceptive efficacy. In: Hatcher R, Trussell J, Nelson AL, et al., editors. Contraceptive technology. 20 rev ed. New York: Ardent Media; 2011. p. 779–863.
7. Trussell J. Contraceptive failure in the United States. Contraception. 2011;83(5):397–404. https://doi.org/10.1016/j.contraception.2011.01.021. Epub 2011 Mar 12. PMID: 21477680; PMCID: PMC3638209
8. Choi J, Chan S, Wiebe E. Natural family planning: physicians' knowledge, attitudes, and practice. J Obstet Gynaecol Can. 2010;32(7):673–8. https://doi.org/10.1016/s1701-2163(16)34571-6.
9. Davidson AV, Butler FM. Physician dispositions toward noninvasive non-hormonal contraception. Kans J Med. 2023;16:94–104. https://doi.org/10.17161/kjm.vol16.18958. PMID: 37124100; PMCID: PMC10136678
10. Algera E, Leusink P, Gerrits T, Pols J, Ravesloot JH. mHealth technologies for pregnancy prevention: a challenge for patient-centred contraceptive counselling in Dutch general practice. Eur J Gen Pract. 2024;30(1):2302435. https://doi.org/10.1080/13814788.2024.2302435. Epub 2024 Jan 24. PMID: 38264977; PMCID: PMC10810654
11. Duane M, Martinez V, Berry M, Manhart MD. Evaluation of a fertility awareness-based shared decision-making tool. Part 1: Study design and impact on clinician knowledge. PEC Innov.

2022;1:100061. https://doi.org/10.1016/j.pecinn.2022.100061. PMID: 37213746; PMCID: PMC10194193
12. Duane M, Martinez V, Berry M, Gilpatrick S, Manhart MD. Evaluation of a fertility awareness-based shared decision-making tool. Part 2: Patient experiences. PEC Innov. 2023;2:100169. https://doi.org/10.1016/j.pecinn.2023.100169. PMID: 37384150; PMCID: PMC10294094
13. Maman E, Adashi EY, Baum M, Hourvitz A. Prediction of ovulation: new insight into an old challenge. Sci Rep. 2023;13(1):20003. https://doi.org/10.1038/s41598-023-47241-2. PMID: 37968377; PMCID: PMC10651856
14. U.S. Food and Drug Administration. 510(k) Premarket Notification Number K193330; 2024. Available from: https://www.accessdata.fda.gov/scripts/cdrh/cfdocs/cfpmn/pmn.cfm?ID=K193330. Accessed 29 Nov 2024.
15. U.S. Food and Drug Administration. Device Classification Under Section 513(f)(2)(De Novo); Number DEN170052; 2024. Available from: https://www.accessdata.fda.gov/scripts/cdrh/cfdocs/cfpmn/denovo.cfm?id=DEN170052. Accessed 29 Nov 2024.
16. Berglund Scherwitzl E, Lundberg O, Kopp Kallner H, Gemzell Danielsson K, Trussell J, Scherwitzl R. Perfect-use and typical-use Pearl Index of a contraceptive mobile app. Contraception. 2017;96(6):420–5. https://doi.org/10.1016/j.contraception.2017.08.014. Epub 2017 Sep 4. PMID: 28882680; PMCID: PMC5669828
17. Jennings V, Haile LT, Simmons RG, Spieler J, Shattuck D. Perfect- and typical-use effectiveness of the Dot fertility app over 13 cycles: results from a prospective contraceptive effectiveness trial. Eur J Contracept Reprod Health Care. 2019;24(2):148–53. https://doi.org/10.1080/13625187.2019.1581164. Epub 2019 Mar 18
18. Schimmoeller N, Creinin MD. More clarity needed for contraceptive mobile app Pearl Index calculations. Contraception. 2018;97(5):456. https://doi.org/10.1016/j.contraception.2018.01.005. Epub 2018 Mar 3
19. Freundl G, Fehring RJ, Frank-Herrman P, Gnoth C. Study of contraceptive mobile app fails to provide convincing findings. Contraception. 2019;99(5):312. https://doi.org/10.1016/j.contraception.2018.07.141. Epub 2019 Feb 14
20. Duane M, Contreras A, Jensen ET, White A. The performance of fertility awareness-based method apps marketed to avoid pregnancy. J Am Board Fam Med. 2016;29(4):508–11. https://doi.org/10.3122/jabfm.2016.04.160022.
21. Redmond JJ, Jensen ET, Stanford JB, Greene ME, Kennedy E, Urrutia RP. Effectiveness of fertility awareness-based methods for pregnancy prevention during the postpartum period. Contraception. 2022;114:32–40. https://doi.org/10.1016/j.contraception.2022.06.007. Epub 2022 Jun 15
22. Fehring RJ, Schneider M, Barron ML, Pruszynski J. Influence of motivation on the efficacy of natural family planning. MCN Am J Matern Child Nurs. 2013;38(6):352–8. https://doi.org/10.1097/NMC.0b013e3182a1ecc0.
23. Moreau C, Cleland K, Trussell J. Contraceptive discontinuation attributed to method dissatisfaction in the United States. Contraception. 2007;76(4):267–72. https://doi.org/10.1016/j.contraception.2007.06.008. Epub 2007 Aug 28
24. Brewer M, Stevens L. Use of fertility awareness-based methods of contraception: evidence from the National Survey of Family Growth, 2013–2017. Contraception. 2021;104(2):183–7. https://doi.org/10.1016/j.contraception.2021.03.014. Epub 2021 Mar 21
25. Yeh PT, Kautsar H, Kennedy CE, Gaffield ME. Values and preferences for contraception: a global systematic review. Contraception. 2022;111:3–21. https://doi.org/10.1016/j.contraception.2022.04.011. Epub 2022 May 4. PMID: 35525287; PMCID: PMC9232836
26. Dudouet L. Digitised fertility: the use of fertility awareness apps as a form of contraception in the United Kingdom. Soc Sci Humanit Open. 2022;5(1):100261. https://doi.org/10.1016/j.ssaho.2022.100261.
27. Foran T. Contraception and the media: lessons past, present and future. Eur J Contracept Reprod Health Care. 2019;24(1):80–2. https://doi.org/10.1080/13625187.2018.1563067. Epub 2019 Jan 24

28. Kohler T, Guidry JPD, Perrin P, Laestadius L. Oh baby! A content analysis of contraception pins on pinterest. Health Educ Behav. 2023;50(6):783–91. https://doi.org/10.1177/10901981231152238. Epub 2023 Feb 3
29. Pfender EJ, Tsiandoulas K, Morain SR, Fowler LR. Hormonal contraceptive side effects and nonhormonal alternatives on TikTok: a content analysis. Health Promot Pract. 2024:15248399231221163. https://doi.org/10.1177/15248399231221163. Epub ahead of print
30. Starling MS, Kandel Z, Haile L, Simmons RG. User profile and preferences in fertility apps for preventing pregnancy: an exploratory pilot study. Mhealth. 2018;4:21. https://doi.org/10.21037/mhealth.2018.06.02. PMID: 30050917; PMCID: PMC6043758
31. Ayala-Ramirez M, Grewe ME, Kaiser J, Kennedy E, Winn M, Urrutia RP. Understanding the perspective of women who use the Billings Ovulation Method®: a focus group study. BMC Womens Health. 2023;23(1):251. https://doi.org/10.1186/s12905-023-02398-w. PMID: 37161466; PMCID: PMC10170796
32. Stujenske TM, Mu Q, Pérez Capotosto M, Bouchard TP. Survey analysis of quantitative and qualitative menstrual cycle tracking technologies. Medicina. 2023;59(9):1509. https://doi.org/10.3390/medicina59091509.
33. Pyper CM, Knight J. Fertility awareness methods of family planning: the physiological background, methodology and effectiveness of fertility awareness methods. J Fam Plann Reprod Health Care. 2001;27(2):103–9. https://doi.org/10.1783/147118901101195173.
34. Duane M, Stanford JB, Porucznik CA, Vigil P. Fertility awareness-based methods for women's health and family planning. Front Med (Lausanne). 2022;9:858977. https://doi.org/10.3389/fmed.2022.858977. PMID: 35685421; PMCID: PMC9171018
35. Austad K, Chary A, Colom A, Barillas R, Luna D, Menjívar C, Metz B, Petrocy A, Ruch A, Rohloff P. Fertility awareness methods are not modern contraceptives: defining contraception to reflect our priorities. Glob Health Sci Pract. 2016;4(2):342–5. https://doi.org/10.9745/GHSP-D-16-00044. PMID: 27353626; PMCID: PMC4982257
36. Malarcher S, Spieler J, Fabic MS, Jordan S, Starbird EH, Kenon C. Fertility awareness methods: distinctive modern contraceptives. Glob Health Sci Pract. 2016;4(1):13–5. https://doi.org/10.9745/GHSP-D-15-00297. PMID: 27016540; PMCID: PMC4807745
37. Hubacher D, Trussell J. A definition of modern contraceptive methods. Contraception. 2015;92(5):420–1. CrossRef. Medline
38. Hood L, Friend SH. Predictive, personalized, preventive, participatory (P4) cancer medicine. Nat Rev Clin Oncol. 2011;8(3):184–7.

Part III
Hormonal Contraception: Principle, Molecules Route of Administration, Liver Effects and Arterial Safety

Chapter 8
Female Hormonal Contraception: Principles and Molecules

Giuseppe Benagiano, Paola Bianchi, and Marwan Habiba

8.1 Introduction

The great Roman orator and statesman Marcus Tullius Cicero called history the "*witness of the times, the light of truth, the life of memory, the teachers of life*" [1]. It is for this reason that to fully understand the present place of hormonal contraception (HC) and its possible future developments, it is important to go back in time and revisit the path that led to the identification of the compounds, as well as the basic mechanisms that made HC possible.

To carry out this task properly, it is necessary at the outset, to state that the control of human fertility is not a modern quest; rather, it has been sought for millennia. The need is shaped by the unique characteristics of human sexuality. Indeed, the female of *Homo sapiens* is unique (with the exception of a chimpanzee species named *Pan paniscus* or bonobo [2], with which we share 99% of our DNA [3]), in that she is not seasonally receptive to the male, but has a hidden fertile period. The human fertile period was determined in the 1930s, through the famous observations of Ogino [4] and Knauss [5].

The history of contraception in general is totally outside the scope of this essay, and those interested may consult the publication by Riddle and Estes [6].

Here, it is important to mention that over the centuries, efforts to develop methods to prevent pregnancy were made for two distinct purposes: to avoid unwanted pregnancies and to quench population growth. With regard to second objective,

G. Benagiano (✉) · P. Bianchi
Sapienza, University of Rome, Rome, Italy
e-mail: paola.bianchi@uniroma1.it

M. Habiba
Department of Health Sciences, University of Leicester and University Hospitals of Leicester, Leicester, UK

A. R. Genazzani et al. (eds.), *Ethical, Efficacy and Safety Issues in Contraception*, Reproductive Medicine for Clinicians 4,
https://doi.org/10.1007/978-3-032-07322-8_8

warnings were repeated over the centuries about the dangers of human overpopulation. Reference to this can be found as early as the seventh century, when the Syrian Bishop Saint John Damascene proclaimed: "The world is now congested and can no longer contain us" [7].

At any rate, according to Short [8], the first analytic approach to issues related to population growth was that of the Scottish economist, Adam Smith, the pioneer of Political Economy, who, in 1776, published his famous book *The Wealth of Nations* [9]. In the book, he exposed the inherent flaw in the Economy, which as a human artefact, offers unlimited power, but no feedback controls to self-interest. He argued that this greed will ultimately run counter to the inherent ecological constraints of the planet, and population growth will become a problem.

Interestingly, in a 1964 review, Pincus and Bialy highlighted the emphasis being placed at the time on the "problem" of population growth which they describe as especially acute in some of the newly emerging and some of the older underdeveloped nations [10].

The point of view expressed by Short does not seem totally correct: In fact, Adam Smith was not critical of market forces driving the Economy; rather, he was a proponent of what is now termed with a French expression "Laissez-faire" economics and minimal government. He saw population growth as a measure of a healthy economy and was neither for or against population growth; rather, he used it in the way we measure the Gross Domestic Product (GDP) today.

In the eighteenth century, well before the birth of GDP, looking at the sign of the balance of trade was a way to take the pulse of a nation's economy. Adam Smith rejects this measure and instead suggests that we should look at population growth. Nations that are able to produce enough to support the life of a growing population have growing economies; nations with constant population have stagnant economies, and nations that face a declining population have contracting economies.

Leaving aside these considerations, a real movement against overpopulation started when, in 1798, the Rev. Thomas Robert Malthus anonymously published an "*Essay on the Principle of Population*" [11] stating that the impact of population growth in Britain is far greater than its ability to produce livelihood. He reasoned that, if uncontrolled, population grows geometrically, whereas means of subsistence increase arithmetically. It must be stressed that Malthus condemned both abortion (an "*improper art that hides the consequences of irregular relationships*") and contraception (amounting to "*promiscuous concubinage*").

Finally, at the end of the nineteenth century, Sigmund Freud endorsed contraception in its modern meaning as a tool allowing free decision-making by couples. He wrote: "*It would be one of the greatest triumphs of humanity … if the act responsible for procreation could be raised to the level of a voluntary and intentional behavior in order to separate it from the imperative to satisfy a natural urge*" [12].

Against this background, we will retrace the path that led from the first hormonal contraceptives to the present days in order to illustrate the thinking (and errors) that made progress possible. We believe that this is the best way to better understand how the growing and emerging knowledge of the active substances and their role in reproductive endocrinology led to the development of the range of methods currently available that can induce temporary, reversible suppression of fertility.

8.2 The Early History

According to Kirsch and Ogas [13], the first step in acquiring knowledge that would eventually lead to the development of hormonal contraception was made almost 160 years ago when an anonymous Swiss veterinarian wanted to help a peasant who complained that "*Meine Kuh hat kein Kalb*" (My cow has no calf). He had the idea of exploring the animal's ovaries and found that by inserting a hand in the rectum of the cow, it was possible to break a structure in the ovary (today we know that it was the corpus luteum) and make the animal fertile again. We traced this practice to the description by Graber-Kölliken, who reported on restoring the estrus cycle in cows by inserting a hand in the rectum to cause manual enucleation of the ovarian yellow body. His first case in 1892 was a success, but the two subsequent cases died from internal bleeding [14]. So, paradoxically, the first step may have been through finding how to reset animal fertility.

Then, in 1897, Erwin Zschokke [15], Professor of Veterinary Pharmacology in Zürich, published an article explaining the procedure and mentioned that no new follicles are found in the ovaries of cows in the presence of a corpus luteum. The implication is that the corpus luteum induces a temporary, reversible physiologic infertility.

This observation started a process that within half a century would lead to the commercialization of the first hormonal contraceptives.

As aptly described by Djerassi [16], "*the least-known character in the history of the Pill*" was the Austrian physiologist Ludwig Haberlandt, who described his work in an almost completely forgotten book published in 1931 [17] (Fig. 8.1). Haberlandt stated that—to his knowledge—the first ever human experiments were conducted in 1924 in Germany by Rübsamen [18] who administered a corpus luteum extract to two women to block ovulation. Following the injection, there was a period of amenorrhea, interpreted as proof that infertility had been induced. Haberlandt also vaguely mentions information that in Russia "*hormonal sterilizations are already carried out with placenta extracts.*"

Haberlandt claims that he was the first to work experimentally since 1919 on ways to induce temporary infertility in female rabbits and guinea pigs by transplanting ovaries from a pregnant counterpart animal [19] (see Fig. 8.2). His further experiments were then presented in a second publication [20].

For his interest in applying the techniques to humans, Ludwig Haberlandt came under strong criticism by physicians accusing him of endangering future mothers and their offspring. As an example, in 1924, he replied to repeated attacks by A. Greil. In his rebuttal, he started by reminding his critic that "I have already repeatedly rejected his repeatedly expressed concerns about possible damage to future offspring and have also refuted them experimentally." He went on to explain

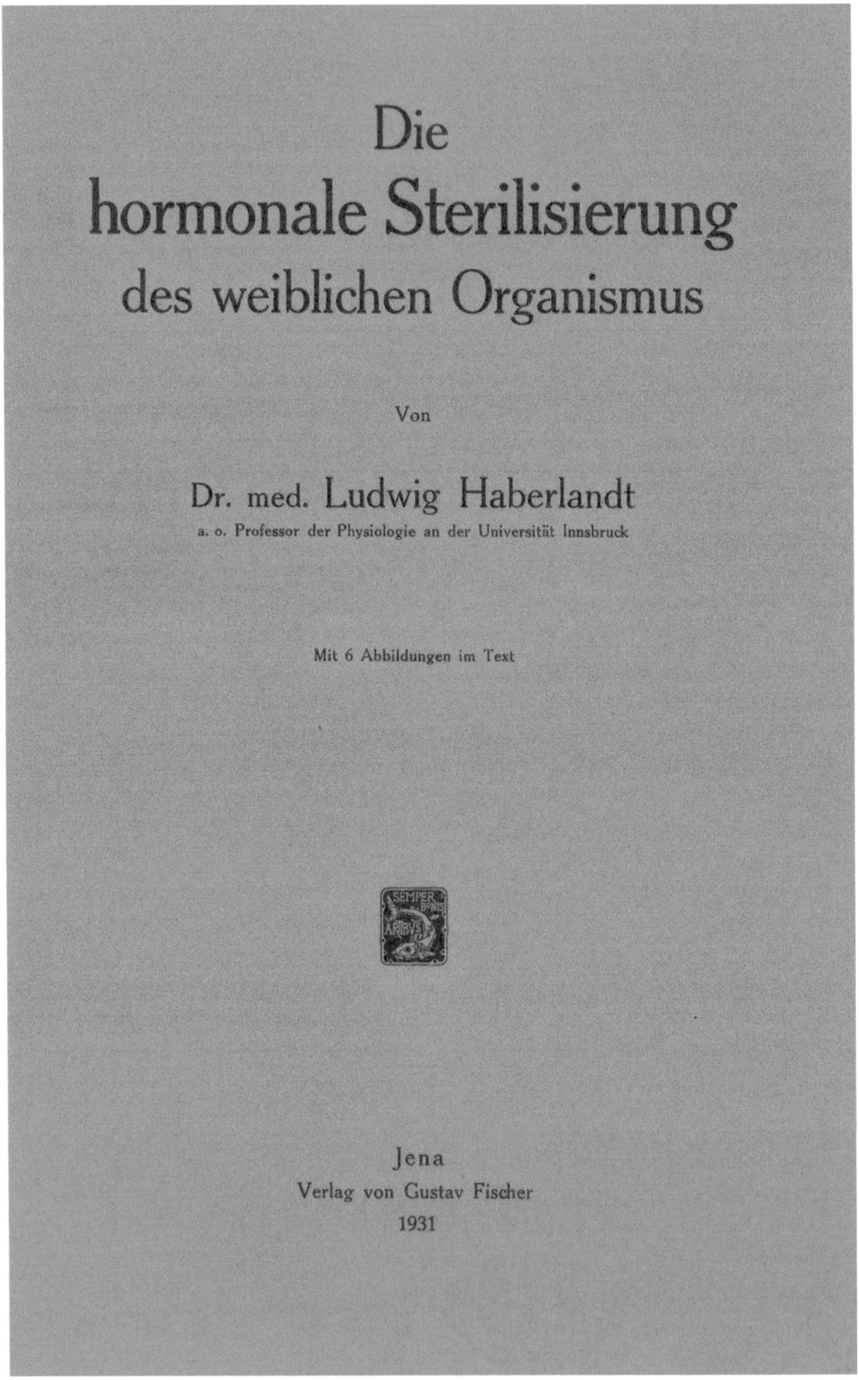

Die
hormonale Sterilisierung
des weiblichen Organismus

Von

Dr. med. Ludwig Haberlandt
a. o. Professor der Physiologie an der Universität Innsbruck

Mit 6 Abbildungen im Text

SEMPER BONIS ARTIBVS

Jena
Verlag von Gustav Fischer
1931

Fig. 8.1 (**a**) The title page of the book by Haberlandt (1931) [17]

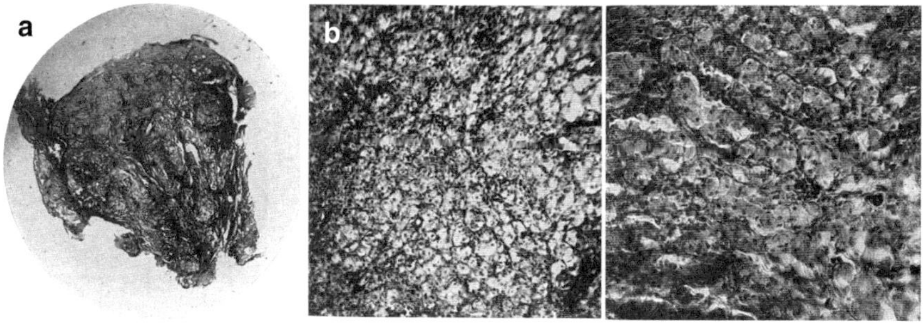

Fig. 8.2 (**a**) The ovary that was obtained from a pregnant rabbit and transplanted in the subcutaneous tissue of a parous rabbit [17]. (**b**) Higher magnification of sections obtained from the ovary [17]

that he was able to determine that the rabbits were temporarily hormonally sterilized by implanting the ovaries of animals of the same species, or by injections of ovarian or placenta extracts. However, they remained completely healthy and delivered completely normal and fully mature pups after the end of the blocking effect. The pups which were born after the correct gestation period continued to develop normally. Since A. Greil apparently rejected the existence of an internal secretion by the corpus luteum and theca interna cells, it should not be a surprise that he regarded the sterility to be a "toxic" rather than a hormonal effect [21]. Such an attitude sounds very much like the popular modern saying "I know: don't confuse me with facts."

Given this climate, the fact that he was in favor of applying temporary sterilization for medical conditions, like tuberculosis, heart disease, Graves' disease, and also for eugenic purposes, must have contributed to the development of a hostile climate in conservative catholic Austria, where many opposed the growing popularity of eugenics [22]. Indeed, when Haberlandt envisaged the possibility of starting clinical trials with ovarian extracts, his colleagues repeated the accusation that he was endangering "unborn life." The truth is that both his ideas and his experiments went against the moral, ethical, religious, and political agendas of that time. Hostility grew to the point that he was forced to move out of Austria and settle in Budapest [23].

In Hungary, in spite of all opposition, he began trials in animals in 1930 with substantial help from Gedeon Richter Pharmaceutical Company (Richter was a skilled pharmacist). He called his biological extract *Infecundin* and started a series of animal trials with the preparation that the company produced for him. The results were published in 1931 in the already mentioned book [17] in which he clearly stated that his research could be usefully applied to human females. He stated: "*Without any doubt, practical applications of the temporary hormonal sterilization of a woman represent a contribution to making the ideal dreamed by Sigmund Freud a reality*" (see [12]).

Sadly, he died, probably by suicide, the following year, leaving his work unfinished. No research directly relevant to contraception was carried out for the following two decades. Even his work seemed to have been forgotten for almost half a century, till Simmer [24] reminded the scientific community that the possibility of developing hormonal contraception had been conceived "as early as 1919 by the physiologist Ludwig Haberlandt in Innsbruck." Haberlandt's work was also praised by Müller-Jahncke [25] who stressed that after his death, his clinical trials were not only stopped, but his work was totally forgotten until the 1950s. Haberlandt's pioneering work was also recognized by Djerassi [26].

8.3 The Identification of the Hormones Capable of Blocking Female Fertility

The next step in the development of HC was the isolation, Identification, and synthesis of reproductive steroid hormones.

A proper reconstruction of the path leading to the identification of the substances governing female reproduction must start with the classic description during the second half of the seventeenth century by Reinier (Regnerus or Reignier) de Graaf [27] (see Fig. 8.3), "*de mulierum organis generationi inservientibus*" (of the female reproductive system). He made two experimental observations: (a) in cows the presence and number of corpora lutea in the ovaries correlated with pregnancy and the number of fetuses; (b) the removal of the ovaries during pregnancy caused parturition. This meant that the corpus luteum was somehow involved in maintaining gestation. The term corpus luteum is attributed to Marcello Malpighi (1628–1694) [28], but its first description was provided by Volcher Coiter in the sixteenth century [29].

However, it took two and a half centuries before additional progress was made: According to Frobenius [30], the first researcher who, at the beginning of the twentieth century, provided experimental proof for an endocrine function of the corpus luteum was the gynecologist Ludwig Fraenkel [31]. Apparently, he had been inspired by the work of the anatomist Gustav Jacob Born [32] to conduct experiments on the rabbit. This work established the important role of the corpus luteum in nidation and in maintaining pregnancy until midgestation.

Ovarian products and extracts were used since the latter part of the nineteenth century for the treatment of various conditions, including the menopause, amenorrhea, and dysmenorrhea. According to Mossé [33] and Fraenkel [34], the first use of a corpus luteum extract in women was in the cases reported by Lebreton in 1899 [34]. Additional cases were reported by Burnman [28] and Dannreuther [35].

This new knowledge was then applied by Ludwig Haberlandt, who—as we have seen—was the first to demonstrate that substances present in the ovary (more specifically, in the corpus luteum) were capable of rendering animals temporarily infertile [17]. He argued for trials in women, but his untimely death put a stop to any further work on contraception for more than 15 years.

There was, however, a parallel line of research that indirectly created the basis for further work: the isolation of female hormones, followed by the identification of their structure.

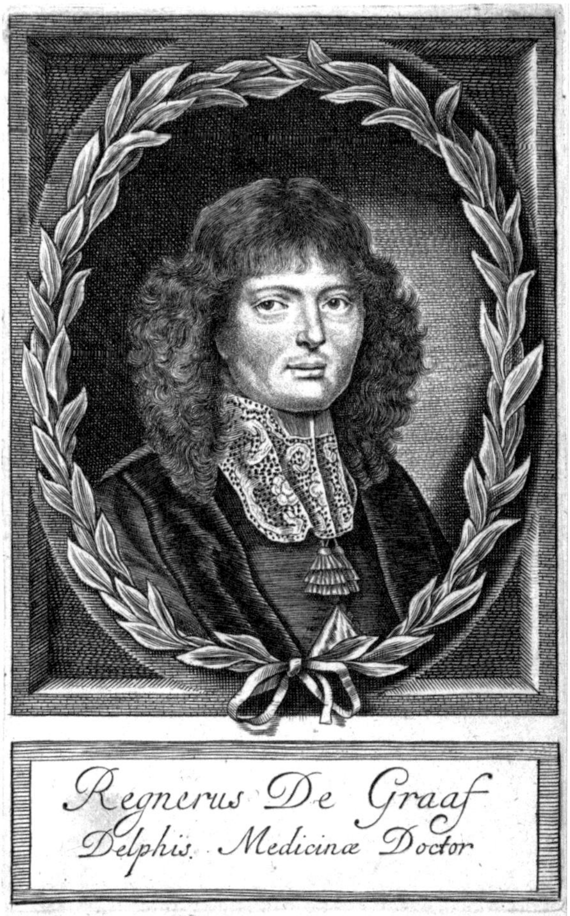

Fig. 8.3 Regnier de Graaf, the first scientist to describe the anatomy of the ovaries

8.3.1 Progesterone

According to Ali et al. [36], the search for the hormone of the corpus luteum started when a young doctor, Willard Allen, met George Corner, Professor of Anatomy at the University of Rochester Medical School. In 1929, they reported the "progestational" proliferative effect of a corpus luteum extract on the endometria of castrated mature female rabbits, a reaction not observed using follicular fluid or placental extracts [37]. Their work led to the development of the Corner-Allen bioassay, which relied on examination of the endometrium of ovariectomized rabbits that were injected with the substance of interest.

The history of the investigations that made it possible to identify the molecule we call progesterone, its structure and activity, has been aptly described by Frobenius [30], who summarized it as follows: *In 1934, after a dramatic neck-and-neck scientific race, four research groups independently from each other reported on the successful isolation of the pure substance.* The four groups were as follows: one from the United States [38, 39]; two from Germany (today both the cities where work took place are in Poland) [40, 41]; one from Switzerland [42].

Two additional recent reconstructions of the history of progesterone were also made by Di Renzo et al. [43] and Bulletti et al. [44].

According to these historical essays, it was the already-mentioned semiquantitative Corner-Allen Test [37], which made it possible to evaluate the biological activity of corpus luteum extracts during the progressive purification procedure leading to the isolation of progesterone.

8.3.2 Estrogens

Huffman et al. [45] provided an excellent historical overview of the work leading to the isolation of estrogens. Eighty years later, Santen and Simpson published a "History of Estrogen" [46] in which they recounted the purification, structure, synthesis, biologic actions, and clinical implications of estrogens.

The first step in identifying estrogens was accomplished in the early 1920s by another Allen, Edgar (unrelated to Willard), who with Edward Adelbert Doisy began researching where the "primary ovarian hormone" was produced. In 1923, they published a report in which they determined the localization, extraction, and partial purification of this substance, as well as its effect in test animals [47].

The purification procedure was made possible by two observations: the first is that in the estrous cycle of mice, the development of ovarian follicles precedes the appearance of cornified cells in the vagina; the second is that the injection into ovariectomized mice of extracts from sow ovaries resulted in the production of cornified cells in the vagina [48]. Applying this test to the progressive purification of extracts of huge quantities of human pregnancy urine, Doisy isolated first estrone (initially named *Theelin*) [49], then estriol (initially named *Theelol*) [50]. Preliminary data on the isolation of estradiol (initially named D*ihydrotheelin*) by Doisy's group was published some 5 years later [50]. They wrote: "*Although we have not yet accumulated sufficient material for complete analysis, our results indicate the identity of the hormone with dihydro-theelin.*" Final results were then published in 1940 when estradiol was isolated from human placentas [45].

For completeness, it must be mentioned that in 1989 Diczfalusy [51] stated that estriol was first identified by Marrian [52], who described the isolation from human urine of a substance called "Estrin." For the record, Marrian mentioned that "*Doisy also described the preparation of an active crystalline substance at the Physiological Congress in Boston last summer. So far, however, no details of Doisy's work have reached the author.*" He also mentioned the work of Butenandt [53, 54], who—as we have seen—led one of the four groups which isolated progesterone. Butenandt, however, was working on the purification of a compound he called "Progynon." When he was told of the progress made by Doisy and his group, he rushed to "claim priority." It was in 1929 when he published a brief note in which he stated: "*The present note about the feminine sex hormone appears because I learned from a participant at the 13th Physiological Congress in Boston (August 1929) that E. A. Doisy made a brief report there that he had succeeded in obtaining from pregnant women urine a highly effective substance (around 8 million units per gram). I don't know anything about the presentation or the physical and chemical properties of Doisy's preparation. A few months ago, our own work, which was carried out with the support of the Not-gemeinschaft der deustchen Wissenschaften, led to the isolation of a crystallized substance with an equally high physiological effectiveness; its chemical examination is currently being carried out*" [52].

Butenandt then published his results in a second article, also in 1929 [54], in which he mentioned possible crude formulas for his "*Progynon.*" The two formulae that he considered most likely were $C_{23}H_{28}O_3$, or $C_{24}H_{32}O_3$; the crude formula of estrone is $C_{18}H_{22}O_2$; that of estradiol is $C_{18}H_{24}O_2$; and that of estriol is $C_{18}H_{24}O_3$. The formulae proposed were inaccurate in terms of atoms of carbon and hydrogen, but coincided with estriol for the atoms of oxygen. Whether this is sufficient to claim "priority" is a topic for a historical debate.

In 1931, Marrian and Butenandt, in a brief, polemical note in Science [55], agreed that Doisy and his coworkers were the first to isolate Theelin (estrone), but insisted that Butenandt and Marrian were independently the first to isolate Theelol (estriol). They wrote: "*A year ago when the presence in urine of two distinct oestrus-producing substances was clear to us, we were considerably puzzled over the relationship between them ... At the same time, it was shown that both substances occur together in urine, and that by distillation in a high vacuum with potassium bisulphate, $C_{18}H_{24}O_3$ (estriol) could be converted into $C_{18}H_{22}O_2$.*" They complained that Doisy had not properly acknowledged their work. In an immediate reply, Doisy and Thayer [56] rebutted by affirming that several of the statements "can hardly be substantiated if one refers to our original papers." In the end, in 1939, the Nobel Committee granted the Nobel Prize for Chemistry to Butenandt "for his work on sex hormones," implicitly agreeing that he was also instrumental in isolating other steroid hormones, including estriol.

8.4 The Birth of Hormonal Contraception

Following the identification of the hormones governing the female menstrual cycle, research efforts began to explore their administration to produce reversible, temporary infertility.

Kurzrock, in the United States, was the first to rediscover the work of Haberlandt and advocate that the administration of estrone, by inhibiting ovulation, could represent a valid method of hormonal sterilization, concluding that "*the potentialities of hormonal sterilization are tremendous*" [57]. Shortly after, Lyon showed that cyclical ethinyl-estradiol (0.05 mg per day from day 4–5 to day 25) can inhibit ovulation and advocated its use for the treatment of dysmenorrhea [58].

Nonetheless, it took over 10 years after Haberlandt carried out his pioneering work for Sturgis and Albright [59] to specifically study the contraceptive potential of a dose of an estrogen capable of inhibiting ovulation.

Notwithstanding these early attempts at utilizing estrogens, the first systematic efforts to achieve hormonal contraception were made using progesterone. It is widely known that it was the mammalian biologist Gregory Goodwin Pincus who, in collaboration with John Rock, Celso-Ramon Garcia, and Min-Chueh Chang, led the development and field testing in Puerto Rico of the first combined oral contraceptive (COC) [60].

It is important to stress that Pincus' work was inspired by Margaret Sanger, a pioneer in advocating the development of contraceptive methods who, in 1922, wrote: "*No woman can call herself free who does not own and control her body. No woman can call herself free until she can choose consciously whether she will or will not be a mother*" [61]. Sanger's views on contraception were tainted by her advocacy of eugenics; indeed, her early motivation stemmed from her view that birth control is, in her words, "*not merely of eugenic value, but is practically identical with the final aims of Eugenics.*" She also wrote: "*the most urgent problem today is how to limit and discourage the over-fertility of the mentally and physically defective.*" Details of Sanger's life and achievements can be found in the already mentioned Kirsch & Ogas book "*The Drug Hunters*" [13]. By associating fertility regulation with eugenics, paradoxically she may have involved fertility regulation in the growing controversy over this doctrine [23] and contributed to the continuing rejection of contraception in those days.

Margaret Sanger was able to secure a grant from the Planned Parenthood Federation to support Pincus' research into animal fertilization. The goal, however, was to develop a hormonal contraceptive. With this in mind, Sanger acted as a go-between with Katharine Dexter McCormick, an aristocratic very wealthy Mayflower American, who provided almost all the funding for the work on contraception by the Boston Group led by Pincus [13].

At the end of the nineteenth century, Beard [62], followed by Prenant [63], made the observation that no ovulation occurs during pregnancy. Then, in 1936, Selye et al. [64] documented that the daily administration of 4 mg of the newly isolated hormone, progesterone, to normally cycling female rats caused immediate cessation of estrus cycles, ovarian atrophy, and hypertrophy of the pituitary. In 1953, Pincus and Chang carried out a similar investigation and found that ovulation in rabbits can be prevented by the subcutaneous or intravaginal administration of high-dose progesterone [65]. In a further study in rats, the Boston group documented that single injections of 5–50 mg of progesterone inhibit the occurrence of estrus in a way proportional to the dosage used [66].

This work represented the scientific basis for the use of progesterone as a contraceptive in women.

Initially, in their systematic work, the Boston Group led by Gregory Pincus used the natural hormone progesterone (300 mg per day on cycle day 5–25), to mimic what happens naturally during pregnancy when increasing circulating levels of progesterone prevent follicular maturation.

In clinical practice, however, progesterone could not be utilized for two main reasons:

- It has a low activity when given orally because of negligible water solubility and, as a consequence, its poor absorption with a further decrease in bioactivity due to the so-called first-pass metabolism effect (inactivation by liver through quick degradation) [67]. Greenblatt [68] attempted without real success to increase its activity by administering it sublingually; subsequently, Bicker compared various routes of administration and concluded that it could be used orally [69], a statement rejected by Greenblatt et al. [70]. In their experiments with rabbits, Pincus et al. [65] found that progesterone could be administered orally, but failed to suppress ovulation in 12 39% of subjects when administered to women, depending on the test used.
- At therapeutic doses, it causes breakthrough bleeding[1] (shortening of the cycle). However, it was later discovered that synthetic progestins may produce the same adverse effect, and for this reason, it was decided to combine a progestin with an estrogen.

Progesterone was definitively abandoned when Pincus and his collaborators discovered that synthetic progestins, such as norethisterone and norethynodrel, were at least 10–15 times more potent when given orally.

8.4.1 *The Chemical Synthesis of Progesterone*

Following its initial discovery, progesterone was isolated from the corpora lutea of animals, but the yield was small and prohibitively expensive. In order to obtain the quantities necessary to satisfy the needs of the scientific and medical communities', progesterone had to be chemically synthesized.

As recounted by Djerassi [71], "*until the mid-40s, all the progesterone needed for biological and clinical purposes was prepared in one way or another from cholesterol through three of his oxidation products.*" Unfortunately, the yield was very low, and the price was, therefore, very high.

In 1936, an American chemist, Russell Marker decided to dedicate all his efforts to devise a method for producing the hormone on an industrial scale.

His approach was novel and genial. Kirsch and Ogas [13] described Marker's work in detail, but erroneously mentioned that "*instead of assembling the 4 rings one by one, Marker started looking for naturally-occurring complex substances from which progesterone could be obtained by degradation, not synthesis. In other words, he looked for large molecules from which to 'cut out' progesterone.*" The

[1] This term, first utilized by Pincus and his group, and commonly utilized today in trials of hormonal contraceptives, is defined (Webster Dictionary) as "an abnormal flow of blood from the uterus that occurs between menstrual periods especially due to irregular sloughing of the endometrium in women on contraceptive hormones."

procedure became known as the Marker Degradation [72]. The statement by Kirsch and Ogas is incorrect since, in fact, the synthetic procedure involved removing the cholesterol side chain [71].

The class of molecules he selected were the *phytosterols*, plant sterols structurally similar to cholesterol that are today utilized to lower cholesterol absorption [73]. Initially, he focused on diosgenin that he extracted from Sarsaparilla roots (plants of the genus *smilax*). Having devised the method for producing large quantities of progesterone, Marker needed a pharmaceutical company to make large-scale production a reality. Intriguingly, none of the major companies he approached in the United States was interested. Marker then resigned from his academic position at Penn State University and set up his own private lab in an old pottery shed in Mexico City where he produced a crude extract which he took back to the United States, and from this, he produced 3 kg of progesterone.

Then, in 1943, Marker moved back to Mexico and in collaboration with Emeric Somlo and Federico Lehman of Laboratorios Hormona founded the Syntex company. Despite considerable success and the production of 30 kg of progesterone, he left the company in 1945 because of a serious disagreement around its finances [72]. At this stage, Marker turned his attention to *saponins* [74], a family of natural products that consist of a steroid or triterpene skeleton as part of their core structures [75]. In 1947, he isolated and characterized a part of the saponin molecule, *sapogenin* [76], and used it to synthesize progesterone (see Fig. 8.4).

Of great importance, using the same source material, it was possible—as we will see—to also obtain synthetic progestins.

After leaving Syntex, Marker went on to form another company, Botanicamex, in Texcoco, and then worked with Gedeon Richter. Soon, however, he left Mexico, and until the end of his days, Russell Marker spent most of his time on eighteenth-century silversmithing.

8.4.2 *Creating Orally Active Synthetic Progestins*

The great interest in clinical applications of progesterone led to the development of a large number of synthetic compounds with progestogenic activity. In 1951, a genial chemist, Carl Djerassi, who worked at Syntex, synthesized the first orally active progestin, 17-ethinyl-19-nortestosterone (known in the United States as *norethindrone* and as *norethisterone* elsewhere). It is widely used even today. The

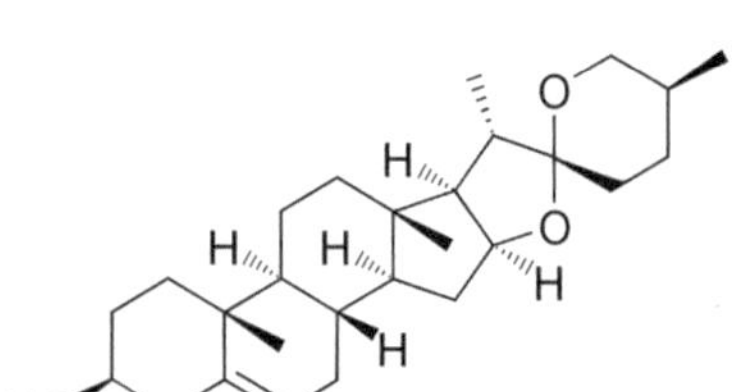

Fig. 8.4 Sapogenin, the starting material for the industrial synthesis of progesterone

following year, Frank B. Colton, a chemist working at G.D. Searle & Co synthesized the second orally active progestin, *norethynodrel* [77], and the Company filed a patent on 31 August 1953, before Djerassi published the result in 1954 [78]. As shown in Fig. 8.5, the two steroids differ only by the location of the double bond in ring "A." In addition, according to Djerassi: "mild treatment of Colton norethynodrel with acid, or just with human gastric juice converts it into our norethindrone. Our patent was thus circumvented in the bottle or in the tablet, though not in the stomach." Apparently, the fine legal point of whether or not "synthesis in the stomach" represents an infringement of a patent was never tested in court [71].

In a 1955 review, Djerassi recalled: "*Contrary to predictions, orally effective steroid ovulation inhibitors became the most widely used method of reversible birth control in most parts of the world some 40 years after their first synthesis*" [79].

8.4.3 *Designing the First Combined Hormonal Contraceptive*

The search for contraception was inspired by the observation, first made by Makepeace et al. in 1937 [80], that progesterone inhibited ovulation in the rabbit and the subsequent demonstration of the effectiveness of synthetic progestins in animals. As will be described in detail in Sect. 10.4.4, this led, in 1956, to the first human study which was undertaken at the Free Hospital for Women in Brookline (now merged into Brigham and Women's Hospital, Boston, Massachusetts) by John Rock. At the time, research into contraception was illegal in much of the United States, including in Massachusetts (under the Comstock "chastity" Law which was passed in 1873, and remained in force for part of the following century [81]). Thus, the research was conducted under the auspices of enhancing fertility through a "rebound effect" following ovulation suppression. Early clinical observations that compared the effect of norethisterone 10 mg per day, norethynodrel 10 mg per day, and norethandrolone (17-ethyl-19-nortestosterone) 10–50 mg per day revealed a higher incidence of breakthrough bleeding with norethisterone and norethandrolone. Better cycle control when using norethynodrel was attributed to the presence of a coexisting "intrinsic estrogenic activity," because of contamination with the

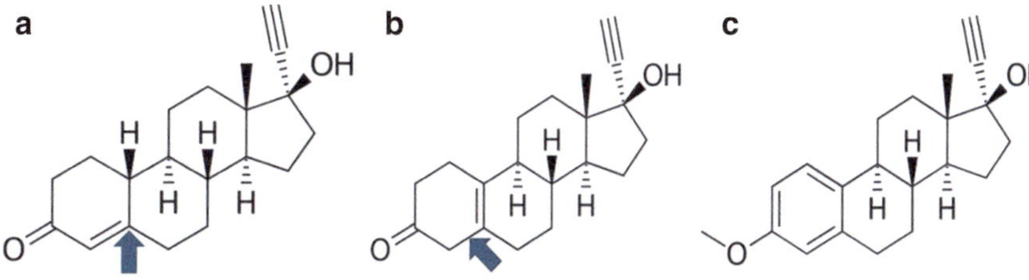

Fig. 8.5 The two first synthetic progestins (**a** and **b**) and estrogen (**c**) utilized in hormonal contraception. (**a**) Norethisterone. (**b**) Norethynodrel (noretynodrel). (**c**) Mestranol (estrogenic component)

estrogen, ethinyl-estradiol-3-methyl-ether (mestranol) (Fig. 8.5c), due to the synthetic procedure utilized. Surprisingly, the use of pure norethynodrel caused an increase in the incidence of breakthrough bleeding, forcing the conclusion that better cycle control was due to the presence of the estrogen contaminant (from 1% to 3%) [82–85].

Further improvement in cycle control was achieved through doubling the dose of norethisterone and norethynodrel to be administered from day 5 to 25. The addition of the estrogen to the pure progestins resulted in a further reduction of the incidence of breakthrough bleeding, but caused an increased incidence of breast symptoms, nausea, vomiting, and cramps [86].

In the end, the better cycle control using norethynodrel led to the development of a commercial product, *Enovid 10 mg*, which gained FDA approval for the regulation of menstruation in 1957. It was licensed featuring a "warning" that it "prevented pregnancy"!

As mentioned above, it was soon found out that Enovid, in fact, contained 9.85 mg norethynodrel and 0.15 mg of the "contaminating" estrogen, mestranol, and this "mixture" became the standard for a COC. The license was extended to include contraception in 1960, but the manufacturer (G. D. Searle) did not market the 10 mg containing tablet for contraception as the lower dose (containing 5 mg or 2.5 mg norethynodrel) proved equally effective and had fewer side effects. These side effects were known to but dismissed or set aside by the investigators.

So, thanks to a "contaminant" left by the synthetic procedure for norethynodrel, the first COC, based on the inhibitory action of the progestin, was born.

It must be stressed that inhibition of ovulation in humans can easily be obtained also with an estrogen, as reported already in the 1940s by Sturgis and Albright [59] and by the group of Goldzieher [87, 88]. This led to the development of sequential contraceptives, the first of which employed mestranol alone for 15 days followed by mestranol plus chlormadinone for another 5 days [89]. However, sequential regimens were associated with higher failure rate [90], a higher risk of thromboembolism and a higher risk of endometrial hyperplasia and even carcinoma [91, 92]. They were removed from the market in the United States at the request of the Food and Drug administration (US-FDA) in February 1976 and globally in the late 1970s [93, 94].

8.4.4 The First Human Trials of a Hormonal Contraceptive

As we have seen, the first animal experiments of a hormonal preparation were performed by Haberlandt starting from 1919 [19, 20], and the first human studies were apparently carried out in 1924 in Germany by Rübsamen [18]. It must be stressed that for this pioneering work, they utilized a "biological extract," not chemically pure substances.

Then in the 1950s, in collaboration with John Rock and Celso Ramon Garcia, Pincus set up the first clinical field studies in a slum area (Rio Piedras) of Puerto

Rico. The location was chosen because the island, officially a Commonwealth and unincorporated territory of the United States, did not have legislation prohibiting contraception and had a network of birth control clinics funded by the US government with the aim of increasing contraception uptake among the poor. Paradoxically, this included sterilization and even hysterectomies. Women living in poverty had strong incentive for family planning and the network of family planning clinics in Puerto Rico provided Pincus with a highly motivated population that was easy to monitor.

The first clinical trial of synthetic, "pure" substances was carried out some 25 years later by Gregory Pincus and his collaborators. Following testing of progesterone and 45 synthetic derivatives in rabbits and rats, norethisterone and norethynodrel emerged as the most potent preparations when given orally. Over the years, norethisterone has become one of the preferred progestins for a variety of indications, whereas norethynodrel has been all but abandoned. Yet, norethynodrel, at the daily dosage of 10 mg, was chosen for clinical field testing, because it was found to be more potent than any of the other compounds when tested in the rat [95]. In view of the abovementioned results obtained with "pure" norethynodrel, the progestin was combined with mestranol, the synthetic estrogen that "contaminated" its initial synthesis, in a dose range 0.23–0.18 mg [86]. The commercial name of this combination was "Enovid 10 mg."

The main trial of Pincus' Group was preceded by preliminary animal experiments to demonstrate the ability of norethynodrel to inhibit ovulation [96]; then, in 1956, Pincus' Group published the first results on the effect on human ovulation of various progestins [97] and started the already-mentioned clinical trial in Puerto Rico [98]. The final results of this investigation were published in 1958 [86]. As to the mechanism of action of their combination, they wrote: "*Presumption of suppression of ovulation is strengthened by the fact that conception did not occur in any instance in which the medication schedule was followed faithfully*" [99].

The pioneering work led by Gregory Pincus was immediately "picked-up" by another group led by Joseph W. Goldzieher in Texas [100] who also started clinical trials of COCs.

As we have seen, in the early days, the inhibition of ovulation was attributed to the action of the progestin, with estrogen added to avoid break-through bleeding. Yet, as already mentioned, since 1947, Goldzieher had presented evidence that, at the daily dose of 60 μg, the synthetic steroid ethinyl-estradiol (EE) was by itself capable of inhibiting ovulation. The evidence was obtained in an investigation in which he administered EE to treat dysmenorrhea [87]. This work led to EE becoming the most widely used estrogenic compound in COC.

A fundamental observation made by Goldzieher and his Group has been the presence of major variations in the bioavailability of orally administered EE, ranging between 25% and 65%, with a half-life varying between 6 and 27 h [101]. They investigated a number of oral contraceptives containing various combinations of norethisterone/ethynyl-estradiol, concluding that the great variability in circulating levels of the two steroids is more important than the observed clinical differences between dosages [102].

Goldzieher will be 105-years-old in September 2024, the last of the founding fathers of the pill still alive as of the day of publication of this chapter.

8.4.5 Types of Hormonal Contraceptives

Today, the classic estrogen-progestin combined contraception can be administered orally (e.g., [103–105]), transdermally (e.g., [106]), intravaginally (e.g., [107, 108], and (although less widely available) as a monthly injectable (e.g., [109]).

These routes have been extensively investigated and compared against each other (e.g., [110, 111]).

Marketing of combined contraceptives was followed by the development of progestin-only contraception; Initially, this was achieved through three-monthly injections of medroxyprogesterone acetate (e.g., [112, 113]) and later norethisterone enanthate (e.g., [114]). At about the same time, the so-called progestin-only "Minipill" was also introduced (e.g., [115]). Two additional routes of administration were subsequently added: through subcutaneous implants (e.g., [116–118]) and via an intrauterine system (e.g., [119, 120]).

The description and a discussion of these modalities falls outside the scope of this chapter and will be discussed in other chapters of this volume.

8.4.6 The Role of Industry

It is an undeniable fact that, after the initial neglect at the time of Russell Marker [13], a major role in the development of hormonal contraception has been played by the pharmaceutical industry.

In the already quoted review, Djerassi mentioned that "*Toward the end of the 1960s, at least 13 international pharmaceutical companies (9 of them in the US) had active research and development programs dedicated to new advances in the field of contraception*" [79].

As a consequence of the major merging of pharmaceutical companies that was initiated toward the end of the previous millennium (for details, see [121]), the majority of the initial pharmaceutical major actors in the development of hormonal contraception no longer exist in their original structure.

The pioneering work was carried out at companies such as **Syntex Corporation** (originally Syntex S.A. in Mexico); **G.D. Searle & Co**. (incorporated into Pfizer in 2003); **Ortho Pharmaceuticals** (merged with McNeal Pharmaceuticals into Ortho McNeil Pharmaceuticals in 1993); **N.V. Organon** (initially located in the Netherlands and owned by Akzo-Nobel; it was purchased by Schering-Plough and its headquarters was transferred to the state of New Jersey. In turn, Schering Plough merged with Merck Sharp & Dohme); **Schering AG** (today part of Bayer); **Upjohn Corp**. (merged with Pharmacia AB to form Pharmacia & Upjohn in 1995, which merged with Monsanto and Searle creating a new Pharmacia in 2000); **Gedeon Richter**, with headquarters in Budapest is where the first contraceptive ovarian extract (*Infecundin*) was produced in 1931. In 1966, the Company marketed the first oral contraceptive manufactured by a country of the "Eastern bloc" under the same trade name.

With the expansion of the contraceptive market, a number of other companies launched their products in developing, as well as in the industrialized world. It is also important to point out that major developments in contraception took place under the auspices of the **Special Program of Research in Human Reproduction**, a UN interagency program located in WHO (for details, see [122] and of the **Population Council** (see [123]). Their importance stems from the fact that they facilitated international scientific collaborations and supported national programs for family planning together with the **United Nations Populations Fund** (UNFPA) and the **International Planned Parenthood Federation** (IPPF). Their contribution was critical to the development of HC.

8.5 The Difficult Way Forward

Hormonal contraceptives have a specific peculiarity that of having been designed for use by young, mostly healthy women. This unique situation contributed to the exceptionally close scrutiny to which COCs were submitted. In addition, as we have seen in the tragic story of Haberlandt (see Sect. 10.2), from the very beginning, research on hormonal contraceptives created conflict, some of which was rooted in religion or tradition.

This is why early researchers took the view that progesterone is safe because of it being a natural compound. Unfortunately, progesterone (and estradiol) could not be used, and synthetic progestins and estrogens were considered potentially harmful.

In spite of the initial socioethical doubts about using COC, the popularity of the pill resulted in a rapid acceleration in use, and their development not only continued, but was even accelerated. Adverse effects were closely scrutinized and, at least in part, were attributed to the dosage, leading to a major effort to reduce the amount of both hormone components, while maintaining efficacy.

It must be stressed that reduction was "real" for the estrogen, since the daily dose of EE was reduced from 50 to 20 (and even 15 μg) and its presence was totally eliminated in the progestin-only pill.

With regard to the progestin, the situation is more complex, because the new compounds introduced over several decades have different progestogenic potency, pharmacodynamics, and risk and benefit profiles, which renders comparisons more challenging.

The adverse events associated with the use of both estrogens and progestins gave rise to public "pill scares." The reason for the existence of these episodes of collective panic is obvious: as stressed above, drugs are used to treat an illness or a medical problem and as such adverse events are—almost unconsciously—considered a possibility. As mentioned, COCs are mostly used by healthy women for prolonged periods of time. This amplifies the importance of reducing any associated risk.

Two of the "pill scares" deserve mention:

The first of these was triggered by the high incidence of thromboembolic events observed with the use of first-generation COCs (containing 50 μg of EE) (e.g., [124, 125]). This led to the abovementioned substantial reduction of the daily dose of EE in modern COCs.

Curiously, the second was also linked to a higher incidence of thromboembolism that was attributed to the progestins, following the introduction of the so-called third-generation pills, which on the one hand were associated with a favorable side effect profile because of their antiandrogenic potency—on the other, they produced a small increased risk of venous thromboembolism [126–128].

Poor risk communication resulted in women abandoning their pills [129]. In the United Kingdom, the "progestin scare" resulted in a higher rate of unwanted pregnancies and of pregnancy terminations [130].

In this context, in a recent publication, Gavina et al. [131] addressed the issue of reducing the dose of estrogen and progestin needed to block ovulation. They utilized a mathematical model based on the so-called optimal control theory. They first used a modified menstrual cycle model in order to identify the minimum total estrogen/progesterone dose, and timing of administration capable of inducing anovulation. According to Gavina et al., using this model, it is possible to correctly predict the mean daily levels of LH and FSH, and of estradiol and progesterone throughout a physiological menstrual cycle and, as a consequence, to calculate the reduction in these hormone levels "caused by exogenous estrogen and/or progesterone."

Their results indicate that it is possible to reduce the total dose by 92% with estrogen monotherapy and 43% in progesterone monotherapy in an approach that can enable personalized contraception. They also suggested that, if using an estrogen for contraception, it would be most effective to deliver it in the midfollicular phase. Finally, they claim that with the combined use of estrogen and progesterone, the doses can be lowered even more. Gavina et al. concluded that their results "may give clinicians insights into optimal formulations and schedule of therapy that can suppress ovulation."

Without in any way detracting from the value of mathematical models in biology, the conclusions of Gavina et al. are problematic:

1. Irrespective of what the model may signal, decades of clinical experience prove that COCs need to be administered daily for a minimum of 3 weeks to obtain a reproducible antifertility effect.
2. To this day, no COC is available that contains estradiol and/or progesterone. In the case of the estrogen, the great majority of products contain EE, orally active and with a pharmacodynamic profile that differs from estradiol. In the case of the progestational component, literally dozens of synthetic molecules have been used experimentally. Only a few are still in use, each has its own pharmacodynamic profile.

3. The concept of "personalizing" the administration of the two hormones has its appeal but is probably impossible to implement at the practical level. In clinical practice, COCs inhibit ovulation irrespective of the woman's cycle length, provided the pill is administered for a minimum of 21 days, so that the "cycle length" is maintained and an early onset of bleeding is avoided. It may be more than absolutely necessary in some cases, but it is the only practical way to proceed given the range of inter- and intra-individual variability.

8.5.1 Reducing the Daily Dosage of the Estrogen

As a consequence of the pill scares of the 1970s [124, 125], a major effort was made by the pharmaceutical industry to reduce the daily dosage of estrogen in their products.

However, it must be recognized that research carried out in China preceded work by Western companies and scientists. The first low-dose combined oral contraceptive was introduced in China in 1967 under the auspices of the National Coordinating Group on Oral Contraception [132, 133].

8.5.2 Utilizing Natural Estrogens

The attempt to decrease the daily dose of EE in COC to reduce estrogen-related adverse effects and risks was followed by attempts at utilizing natural estrogens (see Fruzzetti et al. [134]).

Today, three such compounds are utilized in COC: micronized estradiol, its prodrug estradiol valerate, and estetrol (15α-hydroxy-estriol). They all seem to have a limited impact on the liver, lipid, and carbohydrate metabolism and on hemostasis. Both estradiol and its prodrug seem to also have a more limited impact on the risk of venous thromboembolism.

Stanczyk et al. [135] carried out a comparative analysis of these three natural estrogens, viz-a-viz EE, with particular emphasis on structure–function relationships, receptor-binding affinity, potency, metabolism, pharmacokinetics, and pharmacodynamics. They concluded that, while the binding affinity of EE for estrogen receptor-α is double that of estradiol, the opposite is true for receptor-β. With regard to estetrol, it has a lower binding affinity for both receptors compared to estradiol. There is a major difference between EE and natural estrogens in that the former produces a dramatic increase in estrogen-sensitive hepatic globulins and coagulation factors. In terms of metabolism, both estradiol and EE undergo extensive metabolism; the contrary is true for estetrol, but the latter has the highest bioavailability among the three natural estrogens. Ovulation is constantly blocked with all three compounds, but the daily required dose of estetrol necessary to inhibit follicular maturation is 5–15 times higher compared to estradiol. This is exponentially increased when estetrol is compared to EE (15 mg vs. 0.01–0.035 mg).

In conclusion, COC formulations containing estetrol show promise over the two other natural estrogens due to its lower potency and possibly fewer side effects [135]. In addition, estetrol allows a predictable bleeding pattern with a minimal incidence of unscheduled bleeding.

8.5.3 Families of Progestins

Synthetic progestins are classified into four "families" depending upon the parent molecule, in the majority of cases 19-nor-testosterone or progesterone (see Diagram 8.1) from which they are derived. All four "families" of progestins have been proven effective in COC. Very small structural changes in the parent molecule may induce considerable differences in activity. In hormonal contraceptives, progestins represent the major agent designed for suppressing ovulation, although they are invariably used in combination with an estrogen, usually EE. The development of new generations of progestins with improved selectivity profiles has improved COC but has represented also a great challenge. Steroidal and nonsteroidal progesterone receptor agonists have been synthesized as well, although the latter are still at a very early stage of development.

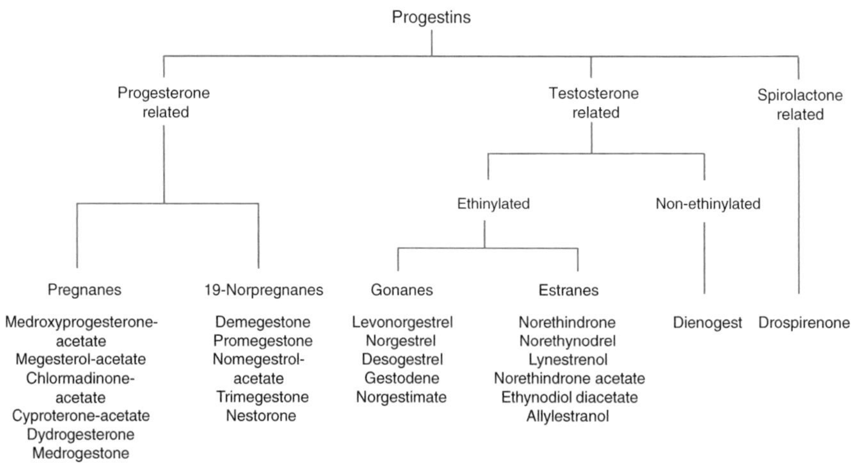

Diagram 8.1 The four families of synthetic progestogens

8.5.4 Focus on the Pharmacologic Profile of Progestins

Toward the end of the last millennium, the focus of research switched from "daily amount" to "pharmacologic profile" of the new progestins being marketed. As a result, the same pharmaceutical companies that praised the low daily dose required for their progestins: 150 μg/day (desogestrel), or even 75 μg/day (gestodene), introduced new combinations with dienogest or drospirenone in which the daily progestin dosage was 20–30 times higher (2 or 3 mg/day).

Today, synthetic progestational compounds utilized in hormonal contraception have different pharmacokinetic and pharmacodynamic properties, depending—among others—on which of the above-mentioned "family" they belong. They allow "personalized" prescription, depending on a subject needs.

Detailed descriptions of these profiles have been published (e.g., [136–141]).

8.5.5 Focus on Safety: C-21 Progestins

In the early 1970s, unexpected findings in toxicological studies carried out in Beagle bitches created a major panic wave in the world of fertility regulation. At the time, canine toxicology was mandated by the US-FDA. A 7-year study of two C-21 progestins, megestrol and chlormadinone with daily doses 1, 10, and 25 times the projected dose of megestrol for humans and about 25 times the human dose of chlormadinone. During the first 4 years of the study, 60 mammary nodules appeared (50 were nonneoplastic and 10 were neoplastic) [142].

Even in those days, however, the use of this model was criticized by many scientists because of species-specific differences in the relative affinities of estrogen and progesterone receptors for contraceptive steroids and the unique sensitivity of Beagles to C-21 progestins. In addition, the nodules found in the Beagle mammary glands were not histologically comparable to mammary tumors in women [143].

Despite the valid scientific criticism of the animal model, as a consequence of these findings, all C-21 progestins were withdrawn from use with one exception: medroxyprogesterone acetate.

It was soon documented that canines respond in a substantially different way than humans to steroid hormones, including developing cystic endometrial hyperplasia and pyometra (severe enough to require hysterectomy!). These effects do not occur in monkeys and rats [144].

An important finding has been that treatment of dogs with synthetic progestins can induce the overproduction of biologically active growth hormone (GH) in the mammary gland. This GH is highly similar to pituitary hormone and originates from foci of hyperplastic ductular epithelium of the canine mammary gland [145].

Medroxyprogesterone acetate in the form of depot-medroxyprogesterone acetate (DMPA) microcrystals (commercially known as Depo Provera) occupies a special place in the history of synthetic progestins because its manufacturer (Upjohn) refused to accept the relevance of the beagle model and continued to market it outside the United States. This led to charges that those promoting the use of Depo Provera were endangering health and even the life of women in the developing world. As an example, in 1980, Minkin [146] affirmed that "*tests with laboratory dogs and monkeys have revealed many serious side effects from the drug.*" He went on describing "*the most major of these side effects,*" concluding "*The continued use of Depo-Provera for birth control is unjustified and unethical.*" These accusations were rebutted one by one in a detailed article [147] showing that DMPA use was safe in humans and that at contraceptive doses it did not increase the risk of cancer, or impair bone mineralization, or damage the liver or the immune system.

The controversy had its cost since it resulted in the US-FDA delaying its approval of Depo Provera for long-acting contraception until 1992. By then, there was ample proof of DMPA's safety, as reviewed by Jordan in 1993. In a review of DMPA toxicology, he concluded: "*All available toxicological and pharmacokinetic data collected throughout the extensive testing of DMPA suggests that DMPA meets the overall safety standards as established by the US Food and Drug Administration*" [148].

Since then, effective, safe, C-21 progestins (such as chlormadinone acetate, megestrol acetate, nomegestrol acetate, trimegestone, segesterone acetate) have been reintroduced, or introduced de novo in COCs.

Regrettably, the controversy continued with product liability litigation against DMPA by women who claimed to have been injured by their use of the drug. None of the cases have survived the manufacturer's summary judgment motions, because the women have been unable to establish by expert and physician evidence that the FDA-approved labeling was inadequate [149].

For the record, the final nail in the coffin of unnecessary and confusing animal testing in the United States came on 20 April 2024, when the US House of Representatives gave final approval to the "*FDA Modernization Act 2.0.*" This new legislation offers the prospect of a dramatic reduction in the use of dogs, primates, and other animals in laboratory tests [150].

8.6 Conclusion

The concept of using hormones to inhibit female fertility was born some 150 years ago and went through a series of progressive steps marked by the classic procedure of "trials and errors." Hormonal control of fertility continues to be an active field of research, with the promise of new agents with new pharmacodynamic properties and new routes of administration. We cannot predict how the field will evolve, but we are confident that new products that better address the needs and safety concerns of women will continue to be developed.

Indeed, "*If there is a will, there is a way.*"

References

1. Cicero Marcus Tullius. De Oratore, II, 9, 32 [*On the Ideal Orator*]. Translated into English with Introduction, notes, appendices, glossary, and indexes by JM May & J Wisse. New York: Oxford University Press; 2001.
2. De Waal FBM, Lanting F. Bonobo: the forgotten ape. Berkley/Los Angeles/London: University of California Press; 1997.
3. Becquet C, Patterson N, Stone AC, Przeworski M, Reich D. Genetic structure of chimpanzee populations. PLoS Genet. 2006;3:e66.
4. Ogino K. Über den konzeptionstermin des weibes und seine anwendung in der praxis [*About the woman's conception date and its application in practice*]. Zentralbl Gynakol. 1932;56:721–32.
5. Knaus H. Die Periodische Fruchtbarkeit und Unfruchtbarkeit des Weibes. Der Weg zur Naturlichen Geburtenregelung [*Periodic fertility and sterility in women: A natural method of birth control*], authorized English translation by D.H. Kitchin and Kathleen Kitchin. Vienna: Wilhelm Maudrich Publisher; 1934.
6. Riddle JM, Estes JW. Oral contraceptives in ancient and medieval times. Am Sci. 1992;80:226–33.
7. Flandrin JL. L'Église et le contrôle des naissances [*The Church and Birth control*]. Paris: Flammarion; 1970.
8. Short RV. Population growth in retrospect and prospect. Philos Trans R Soc Lond B Biol Sci. 2009;364(1532):2971–4.
9. Smith A. An inquiry into the Nature and Causes of the Wealth of Nations. Edited with an Introduction by K. Sutherland. Oxford: Oxford World Classics; 1993.
10. Pincus G, Bialy G. Drugs used in control of reproduction. Adv Pharmacol. 1964;3:285–313.
11. Malthus TR. An Essay on the Principle of Population; or A view of its past and present effects on human happiness; with an Inquiry into our prospects respecting the future removal or mitigation of the evils which it occasions. Selected and introduced by Donald Winch using the text of the 1803 edition as prepared by Patricia James for the Royal Economic Society, 1990, showing the additions and corrections made in the 1806, 1807, 1817, and 1826 editions. Cambridge: Cambridge University Press; 1992.
12. Freud S. Die Sexualität in der Ätiologie der Neurosen [*Sexuality in the etiology of neuroses*]. Wiener Klinische Rundschau. 1898;2:277.
13. Kirsch DR, Ogas O. The drug hunters: the improbable quest to discover new medicines. New York: Arcade Publishing; 2016.
14. Graber-Kölliken von T. Über das adbrücken von gelben körpern in den ovarien [*About the bridging of yellow bodies in the ovaries*]. Schweizer Arch Tierheilkunde. 1898;40:241–4.
15. Zschokke E. Contribution to the pathology of the bovine ovaries. Agricultural Yearbook (Lecture at the Society of Swiss Veterinarians on November 6, 1898). 1898.
16. Djerassi C. Ludwig Haberlandt "Grandfather of the Pill". Wien Klin Wochenschr. 2009;121:727–8.
17. Haberlandt L. Die hormonale Sterilisierung des weiblichen Organismus [*The hormonal sterilization of the female organism*]. Jena: G Fischer; 1931.
18. Rübsamen W. Über Behandlung mit Corpus luteum-Extrakt (Corluten). Verbal report to the Gynäkol. Gesellschaft zum Dresden 22 November 1923. Zentralblatt Gynäkol. 1924;30:266.
19. Haberlandt L. Über hormonale Sterilisierung des weiblichen Tierkörpers. (Vorläufige Mitteilung.) [*On the hormonal sterilization of the female animal body. (Preliminary note)*]. Münch Med Wochenschr. 1921;49:1577–8.
20. Haberlandt L. Über hormonale Sterilisierung weiblicher Tiere durch subcutane Transplantation von Ovarien trächtiger Weibchen [*On the hormonal sterilization of female animals by subcutaneous transplantation of ovaries from pregnant females*]. Pflüger Arch. 1922;194:235–70.

21. Haberlandt L, Erwiderung Auf Greils A. "Einwände gegen die hormonale Sterilisierung nach Haberlandt" [*Response to A. Greil's "Objections to Haberlandt's hormonal sterilization*"]. Zentralbl Gynäkol. 1924;22:1197–8.
22. Haberlandt E, Haberlandt L. A pioneer in hormonal contraception. Wien Klin Wochenschr. 2009;121:746–9.
23. Leon SM. An image of God: the catholic struggle with eugenics. Chicago: University of Chicago Press; 2013.
24. Simmer HH. Zur Geschichte der hormonalen Empfängnisverhütung [*On the beginnings of hormonal contraception*]. Geburtshilfe Frauenheilkd. 1975;35:688–96.
25. Müller-Jahncke WD. Ludwig Haberlandt (1885–1932) und die Entwicklung der hormonalen Kontrazeption [*Ludwig Haberlandt (1885–1932) and the development of hormonal contraception*]. Z Gesamte Inn Med. 1988;43:420–2.
26. Djerassi C. The Pill at 50 (in Germany): Thriving or Surviving? Journal für Reproduktionsmedizin und Endokrinologie/J Reprod Med Endocrinol. 2011;8:14–31.
27. de Graaf Regnier. De mulierum organis generation inservietibus [*Of the female reproductive system*]. Lugduni Batavorum (Leyden), ex. off. Hackiana; 1672 – Jocelyn HD, Setchell BP. Regnier de Graaf on the human reproductive organs. An annotated translation of Tractatus de Virorum Organis Generationi Inservientibus (1668) and De Mulierum Organis Generationi Inservientibus Tractatus Novus (1672). J Reprod Fertil Suppl. 1972;17:1–222.
28. Burnam CF. Corpus luteum extract with suggestions on its use in gynecologic practice. JAMA. 1912;59:698–703.
29. Niswender GD, Juengel JL, Silva PJ, Rollyson MK, McIntush EW. Mechanisms controlling the function and life span of the corpus luteum. Physiol Rev. 2000;80:1–29.
30. Frobenius W. Ludwig Fraenkel: "spiritus Rector" of the Early progesterone research. Eur J Obstet Gynecol Reprod Biol. 1999;83:115–9.
31. Fraenkel L. Die Funktion des Corpus Luteum [*The function of Corpus Luteum*]. Arch Gynäkol. *1903*;68:*438*–546.
32. Frobenius W. Ludwig Fraenkel, das Corpus luteum und der Weg zum Progesteron [*Ludwig Fraenkel, corpus luteum and discovery of progesterone*]. Zentralbl Gynakol. 1998;120:317–23.
33. Mossé P. L'opothérapie ovarienne [*The ovarian opotherapy*]. Gazette des Hopitaux Civils et Militaires. 1899;114:1049–55.
34. Lebreton JA. Opothérapie ovarienne: role du corps jaune [*Ovarian opotherapy: the role of corpus luteum*]. Cpt Rend Hebdom des séances de la soc. de biol. 1899;51:532.
35. Dannreuther WT. Corpus luteum organotherapy in clinical practice, with report of a case of bilateral salpingooophorectomy in which the administration of corpus luteum extract was followed by the reestablishment of menstruation. JAMA. 1914;62:359–62.
36. Ali S, Balachandran K, O'Malley B. 90 Years of progesterone: ninety years of progesterone: the 'other' ovarian hormone. J Mol Endocrinol. 2020;65:E1–4.
37. Corner GW, Allen WM. Physiology of the corpus luteum. II: production of a special uterine reaction (progestational proliferation) by extracts of the corpus luteum. Am J Physiol. 1929;88:326–39.
38. Allen WM, Wintersteiner O. Crystalline progestin. Science. 1934;80(2069):190–1.
39. Wintersteiner O, Allen WM. Crystalline progestin. J Biol Chem. 1934;107:321–36.
40. Slotta KH, Ruschig H, Fels E. Reindarstellung der Hormone aus dem Corpus luteum. (Vorl. Mitteil.). Krystallographische Untersuchungen von A Neuhaus. [*Pure representation of the hormones from the corpus luteum. (Previous communication). Crystallographic studies by A Neuhaus*]. Berlin Dtsch Chem Ges. 1934;67:1270–3.
41. Butenandt A, Westphal U, Hohlweg W. Über das Hormon des Corpus luteum [*On the hormone of the corpus luteum*]. Hoppe-Seyler's Zschr Physiol Chem. 1934;227:84–98.
42. Hartmann M, Wettstein A. Ein krystallisiertes Hormon aus dem Corpus luteum [*A crystallized hormone from the corpus luteum*]. Helv Chim Acta. 1934;17:878–82.
43. Di Renzo GC, Tosto V, Tsibizova V. Progesterone: history, facts, and artifacts. Best Pract Res Clin Obstet Gynaecol. 2020;69:2–12.

44. Bulletti C, Bulletti FM, Sciorio R, Guido M. Progesterone: the key factor of the beginning of life. Int J Mol Sci. 2022;23:14138.
45. Huffman MN, Thayer SA, Doisy EA. The isolation of alpha-dihydrotheelin from human placenta. J Biol Chem. 1940;133:567–71.
46. Santen RJ, Simpson E. History of estrogen: its purification, structure, synthesis, biologic actions, and clinical implications. Endocrinology. 2019;160:605–25.
47. Allen E, Doisy EA. An ovarian hormone: preliminary report on its localization, extraction, and partial purification, and action in test animals. J Am Med Ass. 1923;81:819–21.
48. Veler CD, Thayer S, Doisy EA. The preparation of the crystalline follicular ovarian hormone: theelin. J Biol Chem. 1930;87:357–71.
49. Thayer SA, Levin L, Doisy EA. Characterization of theelol. J Biol Chem. 1931;91:655–65.
50. MacCorquodale DW, Thayer SA, Doisy EA. The crystalline ovarian follicular hormone. Exper Biol Med. 1935;32:1182.
51. Diczfalusy E. The history of steroid contraception: what is past and what is present? In: Michal F, editor. Safety requirements for contraceptive steroids. Scientific basis of fertility regulation. Proceedings of a symposium on improving safety requirements for contraceptive steroids. WHO, Geneva, 1987. Cambridge/New York: Cambridge University Press; 1989. p. 1–18.
52. Marrian GF. The chemistry of oestrin. IV. The chemical nature of crystalline preparations. Biochem J. 1930;24:1021–30.
53. Butenandt A. Über "Progynon" kristallisiertes weibliches Sexualhormon. [*On "Progynon", a crystallized Female sex hormone*]. Naturwissenschaften. 1929;17:879.
54. Butenandt A. Untersuchungen über das weibliche Sexualhormon. Darstellung und Eigenschaften des kristallisierten "Progynon" [*Studies on the female sex hormone. Representation and properties of the crystallized "Progynon"*]. Deutsche Med Wschr. 1929;52:2172–4.
55. Marrian GE, Butenandt A. Oestrus-producing hormones. Science. 1931;74(1926):547.
56. Doisy EA, Thayer SA. The Oestrus-producing hormones. Science. 1932;75(1938):216–7.
57. Kurzrok R. The prospects for hormonal sterilization. J Contracept. 1937;2:27–9.
58. Lyon RA. Relief of essential dysmenorrhea with ethinyl estradiol. Surg Gynec Obstet. 1943;77:651.
59. Sturgis SH, Albright F. Mechanism of estrin therapy in the relief of dysmenorrhea. Endocrinology. 1940;26:68–72.
60. White A. Gregory Goodwin Pincus (1903–1967). Endocrinology. 1968;82:651–4.
61. Sanger M. Woman and the new race. New York: Truth Publishing Co.; 1922.
62. Beard J. The span of gestation and the cause of birth: a study of the critical period and its effects in mammalia. Jena: Gustav Fisher; 1897.
63. Prenant A. La valeur morphologique du corps jaune, son action physiologique et thérapeutique possible [*The morphological value of the yellow body, its possible physiological and therapeutical action*]. Rev Gen Sci Pur Appl. 1898;9:646–50.
64. Selye H, Browne JSL, Collip JB. Effect of large doses of progesterone in the female rat. Proc Soc Exper Biol Med. 1936;84:472–4.
65. Pincus G, Chang MC. The effects of progesterone and related compounds on ovulation and early development in the rabbit. Acta Physiol Lat Am. 1953;3:177–83.
66. Slechta RF, Chang MC, Pincus G. Effects of progesterone and related compounds on mating and pregnancy in the rat. Fertil Steril. 1954;5:282–93.
67. Royer PA, Jones KP. Progestins for contraception: modern delivery systems and novel formulations. Clin Obstet Gynecol. 2014;57:644–58.
68. Greenblatt RB. Sublingual absorption of progesterone and anhydrohydroxy-progesterone: I. Endometrial studies. J Clin Endocrinol Metab. 1944;4:156–8.
69. Bickers W. Progesterone: a comparison of intramuscular, oral and sublingual routes of administration. J Clin Endocrinol Metab. 1949;9:736–42.

70. Greenblatt RB, Barfield WE, Clark S, Brown N. Physiologic effectiveness of oral progesterone. J Clin Endocrinol Metab. 1950;10:886–96.
71. Djerassi C. Progestins in therapy – historical developments. In: Benagiano G, Zulli P, Diczfalusy E, editors. Progestins in therapy, vol. 3. New York: Serono Symposia Publications From Raven Press; 1983. p. 1–12.
72. American Chemical Society, Sociedad Quimica de Mexico. An international historic chemical landmark. The "Marker degradation" and creation of the Mexican steroid hormone industry 1938–1945. An international historic chemical landmark. https://www.acs.org/education/whatischemistry/landmarks/progesteronesynthesis.html. Accessed 15 Apr 2024.
73. Ostlund RE Jr. Phytosterols and cholesterol metabolism. Curr Opin Lipidol. 2004;15:37–41.
74. Bergner P. Dioscorea: wild yam and hormonal synthesis. Medical Herbalism. 2014;4:9.
75. Choo MZY, Chai CLL. Natural products. Annual Reports in Medicinal Chemistry; 2023. https://www.sciencedirect.com/topics/agricultural-and-biological-sciences/sapogenin. Accessed 15 Apr 2024.
76. Marker RE, Lopez J. Steroidal Sapogenins. No. 165. Structure of the Sapogenin Glycosides. J Am Chem Soc. 1947;69:2389–92.
77. Marks L. Sexual chemistry: a history of the contraceptive pill. New Haven/Connecticut/London: Yale University Press; 2010. p. 74–5.
78. Djerassi C, Miramontes L, Rosenkranz G, Sondheimer F, Longo LD. Steroids LIV Synthesis of 19-nor-17alpha-ethynyltestosterone and 19-nor-17alpha-methyl-testosterone, 1954. Am J Obstet Gynecol. 2006;194:289. discussion 290
79. Djerassi C. The mother of the pill. Recent Prog Horm Res. 1995;50:1–17.
80. Makepeace AW, Weinstein GL, Friedman MH. The effect of progestin and progesterone on ovulation in the rabbit. Am J Physiol. 1937;119:512–6.
81. Anthony Comstock's "Chastity" Laws. https://www.pbs.org/wgbh/americanexperience/features/pill-anthony-comstocks-chastity-laws/. Accessed 25 May 2024.
82. Rock J, Pincus G, Garcia CR. Effects of certain 19-nor steroids on the normal human menstrual cycle. Science. 1956;124(3227):891–3.
83. Pincus G. Some effects of progesterone and related compounds upon reproduction and early development in mammals. Acta Endocrinol Suppl. 1956;28:18–36.
84. Rock J, Garcia CR, Pincus G. Synthetic progestins in the normal human menstrual cycle. Recent Prog Horm Res. 1957;13:323–39. discussion 339–46
85. Pincus G, Rock J, Garcia CR. Effects of certain 19-nor steroids upon reproductive processes. Ann N Y Acad Sci. 1958;71:677–90.
86. Pincus G, Rock J, Garcia CR, Rice-Wray E, Paniagua M, Rodriguez I. Fertility control with oral medication. Am J Obstet Gynecol. 1958;75:1333–46.
87. Haus W, Goldzieher JW, Hamblen EC. Dysmenorrhea and ovulation. Correlation of the effect of estrogen on pain, the endometrium and the basal body temperature. Am J Obstet Gynecol. 1947;54:820–8.
88. Goldzieher JW, Martinez-Manautou J, Livingston NB Jr, Moses LE, Rice-Wray E. The use of sequential estrogen and progestin to inhibit fertility. A preliminary report. West J Surg Obstet Gynecol. 1963;71:187–90.
89. Tyler ET. Sequential mestranol-chlormadinone acetate as an oral contraceptive. Obstet Gynecol. 1966;28:787–92.
90. Karrer MC, Smith ER. Two thousand woman-years' experience with a sequential contraceptive. A more effective method of taking a sequential contraceptive. Am J Obstet Gynecol. 1968;102:1029–34.
91. Lyon FA. The development of adenocarcinoma of the endometrium in young women receiving long-term sequential oral contraception. Am J Obstet Gynecol. 1975;123:299–301.
92. Weiss NS, Sayvetz TA. Incidence of endometrial cancer in relation to the use of oral contraceptives. N Engl J Med. 1980;302(10):551–4.
93. The New York Times (1976) February 26, page 31.

94. Kaufman RH, Reeves KO, Dougherty CM. Severe atypical endometrial changes and sequential contraceptive use. JAMA. 1976;236(8):923–6.
95. Pincus G, Chang MC, Zarrow MX, Hafez ESE, Merrill A. Studies of the biological activity of certain 19-nor steroids in female animals. Endocrinology. 1956;59:695–707.
96. Pincus G, Chang MC, Hafez ESE, Zarrow MX, Merril A. Effects of certain 19-nor steroids on reproductive processes in animals. Science. 1956;124(3227):890–1.
97. Garcia CR, Pincus G, Rock J. Effects of certain 19-nor steroids on the normal human menstrual cycle. Science. 1956;124(3227):891–3.
98. Rice-Wray E. Field study with Enovid as contraceptive agent. In: Proceedings, symposium on 19-nor progestational steroids. Chicago: G. D. Searle & Co.; 1957.
99. Pincus G, Garcia CR, Rock J, Paniagua M, Pendleton A, Laraque F, Nicolas R, Borno R, Pean V. Effectiveness of an oral contraceptive; effects of a progestin-estrogen combination upon fertility, menstrual phenomena, and health. Science. 1959;130(3367):81–3.
100. Benagiano G. Joseph W. Goldzieher and the birth of hormonal contraception. Contraception. 2010;82:119–24.
101. Goldzieher JW. Pharmacokinetics and metabolism of ethinyl estrogens. In: Goldzieher JW, Fotherby K, editors. Pharmacology of the contraceptive steroids. New York: Raven Press; 1994. p. 127–54.
102. Brody SA, Turkes A, Goldzieher JW. Pharmacokinetics of three bioequivalent norethindrone/mestranol-50 micrograms and three norethindrone/ethinyl estradiol-35 micrograms OC formulations: are 'low-dose' pills really lower? Contraception. 1989;40:269–84.
103. Bastianelli C, Farris M, Rosato E, Brosens I, Benagiano G. Pharmacodynamics of combined estrogen-progestin oral contraceptives: 1. Effects on metabolism. Expert Rev Clin Pharmacol. 2017;10:315–26.
104. Farris M, Bastianelli C, Rosato E, Brosens I, Benagiano G. Pharmacodynamics of combined estrogen-progestin oral contraceptives: 2. Effects on hemostasis. Expert Rev Clin Pharmacol. 2017;10:1129–44.
105. Bastianelli C, Farris M, Rosato E, Brosens I, Benagiano G. Pharmacodynamics of combined estrogen-progestin oral contraceptives 3. Inhibition of ovulation. Expert Rev Clin Pharmacol. 2018;11:1085–98.
106. Galzote RM, Rafie S, Teal R, Mody SK. Transdermal delivery of combined hormonal contraception: a review of the current literature. Int J Womens Health. 2017;9:315–21.
107. Wieder DR, Pattimakiel L. Examining the efficacy, safety, and patient acceptability of the combined contraceptive vaginal ring (NuvaRing). Int J Womens Health. 2010;2:401–9.
108. Al-Haddad S, Branham KKR, Clare CA. Advances in contraception: vaginal contraceptive rings. Ther Adv Reprod Health. 2023;17:1–10.
109. Hassan EO, El-Nahal N, El-Hussinie M. Once-a-month injectable contraceptives, cyclofem® and mesigyna®, in Egypt: efficacy, causes of discontinuation, and side effects. Contraception. 1999;60:87–92.
110. Gallo MF, Grimes DA, Lopez LM, Schulz KF, d'Arcangues C. Combination injectable contraceptives for contraception. Cochrane Database Syst Rev. 2013;3:CD004568.
111. Vleskó G, Meznerics FA, Hegyi P, Teutsch B, Unicsovics M, Sipos Z, Fehérvári P, Ács N, Várbíró S, Keszthelyi M. Comparison of combined parenteral and oral hormonal contraceptives: a systematic review and meta-analysis of randomized trials. J Clin Med. 2024;13:575.
112. Mukherjea M, Mukherjee P, Biswas R. Long-term contraception with Depo-Provera: a clinical evaluation. Int J Fertil. 1980;25:122–6.
113. Dragoman MV, Gaffield ME. The safety of subcutaneously administered depot medroxyprogesterone acetate (104mg/0.65mL): a systematic review. Contraception. 2016;94:202–15.
114. Melis GB, Strigini F, Fruzzetti F, Paoletti AM, Rainer E, Düsterberg B, Fioretti P. Norethisterone enanthate as an injectable contraceptive in puerperal and non-puerperal women. Contraception. 1981;23:77–88.

115. Zuniga C, Blanchard K, Harper CC, Wollum A, Key K, Henderson JT. Effectiveness and efficacy rates of progestin-only pills: a comprehensive literature review. Contraception. 2023;119:109925.
116. Power J, French R, Cowan F. Subdermal implantable contraceptives versus other forms of reversible contraceptives or other implants as effective methods of preventing pregnancy. Cochrane Database Syst Rev. 2007;2007:CD001326.
117. Moray KV, Chaurasia H, Sachin O, Joshi B. A systematic review on clinical effectiveness, side-effect profile and meta-analysis on continuation rate of etonogestrel contraceptive implant. Reprod Health. 2021;18:4.
118. Rocca ML, Palumbo AR, Visconti F, Di Carlo C. Safety and benefits of contraceptives implants: a systematic review. Pharmaceuticals (Basel). 2021;14:548.
119. Bastianelli C, Farris M, Rosato E, Varliero F, Del Savio MC, Facchinetti F, Grandi G. The use of different doses levonorgestrel-releasing intrauterine system (LNG-IUS): real-world data from a multicenter Italian study. Eur J Contracept Reprod Health Care. 2022;27:16–22.
120. Jensen JT, Lukkari-Lax E, Schulze A, Wahdan Y, Serrani M, Kroll R. Contraceptive efficacy and safety of the 52-mg levonorgestrel intrauterine system for up to 8 years: findings from the Mirena Extension Trial. Am J Obstet Gynecol. 2022;227:873.e1–873.e12.
121. Wikipaedia. List of largest pharmaceutical mergers and acquisitions. https://en.wikipedia.org/wiki/List_of_largest_pharmaceutical_mergers_and_acquisitions. Accessed 15 Apr 2024.
122. Benagiano G, d'Arcangues C, Harris Requejo J, Schafer A, Say L, Merialdi M. The special programme of research in human reproduction: forty years of activities to achieve reproductive health for all. Gynecol Obstet Invest. 2012;74:190–217.
123. Population Council. The International Committee for Contraception Research (ICCR). https://popcouncil.org/project/the-international-committee-for-contraception-research. Accessed 3 June 2024.
124. Inman WHW, Vessey MP, Westerholm B, Engelund A. Thromboembolic disease and the steroidal content of oral contraceptives: a report to the committee on safety of drugs. Br Med J. 1970;2:209.
125. Vessey MP, Inman WH. Speculation about mortality trends from venous thromboembolism disease in England and Wales and their relation to the pattern of oral contraceptive usage. J Obstet Gynaecol Br Commonw. 1973;80:562–6.
126. Poulter NR, Chang CL, Farley TMM, Meirek O, Marmot MG. World Health Organization collaborative study of cardiovascular disease and steroid hormone contraception. Venous thromboembolic disease and combined oral contraceptives: results of international multicentre case control study. Lancet. 1995;346:1575–82.
127. Jick H, Jick SS, Gurewich V, Myers MW, Vasilakis C. Risk of idiopathic cardiovascular death and non-fatal venous thromboembolism in women using oral contraceptives with differing progestogen components. Lancet. 1995;346:1589–93.
128. Spitzer WO, Lewis MA, Heinemann LA, Thorogood M, MacRae KD. Third generation oral contraceptives and risk of venous thromboembolic disorders: an international case-control study. Transnational Research Group on Oral Contraceptives and the Health of Young Women. BMJ. 1996;312:83–8.
129. Furedi A. The public health implications of the 1995 'pill scare'. Hum Reprod Update. 1999;5:621–6.
130. Edouard L. Pill scare: communication conundrum. BMJ Sex Reprod Health. 2009;35:121–2.
131. Gavina BLA, de los Reyes VAA, Olufsen MS, Lenhart S, Ottesen JT. Toward an optimal contraception dosing strategy. PLoS Comput Biol. 2023;19:e1010073.
132. Xiao BL. Some methods of fertility regulation in China. In: Diczfalusy E, Diczfalusy A, editors. Research on the regulation of human fertility. Copenaghen: Scriptor; 1983. p. 54–71.
133. Xiao B. Challenges to the development of new contraceptive technology in the 21st century. Chin Med J. 1999;112:924–9.

134. Fruzzetti F, Fidecicchi T, Gambacciani M. Oestrogens in oral contraception: considerations for tailoring prescription to women's needs. Eur J Contracept Reprod Health Care. 2024;29:93–102.
135. Stanczyk FZ, Winer SA, Foidart JM, Archer DF. Comparison of estrogenic components used for hormonal contraception. Contraception. 2024;130:110310.
136. Capozzi A, Scambia G, Lello S. Clinical pharmacology of progestins. Minerva Obstet Gynecol. 2022;74:364–76.
137. Liu S, Kciuk O, Frank M, Tyson N. Progestins of today and tomorrow. Curr Opin Obstet Gynecol. 2022;34:344–50.
138. Sitruk-Ware R, Nath A. The use of newer progestins for contraception. Contraception. 2010;82:410–7.
139. Sitruk-Ware R. Pharmacological profile of progestins. Maturitas. 2008;61:151–7.
140. Sitruk-Ware R. New progestagens for contraceptive use. Hum Reprod Update. 2006;12:169–78.
141. Benagiano G, Primiero FM, Farris M. Clinical profile of contraceptive progestins. Eur J Contracept Reprod Health Care. 2004;9:182–93.
142. Nelson LW, Weikel JH Jr, Reno FE. Mammary nodules in dogs during four years' treatment with megestrol acetate or chlormadinone acetate. J Natl Cancer Inst. 1973;51:1303–11.
143. Owen LN, Briggs MH. Contraceptive steroid toxicology in the Beagle dog and its relevance to human carcinogenicity. Curr Med Res Opin. 1976;4:309–29.
144. Weikel JH Jr, Nelson LW. Problems in evaluating chronic toxicity of contraceptive steroids in dogs. J Toxicol Environ Health. 1977;3:167–77.
145. Selman PJ, Mol JA, Rutteman GR, van Garderen E, Rijnberk A. Progestin-induced growth hormone excess in the dog originates in the mammary gland. Endocrinology. 1994;134:287–92.
146. Minkin S. Depo-Provera: a critical analysis. Women Health. 1980;8:49–69.
147. Benagiano G, Fraser I. The Depo-Provera debate. Commentary on the article "Depo-Provera, a critical analysis". Contraception. 1981;24:493–528.
148. Jordan A. Toxicology of depot medroxyprogesterone acetate. Contraception. 1994;49:189–201.
149. Green W. The FDA, contraceptive marketing approval and products liability litigation: Depo-Provera and the risk of osteoporosis. Food Drug Law J. 2013;68:115–35. i
150. The "Beagle Freedom Project". FDA Modernization Act promises to spare animals, bring safer and better treatments to patients, and drive down drug prices. https://bfp.org/fda-modernization-act/. Accessed 20 Apr 2024.

Chapter 9
Different Methods and Routes of Administration of Hormonal Contraception

Martin H. Birkhaeuser

9.1 Introduction

In 1957, combined hormonal contraception (CHC) was introduced as a new contraceptive possibility. In 1960, Enovid-10® (G D Searle Co., Skokie, IL, USA) has been launched in the United States as the first contraceptive 'pill'. Since then, 'The Pill' has revolutionized family planning. For the first time, it gave women control over their own fertility. It has been estimated that 50 years later, about 200 million of women worldwide have been using hormonal contraception [1, 2]. The history of the first 50 years of 'The Pill' has been reviewed in 2010 and 2011 among others by Szarewski, Mansour, and Shulman [1] and by Chadwick, Burkman, Tornesi, and Mahadevan [2], the latter addressing specifically risk reduction and non-contraceptive benefits, both being in the centre of discussion still today.

The 'pill' implied profound social, political and economic changes that have been seen as a chance by the majority of humanity, but also as a thread to their convictions by others. From the beginning on, several religious organizations have been seeing the 'pill' more as a thread than as a chance for women and for families. One example is the Encyclica Humanae Vitae [3] published in 1968 by the Vatican, taking position against the use of 'The Pill', another identical position adopted by some evangelical churches particularly in the United States. All these statements recommend the so-called natural methods. However, these methods are often unreliable, particularly in adolescents and in elderly women prone to irregular cycles. In both groups, hormonal contraception, combined or progestin-only, is particularly helpful also because of its non-contraceptive benefits. Combined hormonal contraceptives (CHCs) are still the most widely used form of contraception in the developed world,

M. H. Birkhaeuser (✉)
Division of Gynaecological Endocrinology and Reproductive Medicine, University of Bern, Bern, Switzerland

A. R. Genazzani et al. (eds.), *Ethical, Efficacy and Safety Issues in Contraception*, Reproductive Medicine for Clinicians 4,
https://doi.org/10.1007/978-3-032-07322-8_9

although they are not the only ones available. Ovulation inhibition, and thus contraceptive efficacy, is achieved by the progestin that inhibits luteinizing hormone (LH). Progestins act also through a second mechanism by altering cervical mucus permeability for sperm [4]. Oestrogens are then added to increase contraceptive efficacy and to improve endometrial control. In high dosed pills, exogenous ethinyl-oestradiol (EE) had also to compensate for the deficiency of endogenous oestradiol induced by the progestin.

The benefits of modern CHC are twofold:

1. Protection against pregnancies not desired at a certain time, without compromising a later successful pregnancy
2. Non-contraceptive benefits:

   - Linked to the suppression of follicular maturation, e.g. better bleeding pattern, decrease of PMS, endometriosis, benign breast diseases, and ovarian cancer
   - Linked to anti-androgenic and anti-mineralocorticoid activity (third/fourth generation)

The contraceptive safety observed in users of hormonal contraception in comparison with users of other frequently used methods is presented in Table 9.1. It shows clearly that all CHCs rank among the best and most reliable methods used for protection against a pregnancy not desired at the time of CHC use. Opponents to CHCs are rarely aware of the conceptive probability, under optimal conditions, of about 25% per cycle in younger women. They also neglect the still high fertility rates in women over 35, reaching without contraception approximately 50%. The oldest age at delivery in the twentieth century has been 57 years 120 days, and in historical times 62 years (6 children between 47 and 62 years) [5].

The positions against hormonal contraception adopted by some religious organizations are mainly based on biological, pharmacological and social assumptions of the 1960s which should be looked at differently today because the society and 'The Pill' of the sixties of the last century have not been the same as they are today. In addition, although CHC remains the most common form of contraception in industrialized countries, new contraceptives such as reliable long-acting progestin-only or non-hormonal methods have been developed. They are not discussed in this chapter.

The aim of this chapter is to present a short overview about the important changes of the different molecules and combinations, as well as the different routes of administration and the impact on safety of CHC available today, over 60 years after the first pill has been launched. The classical but today questioned definitions used in the field of CHC are presented in Table 9.2. It has to be noted that two other methods of hormonal contraception, subcutaneous implants and intramuscular injections, are treated in another chapter (Chap. 19).

Table 9.1 Pregnancies observed in users of hormonal contraception in comparison with other frequently used methods (pearl index) [184, 190, 191]

Percent of women with pregnancy		
Method	Lowest expected Pearl index (%)	Typical ('real life') Pearl index (%)
No method (average) women aged 19–26 years: 92 women aged 27–34 years: 86–87 women aged 35–39 years: 82	85	85
Hormonal methods		
Combined hormonal contraception		
Combination pill	0.3	8.7
Patch	0.3	8.0
Vaginal ring	0.3	8.0
Progestin-only methods		
Progestin-only pill	0.5	3.0
Hormonal implant	0.1	0.18
IUD [progestin-loaded]	0.16	0.16
Depot MPA	0.3	0.88
Non-hormonal methods		
Copper IUD	0.3	0.8
Sterilization (female)	0.2	0.3
Sterilization (male)	0.1	0.1
Withdrawal	4	18
Condom (male)	2	12
Condom (female)	5	25
Portio cap	6	6
Diaphragm and spermicide	1	20
Calendar	3	9
Temperature	0.8	3
Symptothermal	0.4	1.8
Billings	5	35

9.2 Composition of CHC

9.2.1 The Oestrogen Component

Oestrogens are C-18 steroids. Their precursors are androgens. The formula of the natural oestrogens oestradiol (E2), oestrone (E1) and oestetrol (E4, foetal oestrogen) as well as the synthetic oestrogen ethinyl-oestradiol (EE) are shown in Fig. 9.1. E2 is the major oestrogen secreted by the ovaries whereas about half of E1 originates from peripheral aromatization of androgens. E2 stays in equilibrium with E1.

E2 is the most potent natural oestrogen. The major obstacle to its use for contraception has been in the 1950s its short half-life of approximately 15 min and its reduced activity with oral administration. The two synthetic oestrogens mestranol

Table 9.2 Classical definitions used in the field of combined hormonal contraception

Low-dose oral contraceptives
Products containing less than 50-μg ethinyl oestradiol
First-generation progestins
Products containing estranes derived from testosterone such as norethindrone, norethynodrel, norethindrone acetate, and ethynodiol diacetate and pregnanes derived from 17-OH progesterone such as medroxyprogesterone acetate and chlormadinone acetate
Second-generation progestins
Products containing gonanes derived from testosterone such as levonorgestrel and norgestrel
Third-generation progestins
Products containing desogestrel, gestodene, norgestimate/norelgestromin and etonogestrel
Fourth-generation progestins
Products containing nonethylated estranes such as drospirenone and dienogest, or pregnanes (19-norprogesterones) such as nestorone, nomegestrol acetate and trimegestone

and ethinyl-oestradiol (EE) present a more favourable pharmacokinetic profile for contraception [6]. Finally, EE has been preferred to mestranol and chosen for oral contraception. Today, EE is the most potent synthetic oestrogen and the only synthetic oestrogen still used in CHC. In EE, an ethinyl group is added to E2 at C17 to increase its oral activity as well as its half-life (12–15 h) significantly. Its main disadvantage is a strong stimulatory effect on hepatic factors such as the coagulation factors. The metabolism of EE varies highly from woman to woman so that the same dose can cause variable side effects.

In CHC, an oestrogen is added to a progestin, initially mainly to increase the contraceptive efficacy of the progestin and to stabilize the endometrium so that breakthrough bleeding is avoided. To be on the safe side for full inhibition of ovulation, the first pills contained in 1960 up to 150 μg EE. However, the oestrogen content (dosage) of the pill is directly related to most side effects and to the increased risk of thrombosis, stroke and mortality. Therefore, EE dosage has been decreased progressively (Fig. 9.2) in the next 40 years to 10% (15 μg) of the initial dose without compromising the contraceptive efficacy by adapting properties and dosage of the progestin component.

Today, it is generally postulated that the lowest dose of EE allowing a stable bleeding pattern should be chosen. However, low und ultra-low EE doses in combination with a modern more potent progestogen might lead to an over-suppression of the endogenous oestradiol production necessary to reach a normal peak bone mass in adolescents with an immature gonadal axis. However, the literature on the effect of ultra-low-dose pills and MPA on bone is contradictory. Most clinical studies performed in adult women with regular cycles found no unfavourable effect of combined oral contraceptives (COCs) with 20 μg EE. In one study, even a week increase of bone mineral density (BMD) has been reported [7]. In a randomized double-blind study (RC) comparing a COC with 20 μg EE in combination with 100 μg levonorgestrel (LNG) to a COC in combination with 30 μg EE with 150 μg LNG, no significant difference between the two pills has been found for bone mineral density (BMD) and bone turnover markers after a treatment duration of 3 years [8]. Similar results have

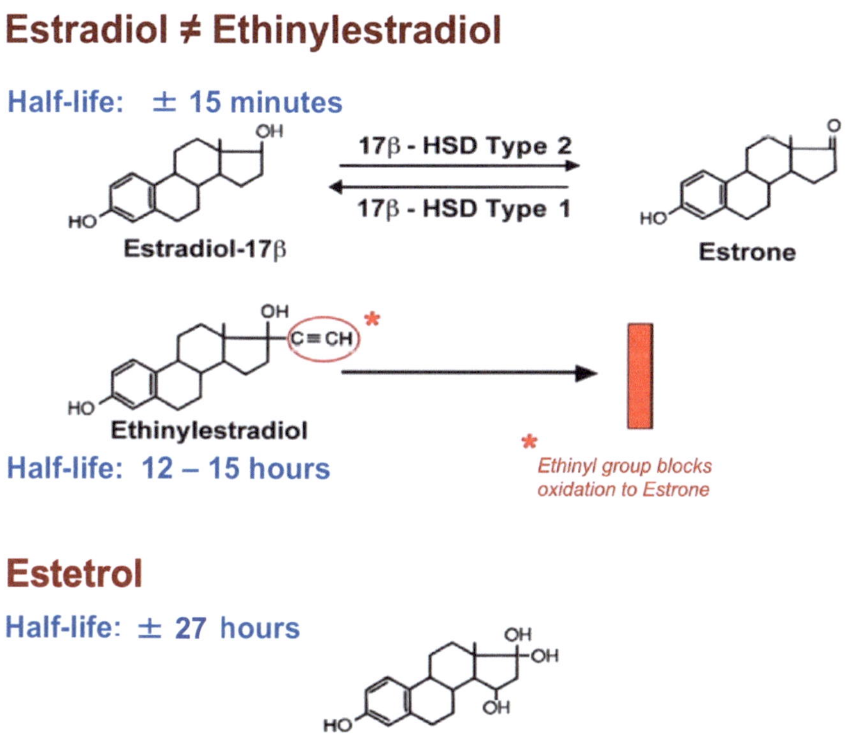

Fig. 9.1 Comparison of the natural oestrogens oestradiol (E2), oestrone (E1) and oestetrol (E4, foetal oestrogen) with the synthetic oestrogen ethinyl-oestradiol (EE)E2 is metabolized to E1In EE, oxidation is blocked by the ethinyl group on position C17 leading to a significantly longer half-life and different metabolic propertiesE4 is the natural native foetal oestrogen

Fig. 9.2 Evolution of combined oral contraception. Decrease of ethinyl-oestradiol dose since 1960

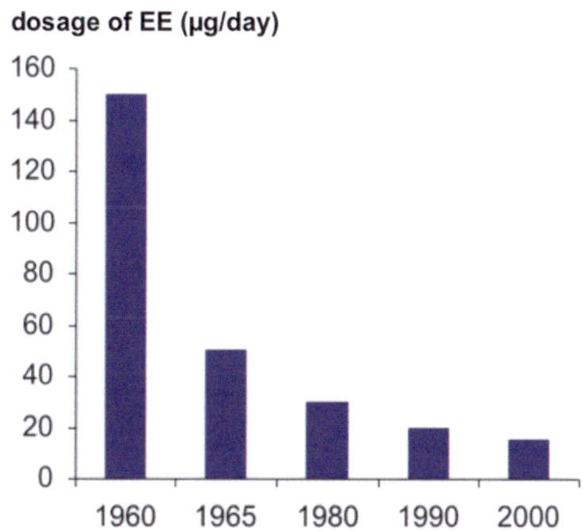

been reported by an RCT comparing the effect of a low-dose 21-day COC containing 20 µg EE and 75 µg gestodene with an ultra-low-dose 24-day COC containing 15 µg EE and 60 µg gestodene on bone turnover and BMD in young, fertile women [9].

In the last decades, contraceptives with micronized oestradiol or oestradiol valerate have been developed. Oestradiol valerate is an oestradiol ester. This ester is known to be significantly better reabsorbed than E2 after oral administration. It is rapidly hydrolyzed to oestradiol. Combinations of several progestins with micronized oestradiol or oestradiol valerate have demonstrated good contraceptive efficacy. More recently, the foetal oestrogen oestetrol (E4) has been introduced as the oestrogen component for menopausal hormone therapy and CHC. The goal of preferring both to EE, micronized oestradiol or oestradiol valerate resp. E4 in CHC, is to reduce the stimulation of liver proteins and therefore serious adverse events such as stroke and thrombo-embolism.

9.2.2 *The Progestin Component*

The progestagens or progestogens include both natural progesterone (P) secreted by ovary and placenta and the synthetic progestins, acting like analogues of P. Synthetic progestins are derived from progesterone or from testosterone and are therefore C-21 and C-19 steroids, respectively (Fig. 9.3) [4, 10–16].

Natural progesterone cannot be used for contraception for several reasons, but the main obstacle is its lack in central inhibitory potential on the gonadal axis.

The breakthrough in hormonal contraception came with the synthesis of progestins allowing a reliable ovulation inhibition. The first two orally active progestins used for contraception were norethynodrel and norethisterone [14].

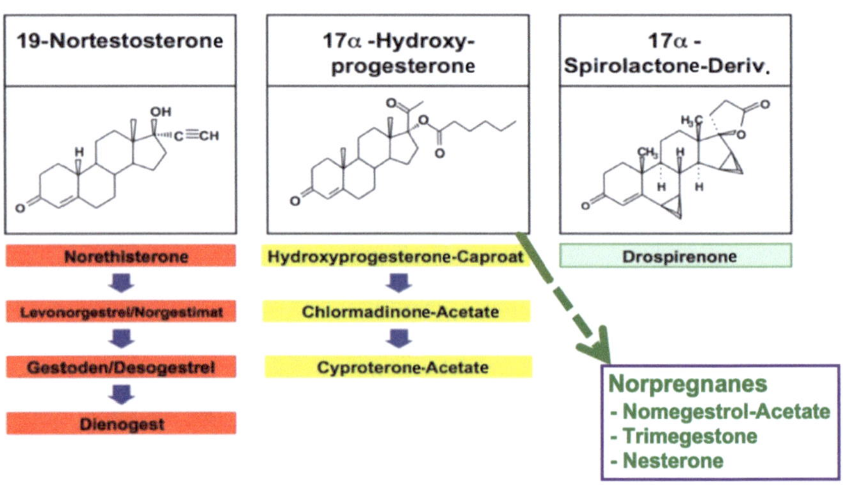

Fig. 9.3 The progestin families used in CHC

The effect of progesterone and of synthetic progestins is mediated by two mechanisms: by a genomic interaction with the progesterone receptor and by a non-genomic interaction with membranic binding sites. There are two isoforms of the progesterone receptor, PRA and PRB. Because synthetic progestins are derived from progesterone (17-α-OH-progesterone derivatives) or testosterone (19-nortestosterone derivatives), they still possess some activities of their steroid family in function of their specific chemical and spatial structures. Natural progesterone and synthetic progestins do not only interact with the progesterone receptors, but also with other steroid receptors, such as androgen receptors (AR) (exerting androgenic of anti-androgenic partial activities), or mineralocorticoid receptors (exerting mineralocorticoid or anti-mineralocorticoid partial activities). Furthermore, some progestins possess an affinity to the glucocorticoid receptor (GR) and may therefore exert a glucocorticoid-like activity [15].

The term 'progesterone' should never be used if synthetic progestins are meant. Progestagens differ considerably in their structure, metabolization and bioavailability as well as their partial effects (Table 9.3). It was therefore a nonsense to postulate a class effect common to all progestogens, as it was done 25–30 years ago in the United States in relation to menopausal hormone therapy (MHT). Today, progestagens are classified in function of their partial activities and their main use (contraception, pre-menopausal substitution, postmenopausal hormone therapy or as anti-androgens).

The advantages of progestins without androgenic partial activity are mainly due to the fact that they induce:

- No weight increase
- No acne
- No negative effects on lipids
- Minimal effect on insulin sensitivity
- Less adverse effects on arterial wall

The effect of ultra-low-dose COC on acne and seborrhoea remains beneficial as it is with older COC if less androgenic progestins are used. However, their thromboembolic risk is slightly higher in some populations (see below).

In part for marketing reasons, progestins have been classified in a first generation, second generation, third generation and fourth generation. Although belonging to the older so-called second generation, NETA (a 19-nortestosterone-derivative) is still one of the most used progestins in CHC, mainly because of its low thromboembolic risk.

First-generation progestins (*pregnanes* and *estranes*) have been largely abandoned due to their androgenic properties that can cause troublesome symptoms [16]. The steric configuration of *retroprogesterones* such as dydrogesterone used in menopausal hormone therapy differs completely from the one of progesterone and all other progestins [4, 10–13]. Whereas in a normal steroid, the rings A-D are laying in the same plane, in dydrogesterone, ring B possesses towards ring C an angle of 60 degrees. As a consequence, dydrogesterone has no central effect and cannot be used in contraception.

Table 9.3 Partial activities and use of progestins compared to natural progestins

	use / Genera-tion	Progestogen	Anti-gonadotrop	Anti-estrogen	Estrogen	Androgen	Anti-androgen	Gluco-corticoid	Anti-mineralo corticoid	Pro Coagulatory
Progesterone	MHT-pref	+	+	+	–	–	+/–	+	+	–
Dydrogesterone (retrosteroid)	MHT-pref	+	–	+	–	–	+/–	–	+/–	–
17a-Hydroxy-Progesterone Derivates										
Medrogestone	MHT	+	+	+	–	–	+/–	–	–	
Chlormadinone acetate	n-a	+	+	+	–	–	+	+	–	–
Cyproterone acetate	AA	+	+	+	–	–	++	+	–	–
Megestrol acetate	cat	+	+	+	–	+/–	+	+	–	+
Medroxyprogesterone acetate		+	+	+	–	+/–	–	+	–	
19-Nor-Progesterone-Derivates										
Nomegestrol acetate		+	+	+	–	–	+/–	–	–	–
Promegestone		+	+	+	–	–	–	–	–	–
Trimegestone		+	+	+	–	–	+/–	–	+/–	–
19-Nortestosterone-Derivates										
Norethisterone = Norethindrone (Norethisterone acetate = NETA)	MHT	+	+	+	+	+	–	–	–	+
Lynestrenol	1	+	+	+	+	+	–	–	–	–
Norethinodrel	out of use	+/–	+	+	+	+	–	–	–	–
Levonorgestrel	2	+	+	+	–	+	–	–	–	–
Norgestimate (active metabolite: Norelgestromin)	2	+	+	+	–	+	–	–	–	–
Desogestrel (active metabolite: 3-keto-desogestrel=Etonogestrel)	3	+	+	+	–	+	–	–	–	–
Gestodene	3	+	+	+	–	+	–	+	+	–
Dienogest	n-a	+	+	+/–	+/–	–	+	–	–	–
Nestorone	n	+	+	+	–	–	–	–	–	–
Spirolonactone Derivate										
Drospirenone	n-a	+	+	+	–	–	+	–	+	–

1 = 1. generation 2 = 2. generation n = newer progestins used in hormonal contaceptives n-a = newer progestins with anti-androgenic partial activity used in hormonal contaceptives

cat: used in cats for contraception

AA = anti-androgen

MHT: used in Menopausal Hormone Therapy

MHT-pref: first choice for use in Menopausal Hormone Therapy

MPA: used for hormonal contraception and for MHT

Based on Refs. [4, 10–13, 15, 16]

9.2.2.1 17-α-OH-Progesterone Derivatives

Oral pregnanes (medroxyprogesterone acetate = MPA, megestrol acetate, medrogestone) are mainly used in hormonal substitution.

17-α-OH-progesterone-derivatives such as cyproterone-acetate (CPA) or chlormadinone acetate (CMA) possess a strong anti-androgenic partial activity and are indicated as anti-androgens. In combination with EE, their contraceptive properties are equivalent to CHC.

Nomegestrol acetate is not a real pregnane, but, because of the profile of its partial activities, it is mostly listed in this group.

Some *norpregnanes* (demegestone, promegestone, trimegestone and nestorone) have been integrated in combination with oestradiol in newer CHC.

9.2.2.2 19-Nortestosterone Derivatives

Although 19-nortestosterone derivatives are derived from the androgen 19-nortestosterone, they loose by the introduction of an ethinyl group in position C-17-α nearly completely their androgenic partial activity in favour of a newly acquired gestagenic activity. Among the nortestosterone derivatives, there are the so-called prodrugs. Prodrugs are rapidly transformed after intake to the active progestagens.

Norethisterone (NET) and Norethistorone Acetate (NETA)
After oral administration, NETA is rapidly hydrolyzed to NET in the intestinal tract and in the liver, so that there is no relevant difference in the pharmacokinetic and pharmacodynamic properties. Of mostly historical interest are the other prodrugs of NET, norethynodrel, lysestrenol and ethynediol diacetate. All three are metabolized to NET after ingestion.

Tibolone (7α-methyl-norethynodrel) with its gestagenic metabolite 7α-methyl-NET (Δ4-isomere) belongs also to this group, but it is only used in menopausal hormone therapy.

Oral bioavailability of NET and NETA is between 40% and 80%. NET is bound in 36% to SHBG and in 61% to albumin. Its terminal half-life is 9.5 h. Of clinical importance is the fact that approximately 0.35% of the absorbed NET is aromatized in the liver to EE [4, 10, 13]. If dosages of 5 or 10 mg NETA are administered orally, the EE levels reached correspond to the intake of 30 or 60 µg EE [17]. This aromatization explains the increased VTE risk in women treated by 5–10 mg NETA [18, 19]. If low doses of ≤1 mg NETA are used, this phenomenon may be neglected. Because of its aromatization to EE, NETA may increase the favourable effect of oestrogens on bone.

NET has no glucocorticoid or anti-mineralocorticoid activity. In combination with an oestrogen, its remaining weak androgenic properties have usually no clinical impact. Transdermal NETA does, in contrast to oral NETA, not compromise carbohydrate metabolism and has only a minimal impact on lipid metabolism.

Levonorgestrel (LNG) and Norgestrel (NG)
LNG is a potent progestin without glucocorticoid or anti-mineralocorticoid activity, but it possesses a certain androgenic activity [4, 10–13, 20]. Therefore, oral administration of LNG alone induces a decrease of SHBG levels. In the combined use of LNG with an oestrogen, the effect on SHBG depends on the dosage of the oestrogen component. Levonorgestrel is bound in 48% to SHBG and in 50% to albumin. The terminal half-life of LNG is 24 h. Transdermal administration of oestradiol and LNG has no impact on lipid metabolism.

NGM is a prodrug and is metabolized in the gastrointestinal tract and in the liver to LNG via LNG-3-Oxim and LNG-17ß-acetate, respectively. The hormonally active metabolites of NGM are LNG and LNG-3-Oxim (NGMN).

NG is a racemate and consists in 50% each of inactive dextronorgestrel and active LNG. In consequence, the hormonal activity of 0.5 mg norgestrel corresponds to the one 0.25 mg norgestimate (NGM) [4, 10, 12, 20]. LNG being the most important metabolite of NGM and NGMN, the partial activities of NGM correspond to the activities of LNG.

In contrast to LNG, NGM and NGMN do not bind to SHBG and CBG. Norelgestromine is contained in the new transdermal contraceptive Evra®.

Desogestrel (DSG)

DSG is a prodrug. Its active metabolite is 3-keto-desogestrel (KDG = etonogestrel). The bioavailability of DSG is 76%. 32% is bound to SHBG and 66% to albumin. In a bioassay, its androgenic potency is 40% of the one of testosterone. The elimination half-life of desogestrel is 1.5 h and of etonogestrel is 21–38 h [21].

Its active metabolite KDG (etonogestrel) has anti-oestrogenic and androgenic, but no glucocorticoid or anti-mineralocorticoid activities [10, 22, 23]. If given alone, DSG can induce slight symptoms of androgenization. However, when DSG is used in combination with an oestrogen, its androgenic partial activity is clinically not relevant [10, 23].

Etonogestrel is contained in the product Nuvaring® where it is combined with EE and in the progestin-only implant Implanon®. *Progestogen-only products confer no increased risk of venous thrombo-embolism* [24].

Gestodene (GSD)

The oral bioavailability of gestodene has been found to range from 87% to 111%, with a mean of 96%. The biological half-life is 12–15 h. GSD has a high affinity to SHBG (binding 64%) and a low affinity to albumin (binding 34%), 2% of GSD are free [25]. GSD possesses the highest potency of all orally administered progestins and has therefore the lowest dosage [4, 10]. GSD has anti-oestrogenic, androgenic, glucocorticoid and weak anti-mineralocorticoid partial activities. The relatively strong androgenic activity of GSD is of no clinical relevance if it is used in a low dosage and in combination with an oestrogen [25, 26].

9.2.2.3 Dienogest and Drospirenone

These so-called 'new' progestins have been designed to have no androgenic or estrogenic actions. Their activity is closer to the physiological hormone progesterone [10, 12]. New progestins having less side-effects based on their activity profile include dienogest (DNG) and the norpregnane derivatives nomegestrol acetate (NOMAc), demegestone, trimegestone (TMG) and nestorone (NES). Drospirenone (DRSP), another new progestin, differs from all other progestins as it is derived from spirolactone. It is essentially an anti-mineralocorticoid steroid with no androgenic effect but a partial anti-androgenic effect. In addition, DNG, TMG and DRSP are characterized by a specific anti-androgenic activity [4, 10, 20, 26–29].

Because the 19-norprogesterones as well as DRSP and DNG are not androgenic, they exert no negative effect on the lipid profile. For the same reason, the new progestins have in combination with an oestrogen a slightly different impact on the hepatic coagulation factors when compared to the older progestins [30].

Dienogest (DNG)

DNG is the only nortestosterone derivative that has no ethinyl, but a cyanomethyl group on position C17α. Although DNG does not bind to SHBG and has only a week affinity to albumin, its bioavailability amounts to high 95%. It possesses a short terminal half-life of 9 h [10, 21, 22, 31]. Its ovulation-inhibitory potency may be compared to the one of progesterone-derivates. On the other hand, its strong progestagenic effect at the endometrium corresponds to the one of nortestosterone derivatives (Table 9.3) [10, 31]. This can be explained by the high DNG serum levels of >50 ng/ml after ingestion of 2 mg DNG with a proportion of 10% of free DNG. It is speculated that for this reason the intracellular concentration of DNG is relatively high, so that in spite of the low binding affinity to the progesterone receptor, the transformation dose corresponds to LNG.

DNG has no androgenic, glucocorticoid or anti-mineralocorticoid partial activities, but it is the only nortestosterone derivative with anti-androgenic properties.

DNG does not modify oestrogen-induced changes of many hepatic serum parameters [10, 31].

To minimize metabolic side effects, DNG has been combined with oestradiol-valerate instead of EE and successfully introduced in clinical routine as a contraceptive pill [32]. To have an optimal bleeding pattern, it is presented in a blister as a multiphasic preparation (Fig. 9.4). E2-V/DNG has a minimal impact on metabolic and haemostatic parameters, and a more favourable effect than EE/LNG on lipid markers [33]. It is expected to have a lower VTE risk than pills with EE. However, clinical data confirming this hypothesis are still missing.

Drospirenone (DRSP)

DRSP belongs to the group of the spirolactones. As a spirolactone derivative, DRSP has a molecular structure that differs from all other progestins [33–37]. In contrast to spironolactone, DRSP has in addition to its anti-mineralocorticoid and anti-androgenic activities also strong progestagenic potencies (Table 9.3). DRSP has no glucocorticoid or androgenic activities and no clinically relevant impact on oestrogen-induced changes of hepatic parameters [33–37]. DRSP has a bioavailability of 66–85% and is, in the serum, only bound to albumin (in 95–97%). Its elimination half-life is 25–33 h [33–37]. The ovulation inhibition dose of drospirenone is 2 mg per day (the new DRSP-POP has 4 mg DRSP per tablet and day).

The strong anti-mineralocorticoid activity leads to a reduction of the sodium and water retention and has a beneficial effect on the development of oedemas. However, this effect is counterbalanced in the longer range by a strong compensatory increase of the plasma-renin activity and serum aldosterone levels [33, 34]. As a side effect, an increase of serum potassium levels may be seen. DRSP is also referred to as a 'fourth-generation' progestin. DRSP is administered together with an oestrogen or alone as an oral progestin-only contraceptive (not discussed in this chapter). In combination with the E2 or E4, DRSP is used also for menopausal hormone therapy (MHT) [38–40].

In combination with EE, with or without supplemental folic acid, DRSP is indicated as a second-line COC. DRSP combined with low-dose EE is indicated for the

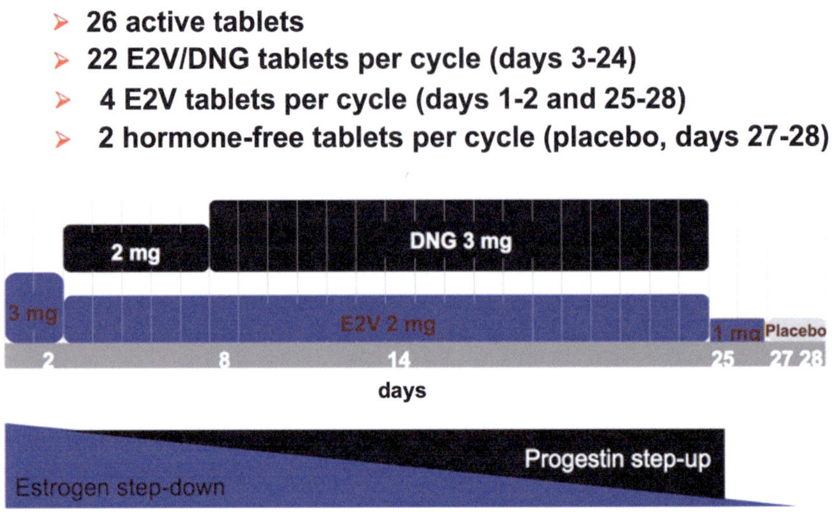

Fig. 9.4 Example of a step-up/step-down COCIn a modern contraceptive pill, DNG has been combined with oestradiol-valerate instead of EE (Qlaira®) [32]. To obtain an optimal bleeding pattern, it is presented in a blister as a multiphasic preparation

treatment of moderate acne, pre-menstrual syndrome (PMS), pre-menstrual dysphoric disorder (PMDD) and dysmenorrhoea [41–44]. Several observations point to an increased VTE risk in pills containing drospirenone and EE [11, 30]. This risk has been estimated by the FDA to an approximately 1.5-fold increase [45]. In 2018, the FDA updated its label dating from 2011 for birth control pills containing DRSP and some other newer progestins to include warnings for stopping use prior to and after surgery, and to warn that such birth control pills may have a higher risk of blood clots [46]. Therefore, COCs containing DRSP and EE should not be used as a first-choice pill, but should be reserved for women with additional indications (see, also below, vascular side effects).

The first COC containing oestetrol (E4) and not EE as the estrogenic component contains 14.2 mg oestetrol (E4) and 3 mg drospirenone (DRSP) in a monophasic 24/4 regimen (approved by EMA in 2022). Its contraceptive efficacy is high (pearl index 0.47 in the European study) [47, 48]. Due to its anti-mineralocorticoid activity, drospirenone opposes oestrogen-induced salt and water retention and maintains or slightly reduces body weight in women using E2/DRSP [39, 44]. DRSP decreases blood pressure in women with arterial hypertension [38, 45, 49]. E2/DRSP has been shown to increase BMD (52) and to decrease the risk of bone fractures in postmenopausal women [50, 51]. E2/DRSP has a favourable influence on cholesterol and triglyceride levels [38, 49, 52]. Data also indicate slightly lower metabolic effects on haemostasis parameters in the liver compared to EE/LNG and EE/DRSP [53]. However, it is still open if these findings can be translated in a lower incidence of venous thrombo-embolism compared to classical pills containing EE. Because clinical long-term data are not yet available (phase 4 studies are not yet published), its FDA labelling is still prudent [54].

9.2.2.4 Norpregnane Derivatives

The 19-norprogesterone derivatives of progesterone (19-norpregnanes) lack a methyl group at position C10 [26]. The 19-norprogesterones are derived from the pregnane structure but have one carbon less as they do not have a radical methyl at C-19 [20]. They are referred to as 'pure' progestational molecules as they bind more selectively to the progesterone receptor. The19-norprogesterones include nomegestrol acetate (NOMAC), an acetylated compound [55], as well as four non-acetylated molecules: demegestone, promegestone, TMG [56] and NES [57].

Unlike nomegestrol acetate and nesterone, trimegestone, demegestone and promegestone all have a double bond between carbons 9 and 10 and a methyl group substituted for the acetate group at carbon 17. TMG and NES are the most potent progestins synthesized to date, followed by two of the older progestins, keto-desogestrel (keto-DSG) and levonorgestrel (LNG). Trimegestone (TMG) and promegestone also have a methyl group on the two-carbon side chain at carbon 17; in trimegestone, the penultimate carbon is also hydroxylated. Nesterone (NES) differs from nomegestrol acetate in the presence of a methylene group at carbon 16 and absence of the methyl group at carbon 6 and the double bond between carbons 6 and 7 [26].

Nomegestrol Acetate (NOMAC)

Nomegestrol acetate (NOMAC) is a potent, highly selective progestogen, which is structurally similar to 19-norprogesterone and characterized as a full agonist at the progesterone receptor. Its affinity for the progesterone receptor (PR) is high and corresponds to about 125% of the affinity of progesterone. It is associated with effective suppression of gonadotropic activity and ovulation in premenopausal women. NOMAC is bound in 97.5–98% to albumin, but does not bind to SHBG. Its bioavailability is 63%; the elimination half-life ranges from 30 to 80 h. NOMAC is formed by adding a double bond between C-6 and C-7 of the hydroxyprogesterone skeleton and deleting the CH3 radical at C-19. These structural changes confer a higher progestational potency to NOMAC, higher than the one of MPA [10, 11, 55, 58]. Except for the absence of the methyl group at carbon 10, the norpregnane derivative nomegestrol acetate is identical to that of the pregnane derivative megestrol acetate. As with other oral contraceptives, there is a potential for interaction with drugs that induce hepatic enzymes. Examples include rifampicin and some anti-epileptic drugs.

NOMAC has no or minimal binding to other steroid receptors, including the androgen, mineralocorticoid and glucocorticoid receptors [10, 58, 59].

Therefore, NOMAC has no androgenic effect [10–12, 64]. Its partial anti-androgenic effect is 20 times lower than that of CPA.

NOMAC has a neutral impact on lipids and carbohydrate metabolism. Older studies suggested that NOMAC-E2 may not have negative effects on haemostatic and other metabolic parameters [60–62]. In normal and cancerous human breast tissue, NOMAC/E2 has shown favourable effects on oestrogen metabolism, and in human breast cancer cell lines in vitro it does not stimulate cell proliferation [63]. A phase 3 study points to less overall impact with NOMAC/E2 on haemostatic, lipid, inflammatory and carbohydrate metabolism parameters than with levonorgestrel 150 μg/EE 30 μg. A recent review [64] postulates that NOMAC/E2 is not associated with increased risk of venous thrombo-embolism, a major safety concern of health-care professionals for women receiving hormonal contraceptives. These clinical real-world findings are promising and suggest incidence levels of VTE, a major safety concern for healthcare professionals, with NOMAC/E2 similar to COCs containing levonorgestrel. However, full publication of results from the pivotal phase 3 trials of NOMAC/E2 is still pending.

Trimegestone (TMG)
TMG is a promegestone prodrug [57]. TMG differs from promegestone by the presence of a hydroxylated carbon on the penultimate carbon of the side chain (C-17). On the ovulation inhibition test, TMG is close in activity to medroxyprogesterone acetate (MPA) [20]. TMG is bound in 98% to albumin. Elimination half-life is estimated to 13.8–15.6 h. In vivo, TMG has a potent progestin activity. TMG has a high affinity for the PR but only 42% for the mineralocorticoid receptor (MR) [65]. TMG has also been demonstrated to have weak anti-androgenic activity and some anti-mineralocorticoid activity [56, 66].

TMG binds to the human PR with an affinity greater than do MPA, norethisterone (NET) or LNG. In contrast, TMG binds with low affinity to the AR, the GR and the MR and has no measurable affinity for the ER.

Most of the clinical experience with this progestin has been collected in the treatment of post-menopausal women [67]. The overall profile of TMG is qualitatively similar to that of P. Although TMG is one of the most potent progestins of the new generation, it is not presently developed as a contraceptive.

Nesterone (NES)
The 19-norprogesterone derivative is one of the most potent progestins, about 100 times more potent than progesterone. This is mainly due to its 19-methyl substitution and the addition of the16-methylene substituent, which enhances binding to the PR [29, 65]. NES is bound in 95% to albumin, but does not bind to SHBG and has a short half-life of 4.5 h if administered by a vaginal ring [68]. The oral bioavailability of NES is only about 10%. For this reason, a subcutaneous implant releasing NES alone has been tested in lactating women in a 2-year study comparing the NES implant to the copper T intrauterine device (T-Cu) [69].

A NES-only vaginal ring is being developed as a contraceptive based on the potent anti-ovulatory effect of this progestin.

9.3 The Importance of Compliance and Its Impact on the Regimen and the Way of Administration of CHC

9.3.1 Reasons for Non-compliance in CHC Users

There is no secret that in general contraceptive compliance is far from ideal in hormonal contraception. The abortion rate remains high even in countries with an easy access to advanced contraceptive technology. Contraceptive compliance is defined as the correct use of a contraceptive method, according to the specific prescriptions given by a medical professional and/or in written form as patient information leaflet. Non-compliance describes a mismatch between the real behaviour of a user and the correct or ideal behaviour [70].

Not only with barrier methods, but also with hormonal contraception the gap between correct and real use is large. Discontinuation rates per year reach up to 50%. Reasons for non-compliance mainly are as follows:

1. Lack of motivation to prevent a pregnancy due to an ambivalence regarding the wish for a child or the feeling/conviction of the female partner that she cannot become pregnant both reduce compliance, as well as sexual and relational problems with the couple [71].
2. Cognitive factors (false information, misconceptions, irrational fears) are not rare. Essential for a good compliance and adherence is an individualized information concerning the method chosen, including its benefits and risks. The decision about the method fulfilling best the needs, preferences, medical indications and counterindications as well as the expectations regarding eventual non-contraceptive benefits has to be taken in a common agreement between doctor and patient. Acceptance, compliance and adherence to the therapy seem to depend strongly on the quality of the counselling received by the patient at the moment of the prescription of the contraceptive method [72]. The inclusion of the partner in the counselling process increases compliance [73].
3. Behavioural errors and mistakes (forgetting, loosing, etc.).
4. In some regions, difficult or lacking access to contraceptive methods is a major problem [71, 74].
5. Last but not least, side effects are one of the most important factors for insufficient compliance and may lead to the interruption of the contraceptive method used.

Women using CHC often mention nausea, irregular bleeding, weight increase, mastalgia, decrease of libido and mood swings or depressive mood [74–76].

9.3.2 How to Improve Compliance in CHC Users

Three strategies to improve compliance can be distinguished [70]:

1. Improving counselling
2. Developing non-oral contraceptive methods which demand a low level of compliant behaviour by the user
3. Improving quality of life by minimizing the negative side effects and maximizing the non-contraceptive health benefits

By combining low-dose EE with less androgenic or even slightly anti-androgenic progestins, some of them possessing in addition weak anti-mineralocorticoid properties, negative side effects have been decreased and non-contraceptive health benefits as well as quality of life increased.

A second effort intends to reduce the VTE risk of CHC. Because of the recognized correlation between the amount of ethinyl-oestradiol (EE) and the thromboembolic risk, a constant lowering of the EE dosage has been targeted. The consecutive decrease of ovulation inhibition can be avoided by the combination of EE with more potent progestagens. Mostly, these more potent progestins are also less androgenic. So, the contraceptive safety has been maintained in presence of even less side effects.

However, the price to pay for these favourable modifications of COC was a less stable bleeding pattern with an increased incidence of spotting and break-through bleedings.

9.3.2.1 Methods Used to Stabilize the Bleeding Pattern in Modern COC

Reduction of the Hormone-Free Interval

Spotting and breakthrough bleedings are more frequent with preparations containing 15 μg or 20 μg than with pills containing 30 μg EE. This is mainly linked to the different proportion between the EE and the progestin components. In the classical pill, 21 tablets containing EE and a progestin are followed by a pill-free interval of 7 days. The reduction of the hormone-free interval to 5 or 4 days is used to re-establish a better bleeding profile [77, 78]. It results in a complete suppression of the ovarian function, a reliable ovulation inhibition and an increase of the contraceptive efficacy in spite of a reduction of the EE dosage to 20 μg or 15 μg. Considering the risk of undesirable side effects, the advantage of lower dosages of EE per day prevails over the small increase of the total dosage of EE per cycle. On the other hand, the short hormone-free interval with its early restart of hormone intake might hinder the completion of the normal bleeding process at the endometrium, favouring again spotting.

The so-called *long-cycle treatment in oral contraception* is an extreme reduction of the hormone-free interval. Regular withdrawal bleedings are avoided by omission of one or more hormone-free intervals [77]. Long-cycle regimens with continuous administration of COCs for 3 or 6 months followed by a hormone-free interval of 7 days may reduce the frequency of menstruations and cycle-dependent complaints due to menses-associated disorders such as hypermenorrhoea, dysmenorrhoea, premenstrual syndrome and menstrual migraine. They may also have beneficial effects in patients with haemorrhagic diathesis, endometriosis, uterine leiomyoma and polycystic ovary syndrome [77]. Long-cycle regimens may be prescribed also to extend COC cycles for postponement of menstruation occurring otherwise at an inconvenient time.

The long-cycle regimen with its continuous use of COCs prevents the cyclic fluctuations of serum levels of EE and a progestin and, hence, the cyclic variations of metabolic serum parameters. Although the long-cycle regimen is initially associated with an elevated rate of irregular bleeding, the total number of bleeding days is lower than during conventional COC treatment. The available data suggest that treatment-related side effects in COCs users according to the long-cycle regimen is similar to that of conventional COC regimens [77, 78]. However, the impact of long-term COC administration in users of the long-cycle regimen on safety, particularly the risk of cancer and cardiovascular disease, has not yet been investigated by clinical trials.

Bi- and Triphasic Instead of Monophasic Regimens

Bi- and triphasic regimens [79, 80] mainly intend to stabilize the bleeding pattern in low- and ultra-low-dose COC with EE, and in COC using E2 as an oestrogen component, pills with three phases provide different amounts of hormones over 3 weeks. Whether three-phase or multiphasic pills lead to more pregnancies is unknown. A typical example is shown in Fig. 9.4.

Studies comparing in a randomized prospective way monophasic to multiphasic regimens are rare. There have been no significant differences in intermenstrual bleeding, amenorrhoea and study discontinuation due to intermenstrual bleeding between the biphasic and monophasic oral contraceptive pills. About half of the included tri- versus monophasic trials reported favourable bleeding patterns, that is less spotting, breakthrough bleeding or amenorrhoea, in triphasic versus monophasic COC users. It is not known if these pills give fewer side effects. No significant differences were found in the numbers of women who discontinued due to medical reasons, cycle disturbances, intermenstrual bleeding or adverse events. The authors of the COCHRANE meta-analysis recommend classical one-phase pills for women starting to use birth control pills [79, 80].

9.3.2.2 Non-oral Ways of Administration

The combined contraceptive transdermal patch and the combined contraceptive vaginal ring release progressively EE and a progestin (norelgestromine and etonogestrel, respectively). Both are safe contraceptive methods, and their side effects are comparable to COC. Patch and ring present the advantage that adherence is easier: no need to remember every day to take a pill.

Due to a wrong analogy to MHT, it is often mistakenly believed that the *non-oral administration* of EE decreases the VTE risk in comparison to COC [81, 82]. However, because there are fundamental metabolic differences between oestradiol and EE, the VTE risk is not decreased by the parenteral administration of EE. In users of the contraceptive patch, it might even be increased [50].

EE is not bound at SHBG. Because of its ethinyl group, the inactivation of EE occurs slowly. Therefore, EE reaches the liver in a low but constant concentration where it modifies many oestrogen-dependent hepatic parameters significantly. One of these is haemostasis. It is generally accepted that such changes are responsible for the increased thrombo-embolic risk of the contraceptive patch and vaginal ring.

9.4 Precautions in Selected Subgroups of Women Using CHC

9.4.1 Women >40 Years

Above the age of 40 years, the number of ovulatory cycles starts to decrease, whereas cycles marked by luteal insufficiency and anovulation increase, leading to an irregular bleeding pattern and first intermittent climacteric symptoms. Fertility becomes less predictable so that the risk for unwanted pregnancies rises. At the same time, due to the higher maternal age, the risk for congenital malformations, spontaneous abortions, perinatal mortality of the child and also the risk of maternal morbidity and mortality increase significantly. The cumulative risk of mortality due to the pregnancy increases in women aged ≥40 years to 245 deaths per 100,000 women and is higher than it is in users of COC (80 deaths per 100,000 women) [83, 84] of the same age. A safe contraception is therefore highly recommended. Because of limited space, only the most relevant aspects are presented here.

If there are no contraindications, healthy non-obese non-smokers without contra-indications may continue low-dose combined oral contraception up to the age of menopause [85–87]. The risk–benefit ratio of CHC is positive in women over 40 years of age if all contraindications are respected. Contraindications such as hypertension, obesity, smoking or dyslipidaemia have to be actively excluded. Particularly in this age group, the risk of a correctly indicated COC is inferior to the risk of an unwanted pregnancy. With the exception of an additional specific non-contraceptive indication, a second-generation progestin should be used. CHC treats also vasomotor symptoms and prevents bone loss.

In women aged ≥40 years, the following rules have to be respected when continuation or initiation of CHC is planned [88]:

- The indication for hormonal contraception has to be re-evaluated every year together with a complete history and a thorough risk–benefit evaluation. Sexual health and quality of life should be included.
- Every year, a clinical and gynaecological examination has to be done, including blood pressure and weight/BMI as well as a laboratory check to exclude haematological, metabolic (in particular diabetes mellitus) and renal disorders.

- Initiation of CHC has a higher risk for many side effects than continuation of the same product, in particular for VTE and obesity [87]; see also FSRH Guideline Contraception for Women Aged Over 40 Years [88].

CHC obscures the passage into post-menopause. Therefore, it is recommended to measure every year serum FSH levels [89, 90]. However, the often-used method to determine serum FSH on day 6 or 7 of the pill-free week is not reliable because in some women, FSH starts only to rise about 2 weeks after stopping the pill. Furthermore, it has always to be kept in mind that only one elevated FSH level is no proof for menopause and may be followed by a fertile cycle. In the menopausal transition, MHT can in no way block ovulation [91]. Definite physiological infertility can only be admitted if two high serum FSH levels (>40 U/l) have been measured at a distance of 6 months.

Because it is nearly impossible to predict when contraception becomes unnecessary, an elegant method—particularly in women with beginning vasomotor symptoms—is the combination of oral or non-oral E2 with a LNG-loaded IUD admitted by FDA and EMA for this indication. In women above the age of 40 years presenting a contraindication for CHC, also progestin-only pills (POP), IUDs, barrier methods or the sterilization of the female or male partner have to be considered.

9.4.2 Adolescents

Combined oral contraceptives (COCs) used regularly and consistently have a more than 99% efficacy to prevent a pregnancy. However, to be effective, COCs have to be taken regularly which is frequently not the case in adolescents. Omission of pills diminishes considerably their effectiveness.

Bitzer has defined the ideal contraception for adolescents as follows [92]: ‘Taking into account the biological and psychosocial changes during the transition from childhood to adulthood, adolescents would need a contraceptive method which ideally would be very effective, independent of compliance, without major health risks during use and no negative impact on the future health of the adolescent, protective against STI, favourable for bone development, with no or only few side effects and having some preventive and therapeutic potential with respect to frequent health problems of adolescent girls’.

For most adolescents, the risk–benefit profile of oral contraceptives is favourable.

Thrombo-embolic events are rare at this age. In adolescents, COCs have a very low health risk which seems to differ marginally with respect to dosage and type of the components. However, in adolescent girls using low-dose or ultra-low-dose COCs (15–20 µg EE daily), the gain in bone density to reach a normal peak bone mass might be reduced compared to users of 30-µg EE pills or untreated controls [93]. This danger prevails particularly in adolescents with immature or instable cycles presenting oligo-amenorrhoea, eating disorders, athletic triad or hypothalamic dysfunction [93, 94]. The same is reported for DPMA. In consequence, COCs containing 15–20 μg EE as well as DPMA should be avoided in adolescents with immature cyclicity before peak bone mass has been fully acquired. For newer hormonal contraceptive methods, good evidence is missing concerning their effect on bone. The supply of sufficient calcium and vitamin D through food or with substitutes and proteins is important for the bone health in women of all ages needing contraception. It should therefore be mentioned when counselling adolescents.

If the needed compliance for COC is not guaranteed, other methods have to be suggested such as contraceptive patches or rings or progestin-only implants. If peak bone mass is not endangered, depo-injections can be chosen.

However, COCs do not protect against sexually transmitted diseases (STI) and may even have an inhibitory effect on the use of condoms. Because the protection against unwanted pregnancies may increase sexual activity, the risk of STI including HPV infection is higher [95]. Specialized counselling with a high degree of confidentiality adapted to the knowledge and needs of the individual adolescent is desirable. It has to stress the importance of the use of condoms in spite of contraception by CHC when partners are changing.

9.5 Selected Side Effects and Underlying Diseases

Contraceptive users are usually medically fit and can use any available contraceptive method safely, but some subgroups presenting special medical conditions need special attention.

9.5.1 Weight Increase in Users of Hormonal Contraception

Weight increase belongs to the most frequently indicated side effects of hormonal contraception [96]. Most studies entering in the actual guidelines [97, 98] report a weight increase of approximately only 1 kg. However, a recent Cochrane review concluded from 49 randomized studies that the available evidence is not sufficient to affirm that hormonal contraception per se has a direct effect on body weight [99]. Hormonal contraception may lead indirectly to a weight increase through a change in eating habits or water retention. Water retention may occur particularly with EE/norelgestromin preparations [100–102] and some EE/LNG combinations [101] and seems to depend on the doses of EE: Low-dose CHC with 15 μg EE induce practically no weight increase [103]. Anti-mineralocorticoid progestins such as drospirenone act on the renin–angiotensin–aldosterone system (RAAS) [104, 105]. Therefore, after the evaluation of the benefit–risk balance, an increased water retention can be reduced by a COC containing a progestagen with an anti-mineralocorticoid activity. The slightly higher VTE risk of anti-mineralocorticoid progestins is discussed below. The replacement of EE by E2 or E2V affects body weight favourably. In users of E2V/dienogest [106–109] or E2/nomegestrolacetate, no increase of body weight has been observed [109].

9.5.2 *Diabetes Mellitus*

Although carbohydrate tolerance and insulin resistance can be influenced by hormonal contraception, the main problem for diabetic women does not consist in metabolic changes due to CHC, but in the increase of the cardiovascular risk (myocardial infarction, stroke) due to an underlying diabetic vascular disease, mainly nephropathy with proteinuria, progressive retinopathy, coronary heart disease or arterial hypertension [97, 98]. A Cochrane review [110] investigated eventual differences in diabetic women using CHC, POC or non-hormonal contraceptive methods in respect to the side effects on the carbohydrate or lipid metabolism as well as to long-term effects such as micro- and macrovascular changes. Unfortunately, the insufficient database of the three included RCTs did not allow to draw differentiated conclusions, but there were no differences after 12 months between the included groups for HbA1c and serum glucose levels neither for the daily amount of insulin needed. Therefore, CHC might be a safe option in diabetic women without an underlying diabetic vascular disease and without pre-existing vascular complications [111]. High contraceptive safety is indispensable in diabetic women where each pregnancy has to be planned and meticulously prepared. However, because an incipient diabetic vasculopathy may be at first clinically silent, hormonal contraceptives, CHC as well as POP, should not be used in diabetic women without strict limitations, even if there are no detectable clinical complications (Table 9.4). UKMEC [97] and WHO [98] class diabetic women without vascular diseases in category 2 (advantages of using CHC usually outweigh the risks), whereas diabetic women with vascular diseases belong to category 3 (theoretical risks of using CHC usually outweigh the advantages [97]).

Particular prudence is recommended in diabetics with additional cardiovascular risk factors such as obesity. CHC should be avoided, but progestin-only contraceptive methods may be used (category 2, Table 9.4 [97]). In diabetic women, UKMEC classes only cupper but not LNG-loaded IUDs in category 1 [97]).

9.5.3 *Vascular Diseases*

Thrombo-embolic, cardiovascular and cerebrovascular events are age-dependent.

Among all users of CHC, women characterized by the following factors have an increased risk for vascular diseases:

- Age >35 years
- Smokers (increases VTE risk significantly)

Table 9.4 Recommendations for contraception in women with an underlying cardiovascular disease

Women with an underlying disease

UKMEC	Definition of category
Category 1	A condition for which there is no restriction for the use of the method
Category 2	A condition where the advantages of using the method generally outweigh the theoretical or proven risks
Category 3	A condition where the theoretical or proven risks usually outweigh the advantages of using the method. The provision of a method requires expert clinical judgement and/or referral to a specialist contraceptive provider, since use of the method is not usually recommended unless other more appropriate methods are not available or not acceptable
Category 4	A condition which represents an unacceptable health risk if the method is used

A Diabetes mellitus

	Cu-IUD	LNG-IUS	IMP	DMPA	POP	CHC
ENDOCRINE CONDITIONS						
Diabetes						
a) History of gestational disease	1	1	1	1	1	1
b) Non-vascular disease						
(i) Non-insulin dependent	1	2	2	2	2	2
(ii) Insulin-dependent	1	2	2	2	2	2 **B**
c) Nephropathy/retinopathy/neuropathy	1	2	2	2	2	3 **A**
d) Other vascular disease	1	2	2	2	2	3 **A**

B Rheumatic diseases

	Cu-IUD	LNG-IUS	IMP	DMPA	POP	CHC
RHEUMATIC DISEASES						
Rheumatoid arthritis	1	2	2	2	2	2
Systemic lupus erythematosus (SLE)						
a) No antiphospholipid antibodies	1	2	2	2	2	2 **B**
b) Positive antiphospholipid antibodies	1	2	2	2	2	4 **A**
Positive antiphospholipid antibodies	1	2	2	2	2	4 **A**

Women ≥ 40 yrs: A: no
B: consultation specialist first

CHC combined hormonal contraception, *POP* progestin-only pill, *DMPA* depot medroxyprogesterone acetate, *LNG-IUS* levonorgestrel-loaded system, *Cu-IUD* copper intrauterine device
Adapted from Refs. [88, 97]

- History of venous blood clot, stroke, heart attack
- Thrombogenic conditions
- Hypertension, diabetes with vascular complications
- Positive family history for blood clot, stroke or heart attack
- Migraine with aura
- Severe liver or gallbladder disease

Obesity and smoking are essential risk factors for venous thrombo-embolic events. Basic VTE risk in non-users of CHC increases with age and BMI. In younger obese women (BMI >30.0), VTE risk is approximately three times higher than in women with normal weight (BMI 20.0–24.9). In obese women aged 40+ years, the risk increases approximately six times [24, 116–118].

In young healthy non-obese women who do not smoke, venous and arterial side effects are extremely rare.

9.5.3.1 Increased Risk for Venous Thrombo-Embolic Events (VTE)

In contrast to the progestogen-only pills, combined oral contraceptives (COCs) increase the risk of venous thrombosis. Because of the hepatic first pass, COCs influence the liver and modify its protein synthesis. The action of oestrogens on oestrogen receptors in the liver leads to regulation of gene expression, as sex hormone receptors are primarily transcription factors [112]. Current CHCs affect several metabolic factors, including haemostatic variables and oestrogen-sensitive liver proteins [113, 114]. These effects may vary depending on the types of oestrogen and progestin used in a specific combination. An oestrogen-related increase in levels of sex hormone-binding globulin (SHBG), corticosteroid-binding globulin, angiotensinogen and apolipoprotein A1, as well as changes in various coagulation and fibrinolytic factors, is observed with CHC use [113, 114]. As a consequence of the different metabolism of synthetic EE compared to natural oestrogens, a particularly powerful hepatic effect is exerted by the synthetic EE, also when EE is administered parenterally [113]. Non-oral formulations containing EE have been wrongly thought to reduce these metabolic changes, but EE retains its strong metabolic effect on the liver in its second hepatic pass [113–115].

Over 20 years ago, it has been shown that the VTE risk depends also on the progestin component of the COC taken by the patient. Among others, Lidegaard et al. [24, 116] had published data showing that newer progestins induce a slightly higher VTE risk than older. Lidegaard had stated in 2011: ‘Compared with non-users of hormonal contraception, current users of oral contraceptives with levonorgestrel had a threefold increased risk of VTE. And those using oral contraceptives with desogestrel, gestodene, drospirenone, or cyproterone a six to sevenfold increased risk’. Two meta-analysis [117, 118] and a statemen of the European Medicines Agency (EMA) [119] confirmed this trend (Fig. 9.5, Table 9.5). However, EMA declared clearly on 11 October 2013 in its report 607314/2013 through its

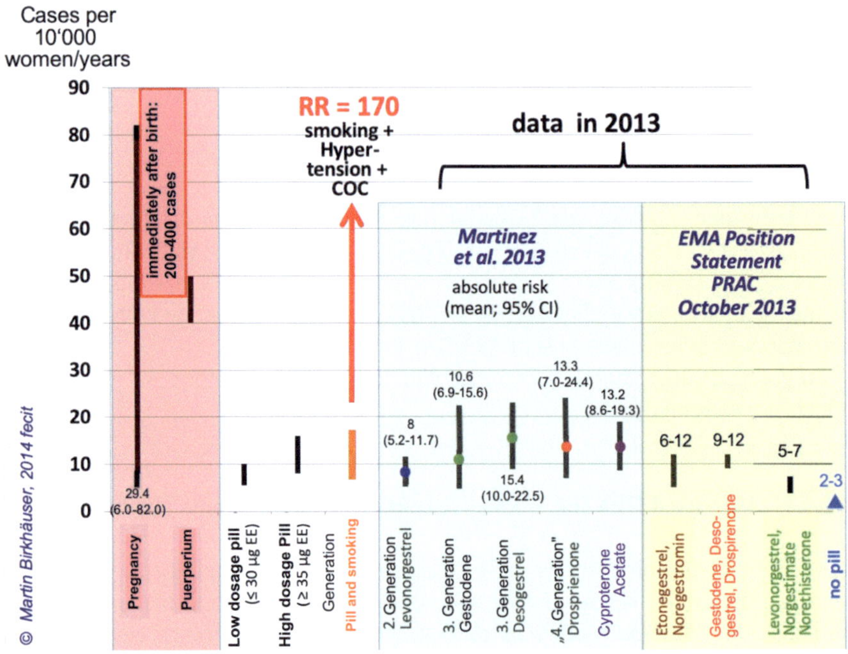

Fig. 9.5 Risk of thrombo-embolic events (VTE) in function of the progestin used in different COCs. (Adapted from Refs. [117, 119])

Table 9.5 Risk of thrombo-embolic events (VTE) in function of the progestin used in different COCs

Results of a systematic review and meta-analysis of venous thrombosis risk among users of combined oral contraception [118]	
Progestin	Risk ratio (95% CI)
Levonorgestrel	1
Cyproterone	2.04 (1.55–2.49)
Desogestrel	1.83 (1.55–2.13)
Dienogest	1.46 (0.57–5.41)
Drospirenone	1.58 (1.12–2.14)
Gestodene	1.67 (1.32–2.10)
Norgestimate	1.14 (0.94–1.32)
Pooled estimates (95% confidence intervals) of unadjusted risk ratios for venous thromboembolism among users of combined oral contraceptives by progestogen type compared with levonorgestrel in published meta-analyses.	
CI = confidence interval	

Dragoman et al. [118]

subcommittee PRAC that 'benefits of all combined hormonal contraceptives (CHCs) continue to outweigh risks'. Furthermore, PRAC stated that

- The risk is lowest with the CHCs containing the progestogens levonorgestrel, norgestimate and norethisterone: It is estimated that each year there will be between 5 and 7 cases of VTE per 10,000 women who use these medicines.
- The risk is estimated to be higher with the progestogens etonogestrel and norelgestromin, with between 6 and 12 cases yearly per 10,000 women.
- The risk is also estimated to be higher with the progestogens gestodene, desogestrel, drospirenone, with between 9 and 12 cases yearly per 10,000 women.
- For CHCs containing chlormadinone, dienogest and nomegestrol, the available data are insufficient to know how the risk compares with the other CHCs, but further studies are ongoing or planned.

For comparison, in women who are not using CHCs and who are not pregnant, there will be around 2 cases of VTE each year per 10,000 women [119]. PRAC points to the fact that, although there are small differences between the CHCs depending on the type of progestogen they contain, the risk of VTE with all CHCs remains small.

Preliminary data show that newer progestins combined with E2, E2-valerate or E4 significantly reduce the hepatic first-pass effect compared with COC containing EE [20, 120], altering less the coagulation system. Unfortunately, randomized clinical phase 3 trials are still missing for COCs using natural oestrogens combined with a newer progestin, so that prospective data describing the VTE risk are not yet available. However, in a pooled analysis of so-called real-life data including 11,616 users of a E_2V/DNG-pill and 18,681 user of an EE/LNG-pill [121], the occurrence of VTE has been investigated. In this analysis, the VTE risk is significantly lower in E_2V/DNG-users than in EE/LNG-users (propensity-score-stratified hazard ratio [HR] 0,46, 95% CI: 0.22–0.98). These data show that the VTE risk is lower in women using a COC with a natural oestrogen (E_2V/DNG) than the risk presented by a classical 'second-generation' pill with synthetic EE (EE/LNG), but the data available do not allow to concude that the increased risk is abolished.

The parenteral administration of CHC does not decrease the VTE risk in a clinically relevant way [122, 123] (see also above).

PRAC recommends that women and prescribers be better informed of the known risk of thrombo-embolism and alert for signs and symptoms [119].

In women possessing a hereditary thrombo-embolic predisposition in her personal or family history (e.g. factor V Leiden, prothrombin mutation, protein S, protein C and anti-thrombin deficiencies), there is a strict contraindication against the prescription of CHC, in adolescents included. The European Medicines Agency's guidelines for investigating haemostasis during the development of steroid contraceptives [115] state that haemostasis testing is critical to identifying risk of VTE of new molecules at an early stage of development [124–127]. The same tests can also be used to assess risk at the individual level, allowing for safer and more personalized contraceptive prescribing. However, routine screening for genetic mutations is not cost-effective [115].

9.5.3.2 Arterial Diseases in Users of CHC

Risk of Cardiovascular Diseases (CVD)

Decisive for an increased risk of arterial diseases is the genetic predisposition. A Cochrane meta-analysis done in a non-selected population (obese women and smokers have not been excluded) showed that the overall risk of arterial thrombosis was 1.6-fold increase in women using COC compared with women who did not use COC [128]. The risk of arterial thrombosis seemed to be twice as high in women taking pills with higher doses of oestrogen but not with low doses. It was highest for pills containing ≥50 μg of EE per day. It did not vary clearly according to progestagen type. When users were compared to non-users, there was no significant difference between users of second- and third-generation COC, respectively, and non-users. The pooled relative risks for second generation versus non-use and third generation versus non-use were 1.1 (95% CI 0.8–1.7) and 1.1 (95% CI 0.7–1.7), respectively. The same Cochrane meta-analysis showed no increased risk of myocardial infarction or ischemic stroke in women using newer COC preparations [128]. Therefore, regarding myocardial infarction and ischemic stroke, prescribing COCs with ≤50 microg of EE to healthy women <35 years having no risk factors for arterial disease seems safe.

In healthy non-smokers of less than 35 years of age, the risk to suffer from a myocardial infarction or a cerebrovascular accident is not increased by COC.

Because risk factors play a major role in the aetiology of cardiovascular diseases, a detailed personal and family history is therefore mandatory before COCs are prescribed.

Very rarely, blood pressure is increased by classical COC. Although the incidence of such an increase is very low, blood pressure has to be measured regularly in pill users. It has to be noted that blood pressure is decreased by the new E4/DRSP pill. In a recent study, E4/DRSP did not modify BP in normotensive women, but a clinically relevant BP decrease was observed in women with a high normal BP [44, 129]. The last UKME recommendations are shown in Table 9.6.

In spite of a current opinion, weight increase as an independent risk factor for CVD is rare in COC users [130]. It depends mainly on the individual predisposition.

It is likely that the COC pill containing levonorgestrel and 30 μg of oestrogen and, as an alternative, the oral combinations of E2 or E2-valerate with a progestin

Table 9.6 Recommendations for contraception in women with an underlying cardiovascular disease

CHC (COC, transdermal patches, vaginal rings):
Recommendations in women with cardio-vascular diseases

UKMEC	Definition of category
Category 1	A condition for which there is no restriction for the use of the method
Category 2	A condition where the advantages of using the method generally outweigh the theoretical or proven risks
Category 3	A condition where the theoretical or proven risks usually outweigh the advantages of using the method. The provision of a method requires expert clinical judgement and/or referral to a specialist contraceptive provider, since use of the method is not usually recommended unless other more appropriate methods are not available or not acceptable
Category 4	A condition which represents an unacceptable health risk if the method is used

CARDIOVASCULAR DISEASE (CVD)		
Hypertension and vascular disease		
a) Adequately controlled hypertension	3 **B**	**Clarification:** For all categories of hypertension, classifications are based on the assumption that no other risk factors for CVD exist. When multiple risk factors do exist, the risk of CVD may increase substantially. **Clarification:** Women adequately treated for hypertension are at reduced risk of acute MI and stroke compared to untreated women. Although there are no data, CHC users with adequately controlled and monitored hypertension should be at reduced risk of acute MI and stroke compared with untreated hypertensive CHC users.
b) Consistently elevated BP levels (properly taken measurements)		
(i) Systolic >140–159 mmHg or diastolic >90–99 mmHg	3 **A**	
(ii) Systolic ≥160 mmHg or diastolic ≥100 mmHg	4 (circled)	
c) Vascular disease	4 (circled)	**Clarification:** This includes coronary heart disease presenting with angina, peripheral vascular disease presenting with intermittent claudication, hypertensive retinopathy and TIA.
Current and history of ischaemic heart disease*	4 (circled)	
Stroke* (history of cerebrovascular accident, including TIA)	4 (circled)	

4 (circled) **ABSOLUTE CONTRA-INDICATION**

Women ≥ 40 years
A: chose alternative contraception, COC contra-indicated
B: chose alternative contraception, except if specialist agrees with COC

Adapted from Refs. [88, 97]

[120, 121] or of E4 and drospirenone [44] are the safest oral forms of hormonal contraception when venous and arterial vascular side effects are considered together. However, although preclinical and first clinical data are promising, solid clinical long-term proofs obtained by RCTs are still missing.

9.5.4 PCOS with and Without Metabolic Syndrome

In close relation to overweight and obesity, the PCOS with and without the metabolic syndrome is the most common reproductive endocrinopathy of women with a prevalence of 6–8% [131]. The metabolic syndrome describes a clustering of metabolic abnormalities that increase together with obesity the cardiovascular and diabetes risk. The main risk factors include glucose abnormalities, dyslipidaemia with low levels of high-density lipoprotein (HDL) cholesterol or raised triglyceride, and raised blood pressure [130]. Insulin resistance is thought to be the main factor linking these various metabolic and clinical disturbances together. The impact of obesity on drug pharmacokinetics is poorly understood. Increased storage of steroid hormones in adipose tissue may lower blood levels of steroid contraceptives reducing their ability to prevent pregnancy [130]. However, the decrease of contraceptive safety of CHC is probably minimal. Because most contraceptive efficacy studies have excluded women above 130% ideal body weight or presenting other risk factors such as diabetes, solid evidence in women suffering from PCOS with and without the metabolic syndrome is scarce.

Hormonal contraceptives, on the whole, do not appear to affect adversely body weight in women with PCOS with and without the metabolic syndrome and may provide non-contraceptive benefits including regulation of menses and a significant reduction in endometrial and ovarian cancer risk. Although studies are limited, the existing literature suggest that modern types of low-dose hormonal contraceptives are safe in this group of women [130, 132]. In patients suffering from severe acne or hirsutism, EE combined with an anti-androgenic progestin may be an efficient treatment, if specific risk factors for VTE are excluded, but it has to be considered that obese females have a baseline-increased risk of thrombosis. Metformin, GLP-1-receptor-agonists and myo-inositol are important therapeutic tools and may be combined with CHCs. Body weight control through a healthy lifestyle is essential. Women with PCOS often have metabolic abnormalities (i.e. obesity, insulin resistance, and metabolic syndrome) that should be evaluated and treated to prevent cardiometabolic consequences later in life.

The attributable risk of CHC due to the oestrogen component can be eliminated by using the progestin only preparations or a progestin-loaded IUD. However, high-dose progestogens such as depot medroxyprogesterone acetate must be avoided. Depot medroxyprogesterone acetate has a glucocorticoid partial activity increasing body weight and truncal fat deposition and may lower glucose tolerance in women with metabolic syndrome.

9.5.5 Migraine

A significant number of women with migraine has to face the choice of reliable hormonal contraception during their fertile life. Combined hormonal contraceptives (CHCs) may be used in the majority of women with headache and migraine.

However, they possess a small, but significant vascular risk translated by an increase of risk for stroke, especially in migraine with aura (MA). This increased risk may also occur in migraine without aura (MO), but with additional risk factors for stroke such as smoking, hypertension, diabetes, hyperlipidaemia and thrombophilia and an age over 35 years [133]. Therefore, migraine with aura is an absolute, migraine without aura a relative contraindication against CHC containing EE.

Guidelines recommend progestogen-only contraception or IUD as an alternative. POP and LNG-loaded IUD do not seem to be associated with an increased risk of venous thrombo-embolism (VTE) and ischemic stroke [133].

Preliminary evidence based on headache diaries in women suffering from migraine suggests that the progestin-only pill containing desogestrel 75 μg has a positive effect on the course of both migraine without and with aura in the majority of women. It reduces the number of days with migraine [133, 134] probably by the maintenance of stable oestrogen levels.

9.5.6 Breast Cancer, Ovarian Cancer and Endometrial Cancer

9.5.6.1 Breast Cancer

The relationship between oral contraceptive use and breast cancer has been the subject of a number of studies, in part contradictory. Because of the low baseline risks in the age group using hormonal contraception (premenopausal women), the risk difference between hormonal contraception users and non-users is small [135, 136]. Meta-analyses have shown a slightly increased risk, ranging from 8% to 24% [137–141]. The recently published data of the Nurses' Health Study II (NHS II) translate the breast cancer risk into absolute numbers. The NHS II, a large prospective cohort study, included 113,187 predominantly premenopausal women at baseline with up to 28 years of follow-up [142]. The study reports

- 127 cases/100,000 person-years in current COC users, compared to
- 91 cases/100,000 person-years in never COC users

This corresponds to 36 excess cases/100,000 person-years among current users. The longer lasted the current use of COC, the higher was the risk increase:

<5 years: median, 2 years; HR, 1.19 (0.95–1.49)
>5 years: median, 8 years; HR, 1.56 (1.23–1.99)

n contrast, two recent Swedish register studies did not find any increased breast cancer risk among current users of CHC [141]. In the NHS II, the risk decreased in past-users: There have been only 95 cases/100,000 person-years in past-users of COC, corresponding to 4 excess cases/100,000 person-years among past-users. In women being >5 years after cessation, no more excess risk is found. Duration of use was not associated with breast cancer risk in past COC users.

The magnitude of the risk increase observed in a recent Danish study was similar and translated into 1 additional case of invasive breast cancer for every 7690 women using hormonal contraception [137]. The risk varied with age. For women younger than 35 years, there was 1 additional case of invasive breast cancer for every 50,000 women using hormonal contraception. It was slightly higher in women approaching perimenopause. British data showed that in adolescent COC users [138], the risk for breast cancer is extremely low. It is estimated at 1:20,000 after 5 years of regular pill use, a risk that lays within the normal incidence.

The data available today do not suggest that the type of the progestin might influence breast cancer risk [143]. The same study reports that current use of progestogen-only methods is associated with a minimally increased risk of developing breast cancer.

Breast cancer remains a contraindication for the use of any form of CHC [144], independent of receptor status or histotypes.

9.5.6.2 Ovarian Cancer and Endometrial Cancer

In healthy women, the use of CHC has consistently shown a significant protective effect on the risk of ovarian cancer. After 15 years of use, the risk reduction is 50%. This reduction is valid for epithelial cancers, but also for various other histotypes. Protection is particularly marked in the perimenopause [145].

The risk of endometrial cancer is reduced by about 50% in ever users of CHCs [145].

9.5.6.3 Women with BRCA1/BRCA2 Mutations

A systematic meta-analysis published in 2023 investigated the impact of contraceptive use on breast and ovarian cancer risk among BRCA1/2-PV carriers [146]. The analysis depended on the outcome measure. Regarding breast cancer risk, the data were limited to COC.

The results were heterogenous depending on the reported outcome measures: breast cancer risk was either increased (HR: 1.55, 95% CI: 1.36–1.76) or unaffected (OR: 1.06, 95% CI: 0.90–1.25) in COC users. In analysis 1, the risk remained increased at 10 years after the last COC use; however, no clear association was identified between breast cancer risk and duration of COC use. The risks for different progestin-only formulations were inconsistent. Dose–response and duration–response relationships were not present, making it very difficult to interpret these findings.

Women with *BRCA mutations*, especially *BRCA1*, are at a very high risk for ovarian cancer. The risk is up to 30–40 times higher than that of the general population [147]. COC use reduced ovarian cancer risk in BRCA mutation carriers, with a HR of 0.62 (95% CI: 0.52–0.74) and an OR of 0.49 (95% CI: 0.38–0.63), This benefit is greater with increasing duration of use, but it seems to vanish over time following the cessation of COC use [147], suggesting a promoter effect.

Considering the importance of the protective effect of CHC on ovarian and endometrial cancer, it is advocated [142, 147] that these benefits outweigh the increasing breast cancer risk in BReast CAncer (BRCA) 1 or 2 pathogenic variant carriers [146] at high risk for both breast and ovarian cancer. CHC is therefore recommended for BRCA1/2-PV carriers without prior risk-reducing surgeries such as ovariectomy.

The genetic predisposition and the non-genetic factors (like prior risk-reducing surgeries, prior breast cancer and age) and patients' preferences should be evaluated before taking a decision about CHC use in BRCA1/2-PV carriers. Finally, patients' preferences to be respected include wish for contraception, reversibility of the treatment, ease of use, reliability and effect on menstrual cycle.

9.5.7 Other Underlying Diseases and Drug Interaction Influencing the Use of CHC

9.5.7.1 Other Underlying Diseases

There are many other underlying diseases having an impact on the use of CHC besides the few selected diseases discussed above, such as follows:

- Ischaemic heart disease, cardiomyopathy and complicated valvular heart disease
- Morbid obesity (BMI $\geq$40 kg/m^2); bariatric surgery within the past 2 years
- Rheumatoid arthritis; systemic lupus erythematosus (SLE) (Table 9.4); systemic sclerosis
- Cystic fibrosis (not a contraindication against CHC; [148])
- Epilepsy [149]
- Gestational trophoblastic neoplasia
- Malignant liver tumours (hepatocellular carcinoma); severe (decompensated) cirrhosis
- Kidney transplant; failure/transplant of other organs
- Sickle cell disease
- Tuberculosis; HIV-related diseases
- Teratogenic drugs

It has to be stressed that this list is not exhaustive and that initiation of CHCs has a different impact on underlying diseases than continuation.

Unfortunately, solid information about the effect of CHC on these underlying diseases and vice versa is scarce. The reason is that most trials of new contraceptive methods deliberately exclude women and subjects with chronic medical conditions. In consequence, there is little direct evidence in a high proportion of women suffering from an underlying disease and seeking contraceptive advice, although some medical conditions are associated with potential or theoretical increased health risks when certain contraceptive methods are used.

It is highly recommended to any GP or family planning specialist confronted to such a question to consult one of the main guidelines developed to offer well-funded recommendations:

- UKMEC has been developed for industrialized countries [97]
- WHOMEC is primarily intended for use in developing countries [98]

9.5.7.2 Drug Interaction

Drug interactions between CHC and some drugs used currently to treat an underlying disease have a practical impact on the choice of the contraceptive method. It is therefore essential that contraceptive providers take a drug history and check for drug interactions prior to provision of hormonal contraception.

The recent update of the FSRH CEU drug interactions with hormonal contraception guidance [150] gives general information about the types of drug interaction that relate to hormonal contraception. Such interactions with drugs could increase or reduce exposure to contraceptive hormones and thus affect contraceptive effectiveness and safety of hormonal contraception. On the other hand, CHC may themselves increase or reduce exposure to other drugs that an individual is taking. Therefore, CHC may affect effectiveness and safety of other drugs.

Well known are the interactions between CHC and anti-epileptics (phenytoin, barbiturates, carbamazepine, topiramate, lamotrigine or oxcarbazepine) in both directions. These anti-epileptics induce two enzymatic groups in the liver: the cytochrome p450-oxidase enzyme system and UDP-glucuronyl transferase enzyme (UGT). Serum concentrations of lamotrigine, for example, decrease by about 50% after 1 month of simultaneous intake of a COC [149]. It has to be noted that, as a general rule, the uninterrupted monophasic administration of CHCs possesses a higher contraceptive safety than the cyclic intake of a pill, when an additional long-term treatment with a drug interacting with CHC is needed (for more information, see Ref. [150]).

The antibiotic rifampicin reduces contraceptive safety by acting on the enterohepatic circulation of EE and progestins [151]. However, available scientific and pharmacokinetic data do not support the hypothesis that all antibiotics lower the contraceptive efficacy of oral contraceptives. Pharmacokinetic evidence demonstrates that plasma levels of COC are unchanged with the concomitant administration of ampicillin, ciprofloxacin, clarithromycin, doxycycline, metronidazole, ofloxacin, roxithromycin, temafloxacin and tetracycline [151]. If a specific information is needed, it is recommended to use online drug interaction checkers available today which give useful information on drug interactions. For up-to-date information on the potential drug interactions between hormonal contraception and other drugs, please refer to Stockley's Drug Interactions website [152]. Stockley's Drug Interactions website includes clinically relevant information on interactions between therapeutic drugs, proprietary medicines, herbal medicines, foodstuffs, drinks, pesticides and drugs of abuse.

For up-to-date information on the potential drug interactions between CHC and anti-retroviral (ARV) drugs, the free online HIV drugs interaction checker of the University of Liverpool may be consulted [153].

9.6 Progestin-Only Contraceptives

Progestin-only contraceptives are available as oral products (the progestin-only pill, POP), and as parenteral forms (levonogestrel IUD, implants and depot injections). Because another chapter of this volume is consecrated to the latter (Chap. 19), the following discussion is limited to the POP and the levonogestrel IUD.

9.6.1 Progestin-Only Pill (POP)

POPs have no increased VTE risk and are therefore an excellent alternative to COC for women where an increased VTE risk exists or is suspected.

9.6.1.1 'Classical' Minipill

The first POP contained levonorgestrel administered as a continuous monotherapy (30 μg per day). Depending on the observation of the very strict compliance demanded, the pearl index of the 'classical' minipill was highly variable (0.4–4.3). Contraceptive safety was not guaranteed if the intake of the pill has been delayed for more than 3 h: the 3 h rule. A strict discipline of the pill intake is mandatory [154]. Irregular bleeding is frequent, and silent menstruation may occur.

The minipill was based on two contraceptive mechanisms:

1. Endometrial changes and impermeability of the cervical mucus for sperm. This effect lasts only 3 (classical minipill) to maximum. 27 h.
2. Ovulation inhibition. However, in the minipill, only 50–60% of all cycles are anovulatory. Therefore, contraceptive safety had to rely on other remaining protective effects, such as cervical mucus thickening and endometrial progestogenic changes. It is less safe than the modern POPs.

Because of its insufficient contraceptive safety, the 'classical' minipill has been largely replaced by newer drugs. The most used newer POPs contain desogestrel [155, 156] or drospirenone [157]. Their pearl index is 0.2–1.4. Ovulation inhibition is the main mechanism of action for the contraceptive efficacy of these new progestin-only pills. Both inhibit ovulation in approximately 97%, in contrast to the classical 'minipill' (50–60%). As second mechanisms of action, both induce progestogenic endometrial changes and cervical mucus thickening.

In some countries, other progestins are approved as a contraceptive monotherapy. In Germany, Chlormadinone fem® (2 mg, Jenapharm) is available. The dosage is 1–2 mg per day. In France, Luteran® (chlormadinone, dosage 5 mg and 10 mg) and Lutenyl® (nomegestrol, dosage 3.75 mg or 5 mg) have been approved. These high-dose French preparations might have a stimulating effect on meningiomata and are therefore actually reviewed by PRAC [158]. The safety of the low-dose German preparation (chlormadinone, 1–2 mg/day) is not questioned by PRAC.

9.6.1.2 Desogestrel-Only Pill

Desogestrel-only [155, 156] is still the most widely used oestrogen-free contraceptive. Its pearl index is 0.2–1.4. depending on adherence. The original preparation is dosed at 75 µg desogestrel/day as are its numerous generics. Desogestrel-only inhibits ovulation. Its ovulation inhibition dose is 60 µg/day. Because the dose of desogestrel of 75 µg/day is only slightly above the ovulation inhibition dose, it is necessary to respect a precise regular intake to guarantee the contraceptive safety. Therefore, the window of oblivion of desogestrel-only is only 12 h. This still means a great progress compared to the 3 h of the traditional minipill. The irregular bleeding pattern is better than in the classical minipill [159], but remains a main disadvantage for many women when compared to COCs.

9.6.1.3 Drospirenone-Only Pill

Drospirenone possesses a long half-life, up to 32–36 h. The ovulation inhibition dose of drospirenone is 2 mg per day, but the new DRSP-only POP [157] contains 4 mg DRSP per tablet and day. Therefore, together with the long half-life, inhibition of ovulation is still maintained when the intake is delayed for up to 24 h. The result is a large 'window of safety'. This flexibility in administration tolerates a delayed intake for up to 4 tablets per cycle. In consequence, the DRSP-only POP has an excellent pearl index of 0.73 [157]. The high contraceptive safety does not decrease in overweight or obese women [161–163]. For the first time in the history of progestin-only-preparations, DRSP-only uses a cyclic regimen: 24 days of continuous DRSP-only administration followed by 4 hormone-free days where a withdrawal bleeding should occur. The aim is to obtain a cyclic and more regular bleeding pattern. In a randomized study, the bleeding pattern of continuous desogestrel-only and cyclic DRSP-only has been compared [159]. Because of the cyclic regimen, the number of women indicating unplanned bleedings/spotting has been significantly lower in the DRSP than in the desogestrel group, at least during the first 6 treatment cycles. Furthermore, there have been less long bleeding episodes >10 days in DRSP 4 mg (24/4) users. Women should be informed that in approximately 45% the expected menstruation will not occur ('silent menstruation').

9.6.2 Intrauterine Devices (IUDs) Releasing LNG

Hormone-free IUDs are introduced into the intrauterine cavity and have a contraceptive effect through their direct activity on the endometrium. They are not discussed in this chapter.

Mainly to obtain a better bleeding pattern and to decrease dysmenorrhoea, a levonorgestrel-releasing IUD (LNG-IUD) has been developed. The hormonal effect was primarily meant to be local. However, the original LNG-IUD (Mirena®) releases during the first year 20 µg and in the following 4 years 15 µg LNG per day [10, 164] so that LNG-IUDs have also a systemic effect corresponding to the oral administration of an equivalent dose of LNG. After the introduction of Mirena®, several other IUDs releasing LNG have been developed. All LNG-IUDs are approved for contraception. In the European Union and in the United Kingdom, Mirena® only obtained the regulatory approval in contraception for up to 8 years. In addition, only Mirena® has been approved for a duration of 5 years for endometrial protection in peri- and postmenopausal women [164].

9.6.3 Safety of POPs and LNG-Releasing IUDs

9.6.3.1 Obesity

There is no significant weight gain during the use of POPs in general. Obese women using DRSP-only POP experienced a weight loss of 0.7 kg on average [165]. In users of the DRSP-only pill, there was no difference in safety when women with a normal BMI have been compared with patients having a BMI of ≥ 30 kg/m^2 [163, 165]. But it has to be recalled that, in overweight or obese women, the basic VTE risk is up to four times higher (odds ratio overweight 2.5, 95% CI 1.7–3.7: OR obesity 3.9, 95% CI 2.2–6.9), as it is seen in normal women [165].

9.6.3.2 Vascular Diseases, Arterial Hypertension, Other Underlying Risk Factors

In CHC, the most feared serious adverse effects are VTE, acute myocardial infarction (AMI) and stroke, particularly in women at risk. In contrast to CHC, POP and LNG-releasing IUD do not seem to be associated with an increased risk of vascular diseases. Two meta-analysis from observational studies reported no increase in risk of MI [166] and of stroke [166] with progestogen-only contraceptives use. However, these results have been based on limited data. These meta-analyses have been confirmed by two newer studies, a meta-analysis [167] and a systematic review [168]. Both analyzed different progestin-only methods and concluded the following:

- There is no increased risk of VTE, AMI and stroke in a general population using POPs, progestin-only implants or LNG-IUDs [167, 168].
- There is no increased risk of VTE, AMI and stroke in women suffering from an underlying disease such as arterial hypertension, lupus erythematosus, smoking, thrombophilia or a history of VTE [167, 168]. In the meta-analysis, the pooled adjusted relative risks (RR) of venous thrombo-embolism, myocardial infarction and stroke for oral versus non-POP users were 1.06 (95% CI 0.70–1.62), 0.98 (95% CI 0.66–1.47) and 1.02 (95% CI 0.72–1.44), respectively [167].

It has to be stressed that the increased VTE risk calculated for the combined DRSP-EE pill should not be confused with the absent VTE risk of the DRSP-only pill. The progestin DRSP administered alone has no known VTE risk. In a coagulatory study, DRSP 4 mg was not associated with any meaningful changes on haemostatic parameters, indicating a lack of effect on haemostasis [169]. In the clinical development program of the DRSP-only pill (>20,000 cycles), there were no cases of VTE despite the fact that, in the American arm, 41% of women had at least one risk factor for VTE, and in European studies, up to 16% [163]. Both arms confirmed the high safety of this formulation of DRSP-only in patients with pre-existing risks. However, long-term data are still missing.

Pre-existing arterial hypertension is one of the most important arterial risk factors for cerebral vascular accidents (CVAs). As stated above, COCs are contraindicated. Exceptions may only be allowed if BP is fully controlled by an efficient anti-hypertensive treatment and if it stays within the normal range [97, 98]. Such an increase of stroke risk does not occur with low- or medium-dose progestin-only methods (POP, implant and LNG IUD) [170]. In the case of the DRSP-only pill, a decrease in systolic levels of 8 mm Hg and diastolic levels of 5 mm Hg was shown in patients with mild hypertension, probably due to the anti-mineralocorticoid properties of DRSP [171].

9.6.3.3 Other Underlying Diseases

Like all progestin-only pills, the DRSP-only pill can also be used without restriction in smokers and/or women over 35 years of age and in cases of heart disease and migraine with aura as well as in nearly all other underlying diseases. Drug interactions are rare and concern mainly antiseizure medications and antibiotics; in case of doubt, the existing international guidelines should be consulted [97, 98, 150–153, 172].

9.6.3.4 Breast Cancer

In a systematic review published in 2016 on the use of progestin and breast cancer risk [173], Samson et al. reported that five of the six studies found no association between progestin-only formulations (including norethindrone oral contraceptives, depot medroxyprogesterone acetate, injectables, levonorgestrel system users, implantable and intrauterine devices) and breast cancer risk.

However, two more recent Swedish nationwide register-based studies among Swedish women 15–34 years of age currently using progestogen-only methods report a small risk increase [141, 284]. These register studies show a slightly increased relative risk of developing breast cancer or breast cancer in situ (RR 1.32 (1.20–1.45)) [174] compared with women who have never used hormonal contraceptives. In contrast, this study could not detect any overall increased risk among current users of combined HC. There were no major differences between the different formulations, except for a slightly lower risk with the depot medroxyprogesterone acetate (DMPA) injectable, in contradiction to other studies. A Danish research letter published online in October 2024 [175] reports a slightly increased breast cancer risk in LNG-IUD users aged 15–49 years (hazard ratio overall 1.4; 95% CI 1.2–1.5) compared to non-users, corresponding to an excess risk of 14 cases per 10,000 women. The risk increased with duration of use. The test for trend was not statistically significant ($p = 0.15$). However, these data have to be confirmed.

This unexpected increased risk in progestogen-only users of POP and LNG-IUD may be explained by a selection bias due to a more liberal prescription of progestogen-only methods to women with risk factors for breast cancer such as history, smoking and obesity. The limitation of all these studies is that the impact of these well-known risk factors on the observed breast cancer risk could not be analyzed because they had not been available in the data basis accessible. Further research is needed.

9.6.4 POP Over the Counter

By the FDA, the risk of adverse events of progestin-only pills (POPs) has been considered to be so low that a POP has been made available over the counter without prescription in 2023. The choice fell on Opill®, a classic norgestrel minipill (0.075 mg norgestrel tablets) [176, 177]. Opill® needs a very strict compliance (the old 3-hour rule). Women who miss a dose by more than 3 h are recommended to use a backup birth control method (such as a condom) and should take the missed dose as soon as possible. The users are informed about common (irregular, lighter or more frequent periods) and less common side effects (nausea, vomiting, headache or fatigue). They are urged to consult their clinician if they are taking antiseizure medications, antibiotics and over-the-counter supplements before starting Opill®.

The two main disadvantages of Opill® may be the difficult 3-hour rule for intake and may include the unfavourable bleeding profiles that are not explained to the user in a professional counselling [178, 179]. Occasionally, ovarian cysts may form, but they are usually asymptomatic and disappear spontaneously. The lack of effect of oestrogen can be counterproductive for women with symptoms of androgenisation, as oestrogen-free pills do not influence SHBG production.

9.7 Ethical Aspects

The United Nations stated in 2024 that continued high fertility in some countries is still the major driver of population growth, while in other countries fertility declines to historically low levels. The reproductive behaviour of women and men is also linked to wider social and economic changes such as improvements in women's educational attainment and labour force participation. Last but not least, overpopulation has an unfavourable impact on climate changes [180, 181].

It has been demonstrated in this chapter that the contraceptive safety of CHC is very high and that in the last 65 years the risk of side effects has significantly decreased so that the benefits of all CHCs outweigh clearly the risks [119, 182]. By blocking the maturation of a fertilizable egg, CHC and modern POPs administering desogestrel or drospirenone are neither abortive nor interceptive.

In the last 60 years, the social, political and economic implications induced by CHCs and particularly by 'the pill' were profound. It was widely well received, and seen as part of the movement of women's liberation launched in the 1960s.

Therefore, the fears formulated by some religions and several social and political groups, best formulated in the 1960s by the Catholic Church [3] cannot be maintained from a medical aspect. Seen from the point of moral theology, 60 years ago, some Christian religions and churches (but not the Jewish and Islamic religions) underlined the negative aspects of the pill for the equilibrium of the traditional family and criticized that women using the pill obtained the full control on procreation. In some churches, still today the opinion prevails that it is a serious error to postulate that a whole married life of otherwise normal relations can justify sexual intercourse which is deliberately contraceptive. More than 60 after the publication of the Encyclical letter Humanae Vitae [3], in a highly different world, it is officially still not allowed to take any action which is specifically intended to prevent procreation (either before, at the moment of, or after sexual intercourse). In the same 60 years, other Christian churches have developed a new understanding of the dignity of woman and of her place in society and accepted the separation of sexual enjoyment from the function of reproduction. Would it not be time for all societies, churches and religions to think less on self-imposed interdictions and more on the much older message of the 'Song of Solomon' in the Old Testament [183]? Shoudn't it be considered that pushing to overpopulation and in certain circumstances poverty by interdicting a modern, safe and efficient hormonal contraception might be unethical, too?

9.8 Discussion

Combined hormonal contraception (CHC) goes back to 1957 [1]. The first combined oral contraceptive (COC) was launched in the United States in1960. It revolutionized family planning by giving women control over their own fertility. In

2011, 50 years later, over 100 million women worldwide used CHCs. Today, CHCs are the most used form of contraception in industrialized countries. The United Nations Population Division postulates to ensure, by 2030, universal access to sexual and reproductive healthcare services, including family planning, information and education, and the integration of reproductive health into national strategies and programmes [180, 181].

Safety of CHC, expressed by its pearl index [184] of 0.5–1.4, is high [1, 2]. A low failure rate depends on a good adherence to the method, particularly important for COC and POP users. Adherence has been facilitated by the introduction of parenteral forms of CHC. In contrast to COCs, non-oral CHCs, such as patches and vaginal rings, guarantee stable steroid blood levels and do not need a daily administration. Non-oral CHCs, particularly the contraceptive patch, are still an underestimated option in contraceptive counselling [185]. However, because of the long half-life of EE, its impact on the coagulation system is not eliminated [6, 50, 186, 187]. Therefore, contraceptive rings and patches containing EE still have an increased VTE risk, similar to the 'pill'.

65 years after the launch of the first COC, the risks of modern COCs have dramatically fallen and the contraceptive safety increased compared to the first COC [1, 180, 181]. Today, structured counselling allows to find a safe contraceptive method for nearly every couple. Non-contraceptive benefits should be respected when a pill is prescribed. These non-contraceptive benefits include a better bleeding pattern, a decrease of PMS, endometriosis, benign breast diseases and ovarian cancer, and depending on the combination chosen, an anti-androgenic activity reduces acne and excessive hair growth. These benefits have to be part of an informed choice [188].

The three main steps in the evolution of CHC to less side effects and lower risks have been the following:

- *Dose reduction of EE*

- In COCs, the classical oestrogen component, ethinyl-oestradiol (EE) has been reduced from initially 150 µg per tablet to 15–20 µg per tablet, decreasing significantly the risk of adverse events, particularly of stroke and deep venous thrombosis (DVT) [1].
- *Introduction of newer progestins with anti-androgenic and anti-mineralocorticoid partial activities*
- Important differences exist among the progestins regarding their side effects whether the associated progestin counterbalances, more or less, the estrogenic metabolic action. Newer progestins possessing favourable partial activities (mainly anti-androgenic and anti-mineralocorticoid) may reduce weight gain and acne, but they do not decrease insulin sensitivity and have no negative effects on lipids. However, these so-called 'third-generation' and 'fourth-generation' progestins induce in combination with EE greater changes of the coagulation system. These newer progestins might therefore increase, if combined with EE, slightly the risk of DVT [24]. The risk of thrombosis is highest in the first year of use, particularly during the first 3 months. The European Medicines Agency con-

firms in 2013 that the benefits of all CHCs continue to outweigh the risks [119], but recommends for pill starters without special indications low-dose COCs containing a 'second-generation' progestin (gonanes derived from testosterone such as levonorgestrel and norgestrel) as first-line preparations. However, it should be evaluated if the actual recommendation to use in starters a CHC containing EE combined with levonorgestrel as a first-line preparation can be maintained in presence of newer and probably safer COCs where EE is replaced by E2 or E4.

- Furthermore, it has to be stressed that among the side effects, not only venous thrombo-embolic events but also the sum of all other positive and negative side effects are decisive for the prescription of oral contraceptives. For example, considering their pharmacological properties, it is likely that the new progestins may have neutral effects on metabolic or vascular risks. However, this hypothesis has to be confirmed in large clinical trials.
- *Replacement of EE by natural oestradiol (E2) or oestetrol (E4)*

- The metabolically highly problematic EE is replaced by natural 17-beta-estradiol (17-beta-E2) or E2-valerate or by the foetal oestetrol (E4). All are used in combination with newer progestins [6, 10–12].

- Although for most of these new COCs, long-term clinical data are still not available, preclinical and pharmacological results suggest that modern pills containing E2 or E4 do not possess the same strong negative hepatic side effects well known for EE, even at a low-dosage. This is of particular interest for the negative action of EE on the coagulation system, responsible for one of the most feared side effects of CHC: the increased risk of VTE [32, 35, 44, 47, 48, 53, 61, 62]. However, in youg women, venous thrombo-embolisms are among the rarer side effects of hormonal contraceptives.

- COCs containing E2, E2-valerate or oestetrol are safe, reliable and demonstrate in pharmacological studies less metabolic side effects than COCs containing EE. However, if these findings can be translated into a lower incidence of venous thrombo-embolism depends on ongoing phase 4 studies trials. Therefore, all preparations with natural oestrogens approved until today keep the warning from an increased VTE risk. But it has to be noted that in a recent 'real-life' comparison, the VTE risk was significantly lower in E_2V/DNG users than in EE/LNG users (propensity-score-stratified hazard ratio [HR] 0,46, 95% CI: 0.22–0.98) [121]. It may be speculated that the VTE risk may be lower also for other COCs with a natural oestrogen than it is in classical 'second-generation' pills with synthetic EE. This leads to the question if the dogma can be maintained that the 'second-generation' pills with EE and LNG should remain the only first-line oral CHC accepted. Newer COCs containing natural oestrogens might be equal or even superior to a second-generation COC as far as the VTE risk is concerned [121].

- Because prospective randomized clinical data and direct comparisons with a 'second-generation' pill are missing, the labelling of FDA [56) as well as of EMA [189] for the contraceptive combination with E4 (contraceptive drospirenone 3 mg and oestetrol 14.2 mg tablets) still contains the warning for thromboembolic disorders and other vascular problems used for EE pills, in spite of the encouraging pre-clinical data. For E4-COCs, reliable clinical trials are still missing.

This chapter illustrates that the classification of progestins in so-called generations, a marketing instrument of the last millenary, should be replaced by the traditional but still actual classification in function of the structural and pharmacological properties of the progestin. It is further stated that the actual dosage limit of low-dose pills is still too high. It is therefore recommended that low-dose pills should be defined as COCs containing ≤35 µg EE.

One of the fundamental issues in developing new contraceptives is safety, another the potential to alter the health of the normal user and of a user who has underlying diseases. Therefore, it has to be kept in mind that most trials of contraceptive methods deliberately exclude women and subjects with chronic medical conditions so that there is little direct evidence for women with an underlying disease. In such women, low-dose COCs (15–35 µg EE, or pills using natural E2, E2-valerate or E4) may only be initiated if the responsible GP or specialist agrees. In women at risk, alternatives to COC, such as POPs or progestin-loaded IUDs, might be preferred. Long-acting hormonal contraceptive methods, such as progestin-only implants or injections or non-hormonal Cu-IUD, are particularly suited for women where the necessary compliance needed for classical CHCs cannot be fulfilled (see Chap. 19). Today, POPs are considered to be so safe by the FDA that the first POP has been approved in the United States for selling over-the-counter without prescription.

It has to be reminded that the observance of an old clinical rule could reduce significantly serious side effects if it would be systematically applied: before prescribing for the first time a CHC, blood pressure, weight, smoking habits and serum cholesterol have to be checked, and re-checked each time that a new episode of CHC use is started.

Finally, ethical considerations should not be neglected in contraceptive counselling. The majority of mankind considers an unlimited growth of the global population to be unethical because it leads to lack of education, impoverishment and to man-made climate changes. Therefore, conservative political groups and religions still promoting marital chastity or unreliable contraceptive methods and not permitting safe CHC to their own members, and worse to the whole society they are living in, are invited to rethink their positions, going in part back to very old dogmata where completely different conditions prevailed.

Declarations

Competing Interests The author(s) has no competing interests to declare that are relevant to the content of this manuscript.

Ethics Approval The author(s) declares that this manuscript does not include primary research with human participants.

The author(s) declares that this manuscript does not include primary studies involving animals.

Literature

1. Szarewski A, Mansour D, Shulman LP. 50 years of "The Pill": celebrating a golden anniversary. J Fam Plann Reprod Health Care. 2010;36(4):231–8.
2. Chadwick KD, Burkman RT, Tornesi BN, Brinda MB. Fifty years of "the pill": risk reduction and discovery of benefits beyond contraception, reflections, and forecast. Toxicol Sci. 2012;125(1):2–9.
3. Encyclical letter Humanae Vitae of the supreme Pontiff Paul VI to his venerable brothers the patriarchs, archbishops, bishops and other local ordinaries in peace and communion with the apostolic see, to the clergy and faithful of the whole catholic world, and to all men of Good will, on the regulation of birth, July 25, 1968. https://www.vatican.va/content/paul-vi/en/encyclicals/documents/hf_p-vi_enc_25071968_humanae-vitae.html. Accessed 15 Jan 2024.
4. Schindler AE, Campagnoli A, Druckmann R, Huber J, Pasqualini JR, Schweppe KW, Thijssen JHH. Classification and pharmacology of progestins. Maturitas. 2003;46(Suppl. 1):S7–S16.
5. Kennedy WJ, 1882, cited in "She said she was in the family way". Pregnancy and infancy in modern Ireland, In: Farrell E, editor. Institute of Historical Research, Univ. of London, School of Advanced Study, 2012. ISBN 978 1 909646 47 6 (PDF edition). Available to download free at http://www.humanities-digital-library.org.
6. Goldzieher JW, Brody SA. Pharmacokinetics of ethinyl estradiol and mestranol. Am J Obstet Gynecol. 1990;163(6Pt 2):2114–9.
7. Kuohung W, Borgatta L, Stubblefield P. Low-dose oral contraceptives and bone mineral density: an evidence-based analysis. Contraception. 2000;61:77–82.
8. Endrikat J, Mih E, Düsterberg B, et al. A 3-year double-blind, randomized, controlled study on the influence of two oral contraceptives containing either 20 μg or 30 μg ethinylestradiol in combination with levonorgestrel on bone mineral density. Contraception. 2004;69:179–87.
9. Nappi C, Di Spiezio SA, Acunzo G, et al. Effects of a low-dose an ultra-low-dose combined oral contraceptive use on bone turnover and bone mineral density in young fertile women: a prospective controlled randomized study. Contraception. 2003;67:355–9.
10. Kuhl. Comparative pharmacology of newer progestagens. Drugs. 1996;51:188–215.
11. Sitruk-Ware R, Nath A. Characteristics and metabolic effects of estrogen and progestins contained in oral contraceptive pills. Best Pract Res Clin Endocrinol Metab. 2013;27(1):13–24. https://doi.org/10.1016/j.beem.2012.09.004.
12. Sitruk-Ware R. Progestogens in hormonal replacement therapy: new molecules, risks, and benefits. Menopause. 2002;9:6–15.
13. Kuhl H. Pharmacology of progestogens. Basic aspects – progesterone derivatives. Menopause Rev. 2001;6:9–1619.
14. Colton FB. Steroids and 'the pill': early steroid research at Searle. Steroids. 1992;57:624–30.
15. Gompel A, Plu-Bureau G. Progesterone and synthetic progestin controversies. AMA Oncol. 2015;1(7):987. https://doi.org/10.1001/jamaoncol.2015.2283.
16. Sitruk-Ware R. Pharmacological profile of progestins. Maturitas. 2008;61:151–7.
17. Öttel M, Holz C. Hybrid progestins: the example of dienogest. In: Sitruk-Ware R, Mishell Jr DR, editors. Progestins and anti-progestins in clinical practice. New York: Marcel Dekker; 2000. p. 163–78.
18. Pollow K, Jucham N, Elger W, Jacobi N, Hoffman G, Mobus V. Dihydrospirorenone (ZK30595), a new progestogen with anti-mineralocorticoid activity: effects on ovulation, electrolyte excretion, and therennin-aldosterone system in normal women. J Clin Endocrinol Metab. 1991;73:873–42.
19. Kuhnz W, Heuner A, Hümpel M, et al. In vivo conversion of norethisterone and norethisterone acetate to ethinyl estradiol in postmenopausal women. Contraception. 1997;56:379–85.
20. Sitruk-Ware R. New progestagens for contraceptive use. Hum Reprod Update. 2006;12(2):169–78. https://doi.org/10.1093/humupd/dmi046. Advance Access publication 16 Nov 2005.

21. Fotherby K. Bioavailability of orally administered sex steroids used in oral contraception and hormone replacement therapy. Contraception. 1996;54(2):59–69.
22. Runnebaum BC, Rabe T, Kiesel L. Female contraception: update and trends. Springer Science & Business Media; 2012. p. 156–63. ISBN 978-3-642-73790-9.
23. Archer DF. Clinical and metabolic features of desogestrel: a new oral contraceptive preparation. Am J Obstet Gynecol. 1994;170(5 part 2):1550–5.
24. Lidegaard Ø, Nielsen LH, Skovlund CW, Skjeldestad FE, Løkkegaard E. Risk of venous thromboembolism from use of oral contraceptives containing different progestogens and oestrogen doses: Danish cohort study, 2001–9. BMJ. 2011;343:d6423. https://doi.org/10.1136/bmj.d6423. PMC 3202015. PMID 22027398.
25. Spona J, Huber J. Pharmacological and endocrine profiles of gestodene. Int J Fertil. 1987;32(Suppl):6–14. PMID 2906347.
26. Kuhl H, Jung-Hoffmann C, Wiegratz I. Gestodene-containing contraceptives. Clin Obstet Gynecol. 1995;38(4):829–40. PMID, 8616979. https://doi.org/10.1097/00003081-199538040-00018. Stanzcyk FZ, Hapgood JP, Winer S, Mishell DR Jr. Progestogens used in postmenopausal hormone therapy: differences in their pharmacological properties, intracellular actions, and clinical effects. Endocr Rev. 2013;34(2):171–208. https://doi.org/10.1210/er.2012-1008:10.1210/er.2012-1008.
27. Dusterberg B, Humpel M, Speck U. Terminal half-lives in plasma and bioavailability of norethisterone, levonorgestrel, cyproterone acetate and gestodene in rats, beagles and rhesus monkeys. Contraception. 1981;24:673–51.
28. Kuhl H. Published online: 14 Mar 2013 https://doi.org/10.1024/0040-5930.58.9.527.
29. Stanczyk FZ. Pharmacokinetics and potency of progestins used for hormone replacement therapy and contraception. Rev Endocr Metab Disord. 2002;3:3211–24.
30. Kuhl H. Effects of progestogens on haemostasis. Maturitas. 1996;24(1–2):1–19. https://doi.org/10.1016/0378-5122(96)00994-2.
31. Archer DF. Clinical and metabolic features of desogestrel: a new oral contraceptive preparation. Am J Obstet Gynecol. 1997;170(5 Pt 2):1550–5.
32. Borgelt LM, Martell CW. Estradiol valerate/dienogest: a novel combined oral contraceptive. Clin Ther. 2012;34(1):37–55. https://doi.org/10.1016/j.clinthera.2011.11.006.
33. Oelkers W. Drospirenone–a new progestogen with antimineralocorticoid activity, resembling natural progesterone. Eur J Contracept Reprod Health Care. 2000;5(Suppl 3):17–24.
34. Oelkers W. Antimineralocorticoid activity of a novel oral contraceptive containing drospirenone, a unique progestogen resembling natural progesterone. Eur J Contracept Reprod Health Care. 2002;7(Suppl 3):19–26. discussion 42–43.
35. Junge W, Mellinger U, Parke S, et al. Metabolic and haemostatic effects of estradiol valerate/dienogest, a novel oral contraceptive. Clin Drug Investig. 2011;31(8):573–84.
36. Rübig A. Drospirenon: a new cardiovascular- active progestin with antialdosterone and antiandrogenic properties. Climacteric. 2003;6(Suppl. 3):49–54.
37. Fuhmann U, Krattenmacher R, Slater EP, Fritzemeier KH. The novel progestin drospirenone and its natural counterpart progesterone: biochemical profile and anti-androgenic potential. Contraception. 1996;54:243–51.
38. Archer DF. Drospirenone and estradiol: a new option for the postmenopausal woman. Climacteric. 2007;10(Suppl 1):3–10.
39. Foidart JM, Faustmann T. Advances in hormone replacement therapy: weight benefits of drospirenone, a 17alpha-spirolactone-derived progestogen. Gynecol Endocrinol. 2007;23(12):692–9.
40. Whitehead M. Hormone replacement therapy with estradiol and drospirenone: an overview of the clinical data. J Br Menopause Soc. 2006;12(Suppl 1):4–7.
41. Ma S, Song SJ. Oral contraceptives containing drospirenone for premenstrual syndrome (Review). Cochrane Database Syst Rev. 2023;6:CD006586. https://doi.org/10.1002/14651858.CD006586.pub5.

42. Harper JC. Use of oral contraceptives for management of acne vulgaris. In: Del Rosso JQ, Touro DO, Henderson NV, Joshua A, Zeichner MD, editors. Dermatologic clinics. New York: Icahn, School of Medicine at Mount Sinai; 2016. Advances in acne management. An issue of dermatologic clinics. E-Book, University Nevada. Elsevier Health Sciences 2016;34(2):129–234. ISBN 978-0-323-41753-2.
43. Davis AR, Westhoff C, O'Connell K, Gallagher N. Oral contraceptives for dysmenorrhea in adolescent girls. A randomized trial. Obstet Gynecol. 2005;106:97–104.
44. Foidart JM, Gemzell-Danielsson K, Kubba A, et al. The benefits of estetrol addition to drospirenone for contraception. AJOG Glob Rep. 2023;3(4):100266. https://doi.org/10.1016/j.xagr.2023.100266. eCollection 2023 Nov.
45. Farris M, Bastianelli C, Rosato E, Brosens I, Benagiano G. Pharmacodynamics of combined estrogen-progestin oral contraceptives: 2. effects on hemostasis. Expert Rev Clin Pharmacol. 2017;10(10):1129–44.
46. FDA drug safety communication: updated information about the risk of blood clots in women taking birth control pills containing drospirenone. Food and Drug Administration. 2019. Archived from the original on 27 April 2019.
47. Gemzell-Danielsson K, Apter D, Zatik J, et al. Estetrol-Drospirenone combination oral contraceptive: a clinical study of contraceptive efficacy, bleeding pattern and safety in Europe and Russia. BJOG. 2022;129(1):63–71.
48. Creinin MD, WesthoW CL, Bouchard C, et al. Estetrol-drospirenone combination oral contraceptive: North American phase 3 efficacy and safety results. Contraception. 2021;104(3):222–8. https://doi.org/10.1016/j.contraception.2021.05.002.
49. Simoncini T, Genazzani AR. A review of the cardiovascular and breast actions of drospirenone in preclinical studies. Climacteric. 2010;13(1):22–33. https://doi.org/10.3109/13697130903437375.
50. Kuhl H. Pharmacology of estrogens and progestogens: influence of different routes of administration. Climacteric. 2005;8(Suppl 1):3–63.
51. Torgerson DJ, Bell-Syer SE. Hormone replacement therapy and prevention of nonvertebral fractures: a meta-analysis of randomized trials. JAMA. 2001;285(22):2891–7.
52. Gaspard U, Endrikat J, Desager JP, et al. A randomized study on the influence of oral contraceptives containing ethinylestradiol combined with drospirenone or desogestrel on lipid and lipoprotein metabolism over a period of 13 cycles. Contraception. 2004;69(4):271–8.
53. Douxfils J, Klipping C, Duijkers I, et al. Evaluation of the effect of a new oral contraceptive containing estetrol and drospirenone on hemostasis parameters. Contraception. 2020;102(6):396–402.
54. FDA instructions for use nextstellis (drospirenone and estetrol tablets) for oral use. Reference ID: 4779634. https://www.accessdata.fda.gov/drugsatfda_docs/label/2021/214154s000lbl.pdf.
55. Paris J, Thevenot R, Bonnet P, Granero M. The pharmacological profile of TX 066 (17 alpha-acetoxy-6-methyl-19-nor-4,6-pregnadiene-3,20-dione) a new oral progestative. Arzneimittelforschung. 1983;33:710–5.
56. Winneker RC, Bitran D, Zhang Z. The preclinical biology of a new potent and selective progestin: trimegestone. Steroids. 2003;68:915–20.
57. Kumar N, Koide SS, Tsong YY, Sundaram K. Nestorone®: a progestin with a unique pharmacological profile. Steroids. 2000;65:629–36.
58. Mueck AO, Sitruk-Ware R. Nomegestrol acetate, a novel progestogen for oral contraception. Steroids. 2011;76(6):531–9.
59. Duc I, Botella J, Bonnet P, Fraboul F, Delansorne R, Paris J. Antiandrogenic properties of nomegestrol acetate. Arzneimittelforschung/Drug Res. 1995;45(1):70–4.
60. Burke A. Nomegestrol acetate-17b-estradiol for oral contraception. Patient Prefer Adherence. 2013;7:607–19.

61. Gaussem P, Alhenc-Gelas M, Thomas J-L, et al. Haemostatic effects of a new combined oral contraceptive, nomegestrol acetate/17β-estradiol, compared with those of levonorgestrel/ethinyl estradiol. Thromb Haemost. 2011;105(3):560–7.
62. Mansour D, Verhoeven C, Sommer W, et al. Efficacy and tolerability of a monophasic combined oral contraceptive containing nomegestrol acetate and 17beta-oestradiol in a 24/4 regimen, in comparison to an oral contraceptive containing ethinylestradiol and drospirenone in a 21/7 regimen. Eur J Contracept Reprod Health. 2011;16(6):430–43.
63. Ruan X, Schneck H, Schultz S, Fehm T, Cahill MA, Seeger H, et al. Nomegestrol acetate sequentially or continuously combined to estradiol did not negatively affect membrane-receptor associated progestogenic effects in human breast cancer cells. Gynecol Endocrinol. 2012;28(11):863–6.
64. Fruzzetti F, Bonassi Machado R, Lete I, et al. A review of the pharmacology, clinical outcomes, and real-world, effectiveness, safety, and non-contraceptive effects of NOMAC/E2. Eur J Obstet Gynecol Reprod Biol. 2022;21:100283.
65. Philibert D, Bouchoux F, Degryse M, Lecaque D, Petit F, Gaillard M. The pharmacological profile of a novel norpregnane progestin (trimegestone). Gynecol Endocrinol. 1999;13:316–26.
66. Zhang Z, Lundeen SG, Zhu Y, Carver JM, Winneker RC. In vitro characterization of trimegestone: a new potent and selective progestin. Steroids. 2000;65:637–43.
67. Grubb G, Spielmann D, Pickar J, Constantine G. Clinical experience with trimegestone as a new progestin in HRT. Steroids. 2003;68:921–6.
68. Fotherby K. Potency and pharmacokinetics of gestagens. Contraception. 1990;41:533–50.
69. Massai MR, Diaz S, Quinteros E, Reyes MV, Herreros C, Zepeda A, Croxatto HB, Moo-Young AJ. Contraceptive efficacy and clinical performance of Nestorone implants in postpartum women. Contraception. 2001;64:369–76.
70. Bitzer J. Familienplanung. In: Riecher-Rössler A, Bitzer J, editors. Frauengesundheit. Elsevier; 2003.
71. Frost JJ, Singh S, Finer LB. Factors associated with contraceptive use and nonuse, United States, 2004. Perspect Sex Reprod Health. 2007;39:48–55.
72. Halpern V, Grimes DA, Lopez L, Gallo MF. Strategies to improve adherence and acceptability of hormonal methods for contraception. Cochrane Database Syst Rev. 2006;1:CD004317.
73. Harper, et al. Adolescent clinic visits for contraception: support from mothers, male partners and friends. Perspect Sex Reprod Health. 2004;36:20–6.
74. Westhoff CL, Heartwell S, Edwards S, et al. Oral contraceptive discontinuation: do side effects matter? Am J Obstet Gynecol. 2007;196:412–8.
75. Rosenberg MJ, Waugh MS. Oral contraceptive discontinuation: a prospective evaluation of frequency and reasons. Am J Obstet Gynecol. 1998;179:577–82.
76. Moreau C, Cleland K, Trussell J. Contraceptive discontinuation attributed to method dissatisfaction in the United States. Contraception. 2007;76(4):267–72.
77. Spona J, Elstein M, Feichtinger W, et al. Shorter pill-free interval in combined oral contraceptives decreases follicular development. Contraception. 1996;54:71–7.
78. Sullivan H, Furniss H, Spona J, Elstein M. Effect of 21-day and 24-day oral contraceptive regimens containing gestodene (60 μg) and ethinyl estradiol (15 μg) on ovarianactivity. Fertil Steril. 1999;72:115–20.
79. Van Vliet HAAM, Grimes DA, Helmerhorst FM, Schulz KF, Lopez LM. Biphasic versus monophasic oral contraceptives for contraception. Cochrane Database Syst Rev. 2006;3:CD002032. https://doi.org/10.1002/14651858.CD002032.pub2.
80. Van Vliet HAAM, Grimes DA, Lopez LM, Schulz KF, Helmerhorst FM. Triphasic versus monophasic oral contraceptives for contraception. Cochrane Database Syst Rev. 2011;11:CD003553. https://doi.org/10.1002/14651858.CD003553.pub3.
81. Black, et al. Clinical risk factors for venous thromboembolus in users of combined oral contraceptive pill. Br J Clin Pharmacol. 2002;53:637–40.

82. Jick SS, Kaye JA, Russmann S, Jick H. Risk of nonfatal venous thromboembolism in women using a contraceptive transdermal patch and oral contraceptives containing norgestimate and 35 microg of ethinyl estradiol. Contraception. 2006;73:223–8.
83. Henshaw SK. Unintended pregnancy in the United States. Fam Plann Perspect. 1998;30:24–9.
84. Piccinino LJ, Mosher WD. Trends in contraceptive use in the United States: 1982–1995. Fam Plann Perspect. 1998;30:4–10.
85. Casper RF, Dodin S, Reid RL, Study Investigators. The effect of 20 μg ethinyl estradiol/l mg norethindrone acetate (Minnestrin TM), a low-dose oral contraceptive, on vaginal bleeding patterns, hot flashes, and quality of life in symptomatic perimenopausal women. Menopause. 1997;4:139–47.
86. FSRH guideline contraception for women aged over 40 years. August 2017 (Amended September 2019) | FSRH. https://fsrh.org/Public/Documents/fsrh-guidance-contraception-for-women-aged-over-40-years-2017.aspx. Accessed 4 May 2024.
87. Cochrane RA, Gebbie AE, Loudon JC. Contraception in obese older women. Maturitas. 2012;71:240–7.
88. FSRH. Guideline contraception for women aged over 40 years. August 2017 (Amended July 2023). https://www.fsrh.org/standards-andguidance/documents/fsrh-guidance-contraception-for-women-aged-over-40-years-2017/. Accessed 4 May 2024.
89. Castracane VD, Gimpel T, Goldzieher JW. When is it safe to switch from oral contraceptives to hormonal replacement therapy? Contraception. 1995;52:371–6.
90. Creinin MD. Laboratory criteria for menopause in women using oral contraceptives. Feritil Steril. 1996;66:101–4.
91. Gebbie AE, Glasier A, Sweeting V. Incidence of ovulation in perimenopausal women before and during hormone replacement therapy. Contraception. 1995;52:221–2.
92. Bitzer J. Oral contraceptives in adolescent women. Best Pract Res Clin Endocrinol Metab. 2013;27(1):77–89.
93. Birkhaeuser M. In: Meriggiola MC, Gemzell-Danielsson K, editors. Hormonal contraception and bone, in female and male contraception. © Springer Nature Switzerland AG; 2021. ISBN 978-3-030-70931-0. p. 361–297. https://doi.org/10.1007/978-3-030-70932-7.
94. Hartard, et al. Age at first oral contraceptive use as a major determinant of vertebral bone mass in female endurance athletes. Bone. 2004;35:836–41.
95. de Villiers. Relationship between steroid hormone contraceptives and HPV, cervical intraepithelial neoplasia and cervical carcinoma. Int J Cancer. 2003;103:705–8.
96. Gaudet LM, Kives S, Hahn PM, Reid RL. What women believe about oral contraceptives and the effect of counseling. Contraception. 2004;69:31–6.
97. FSHR. UK Medical Eligibility Criteria for Contraceptive use (UKMEC). 2016 (amended September 2019). https://www.fsrh.org/documents/ukmec-2016/ Copyright ©Faculty of Sexual and Reproductive Healthcare 2006 to 2019.
98. WHO. Medical Eligibility Criteria for Contraceptive Use, 5th edition 2015 (WHOMEC). https://www.who.int/reproductivehealth/publications/family_planning/MEC-5/© World Health Organization 2015 ISBN 978 92 4 154915 8.
99. Gallo M, Lopez L, Grimes DA, Schulz KF, Helmerhorst FM, Gallo MF, et al. Combination contraceptives: effects on weight. Cochrane Syst Rev. 2014;29:CD003987.
100. Piccoli A, Crosignani P, Nappi C, Ronsini S, Bruni V, Marelli S. Effect of the ethinylestradiol/norelgestromin contraceptive patch on body composition. Results of bioelectrical impedance analysis in a population of Italian women. Nutr J. 2008;7:1–9.
101. Burkman RT. The transdermal contraceptive patch: a new approach to hormonal contraception. Int J Fertil Womens Med. 2002;47(2):69–76.
102. Burkman RT. Transdermal hormonal contraception: benefits and risks. Am J Obstet Gynecol. 2007;197(134):e1–6.
103. Burkman RT, Fisher AC, LaGuardia KT. Effects of low-dose oral contraceptives on body weight: results of a randomized study of up to 13 cycles of use. J Reprod Med. 2007;52:1030–4.

104. Oelkers WK. Effects of estrogens and progestogens on the renin-aldosterone system and blood pressure. Steroids. 1996;61:166–71.
105. Derkx FHM, Stuenkel C, Schalekamp MPA, et al. Immunoreactive renin, prorenin, and enzymatically active renin in plasma during pregnancy and in women taking oral contraceptives. J Clin Endocrinol Metab. 1986;63:1008–15.
106. Paoletti AM, Lello S, Di Carlo C, Orrù M, Malune ME, Neri M, et al. Effect of Estradiol valerate plus dienogest on body composition of healthy women in the menopausal transition: a prospective one-year evaluation. Gynecol Endocrinol. 2016;32:61–4.
107. Dal'Ava N, Bahamondes L, Bahamondes MV, de Oliveira Santos A, Monteiro I. Body weight and composition in users of Levonorgestrel-releasing intrauterine system. Contraception. 2012;86:350–3.
108. Heinemann LAJ, Lewis MA, Spitzer WO, et al. Thromboembolic stroke in young women. A European casecontrol study on oral contraceptives. Contraception. 1998;57:29–37.
109. Neri M, Malune ME, Corda V, Piras B, Zedda P, Pilloni M, et al. Body composition and psychological improvement in healthy premenopausal women assuming the oral contraceptive containing micronized estradiol (E2) and nomegestrol acetate (NOMAC). Gynecol Endocrinol. 2017;33:958–62.
110. Visser J, Van Oel C, Van Vliet H, Radder J. Hormonal versus non-hormonal contraceptives in women with diabetes mellitus Type 1 and 2. Cochrane Database Syst Rev. 2006;18:CD003990.
111. Gourdy P. Diabetes and oral contraception. Best Pract Res Clin Endocrinol Metab. 2013;27:67–76.
112. Eyster KM. The estrogen receptors: an overview from different perspectives. Methods Mol Biol. 2016;1366:1–10.
113. Sitruk-Ware R. Hormonal contraception and thrombosis. Fertil Steril. 2016;106:1289–94.
114. Sitruk-Ware R, Nath A. Metabolic effects of contraceptive steroids. Rev Endocr Metab Disord. 2011;12:63–75.
115. European Medicines Agency. Guideline on clinical investigation of steroid contraceptives in women. 2004; EMEA/CPMP/EWP/519/98 Rev 1. https://www.tga.gov.au/sites/default/files/2024-06/guideline-clinical-investigation-steroid-contraceptives-women-ema.pdf.
116. Lidegaard O, Lokkegaard E, Svendsen AL, et al. Hormonal contraception and risk of venous thromboembolism: national follow-up study. BMJ. 2009;339:b2890–7.
117. Martinez F, Isabel Ramirez I, Ezequiel P-CE. Venous and pulmonarythromboembolism and combined hormonal contraceptives. Systematic review and meta-analysis. Eur J Contracept Reprod Health Care. 2012;17:7–29.
118. Dragoman MV, Tepper NK, Fu R, Curtis KM, Chou R, Gaffield ME. A systematic review and meta-analysis of venous thrombosis risk among users of combined oral contraception. Int J Gynecol Obstet. 2018;141:287–94.
119. European Medicines Agency. Pharmacovigilance risk assessment committee (PRAC) October 2013, Tech Rep. EMA/607314/2013, EMA, released on 11 Oct 2013.
120. Junge W, Mellinger U, Parke S, Serrani M. Metabolic and haemostatic effects of estradiol valerate/dienogest, a novel oral contraceptive. a randomized, open-label, single-centre study. Clin Drug Investig. 2011;31:573–84.
121. Bauerfeind A, et al. Venous thromboembolic risk of estradiol valerate-dienogest compared with ethinyl estradiol-levonorgestrel combined oral contraceptives. Obstet Gynecol. 2024;143(3):431–4.
122. Elliott TC, Montoya CC. How does VTE risk for the patch and vaginal ring compare with oral contraceptives? J Fam Pract. 2008;57:680–5.
123. Lidegaard Ø, Nielsen LH, Skovlund CW, Lokkegaard E. Venous thrombosis in users of non-oral hormonal contraception: follow-up study, Denmark 2001–10. BMJ. 2012;344:e2990.
124. Morimont L, Haguet H, Dogné J-M, Gaspard U, Douxfils J. Combined oral contraceptives and venous thromboembolism: review and perspective to mitigate the risk. Front Endocrinol (Lausanne). 2021;12:769187. https://doi.org/10.3389/fendo.2021.769187.

125. Douxfils J, Morimont L, Delvigne AS, et al. Validation and standardization of the ETP-based activated protein C resistance test for the clinical investigation of steroid contraceptives in women: an unmet clinical and regulatory need. Clin Chem Lab Med. 2020;58:294–305.
126. Douxfils J, Bouvy C, Morimont L. Evaluation of activated protein C resistance using thrombin generation test. Methods Mol Biol. 2023;2663:211–24.
127. Morimont L, Creinin MD, Gaspard U, Foidart JM, Douxfils J. Hormonal therapies and venous thrombosis: estrogen matters! Res Pract Thromb Haemost. 2023;7:100021. https://doi.org/10.1016/j.rpth.2022.100021. eCollection 2023 Jan.
128. Roach RE, Helmerhorst FM, Lijfering WM, Stijnen T, Algra A, Dekkers OM. Combined oral contraceptives: the risk of myocardial infarction and ischemic stroke. Cochrane Database Syst Rev. 2015;8:CD011054. https://doi.org/10.1002/14651858.CD011054.pub2.
129. Costescu D, Creinin MD, Douxfils J et al. The impact of the combined oral contraceptive Estetrol 15 mg/Drospirenone 3 mg (E4/DRSP) on blood pressure: pooled aa from two phase III clinical trials. Abstract Volume 80th Annual Clinical and Scientific Conference, JOGC MAI 2024, p. 4.
130. Skouby SO. Hormonal contraception in obesity, the metabolic syndrome, and diabetes. Ann NY Acad Sci. 2010;1205:240–4.
131. The Rotterdam ESHRA/ASRM-Sponsered PCOS Consensus Workshop Group. Revised 2003 Consensus on diagnostic criteria and long-termhealth risk related to polycystic ovary syndrome. Fertil Steril. 2004;81:19–25.
132. Verhaeghe J. Hormonal contraception in women with the metabolic syndrome: a narrative review. Eur J Contracept Reprod Health Care. 2010;15:305–13.
133. Nappi RE, Merki-Feld GS, Terreno E, et al. Hormonal contraception in women with migraine: is progestogen-only contraception a better choice? J Headache Pain. 2013;14:66–71.
134. Merki GS. Kontrazeption bei Frauen mit Migräne. Schweizerische Ärztezeitung / Bulletin des médecins suisses / Bollettino dei medici svizzeri. 2000;81:1182–4.
135. Cancer Research UK. Does the contraceptive pill increase risk of cancer? https://www.cancerresearchuk.org/about-cancer/causes-of-cancer/hormones-and-cancer/does-the-contraceptive-pill-increase-cancer-risk.
136. ACOG. Hormonal contraception and risk of breast cancer. Practice Advisory, January 2018, Reaffirmed Oct 2023. https://www.acog.org/clinical/clinical-guidance/practice-advisory/articles/2018/01/hormonal-contraception-and-risk-of-breast-cancer.
137. Mørch LS, Skovlund CW, Hannaford PC, Iversen L, Fielding S, Lidegaard Ø. Contemporary hormonal contraception and the risk of breast cancer. N Engl J Med. 2017;377(23):2228–39.
138. Kubba. Breast cancer and the pill. J R Soc Med. 2003;96:280–3.
139. Zhu H, Lei X, Feng J, Wang Y. Oral contraceptive use and risk of breast cancer: a meta-analysis of prospective cohort studies. Eur J Contracept Reprod Health Care. 2012;17:402–14.
140. Kahlenborn C, Modugno F, Potter DM, Severs WB. Oral contraceptive use as a risk factor for premenopausal breast cancer: a meta-analysis. Mayo Clin Proc. 2006;81:1290–302.
141. Gisch JM, Coeytaux RR, Urrutia RP, Havrilesky LJ, Moorman PG, Lowery WJ, et al. Oierral contraceptive use and risk of breast, cervical, colorectal, and endometrial cancers: a systematic review. Cancer Epidemiol Biomarkers Prev. 2013;22:1931–43.
142. Burchardt NA, Eliassen AH, Shafrir AL, et al. Oral contraceptive use by formulation and breast cancer risk by subtype in the Nurses' Health Study II: a prospective cohort study. Am J Obstet Gynecol. 2022;226(821):E1–821.
143. Hultstrand JN, Gemzell-Danielsson K, Kopp Kallner H, et al. Hormonal contraception and risk of breast cancer and breast cancer in situ among Swedish women 15–34 years of age: a nationwide register-based study. Lancet Reg Health Eur. 2022;21:100470. Published online 29 July 2022. https://doi.org/10.1016/j.lanepe.2022.100470.
144. Gompel A, Ramirez I, Bitzer J, European Society of Contraception Expert Group on Hormonal Contraception. Contraception in cancer survivors – an expert review Part I. Breast and gynaecological cancers. Eur J Contracept Reprod Health Care. 2019;24(3):167–74.

145. Beral V, Doll R, Hermon C, et al. Ovarian cancer and oral contraceptives: collaborative reanalysis of data from 45 epidemiological studies including 23,257 women with ovarian cancer and 87,303 controls. Lancet. 2008;371:303–14.
146. van Bommel MHD, IntHout J, Veldmate G, et al. Contraceptives and cancer risks in *BRCA1/2* pathogenic variant carriers: a systematic review and meta-analysis. Hum Reprod Update. 2023;29:197–217.
147. Grandi G, Sammarini M, Chiara Del Savio M, Toss A, Facchinetti F. Combined hormonal contraceptives in BRCA gene mutation carriers: why not? Eur J Contracept Reprod Health Care. 2019;24:417–9.
148. Fitzpatrick, et al. Use of oral contraceptives in women with cystic fibrosis. Chest. 1984;86:863–7.
149. Crawford P. Best practice guidelines for the management of women with epilepsy. Epilepsia. 2005;46(Suppl.9):117–24.
150. Faculty of Sexual & Reproductive Healthcare. Clinical guidance: drug interactions with hormonal contraception. May 2022. https://www.fsrh.org/Common/Uploaded%20files/documents/drug-interactions-with-hormonal-contraception-5may2022.pdf. Accessed 4 May 2024)
151. Archer JSM, Archer DF. Oral contraceptive efficacy and antibiotic interaction: a myth debunked. J Am Acad Dermatol. 2002;46:917–23.
152. Stockley's drug interactions. https://gvhealth.libguides.com/c.php?g=923171&p=6663846.
153. HIV drug interactions. https://www.hiv-druginteractions.org/.
154. Fachinformation Jenapharm 28 mini® 30 Mikrogramm coated tablets. Released January 2021. https://www.fachinfo.de/fi/pdf/014460/28-mini-0-030-mg-ueberzogene-tabletten. Downloaded 24 Jan 2024.
155. Cerazette® Summary of product characteristics 2020. May 2020. Accessed 31 March 2024 at: https://www.medicines.org.uk/emc/product/1698/smpc#gref.
156. Cerazette Organon Fachinformation. https://www.organon.com/germany/wp-content/uploads/sites/38/2021/10/Cerazette.pdf. Accessed 31 Mar 2024.
157. Fachinformation Slinda (Drospirenon). https://compendium.ch/product/1485130-slinda-filmtabl-4-mg/mpro. Accessed 31 Mar 2024.
158. Birkhaeuser M, Boettcher BA, Germeyer A, Neulen J, et al. Progestins and Meningeomata – is there a relation? [Gibt es einen Zusammenhang?]. Frauenarzt. 2022;2:105–7.
159. Palacios S, Colli E, Regidor P-A. Bleeding profile of women using a drospirenone-only pill 4 mg over nine cycles in comparison with desogestrel 0.075 mg. PloS One. 2020;15(6):e0231856.
160. Römer T, Bitzer J, Christian Egarter C, et al. Oral progestins in hormonal contraception: importance and future perspectives of a new progestin only-pill containing 4 mg Drospirenone. Geburtsh Frauenheilk. 2021;81(9):1021–30.
161. Regidor P-A, Colli E. Drospirenone 4 mg in a 24/4 regimen maintains inhibition of ovulation even after a 24-h delay pill intake - pharmacological aspects and comparison to other progestin-only pills. Eur Rev Med Pharmacol Sci. 2022;26:1994–9.
162. Palacios S, Colli E, Regidor P-A. Multicenter, phase III trials on the contraceptive efficacy, tolerability and safety of a new drospirenoneonly pill. Acta Obstet Gynecol Scand. 2019;98:1549–57.
163. Kimble T, Burke AE, Barnhart KT, Archer DF, Colli E, Westhoff CL. A 1-year prospective, open-label, single-arm, multicenter, phase 3 trial of the contraceptive efficacy and safety of the oral progestin-only pill drospirenone 4 mg using a 24/4-day regimen. Contraception X. 2020;2:100020.
164. Swissmedic. Mirena®. information leaflet. https://www.swissmedicinfo.ch/ShowText.aspx?textType=FI&lang=DE&authNr=52996. Downloaded 15 Mar 2024.
165. Creinin MD, Angulo A, Colli E, Archer DF. The efficacy, safety, and tolerability of an estrogen-free oral contraceptive drospirenone 4 mg (24/4-day regimen) in obese users. Contraception. 2023; https://doi.org/10.1016/j.contraception.2023.110136. Epub 2023 Aug 5.

166. Chakhtoura Z, Canonico M, Gompel A, et al. Progestogen-only contraceptives and the risk of acute myocardial infarction: a meta-analysis. J Clin Endocrin Metab. First published ahead of print February 2, 2011. https://doi.org/10.1210/jc.2010-2065.
167. Glisic M, Shahzad S, Tsoli S, Chadni M, Asllanaj E, Rojas LZ, Brown E, Chowdhury R, Muka T, Franco OH. Association between progestin-only contraceptive use and cardiometabolic outcomes: a systematic review and meta-analysis. Eur J Prev Cardiol. 2018;25(10):1042–52. https://doi.org/10.1177/2047487318774847. Epub 2018 May 10. PMID: 29745237; PMCID: PMC6039863.
168. Tepper NK, Whiteman MK, Marchbanks PA, James AH, Curtis KM. Progestin-only contraception and thromboembolism: a systematic review. Contraception. 2016;94(6):678–700. https://doi.org/10.1016/j.contraception.2016.04.014. Epub 2016 May 3.
169. Regidor PA, Coli E, Schindler AE. Drospirenone as estrogen-free pill and hemostasis: coagulatory study results comparing a novel 4 mg formulation in a 24–4 cycle with desogestrel 75 µg per day. Gynecol Endocrinol. 2016;32:749–51.
170. Bushnell C, McCullough L. Stroke prevention in women: synopsis of the 2014 American Heart Association/American Stroke Association guideline. Ann Intern Med. 2014;160(12):853–7. https://doi.org/10.7326/M14-0762. PMID: 24935489; PMCID: PMC4255708.
171. Palacios S, Colli E, Regidor PA. Efficacy and cardiovascular safety of the new estrogen-free contraceptive pill containing 4 mg drospirenone alone in a 24/4 regime. BMC Women's Health. 2020;20:218. https://doi.org/10.1186/s12905-020-01080-9.
172. FSRH Guideline (August 2022) Progestogen-only pills. BMJ Sex Reprod Health. 2022;48(Suppl 1). https://doi.org/10.1136/bmjsrh-2022-PoP.
173. Samson M, Porter N, Orekoya O, et al. Progestin and breast cancer risk: a systematic review. Breast Cancer Res Treat. 2016;155(1):3–12. https://doi.org/10.1007/s10549-015-3663-1.
174. Hultstrand NJ, Kristina Gemzell-Danielsson K, Helena Kopp Kallner H, et al. Hormonal contraception and risk of breast cancer and breast cancer in situ among Swedish women 15–34 years of age: a nationwide register-based study. Lancet Reg Health Eur. 2022;21:100470. https://doi.org/10.1016/j.lanepe.2022.100470. eCollection 2022 Oct.
175. Steinrud Mørch L, Meaidi A, Corn G, et al. Research letter. Breast cancer in users of levonorgestrel-releasing intrauterine system. JAMA. 2024;332(18):1578–80. https://doi.org/10.1001/jama.2024.18575.
176. Erin F, Mugdha M, Simon MA. Over-the-counter oral contraceptives are birth control pills hat can be obtained without a prescription. JAMA. Patient page over-the-counter progestin-only oral contraceptives. Published Online: 15 Sept 2023. https://doi.org/10.1001/jama.2023.17781.
177. HRA Pharma. Opill (norgestrel 0.075 mg tablets) for Rx-to-OTC switch. https://www.fda.gov/media/167893/download.
178. AWMF. AWMF guideline hormonal contraception 2020. Accessed 6 July 2020 at: https://www.awmf.org/leitlinien/detail/II/015-015.html.
179. Shoupe D. The progestin revolution: progestins are arising as the dominant players in the tight interlink between contraceptives and bleeding control. Contraception and Reprod Med. 2021;6:3–11.
180. United Nations Population Division. World contraceptive use. 2017. http://www.un.org/esa/population/publications/contraceptive2009/contraceptive2022.htm. Accessed 17 Mar 2024.
181. The United Nations Population Division, SDG Indicator 3.7.1 on contraceptive use. https://www.un.org/development/desa/pd/data/sdg-indicator-371-contraceptive-use. Accessed 17 Mar 2024.
182. Lello S, Cavani A. Ethynilestradiol 20 mcg plus Levonorgestrel 100 mcg: clinical pharmacology. Int J Endocrinol. 2014;102184 https://doi.org/10.1155/2014/102184. Epub 2014 Nov 16.
183. The Bible, King James Version, Book 22, Song of Solomon, Chap. 1–8.
184. Pearl-Index. https://www.profamilia.de/themen/verhuetung/pearl-index/. pro familia, Downloaded 28 July 2024.

185. Gemzell-Danielsson K, Farris M, Kopp-Kallner H, et al. Statement on transdermal contraception as an underused option for unmet needs in contraception: the importance of structured counselling. Gynecol Reprod Endocrinol Metab. 2023;4(2–3):48–54.
186. Wiegratz I, Kuhl H. High estrogenic impact on the liver by transdermal contraceptive patch. Expert Rev Obstet Gynecol. 2007;2:15–8.
187. Magnusdottir SD, Bjarnadottir RI, Sigurdardottir K, Önundarson PT, Dieben TOM. The contraceptive vaginal ring (NuvaRing) and hemostasis: a comparative study. Contraception. 2004;69:461–7.
188. Genazzani AR, Fidecicchi T, Domenico Arduini D, et al. Hormonal and natural contraceptives: a review on efficacy and risks of different methods for an informed choice. Gynecol Endocrinol. 2023;39(1):2247093. https://doi.org/10.1080/09513590.2023.2247093.
189. ema.europa.eu. Drovelis: EPAR - product information summary of product characteristics annex I https://www.ema.europa.eu/en/documents/product-information/drovelis-epar-product-information_en.pdf.
190. Raith-Paula E, Frank-Herrmann P, Freundl G, Strowitzki T. Natürliche Familienplanung heute. Modernes Zykluswissen für Beratung und Anwendung. Berlin, Heidelberg: Springer; 2013. ISBN 978-3-642-29783-0, S. 164–165.
191. Trussel J. Contraceptive efficacy Glob. libr. womens med; 2014; ISSN: 1756-2228. https://doi.org/10.3843/GLOWM.10375. Last updated: February 2014.

Chapter 10
Impacts of Hormonal Contraception on Liver

Coralie Fontaine, Anna Gosset, Marine Adlanmerini, Françoise Lenfant, and Jean-Francois Arnal

10.1 Introduction

Hormonal contraception is extensively used worldwide, primarily as combined oral contraceptives (COCs) that combine an estrogen and a progestin. The liver, as a central organ in hormone metabolism and detoxification, is notably impacted by these compounds due to its role in processing and metabolizing estrogens and progestins. Estrogens, especially the synthetic ethinyl estradiol (EE) used in most COCs, can significantly alter hepatic functions, leading to various effects that may have clinical consequences. These effects include changes in liver enzyme activity, lipid metabolism, coagulation profiles, and immune modulation, each carrying potential risks for liver health, especially with long-term use [11]. Newer contraceptives using estetrol (E4), a natural estrogen produced in the fetal liver, have less impact on liver functions than classical estrogens-based COCs (EE, estradiol (E2), etc.) [5, 8]. As a result, E4-based contraceptives may offer effective contraception with reduced risks of subsequent hepatic complications, particularly advantageous for women with venous thromboembolism risk.

C. Fontaine · A. Gosset · M. Adlanmerini · F. Lenfant · J.-F. Arnal (✉)
Université. de Toulouse III/Faculté de Santé – Médecine/INSERM U1297 – I2MC – équipe 4/CHU de Toulouse, Toulouse, France
e-mail: coralie.fontaine@inserm.fr; anna.gosset@inserm.fr; marine.adlanmerini@inserm.fr; francoise.lenfant@inserm.fr; jean-francois.Arnal@univ-tlse3.fr

A. R. Genazzani et al. (eds.), *Ethical, Efficacy and Safety Issues in Contraception*, Reproductive Medicine for Clinicians 4,
https://doi.org/10.1007/978-3-032-07322-8_10

10.2 Pharmacokinetics and Metabolism of Estrogens in the Liver

The liver plays a central role in estrogen metabolism and excretion, managing both endogenous and exogenous estrogens. Following hepatic conjugation, estrogens are excreted through urine and bile, the two primary routes of steroid elimination. Biliary excretion of estrogens can involve their temporary storage in the gallbladder, followed by passage into the intestines, where they may undergo deconjugation and reabsorption. This process, known as enterohepatic circulation, allows estrogens to re-enter the bloodstream, extending their biological activity. This cycle also highlights a unique hepatic function that prolongs estrogen exposure and potentially increases the risk of liver stress or damage when synthetic estrogens are used long term.

In nonpregnant women, the primary active estrogens are estradiol (E2) and estrone (E1), with E2 displaying significantly higher estrogenic activity. More than 95% of circulating E2 is directly secreted by the ovaries, while the remaining portion is produced by peripheral tissues [16]. During pregnancy, estrogen metabolism shifts markedly to accommodate increased production primarily by the fetoplacental unit. This unit produces significant amounts of E1, E2, and estriol (E3), with a smaller amount of estetrol (E4), a unique estrogen primarily synthesized by the fetal liver [17]. While the metabolic pathways remain similar, the volume of estrogens produced is substantially higher to meet pregnancy's requirements. This hormonal surge underscores the liver's adaptive capacity during pregnancy to cope with the heightened metabolic load on hepatic pathways.

The liver metabolizes estrogens extensively through the cytochrome P450 (CYP) enzyme system, particularly CYP3A4, CYP1A2, and CYP2C9. CYP3A4 is notably responsible for the hydroxylation of both endogenous and exogenous estrogens [16]. In particular, CYP3A4 catalyzes the 2-hydroxylation of estrone and estradiol, a critical pathway for estrogen metabolism. This process converts estrogens into catechol estrogens, which are subsequently inactivated or conjugated for excretion. Additionally, CYP1A2 and CYP2C9 play roles in estrogen hydroxylation, contributing to the liver's ability to regulate estrogenic activity and maintain hormonal balance. The metabolism of synthetic estrogens, such as EE, also largely involves the liver's cytochrome P450 enzymes, particularly CYP3A4, which catalyzes hydroxylation reactions. Additionally, EE undergoes conjugation with sulfotransferase (SULT1E1) and UDP-glucuronosyltransferase (UGT1A1) enzymes. These pathways contribute to EE's enterohepatic circulation, by which it re-enters the bloodstream after initial liver processing, extending its bioavailability and exposure in the body [14, 21]. In comparison, natural E2 is more rapidly metabolized and cleared from the liver. The structural difference, primarily the ethinyl group in EE, inhibits rapid degradation, allowing for prolonged activity but also elevating the risk of hepatotoxicity. This prolonged hepatic exposure intensifies EE's interaction with hepatic enzymes, not only affecting drug clearance but also potentially interacting with other drugs metabolized by the liver [14]. Furthermore, hormonal contraception can interact with other medications that act on CYP3A4, either as inducers or inhibitors. CYP3A4 inducers like rifampin and carbamazepine can accelerate EE metabolism, reducing its contraceptive efficacy and increasing breakthrough bleeding [14]. Conversely, CYP3A4 inhibitors like itraconazole increase EE plasma levels, heightening the risk of adverse events, including liver and vascular complications. Such interactions underscore the need for caution and thorough monitoring when COCs are prescribed alongside other medications metabolized through similar pathways [14].

After CYP-mediated hydroxylation, estrogens undergo further conjugation in the liver, where they are converted into glucuronide and sulfate forms. These conjugated estrogens are then excreted either into the bile or urine. Biliary excretion facilitates the cycling of estrogens through enterohepatic circulation, where conjugated estrogens are temporarily stored in the gallbladder, passed into the intestine, and potentially deconjugated by intestinal flora. This process allows estrogens to be reabsorbed, thus maintaining their systemic levels for longer periods, a cycle that particularly prolongs the activity of synthetic EE. Once estrogens are conjugated, their excretion and distribution rely on transport proteins. Sex hormone–binding globulin (SHBG) is a glycoprotein primarily synthesized in the liver, and it plays a central role in regulating the bioavailability of sex hormones [2, 13]. SHBG binds these hormones in the bloodstream, reducing their free and biologically active forms. When SHBG levels are high, a greater proportion of estrogens are bound and thus inactive, while lower SHBG levels allow more free estrogen to interact with target tissues. In premenopausal blood, approximately 38% of E2 is bound with high affinity to SHBG and 62% is loosely bound to albumin and about 2% of E2 is in a free form [20]. Estrogens themselves have a stimulatory effect on SHBG synthesis in the liver, whereas androgens tend to reduce SHBG production. This balance between SHBG levels and hormone activity is crucial for maintaining hormonal homeostasis, particularly in women using hormonal contraception. Importantly, increased SHBG levels have been associated with a higher incidence of venous thromboembolism events (VTE) in COC users [12, 19]. Synthetic estrogens such as EE are known to elevate SHBG levels more significantly than natural E2, while E4 has a minimal effect on SHBG levels. In addition, SHBG does not change E4 plasma distribution and its availability to target tissues [7, 8]. Considering the impact of SHBG levels on the incidence of VTE in COC users [12, 19], this differential effect of E4 on SHBG levels could be an important benefit in at-risk populations.

10.3 Coagulation Effects and Thromboembolic Risk

Liver function is closely linked to the hemostatic system as hepatocytes produce the majority of factors involved in the clotting and fibrinolytic systems. Accordingly, one of the most significant hepatic impacts of combined oral contraceptives (COCs), especially those containing EE, is their effect on coagulation factors, which increases the risk of venous thromboembolism (VTE). Deep vein thrombosis is characterized by blood clot formation in the veins and can lead to serious and potentially fatal conditions, the first of which is pulmonary embolism (PE). Among women, both the dose of EE and the type of progestogen used in COCs are key determinants of this increased VTE risk. For women of reproductive age who do not use COCs, the incidence of VTE is estimated at around 2 per 10,000 woman-years. However, women using COCs containing EE experience a 3- to 6-fold increase in VTE risk, translating to an incidence rate of approximately 5–12 per 10,000 woman-years, depending on the type of progestogen and estrogen dose used. These findings have been consistent across various studies, including those conducted by regulatory agencies like the U.S. Food and Drug Administration (FDA) and the European Medicines Agency (EMA), both of which have issued warnings and guidelines regarding the risks of VTE associated with COC use [11].

The mechanism of thrombosis is complex and involves multiple alterations across the hemostatic system. Classical estrogens, including CEE, EE, E2, are known to increase the hepatic synthesis of several coagulation factors, particularly Factors II, VII, IX, and X. This increase in clotting factors is considered as one of the main contributors to the heightened risk of VTE associated with COCs. These coagulation factors play essential roles in the blood clotting cascade, and their increased synthesis shifts the hemostatic balance toward a pro-thrombotic state, thus raising the likelihood of clot formation in veins. This pro-thrombotic shift is further influenced by the dose of estrogen in COCs, with higher doses of EE or other classical estrogens directly correlating with an increased risk of VTE. When estrogen levels are elevated, hepatic protein synthesis is stimulated, leading to higher plasma levels of pro-coagulant factors as well as reductions in natural anticoagulants like protein S and antithrombin. This dual effect enhances the body's clotting potential, making thrombus formation more likely, especially in women with other risk factors such as obesity, smoking, or a genetic predisposition to clotting disorders. Interestingly, E4 displays a specific transcriptional program in the liver, which differs from those induced by E2 [3]. This underlines the fact that each estrogen ligand induces a highly specific profile of gene regulation in the liver, consistent with the differential action of E4, E2, and EE on hepatic coagulation factors in humans (Fig. 10.1). Indeed, unlike classical estrogens such as E2 and EE, E4 does not induce the synthesis of hepatic coagulation factors in humans, as the changes in hemostasis markers were significantly lower in the E4 15 mg/drospirenone (DRSP) 3 mg group compared to the ethinyl estradiol (EE)/DRSP group and were consistently equivalent to or lower than those observed in the EE/levonorgestrel (LNG) group [6]. Additionally, in postmenopausal women treated with E4 alone once daily over 12 weeks, its impact on hemostasis markers was minimal and similar to placebo [6]. Parameters such as fibrinogen, prothrombin, prothrombin fragment 1 + 2, D-dimer, factor VIII activity, protein C, protein S, antithrombin, and tissue factor pathway inhibitor showed no significant deviations from baseline compared to placebo. Furthermore, E4 demonstrated a limited effect on the normalized activated protein C sensitivity ratio (nAPCsr), a key parameter associated with thrombotic risk [6]. Compared to contraceptive combinations containing EE, including the EE/LNG combination recognized by the EMA as the safest option, E4 exhibited a lower

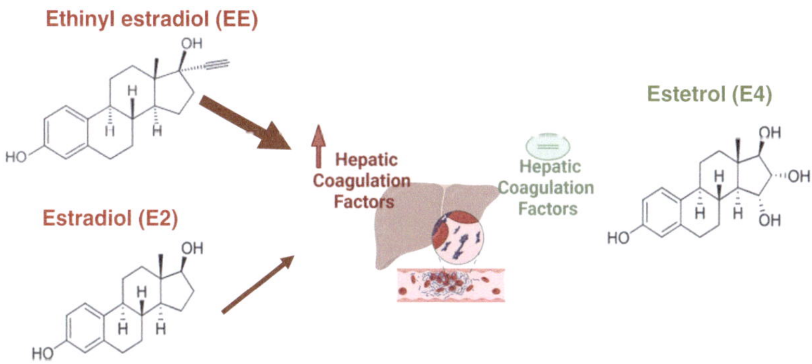

Fig. 10.1 Differential action of ethinyl-estradiol (EE), estradiol (E2), and estetrol (E4) on hepatic coagulation factors in humans. Combined oral contraceptives (COCs), particularly those containing EE, increase the hepatic synthesis of coagulation factors, promoting a pro-thrombotic state and raising the risk of venous thromboembolism (VTE). In contrast, E4 does not induce the synthesis of these hepatic coagulation factors, unlike classical estrogens such as E2 and EE, highlighting its distinct safety profile regarding VTE risk

impact on nAPCsr and other critical hemostatic markers [4, 9, 10]. Altogether, E4 appears to a distinct safety profile regarding VTE risk, compared to EE and E2.

Despite the literature looking at the effect of estrogens on coagulation activity, the full biological impact of COCs on the hemostatic system remains incompletely understood. There is effectively still a lot to learn about how various progestogens combined with estrogens in COCs might modulate these effects, as progestogens can either amplify or counteract estrogen's pro-thrombotic actions depending on their specific properties. Progestins have variable effects on clotting factors and, in addition, these effects likely vary with progestin type, potency, dose, and route of administration [18]. For instance, third- and fourth-generation COCs that contain progestins such as desogestrel or DRSP, when combined with EE, further amplify this risk by altering clotting profiles more profoundly than earlier COCs containing levonorgestrel [18]. The risk of VTE with COCs use is further influenced by several factors, including individual risk factors such as age, smoking, obesity, and a personal or family history of VTE. While some of these individual risk factors are difficult to mitigate, the prescription of safer COC has emerged as the preferred option among clinical practice [11].

10.4 Immunomodulatory Effects and Hepatic Inflammation

The liver plays a central role in immunological homeostasis but COCs, through their immunomodulatory effects, can disrupt this balance, particularly through the pro-inflammatory actions of EE. This immune modulation is evidenced by altered cytokine profiles, including increased pro-inflammatory cytokines such as interleukin-6 (IL-6) and tumor necrosis factor-alpha (TNF-α), which contribute to hepatic inflammation [15]. Estrogen-induced cholestasis (EIC) is one notable hepatic complication, where estrogen affects bile acid transport, leading to toxic bile acid accumulation and subsequent inflammation in the liver. The pathogenesis of EIC in COC users involves estrogen's suppression of bile acid transport proteins such as the bile salt export pump (BSEP) and multidrug resistance protein 3 (MDR3) [22]. By impairing these transporters, estrogens promote bile acid retention in hepatocytes, which can lead to cholestatic symptoms and potential liver injury due to the accumulation of toxic bile acids [22]. These pathological changes are accompanied by inflammatory responses that exacerbate liver injury. Additionally, elevated levels of alkaline phosphatase (ALP), alanine aminotransferase (ALT), and aspartate aminotransferase (AST) are common biochemical markers observed in patients with EIC [22]. In COC users, EIC can thus manifest as decreased bile flow and impaired hepatobiliary transport, resulting in jaundice, pruritus, and in severe cases, hepatic injury. This effect is more pronounced in women predisposed to bile acid metabolism disorders and underscores the need for caution when prescribing COCs to those with a history of cholestatic liver disease.

10.5 Newer Estrogens and Safer Contraceptive Options

In recent years, E4 has emerged as a promising estrogen for COC with a more favorable safety profile. Clinical studies have demonstrated that E4-containing contraceptives have less effect on liver, suggesting a reduced risk of cholestasis, thrombosis, and inflammation compared to EE-based contraceptives [6]. While classical estrogens (such as E2) exert their actions via both activation of nuclear and membrane (ERα), E4 presents a specific profile of ERα activation: E4 binds and activates nuclear ERα but does not induce the activation of membrane ERα signaling pathways [1] (Fig. 10.2). This distinct profile of ERα activation, uncoupling nuclear and membrane activation, is unique. Although additional molecular studies are requested to further delineate the complex interactions between the extranuclear/membrane ERα and nuclear ERα, it is likely that the absence of ERα MISS activity contributes, at least in part, to the limited impact of E4 on the liver that has been observed in several studies and which is very different from others estrogens in both mouse [3] and human [6]. Indeed, unlike classical estrogens such as E2 and EE, E4 does not induce the synthesis of hepatic coagulation factors in humans and thus E4 presents a safer profile regarding VTE risk. This selective receptor activity of E4 could be particularly beneficial for women at higher risk of liver disease or metabolic conditions, as it allows effective contraception without the extensive hepatic side effects commonly associated with EE. As research continues, E4 may serve as a model for developing future contraceptives that balance efficacy with minimized systemic impact, thereby expanding safe contraceptive options.

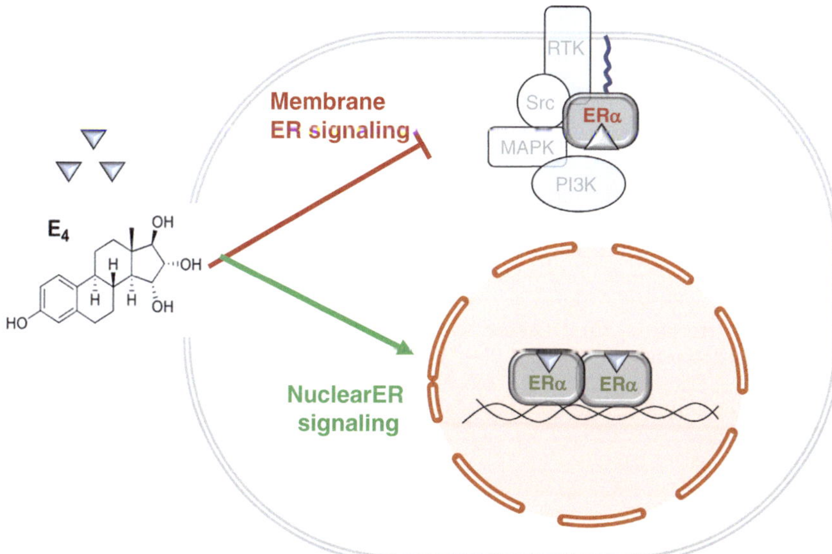

Fig. 10.2 The specific pharmacological profile of estetrol (E4). Estetrol (E4) is an estrogen that activates the nuclear estrogen receptor (ER) α signaling pathway but does not activate membrane ERα signaling pathway in specific tissues. This unique molecular mode of action of E4 is distinct from estradiol (E2). (With permissions from Arnal J.F. et al. Physiol Rev, 2017; 97(3):1045–87. doi:10.1152/physrev.00024.2016)

10.6 Conclusion

In conclusion, while COCs remain a popular and effective contraceptive method, their impact on liver function, particularly through the actions of EE, presents notable health risks. These risks include increased VTE and cholestasis which are particularly significant for long-term users or those with pre-existing hepatic conditions. Newer estrogens, like E4, appear to offer an effective contraception with fewer hepatic side effects, representing a potential paradigm shift in HC safety. Continued research into these alternatives is essential to enhance contraceptive safety and provide personalized options that better accommodate individual health profiles. In addition, while COCs are generally administered orally, alternative delivery methods, including vaginal and transdermal routes, are also used to potentially minimize hepatic first-pass effects and reduce associated risks.

Declarations

Competing Interests The author(s) has no competing interests to declare that are relevant to the content of this manuscript.

Ethics Approval The author(s) declares that this manuscript does not include primary research with human participants.

The author(s) declares that this manuscript does not include primary studies involving animals.

References

1. Abot A, Fontaine C, Buscato M, Solinhac R, Flouriot G, Fabre A, Drougard A, et al. The uterine and vascular actions of estetrol delineate a distinctive profile of estrogen receptor α modulation, uncoupling nuclear and membrane activation. EMBO Mol Med. 2014;6(10):1328–46. https://doi.org/10.15252/emmm.201404112.
2. Bourebaba N, Ngo TH, Śmieszek A, Bourebaba L, Marycz K. Sex hormone binding globulin as a potential drug candidate for liver-related metabolic disorders treatment. Biomed Pharmacother. 2022;153(septembre):113261. https://doi.org/10.1016/j.biopha.2022.113261.
3. Buscato M, Davezac M, Zahreddine R, Adlanmerini M, Métivier R, Fillet M, Cobraiville G, et al. Estetrol prevents western diet-induced obesity and atheroma independently of hepatic estrogen receptor α. Am J Physiol Endocrinol Metab. 2021;320(1):E19–190. https://doi.org/10.1152/ajpendo.00211.2020.
4. Douxfils J, Klipping C, Duijkers I, Kinet V, Mawet M, Maillard C, Jost M, Rosing J, Foidart J-M. Evaluation of the effect of a new oral contraceptive containing estetrol and drospirenone on hemostasis parameters. Contraception. 2020;102(6):396–402. https://doi.org/10.1016/j.contraception.2020.08.015.
5. Gemzell-Danielsson K, Cagnacci A, Chabbert-Buffet N, Douxfils J, Foidart J-M, Kubba A, Lasa LIL, et al. A novel estetrol-containing combined oral contraceptive: European expert panel review. Eur J Contracept Reprod Health Care. 2022;27(5):373–83. https://doi.org/10.1080/13625187.2022.2093850.
6. Gérard C, Arnal J-F, Jost M, Douxfils J, Lenfant F, Fontaine C, Houtman R, et al. Profile of estetrol, a promising native estrogen for oral contraception and the relief of climacteric symptoms of menopause. Expert Rev Clin Pharmacol. 2022;15(2):121–37. https://doi.org/10.1080/17512433.2022.2054413.
7. Hammond GL, Hogeveen KN, Visser M, Coelingh Bennink HJT. Estetrol does not bind sex hormone binding globulin or increase its production by human HepG2 cells. Climacteric. 2008;11(Suppl 1):41–6. https://doi.org/10.1080/13697130701851814.
8. Klipping C, Duijkers I, Mawet M, Maillard C, Bastidas A, Jost M, Foidart J-M. Endocrine and metabolic effects of an oral contraceptive containing estetrol and drospirenone. Contraception. 2021;103(4):213–21. https://doi.org/10.1016/j.contraception.2021.01.001.
9. Kluft C, Zimmerman Y, Mawet M, Klipping C, Duijkers IJM, Neuteboom J, Foidart J-M, Bennink HC. Reduced hemostatic effects with drospirenone-based oral contraceptives containing estetrol vs. ethinyl estradiol. Contraception. 2017;95(2):140–7. https://doi.org/10.1016/j.contraception.2016.08.018.
10. Mawet M, Maillard C, Klipping C, Zimmerman Y, Foidart J-M, Coelingh Bennink HJT. Unique effects on hepatic function, lipid metabolism, bone and growth endocrine parameters of estetrol in combined oral contraceptives. Eur J Contracept Reprod Health Care. 2015;20(6):463–75. https://doi.org/10.3109/13625187.2015.1068934.
11. Nguyen AT, Curtis KM, Tepper NK, Kortsmit K, Brittain AW, Snyder EM, Cohen MA, Zapata LB, Whiteman MK, Contributors. U.S. Medical Eligibility Criteria for Contraceptive Use, 2024. MMWR. Recommendations and reports: morbidity and mortality weekly report. Recommendat Rep. 2024;73(4):1–126. https://doi.org/10.15585/mmwr.rr7304a1.
12. Odlind V, Milsom I, Persson I, Victor A. Can changes in sex hormone binding globulin predict the risk of venous thromboembolism with combined oral contraceptive pills? Acta Obstetricia Et Gynecologica Scandinavica. 2002;81(6):482–90.
13. Pugeat M, Nader N, Hogeveen K, Raverot G, Déchaud H, Grenot C. Sex hormone-binding globulin gene expression in the liver: drugs and the metabolic syndrome. Mol Cell Endocrinol. 2010;316(1):53–9. https://doi.org/10.1016/j.mce.2009.09.020.
14. Rodrigues AD. Drug interactions involving 17α-ethinylestradiol: considerations beyond cytochrome P450 3A induction and inhibition. Clin Pharmacol Ther. 2022;111(6):1212–21. https://doi.org/10.1002/cpt.2383.

15. Soria-Jasso LE, Cariño-Cortés R, Muñoz-Pérez VM, Pérez-Hernández E, Pérez-Hernández N, Fernández-Martínez E. Beneficial and deleterious effects of female sex hormones, oral contraceptives, and phytoestrogens by immunomodulation on the liver. Int J Mol Sci. 2019;20(19):4694. https://doi.org/10.3390/ijms20194694.
16. Stanczyk FZ. Metabolism of endogenous and exogenous estrogens in women. J Steroid Biochem Mol Biol. 2024;242(septembre):106539. https://doi.org/10.1016/j.jsbmb.2024.106539.
17. Stanczyk FZ, Archer DF. Biosynthesis of estetrol in human pregnancy: potential pathways. J Steroid Biochem Mol Biol. 2023;232(septembre):106359. https://doi.org/10.1016/j.jsbmb.2023.106359.
18. Trenor CC, Chung RJ, Michelson AD, Neufeld EJ, Gordon CM, Laufer MR, Jean Emans S. Hormonal contraception and thrombotic risk: a multidisciplinary approach. Pediatrics. 2011;127(2):347–57. https://doi.org/10.1542/peds.2010-2221.
19. Wang S, Wang Y, Ming Bai Y, Peng DZ, Lei P, Zhou B, Zhang P, Zhang Z. Causal inference of sex hormone-binding globulin on venous thromboembolism: evidence from Mendelian randomisation. Thromb J. 2023;21(1):109. https://doi.org/10.1186/s12959-023-00553-9.
20. Watanabe S, Tani T, Watanabe S, Seno M. Transport of steroid hormones facilitated by serum proteins. Biochimica Et Biophysica Acta. 1991;1073(2):275–84. https://doi.org/10.1016/0304-4165(91)90132-z.
21. Zhang H, Cui D, Wang B, Han Y-H, Balimane P, Yang Z, Sinz M, David Rodrigues A. Pharmacokinetic drug interactions involving 17alpha-ethinylestradiol: a new look at an old drug. Clin Pharmacokinet. 2007;46(2):133–57. https://doi.org/10.2165/00003088-200746020-00003.
22. Zu Y, Yang J, Zhang C, Liu D. The pathological mechanisms of estrogen-induced cholestasis: current perspectives. Front Pharmacol. 2021;12:761255. https://doi.org/10.3389/fphar.2021.761255.

Part IV
Combined Hormonal Contraception: Effects on Veins, Endometriosis, Adenomyosis, Myoma, Bone and Collagen

Chapter 11
Cardiovascular Safety: The Point of View of the Veins

Jonathan Douxfils and Charlotte Beaudart

11.1 Introduction

Combined oral contraceptives (COCs) are among the most popular contraceptive methods worldwide, recognized not only for their effectiveness but also for their potential to alter vascular health [1]. Early reports identified a concerning association between COC use and venous thromboembolism (VTE), a condition that includes deep vein thrombosis (DVT) and pulmonary embolism (PE) [2]. The risk of VTE is especially pertinent for young women, as this population is generally at low baseline risk for thrombotic events [3]. Epidemiological studies have demonstrated that COC use increases the risk of VTE three to six times over that of non-users, which translates to an incidence of about 5–12 cases per 10,000 woman-years, depending on the progestogen and estrogen components used in the contraceptive [4].

The increased VTE risk linked to COCs is largely influenced by the estrogen component, traditionally ethinylestradiol (EE), which has been shown to modulate coagulation factors, promoting a pro-thrombotic state [5]. Hemostatic changes

J. Douxfils (✉)
Research Unit in Clinical Pharmacology and Toxicology (URPC), NAmur Research Institute for LIfe Sciences (NARILIS), Faculty of Medicine, University of Namur, Namur, Belgium

QUALIresearch, QUALIblood s.a., Liège, Belgium

Department of Biological Hematology, Centre Hospitalier Universitaire Clermont-Ferrand, Hôpital Estaing, Clermont-Ferrand, France
e-mail: jonathan.douxfils@unamur.be; jonathan.douxfils@qualiblood.eu

C. Beaudart
Research Unit in Clinical Pharmacology and Toxicology (URPC), NAmur Research Institute for LIfe Sciences (NARILIS), Faculty of Medicine, University of Namur, Namur, Belgium
e-mail: charlotte.beaudart@unamur.be

A. R. Genazzani et al. (eds.), *Ethical, Efficacy and Safety Issues in Contraception*, Reproductive Medicine for Clinicians 4,
https://doi.org/10.1007/978-3-032-07322-8_11

induced by EE, such as elevated coagulation factors and reduced anticoagulants, create a more thrombogenic environment, thereby enhancing VTE risk [5]. Efforts to mitigate this risk have led to the gradual reduction of estrogen doses from 150 μg in early formulations to as low as 10 μg in some modern pills [6, 7]. Progestogen compounds have also evolved, with third-generation COCs (e.g., containing desogestrel or gestodene) and newer COCs (e.g., drospirenone-based) intended to reduce androgenic side effects like acne and weight gain [8, 9]. Yet, these adjustments introduced increased VTE risks, particularly with progestogens that lack the androgenic properties observed to offset some of the pro-thrombotic effects of EE [10].

In recent years, a renewed focus has been placed on using natural estrogens, such as estradiol (E2) and estetrol (E4), due to their potential to offer effective contraception with a lower thrombotic risk profile [11–16]. Data suggest that E2- and E4-based COCs may have a reduced impact on coagulation pathways compared to EE-based formulations [15–18]. Recent studies highlight that women using E2-based COCs experience a 33% lower VTE risk compared to those using EE-based COCs, even when paired with progestogens like levonorgestrel, which has a more favorable safety profile [14]. Additionally, the newer estetrol (E4), combined with drospirenone, has demonstrated minimal effects on coagulation proteins, suggesting a safer profile in comparison with traditional EE-containing options [12, 13, 15, 16].

11.2 Impact of Combined Oral Contraceptives on Hemostasis

Combined oral contraceptives induce significant changes across the hemostatic system, leading to a shift toward a prothrombotic state [5]. These contraceptives affect various hemostatic pathways, altering the balance of procoagulant, anticoagulant, and fibrinolytic factors (Table 11.1). One prominent impact of COCs is the increase in procoagulant factors, which includes elevated levels of fibrinogen, prothrombin, and factors VII, VIII, IX, X, and XII [5]. These increases contribute to a heightened capacity for clot formation, positioning users at a higher risk for thrombotic events [16, 19]. These changes are further modulated by the specific estrogen and progestin components in the COC [1, 5, 10, 20, 21]. Ethinylestradiol, the synthetic estrogen commonly used in COC, is known for its strong influence on hepatic protein synthesis, leading to substantial shifts in coagulation factors [22]. Natural estrogens, such as estradiol, have been observed to exert a lesser effect on these factors, even when associated with progestins usually associated with important impact on the hemostatic system [13, 16–18, 23–25].

COCs also alter anticoagulant pathways by reducing levels of antithrombin and proteins C and S [5]. This reduction in anticoagulant factors further influences the balance toward a procoagulant state, as the endogenous anticoagulant capacity is diminished. Specifically, protein S, a crucial cofactor for activated protein C (APC),

Table 11.1 Changes in hemostasis according to the type of oral contraceptive

	Progestins	High estrogen pills (>35mcg EE ± [progestins])	Second generation (≤35 mcg of EE + LNG/ NET(A)/NGM)	Third generation	Drospirenone and cyproterone acetate	Natural/novel estrogen(s) and progestins
Coagulation factors						
Fibrinogen [7, 17, 23, 25, 75–88]	CMA: ↑	EE: ↑↓ EE + LNG: ↑ EE + NET: ↑ EE + NETA: ↑	EE + LNG: ↑ EE + NET: ↑ EE + NETA: ↑ EE + NGM: ↑	EE + DSG: ↑ EE + GSD: ↑(↓ [79])	EE + DRSP: ↑	E2V + DNG: ↑ E2 + NOMAC: =
Prothrombin [20, 23, 25, 75, 84, 89]	CMA: ↑	EE: ↓	EE + LNG: ↑ EE + NET: ↑	EE + DSG: ↑	EE + CPA: ↑ EE + DRSP: ↑	E2 + NOMAC: = / ↑ E4 + DRSP: ↑
Factor V [20, 90]	LNG: =/↑ DSG: =		EE + LNG: =	EE + DSG: ↓	EE + DRSP: ↓	
Factor VII [7, 17, 18, 24, 75, 80, 81, 83–87, 89, 91–94]	CMA: = LNG: ↓ DSG: ↓	EE: ↑↓ EE + NET: ↑	EE + LNG: ↓ ↑ EE + NET: ↑ EE + NGM: ↑	EE + DSG: ↑ EE + GSD: ↑	EE + CPA: ↑ EE + DRSP: ↑	E2V + DNG: = / ↑ E2 + NOMAC: =
Factor VIII [17, 18, 20, 23, 29, 82, 84, 86, 89, 95]	CMA: =/↓	EE + LNG: ↑	EE + LNG: =/↑ EE + NET: ↑ EE + NGM: ↑	EE + DSG: ↑ EE + GSD: ↑	EE + DRSP: ↑	E2V + DNG: = E2 + NOMAC: =
Factor IX [90, 96]			EE + LNG: ↑	EE + DSG: ↑		
Factor X [7, 20, 75, 76, 81, 83, 93, 95]		EE: ↑↓ EE + NETA: ↑ EE + LNG: ↑	EE + LNG: ↑ EE + NETA: ↑	EE + DSG: ↑ EE + GSD: ↑	EE + DRSP: ↑	
Factor XI [90]	LNG: ↑ DSG: =		EE + LNG: ↑	EE + DSG: ↑		
Kallikrein [97–99]		EE + DSG: =/↑† EE + LNG: =/↑† EE+ NET: =/↑	EE + DSG: =/↑† EE + LNG: =/↑†			

(continued)

Table 11.1 (continued)

	Progestins	High estrogen pills (>35mcg EE ± [progestins])	Second generation (≤35 mcg of EE + LNG/ NET(A)/NGM)	Third generation	Drospirenone and yproterone acetate	Natural/novel estrogen(s) and progestins
Factor XII [97–99]		EE + DSG: ↑ EE + LNG: ↑ EE+ NET: ↑				
Anticoagulant factors/system						
Antithrombin antigen/activity [7, 17, 20, 23, 25, 29, 76, 79, 82–84, 86–88, 93, 100, 101]	CMA: =	EE: ↓ EE + NETA: ↓	EE + LNG: =/↓ EE + NETA: ↓ EE + NGM: ↓	EE+ DSG: ↓ (=/↑ [87, 101]) EE + GSD: ↓	EE + CPA: ↓ EE + DRSP: ↓ (↑ [87])	E2V + DNG: = E2 + NOMAC: = E4 + DRSP: =
Protein C [17, 18, 20, 24, 25, 29, 80, 82, 86–88, 95, 100, 102]		EE + LNG: ↑	EE + LNG: =/↑ EE + NET: ↑ EE + NGM: ↑	EE + DSG: =/↑ EE + GSD: ↑	EE + CPA: ↑ EE + DRSP: ↑	E2V + DNG: = / ↑ E2 + NOMAC: = E4 + DRSP: =
Protein S total and free/activity [17, 18, 20, 23, 25, 79, 82–84, 86–89, 91–93, 95, 100, 102–104]	CMA: ↑ DSG: ↑		EE + LNG: ↓/=/↑ EE + NET: ↓ EE + NGM: ↓	EE+ DSG: ↓ EE + GSD: ↓	EE + CPA: ↓ EE + DRSP: ↓	E2V + DNG: = E2 + NOMAC: =/↑ E4 + DRSP: =
Tissue factor pathway inhibitor [20, 23, 25, 84, 104, 105]	CMA: = LNG: ↑		EE + LNG: ↓ EE + NET: ↓ EE + NGM: ↓	EE + DSG: ↓ EE + GSD: ↓	EE + CPA: ↓ EE + DRSP: ↓	E2 + NOMAC: =/↓ E4 + DRSP: ↓
APCsr (aPTT-based) [18, 82, 84, 85, 88, 106]	CMA: =	EE + [progestogen]: ↓	EE + LNG: ↓ EE + NET: ↓ EE + NGM: ↓	EE + DSG: ↓ EE + GSD: ↓	EE + CPA: ↓ EE + DRSP: ↓	E2V + DNG: = E2 + NOMAC: = E4 + DRSP: =
APCsr (ETP-based) [10, 13, 18, 20, 21, 23, 25, 32, 82, 107, 108]		EE + LNG: ↑	EE + LNG: ↑ EE + NGM: ↑	EE + DSG: ↑ EE + GSD: ↑	EE + CPA: ↑ EE + DRSP: ↑	E2V + DNG: =/↑ E2 + NOMAC: ↑ E4 + DRSP: =
Fibrinolytic markers/system						
Tissue plasminogen activator activity/antigen* [78, 82–86, 91, 102, 109]	CMA: = LNG: ↑	EE + LNG: ↑	EE + LNG: ↑ EE + NGM: ↑	EE + GSD: ↑ EE + DSG: ↑	EE + DRSP: ↑	E4 + DRSP: =* (antigen)

Plasminogen [23, 79, 81, 82, 85, 86, 88, 91, 93, 95, 102, 109]	LNG: ↓	EE + LNG: ↑	EE + LNG: ↑ EE + NET: ↑ EE + NGM: ↑	EE + DSG: ↑ EE + GSD: ↑	EE + CPA: ↑ EE + DRSP: ↑	E2 + NOMAC: ↑
α2-antiplasmin [76, 88]		EE + NETA: ↓	EE + LNG: ↑ EE + NET: ↑ EE + NETA: ↓	EE + DSG: ↑	EE + CPA: ↑ EE + DRSP: ↑	
Plasmin - α2-antiplasmin complex [78, 82, 85, 86, 109]		EE + LNG: ↑	EE + LNG: ↑ EE + NGM: ↑	EE + DSG: ↑ EE + GSD: ↑	EE + DRSP: ↑	
Plasminogen activator inhibitor–1 antigen/activity [23, 24, 78, 80–83, 85–88, 102, 109]		EE + LNG: ↓	EE + LNG: ↓ EE + NET: ↓ EE + NGM: ↓	EE+ DSG: ↓ EE + GSD: ↓	EE + CPA: ↓ EE + DRSP: ↓	E2V + DNG: ↓ E2 + NOMAC: ↓
Coagulation activation markers						
D-dimer [17, 18, 24, 25, 78, 81, 83, 84, 87, 88, 93, 100, 109]	CMA: =		EE + LNG: ↑ EE + NET: ↑ EE + NGM: ↑	EE+ DSG: ↑ EE + GSD: ↑	EE + CPA: =/↑ EE + DRSP: ↑	E2V + DNG: = E2 + NOMAC: = / ↓ E4 + DRSP: ↓
Fibrinopeptide A [77]			EE + LNG: ↑	EE + DSG: = EE + GSD: ↑		
Prothrombin fragment 1 + 2 [17, 18, 23–25, 83–85, 92, 94, 100, 110]	CMA: = DSG: ↓ LNG: ↓		EE + LNG: ↑ EE + NET: ↑	EE + DSG: ↑ EE + GSD: ↑	EE + CPA: ↑ EE + DRSP: ↑	E2V + DNG: = E2 + NOMAC: = E4 + DRSP: =
Thrombin-antithrombin complex [80, 87, 101]				EE + DSG: ↑ EE + GSD: ↑	EE + DRSP: ↑	

Abbreviations: *APC* Activated Protein C, *aPTT* activated Partial Thromboplastin Time, *CMA* chlormadinone acetate, *CPA* cyproterone acetate, *DNG* dienogest, *DRSP* drospirenone, *DSG* desogestrel, *E2* estradiol, *E2V* estradiol valerate, *E4* estetrol, *EE* ethinylestradiol, *GSD* gestodene, *LNG* levonorgestrel, *NET* norethisterone, *NETA* norethisterone acetate, *NGM* norgestimate, *NOMAC* nomegestrol acetate, ↑ increase, ↓ decrease, = no change is significantly reduced in users of COCs [5]. This reduction in protein S levels is particularly pronounced in formulations containing third- and fourth-generation progestins, such as desogestrel, gestodene, and drospirenone, compared to second-generation progestins like levonorgestrel. Table 11.1 provides a comprehensive overview, showing that these newer progestins are associated with a marked increase in APC resistance, a state in which the anticoagulant effects of APC are less effective, thus increasing thrombotic risk [26–28].

Additionally, COCs impact fibrinolysis, the process responsible for breaking down clots. While COCs increase levels of plasminogen and tissue plasminogen activator (t-PA), they concurrently reduce the levels of plasminogen activator inhibitor-1 (PAI-1) [5]. At first glance, these changes may suggest enhanced fibrinolytic activity; however, COCs also raise thrombin-activatable fibrinolysis inhibitor (TAFI) levels [5]. TAFI inhibits fibrinolysis by preventing plasminogen from binding to fibrin, thus limiting clot breakdown. The net effect of these changes is a complex balance where fibrinolytic activity is not markedly increased despite higher plasminogen and t-PA levels, due to the counteracting rise in thrombin activable fibrinolysis inhibitor (TAFI). This nuanced effect on fibrinolysis indicates that while clot formation potential is increased, clot breakdown does not proportionately rise, further reinforcing a prothrombotic profile.

The association between APC resistance and thrombotic risk in COC users is one of the most extensively studied outcomes [1, 12, 17, 21, 23–26, 29–32]. Acquired APC resistance, frequently seen in COC users, differs from genetic APC resistance (such as in carriers of the factor V Leiden mutation) in that it arises from reductions in anticoagulant factors influenced by the hormonal components of COCs and not from a genetic mutation in the Factor V (FV) of the coagulation, that is, FV Leiden [33, 34]. This acquired resistance is more pronounced with certain EE-containing formulations, notably those containing drospirenone, cyproterone acetate, or desogestrel, as indicated in Table 11.1. The endogenous thrombin potential (ETP)-based APC resistance assay [26, 35], used to measure thrombin generation in the presence of APC, has shown that these COCs lead to higher resistance levels [28, 36] (Figs. 11.1 and 11.2). This assay is particularly sensitive to changes in protein S and TFPI, two factors significantly impacted by COC use [37]. The combination of reduced TFPI and lower protein S activity contributes to the inability of APC to exert its full anticoagulant effect, increasing thrombotic susceptibility.

COC-induced shifts in the hemostatic balance are dose-dependent, particularly with respect to the estrogen component. Higher doses of ethinylestradiol (over 35 μg) are associated with more significant changes in coagulation markers, while lower doses or alternative estrogens, such as estetrol, exhibit a reduced impact on the hemostatic system as observed by the comparison of the effect of EE/drospirenone versus E4/drospirenone on the coagulation [13, 38]. Estetrol, for example, does not metabolize into estrone [39], an estrogen able to induce hepatic protein synthesis [40], resulting in a more balanced profile with a lower risk of thrombotic complications. This characteristic positions estetrol as a potentially safer estrogenic component in terms of hemostatic impact [12, 13, 15, 16, 36, 38, 41–43]. Despite this, all COCs, regardless of dose or specific formulation, maintain an inherent

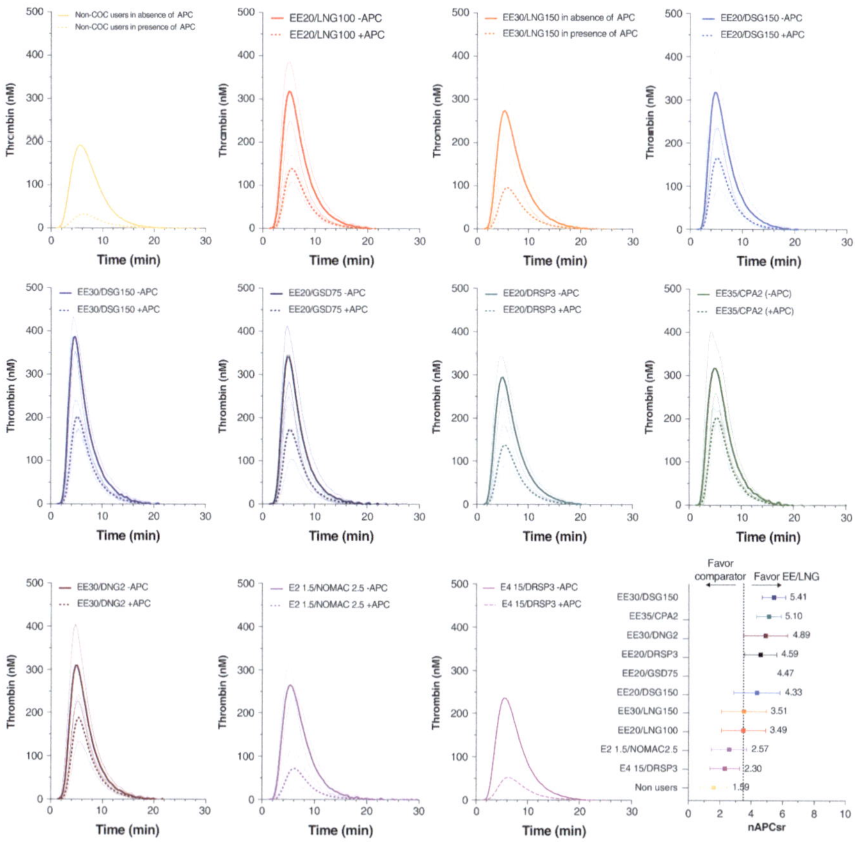

Fig. 11.1 Thrombin generation curves in absence (continuous line) and in presence of APC (dotted lines) of a healthy pooled plasma (top left panel) and women using combined oral contraceptives containing either ethinylestradiol (EE) with different progestins or natural estrogens like estradiol (E2) or estetrol (E4) with different progestins. The area under the curve represents the endogenous thrombin potential (ETP) parameter. The higher the ETP for a specific condition, that is, tests realize in presence or in absence of protein C (APC), the higher the risk of VTE. This test can reveal both the impact of COCs on procoagulant factors (solid line) and on activated protein C (dotted line). The normalized APC sensitivity ratio (nAPCsr) is computed from these curves and represents the ratio of the ETP in presence and absence of APC compared to the same ratio in non-COC users. As for the ETP, the higher the nAPCsr, the higher the risk of VTE (bottom right panel). *Abbreviations: APC, activated protein C; DRSP, drospirenone; DSG, desogestrel; EE, ethinylestradiol; E4, estetrol; HPP, healthy pooled plasma; LNG, levonorgestrel*

prothrombotic effect, emphasizing the importance of individual risk assessment when prescribing these contraceptives [1, 5, 44, 45].

Overall, COCs generate a complex shift toward a prothrombotic state through multiple pathways in the hemostatic system. By increasing procoagulant factors, decreasing key anticoagulant factors, and modulating fibrinolysis, COCs alter the delicate hemostatic balance in a way that predisposes users to thrombotic events. This effect is most pronounced with formulations containing EE, especially when

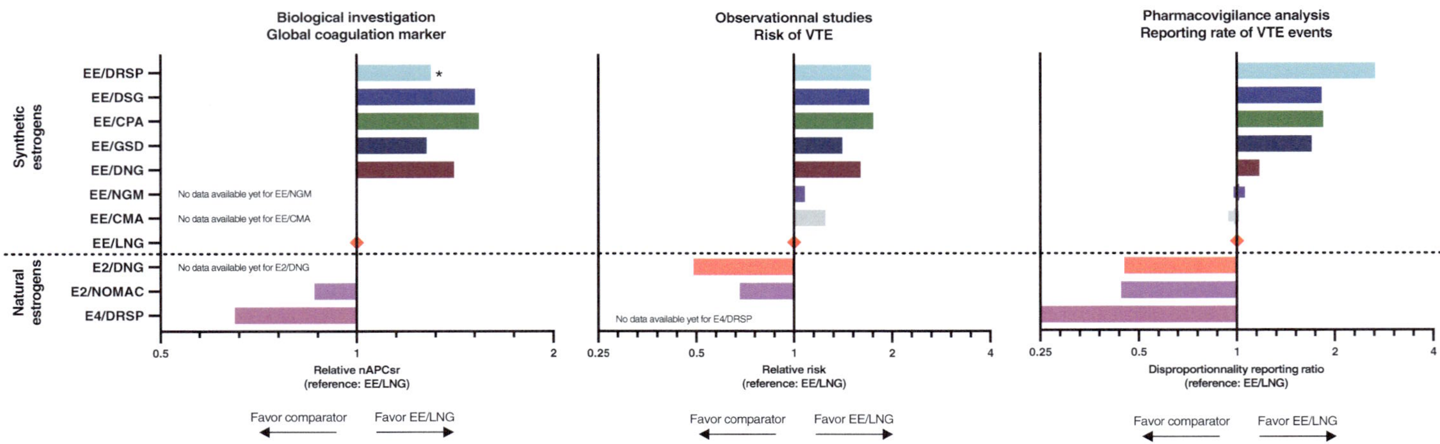

Fig. 11.2 Impact of combined oral contraceptives (COCs) on venous thromboembolism (VTE) risk across biological, observational, and pharmacovigilance data. All panels present data normalized to provide a consistent relative evaluation versus the reference product, ethinylestradiol/levonorgestrel (EE/LNG). The left panel shows the global coagulation parameter (nAPCsr), where a lower nAPCsr indicates a lower thrombotic risk, with COCs containing natural estrogens consistently showing the lowest values compared to synthetic estrogens. The center panel presents the relative risk of VTE based on observational studies, where COCs with natural estrogens demonstrate the lowest relative risk. The right panel illustrates disproportionality reporting rates for VTE from EudraVigilance (2004–2024), a pharmacovigilance database, where natural estrogens again show the lowest VTE reporting rates. These data collectively highlight the consistent safety profile of COCs containing natural estrogens across biological (nAPCsr), observational studies, and pharmacovigilance (EudraVigilance) evidence. Data have been extracted and normalized when appropriate [1, 4, 11, 12, 14, 48, 53, 74]. * *For nAPCsr data with EE/DRSP, only 20 mcg of EE / 3 mg DRSP have been collected so far. As the dose of EE highly influenced nAPCsr, nAPCsr results with EE 30 mcg / DRSP 3 mg are expected to be similar to EE/DSG, reflecting what is observed in observational and pharmacovigilance data. Abbreviations: CMA, chlormadinone acetate; COC, combined oral contraceptives; CPA, cyproterone acetate; DNG, dienogest; DRSP, drospirenone; DSG, desogestrel; EE, ethinylestradiol; E2, estradiol; E4, estetrol; GSD, gestodene; LNG, levonorgestrel; nAPCsr, normalized activated protein C sensitivity ratio; NGM, norgestimate; VTE, venous thromboembolism*

associated with third- or fourth-generation progestins, underlining the necessity for healthcare providers to carefully evaluate the thrombotic risk of patients considering COC therapy.

11.3 Risk of Thrombotic Events with Combined Oral Contraceptives

The epidemiology of VTE risk associated with COCs has evolved substantially, driven by concerns from both the European Medicines Agency (EMA) and the US Food and Drug Administration (FDA) [3, 46]. Both agencies have consistently emphasized the need to mitigate VTE risks due to the widespread use of COCs among healthy young women. Early regulatory assessments attributed VTE risk mainly to EE doses and the progestin component, recognizing that higher estrogen doses and specific progestins correlate with elevated VTE risk. Consequently, the EMA suggested COC formulations to be reduced to 20–30 μg EE, with second-generation progestins like levonorgestrel or norethisterone recommended as first-line options [3]. These combinations were associated with the lowest risk levels, with VTE incidence estimated at 5–7 per 10,000 women per year (Table 11.2). In contrast, higher VTE incidences were documented with third- and fourth-generation progestins, such as desogestrel and drospirenone, due to their relatively weak androgenic activity [1].

The Cochrane meta-analysis by de Bastos et al. [4] provided one of the earliest comprehensive reviews on the topic, pooling data from multiple studies to assess the impact of various COC formulations on VTE risk. This review estimated that COCs with newer progestins, such as desogestrel, gestodene, and drospirenone, were associated with a 1.5 to two-fold increase in VTE risk compared to those with second-generation progestins like levonorgestrel. These findings highlighted the need to avoid higher-risk COC formulations, especially for women with additional VTE risk factors, such as obesity or a family history of thrombosis. Although the work of de Bastos was instrumental in setting the groundwork for VTE risk stratification in COC users, it did not account for the natural estrogen formulations and more recent studies that emerged thereafter [47–52].

Furthermore, another large study not included in the de Bastos's meta-analysis further confirmed these estimates. This study by Vinogradova et al. has been conducted using two large primary care databases in the UK, that is, QResearch and CPRD [53]. Their nested case-control analysis revealed that the risk of VTE varies significantly depending on the type of progestogen combined with EE. Notably, newer progestogens like desogestrel, drospirenone, and cyproterone were associated with higher VTE risks compared to second-generation progestogens such as levonorgestrel and norethisterone. These findings underscore the importance of progestogen selection in mitigating VTE risk and align with the broader evidence advocating for safer contraceptive formulations, particularly those containing natural estrogens or second-generation progestogens, to improve the overall safety profile of COCs.

Table 11.2 Estimated risk of venous thromboembolism events (VTE) with combined oral contraceptives (COC)

Risk group	Estimated risk of VTE	Reference
Non-pregnant non-user	2/10000 WY	EMA/739865/2013 [3]
Pregnant and postpartum women	20/10000 WY	30-year population-based study [111]
User of COC containing EE + LNG EE + NETA EE + NGM	5–7/10000 WY	EMA/739865/2013 [3]
User of COC containing EE + GSD EE+ DSG EE+ DRSP	9–12/ 10,000 WY	EMA/739865/2013 [3]
User of COC containing EE + CMA	6–9/10000 WY	RIVET-RCS [112]
User of COC containing EE + DNG	Incidence rate ratio for VTE compared to LNG-COC of 1.28	EURAS OC study [113]
User of COC containing E2V + DNG	7.0/10000 WY versus 3.5 in non-user and 9.9 in LNG/EE users	INAS-SCORE study [48]
User of COC containing E2/NOMAC	2.0/10000 WY versus 1.8 in non-user and 3.0 in LNG/EE users	PRO-E2 [49]
User of COC containing E4/DRSP	Pending	PASS required by the EMA and FDA (INAS-NESS and INAS-SEECS studies)

Abbreviations: *CMA* chlormadinone acetate, *COC* combined oral contraceptives, *DNG* dienogest, *DRSP* drospirenone, *DSG* desogestrel, *EE* ethinylestradiol, *EMA* European Medicines Agency, *EURAS* European Actie Surveillance Study, *E2* 17β-estradiol, *E2V* estradiol valerate, *E4* estetrol, *GSD* gestodene, *INAS-CELINA* International Active Surveillance Study: Choice of Estrogen and Long-term Investigation of Nomegestrol Acetate, *INAS-SCORE* International Active Surveillance study "Safety of Contraceptives: Role of Estrogens", *LNG* levonorgestrel, *NETA* norethisterone acetate, *NGM* norgestimate, *PASS* post authorization safety study, *VTE* venous thromboembolism

11.4 Epidemiological Investigations on Natural Estrogens and VTE Risk

A series of studies by Lidegaard [47], Dinger [48], Reed [49], Schink [50], and Heikinheimo [51] provided further insights related to the risk of VTE associated with natural estrogens. The nested case-control study by Schink that used German claims data reported that levonorgestrel with low-dose EE remains the safest option for EE-containing pills [50]. This study also indicated a substantial increase in VTE risk with COCs containing progestins like dienogest, cyproterone acetate, and desogestrel, further highlighting the role of progestin selection in VTE risk modulation [36]. Even if the data are sparse, this study also showed a trend toward a reduction in the rate of VTE with natural estrogens.

The INAS-SCORE [48] and the PRO-E2 [49] studies marked a notable advancement in evaluating VTE risk with natural estrogen-based COCs. These large-scale prospective studies compared COCs containing dienogest or nomegestrol acetate in combination with E2 with a traditional levonorgestrel-EE COC. The INAS-SCORE study was then pooled with the INAS-OC study, another large scale prospective, observational cohort study [52]. Findings showed that E2-based COCs had a comparable or lower VTE risk profile compared to EE-levonorgestrel, suggesting a favorable alternative to EE-based contraceptives. The lower effect of E2 on hepatic protein synthesis likely contributes to this reduced risk [17, 18, 23, 24]. These studies underscored the potential of natural estrogens like E2 to provide effective contraception with a safer thrombotic profile, sparking further research into alternative estrogen formulations.

The study by Heikinheimo, based on Finnish registry data, took a broader view by examining various types of hormonal contraception [51]. The Finnish data supported previous findings, showing that COCs with third-generation progestins and EE doses of 30 μg or higher presented an increased VTE risk, especially with progestins like drospirenone and desogestrel. The authors noted that preparations combining low-dose EE with second-generation progestins like levonorgestrel had the lowest VTE incidence rates. They also highlighted that progestin-only contraceptives did not significantly increase VTE risk, which may be suitable for women with underlying risk factors. Finally, their study contributed to the growing body of evidence on natural estrogens, revealing that E2-containing COCs likely have a reduced impact on VTE risk relative to EE-based alternatives.

These recent results with E2-containing COCs, which had been unavailable in de Bastos systematic review and meta-analysis, were integrated in a meta-analysis [14]. This updated meta-analysis provided compelling evidence that natural estrogen-based COCs are associated with a significantly lower VTE risk than EE-based counterparts. Specifically, we found a 33% reduction in VTE risk among users of E2-based COCs, which they attributed to the lower hepatic impact of natural estrogens [14] (Fig. 11.2). This comprehensive assessment underscored the potential for natural estrogens in reducing thrombotic complications, positioning them as a safer alternative for all women desiring effective and safe hormonal contraception. Adjusted data even show a 49% reduction of the risk of VTE (Pooled HR from imposed EMA PASS: 0.51 (95% CI 0.29–0.90). This updated analysis also reinforced previous findings, confirming a 1.5- to two-fold increased VTE risk in EE-based COCs with third- and fourth-generation progestins compared to those with second-generation options like levonorgestrel [14]. The cumulative evidence provided by this meta-analysis suggests that a shift in clinical practice toward prescribing natural estrogen formulations could markedly improve safety outcomes in contraceptive users. Considering these findings, there is a strong case for re-evaluating contraceptive guidelines to prioritize COC options with reduced VTE risk. Moreover, the studies collectively emphasize the need for individualized contraceptive counseling, especially for women with known or potential risk factors for thrombosis.

11.5 Data from Adverse Events Spontaneous Reporting Systems

Prospective observational post-authorization safety studies (PASS), as those described above, are often seen as pharmacovigilance tools used to document and monitor the clinical utility of new drugs when safety concerns arose or when a referral has been issued for a particular therapeutic drug class [54, 55]. For example, in the 2013 referral form of the EMA, a PASS has been imposed on the marketing authorization holder of EE-chlormadinone acetate to document the risk of VTE associated with this product [3]. A similar procedure has then been applied to other new COCs reaching the market, for example, E2-dienogest and E2-nomegestrol acetate. Following the conducting of these PASS, recent guidelines should argue for the use of natural estrogens and emphasize the safer profile of natural estrogens like E2 and the new generation estrogen, E4 [41].

Estetrol, a native estrogen used in combination with drospirenone, represents a promising development in the contraceptive area [39]. Estetrol offers several advantages as an estrogen component in COCs, especially when compared to synthetic estrogens like EE. Estetrol is classified as a Native Estrogen with Selective Action in Tissues (NEST), which means it selectively activates specific estrogen receptors. This unique mechanism allows E4 to have a minimal impact on liver function and associated clotting factors, reducing the risk of VTE compared to EE-based contraceptives. Additionally, E4 provides a consistent bleeding pattern and, with a high bioavailability and longer half-life, maintains effective cycle control, enhancing user satisfaction. Current clinical experience and pharmacological data gathered during the drug development suggest that this combination has a potentially lower risk of VTE thanks to a less pronounced effect on coagulation factors and the hemostatic system compared to EE-levonorgestrel and EE-drospirenone [13, 56–59]. This combination has been evaluated through rigorous phase-2 and phase-3 clinical trials, which have shown favorable outcomes in terms of efficacy and safety, especially concerning the VTE risk [13, 56–59].

The existing pre-clinical and clinical data on E4-DRSP already suggest a favorable risk-benefit ratio. However, due to legally binding concerns, even if current data were already reassuring, agencies applied similar strategy than with E2-based pills and asked the conduction of a PASS to assess the risk of VTE associated with this new COC among other objectives, that is, the INAS-NEES and the INAS-SEECS studies. Results of these PASS are expected to be available in 2027 at the earliest but in light of the potentially safer profile of E4 compared to synthetic estrogens, there is an ethical concern to analyze all available data to allow regulators, clinicians, and patients having access to safest contraceptive methods.

Interestingly, a prospective observational PASS is not the only pharmacovigilance tool that can be used to assess the real-life safety of newly marketed products and detect signals. Indeed, while these studies are of interest for documenting the safety profile of new drugs, they may be subject to several bias like selection bias, channeling bias, protopathic bias, or lack of adjustment for confounding factors

[54]. Analysis of pharmacovigilance database like EudraVigilance or Food and Drug Administration's Adverse Event Reporting System (FAERS) permits to further complement the experience we have with new drugs and allow the conduct of disproportionality reporting rate (DPRR) studies using individual case safety report (Box 11.1). Such databases play a critical role in the ongoing assessment of drug in real-world settings to quickly react to potential safety breakdown. They allow for the monitoring of adverse drug reactions and could provide additional reassurance about the potential risk associated with new agents like E4-containing COCs compared to older ones containing other estrogens like EE or E2 [60]. These databases gather real-world adverse event reports, helping to identify potential risks that might not fully emerge during clinical trials. In recent years, studies by Xu et al. and Didembourg et al. have used FAERS and EudraVigilance, respectively, to assess VTE risk across various COC formulations.

Their findings provide critical insights into the safety profiles of different formulations, particularly those containing synthetic versus natural estrogens.

Box 11.1 Explanation of Disproportionality Reporting Ratio Method for Analyzing Signal of Adverse Events in Pharmacovigilance Databases
Disproportionality analysis is a set of statistical signal detection techniques based on comparison of reporting proportions between the study drug and all drugs of a particular class in the spontaneous reporting database combined [60]. This statistical method relies on the principle that when a signal detection report identifies a specific adverse event linked to a medicinal product, this adverse event is reported more frequently in connection with this product, compared to other medications. This higher frequency of reporting for ADRs associated with the drug is reflected in a table based on the total number of individual cases recorded in a pharmacovigilance database.

According to the 2007 EMA guidelines [60], the proportional reporting rate (PRR) was computed as follows:

$$\text{PRR} = \frac{A/(A+B)}{C/(C+D)}$$

Where:

- (A) Represents the number of individual cases reporting the venous thrombotic event associated with the study drug.
- (B) Represents the number of individual cases reporting other events associated with the study drug.
- (C) Represents the number of individual cases reporting the venous thrombotic event associated with all other medicinal products of the therapeutic class.

(continued)

Box 11.1 (continued)

- (*D*) Represents the number of individual cases reporting other events associated with all other medicinal products of the therapeutic class.

Firstly, for each product or molecule, both the number of all adverse event extracted from the selected reaction groups (A + B) and the number of "adverse events of interest" (A) were extracted. To estimate the importance of "adverse events of interest" reported in the class itself, a ratio was made as follows:

$$\frac{N^{\circ}\text{“}adverse\ events\ of\ interest\text{”}\ of\ the\ selected\ drug}{N^{\circ}\ all\ adverse\ events\ of\ the\ selected\ drug} = \frac{(A)}{(A+B)}$$

Secondly, the number of all adverse event of all analyzed classes minus the number of all adverse event of the selected drug (C + D) was computed. Also, the number of "adverse events of interest" of all analyzed classes minus the number of "adverse events of interest" of the selected drug (C) was calculated.

$$\frac{\begin{array}{l}\text{N}^{\circ}\ \text{all “adverse events of interest” for the therapeutic class}\\ -\text{N}^{\circ}\text{“adverse events of interest” of the selected drug}\end{array}}{\begin{array}{l}N^{\circ}\ all\ adverse\ events\ for\ the\ therapeutic\ class\\ -N^{\circ}\ all\ adverse\ events\ of\ the\ selected\ drug\end{array}} = \frac{(C)}{(C+D)}$$

Xu et al. conducted an analysis of the FAERS database, focusing on Yasmin®, a widely used COC that combines EE and drospirenone. The study aimed to assess adverse events reported for Yasmin® over nearly two decades. The results revealed significant signals for VTE, with elevated reporting odds ratios (RORs) and proportional reporting ratios (PRRs) for thrombotic events. This highlights Yasmin®'s potentially higher risk profile compared to other COCs. Additionally, the study identified adverse events across multiple organ systems, including hepatobiliary disorders and psychiatric issues. Demographic data showed that most reports involved females aged 18–45, the primary users of Yasmin®. Although relying on these data exclusively to draw definitive conclusions is misleading [61], these findings underscore the value of FAERS in identifying safety concerns for specific products, particularly those widely prescribed to at-risk populations.

Complementing Xu's product-specific focus, Didembourg et al. used the EudraVigilance database to perform a comparative analysis of VTE risks across various COC formulations. Their study specifically contrasted synthetic estrogen-based formulations, such as those containing EE, with natural estrogen-based alternatives, including E2 and E4. The results demonstrated a markedly lower PRR for VTE with E2- and E4-based COCs compared to their EE counterparts. For instance, the E4-DRSP combination had a proportionality reporting rate of 0.12, comparable to the rate observed for progestin-only pills, which are known for their minimal to no impact on coagulation [4, 62–64]. Conversely, EE-drospirenone exhibited the highest PRR (2.23), indicating a significantly elevated risk of thrombotic events. Compared to the established gold standard, EE-levonorgestrel, natural estrogen-based formulations consistently showed safer profiles, reinforcing their potential as preferable alternatives for patients with heightened VTE risk (Fig. 11.2).

The results of these studies highlight the strengths of pharmacovigilance databases in identifying and quantifying real-world safety signals. FAERS and EudraVigilance enable large-scale analyses across diverse populations and clinical contexts, offering a broader understanding of drug safety beyond the controlled conditions of clinical trials. Xu's study demonstrates the utility of such databases in pinpointing safety concerns for individual products, while Didembourg's work underscores their comparative strength in evaluating relative risks among therapeutic alternatives. Together, these findings illustrate the complementary capabilities of pharmacovigilance tools in addressing both product-specific and class-wide safety questions.

However, the studies also reveal the limitations inherent to pharmacovigilance databases. Both FAERS and EudraVigilance rely on spontaneous reporting systems, which are subject to underreporting and reporting biases [61]. Serious events like VTE are more likely to be reported than minor adverse effects, potentially skewing the perceived risk. Additionally, these databases lack population exposure data, preventing the calculation of true incidence rates. Disproportionality measures such as RORs and (D)PRRs provide relative frequencies rather than absolute risk estimates. These limitations necessitate cautious interpretation of findings, as highlighted in Creinin et al. critique of Xu study, which raised concerns about methodological flaws and the need for standardized reporting frameworks such as READUS-PV [61].

Despite these challenges, the insights gained from these studies have significant implications for clinical practice. The elevated VTE risk associated with EE-based formulations like EE-drospirenone underscores the need for careful patient selection and monitoring. Conversely, the favorable safety profiles of E2- and E4-based formulations suggest that these natural estrogen options should be prioritized, particularly for patients with elevated baseline VTE risk. The findings also highlight the need for improved reporting practices and adherence to methodological guidelines to enhance the reliability and utility of pharmacovigilance data.

11.6 Discrete Choice Experiments in COCs: What Do Women Want and Know?

The application of discrete choice experiments (DCEs) to assess preferences for COCs provides valuable insights into the multifaceted nature of women's decision-making processes regarding contraceptive use. By examining the trade-offs women are willing to make among various attributes, DCEs offer a robust framework for understanding how preferences align with real-world choices and unmet needs. These DCEs complement earlier sections of this publication, which highlighted the evolving landscape of contraceptive options and the critical need for patient-centered approaches in reproductive healthcare.

Studies consistently highlight that women prioritize contraceptive methods that balance efficacy, safety, and side effect profiles. For example, women value attributes such as longer duration of effectiveness, minimal interference with menstruation (e.g., lighter or less painful periods), and reduced risk of serious adverse effects like VTE [65–67]. Additionally, preferences often vary based on demographic and life course factors. Younger women or those in earlier reproductive stages may emphasize reversibility and minimal side effects, while older women or those who have completed their families may prioritize permanence and convenience [66, 68]. These trends underscore the importance of integrating women's individual preferences into contraceptive counseling, as discussed in the introductory sections of this manuscript.

Discrete choice experiments conducted in diverse populations reveal critical trends in contraceptive preferences. High efficacy remains a dominant factor in contraceptive selection. Preferences for methods with failure rates below 1% are significantly higher than those with greater risk, reflecting a universal desire for reliability [66, 67]. Concerns about safety, particularly hormonal side effects and VTE risk, influence women's choices, with natural estrogens like E2 and E4 emerging as favorable alternatives due to their lower thrombotic risk profiles compared to EE [11, 14]. These findings build on the discussion of hormonal safety profiles in earlier sections, emphasizing the ongoing advancements in contraceptive technology to address these concerns.

Many women prefer methods that reduce or eliminate menstrual bleeding and associated pain. However, perceptions of safety regarding amenorrhea vary. While some women view amenorrhea as a benefit, others express concerns about its long-term health implications, indicating a need for individualized counseling to address misconceptions [67, 69]. Attributes such as frequency of administration and ease of use (e.g., monthly patches or annual injections) significantly impact choices. Women often favor methods that minimize disruptions to daily life, demonstrating the importance of convenience in contraceptive adherence [66]. These considerations align with the broader themes of user-friendly contraceptive design and accessibility discussed previously.

Preferences are also shaped by sociocultural and demographic factors. Studies among women in low-resource settings underscore the importance of affordability and accessibility, while those in high-resource settings highlight concerns about autonomy and informed choice [69, 70]. Healthcare providers play a pivotal role in shaping preferences. However, discrepancies between provider recommendations and patient priorities can create barriers. For example, providers often emphasize medical efficacy, while women may prioritize lifestyle compatibility or fear of side effects [67]. Bridging these gaps, as outlined in earlier sections, remains a critical goal for improving patient-provider communication.

Contraceptive preferences are not static but evolve with changing life circumstances, such as relationship status, fertility goals, and health status. Evidence shows that up to 46% of women may change their preferred contraceptive method within a year, particularly in response to life events such as pregnancy or shifts in marital status [68]. This underscores the need for family planning programs to ensure access to a wide range of methods to accommodate dynamic preferences [68]. These findings tie back to the discussion on the importance of flexibility and adaptability in contraceptive offerings.

To address the diverse and evolving needs of women, contraceptive counseling must adopt a patient-centered approach. Providers should prioritize eliciting individual preferences and concerns, offering tailored recommendations that align with women's values. Comprehensive counseling that includes discussions about newer options, such as E2- and E4-based COCs, can enhance satisfaction and adherence by mitigating concerns about safety and side effects [14].

Importantly, the perception of the risk of VTE may be biased by the lack of literacy of COC's users. Women frequently remain unaware that they may be carriers of inherited or acquired coagulopathies, significantly increasing their risk of thrombotic events when using COCs. Coagulopathies such as factor V Leiden, prothrombin G20210A mutation, or protein S deficiencies are present in approximately 7–8% of the population, with the majority of carriers undiagnosed until the occurrence of a thrombotic event. The use of COCs exacerbates the prothrombotic risk by altering coagulation pathways, creating a supra-additive effect in individuals with these underlying conditions. For example, women with inherited thrombophilia have been reported to face a 34- to 45-fold increased risk of VTE when on COCs compared to non-users [71, 72].

Given these complexities, there remains a critical need for further research to explore the interplay between patient preferences and practitioner recommendations. Discrete choice experiments provide a unique opportunity to harmonize these perspectives, but future studies must explicitly incorporate the views of prescribers alongside those of users. Such research is essential to identify and address potential misalignments, ensuring that contraceptive counseling and healthcare strategies reflect both medical expertise and the lived experiences of women. A deeper understanding of these dynamics will ultimately support the development of holistic, patient-centered approaches that reconcile safety, efficacy, and user acceptability in contraceptive care.

11.7 Risk Mitigation of VTE in Women on COC

To mitigate this risk, individualized risk assessments must become a cornerstone of contraceptive counseling. Standard screening practices, which rely heavily on familial history of VTE, are insufficiently predictive of thrombophilic conditions. Advanced phenotypic assessments such as the endogenous thrombin potential (ETP)-based activated protein C (APC) resistance assay offer a promising solution.

This test captures a comprehensive view of the coagulation process by quantifying thrombin generation and assessing the influence of anticoagulant pathways, including protein S and tissue factor pathway inhibitor levels, which are significantly altered in COC users (Fig. 11.1).

The ETP-based APC resistance assay has shown higher sensitivity to COC-induced hemostatic changes compared to traditional assays. It not only identifies women with inherited thrombophilia but also detects acquired APC resistance induced by hormonal contraceptives. Recent advancements in standardizing this assay, as demonstrated by our group [26], have reduced inter-laboratory variability [73], making it a reliable tool for clinical decision-making. Importantly, this method provides actionable insights into the thrombotic risk profile of individual patients, enabling healthcare providers to recommend safer contraceptive options, such as progestin-only pills or COCs containing natural estrogens like E2 or E4, which have a reduced impact on coagulation (Fig. 11.1 and Table 11.1).

The integration of such personalized screening tools into routine practice could dramatically reduce the incidence of VTE associated with COC use. By identifying high-risk individuals before prescribing COCs, clinicians can proactively minimize adverse outcomes. Furthermore, incorporating these insights into public health strategies and educational programs may increase awareness of coagulopathies, empowering women to make informed choices about their contraceptive, pregnancy, and other hormonal options. This patient-centered approach aligns with modern principles of precision medicine and holds the potential to transform contraceptive safety at the individual level.

11.8 Clinical Implications and Recommendations for Contraceptive Choices

The risk of VTE remains a significant factor in contraceptive safety. Current evidence robustly supports the safety of natural estrogens like E2 and E4 over EE, both in reducing thrombotic risks and minimizing disruptions to hepatic protein synthesis. As more healthcare providers recognize the benefits of natural estrogens, patient outcomes may improve, with a corresponding reduction in VTE incidence among contraceptive users. Further studies should continue to compare long-term safety outcomes to strengthen E2 and E4 roles in contraception, but the data so far indicates a paradigm shift in the prescription of safer COCs.

The evidence underscores the need for a tailored, patient-centered approach in contraceptive counseling to mitigate the risks associated with COCs. The heightened thrombotic risk linked to COCs, especially in women with undiagnosed coagulopathies, highlights the critical importance of individualized risk assessment. Traditional methods of screening, such as assessing familial history of VTE, are insufficient for detecting inherited or acquired thrombophilic conditions. Conditions like factor V Leiden, prothrombin G20210A mutation, and protein S deficiencies often remain undiagnosed, placing these women at a significantly elevated risk of thrombotic events when using COCs. The application of advanced tools, such as the ETP-based APC resistance assay, represents a pivotal development in risk stratification. This assay provides a phenotypic measure of coagulation potential and is more sensitive to the hemostatic changes induced by COCs than traditional assays. It can detect acquired APC resistance and identify individuals who are at a particularly high risk of thrombotic complications, even in the absence of overt familial risk factors.

Natural estrogen-based COCs, such as those containing E2 or E4, offer an effective and safer alternative to synthetic EE. These formulations not only exhibit a reduced impact on coagulation pathways, including lower activation of coagulation factors and diminished resistance to APC, but also provide comparable efficacy and improved tolerability profiles. Studies have demonstrated a 33–49% reduction in VTE risk among women using natural estrogen-based COCs compared to traditional EE formulations, including EE-levonorgestrel. Given their robust safety and efficacy profiles, natural estrogen-based COCs could be considered as a first-line therapy for all women. For women with identified risk factors or detected APC resistance, non-estrogenic options, such as progestin-only pills or non-hormonal methods, should remain the gold standard.

Counseling should emphasize the importance of individualized contraceptive choices and address common misconceptions regarding hormonal contraception and coagulopathies. Patients should be informed about the potential for undiagnosed coagulopathies and the available screening methods to assess individual risks. Tools like the ETP-based APC resistance assay should thus be integrated into routine practice to ensure that women receive contraceptive options aligned with their thrombotic risk profiles. This tool's ability to provide actionable nAPCsr results within a defined reference range adds significant value to clinical decision-making.

Beyond clinical settings, public health initiatives must focus on raising awareness about the interplay between coagulopathies and contraceptive use. Educational campaigns should target both patients and providers, emphasizing the importance of advanced risk stratification tools and the availability of safer contraceptive alternatives. By incorporating these strategies into public health guidelines, the broader population can be empowered to make informed decisions about contraceptive use.

This patient-centered approach aligns with modern precision medicine principles, emphasizing individualized care based on a thorough understanding of a patient's unique risk factors. By integrating advanced screening tools, safer formulations like natural estrogen-based COCs, and comprehensive counseling, clinicians can improve the safety and efficacy of contraceptive choices, reducing the incidence of VTE and enhancing patient outcomes.

Declarations

Competing Interests The author(s) has no competing interests to declare that are relevant to the content of this manuscript.

Ethics Approval The author(s) declares that this manuscript does not include primary research with human participants.

The author(s) declares that this manuscript does not include primary studies involving animals.

References

1. Morimont L, Haguet H, Dogne JM, Gaspard U, Douxfils J. Combined Oral contraceptives and venous thromboembolism: review and perspective to mitigate the risk. Front Endocrinol (Lausanne). 2021;12:769187. https://doi.org/10.3389/fendo.2021.769187.
2. Barritt DW, Jordan SC. Clinical features of pulmonary embolism. Lancet. 1961;1(7180):729–32. https://doi.org/10.1016/s0140-6736(61)92891-4.
3. European Medicines Agency: Assessment report for combined hormonal contraceptives containing medicinal products — Procedure number: EMEA/H/A-31/1356. 2014. https://www.ema.europa.eu/en/documents/referral/combined-hormonal-contraceptives-article-31-referral-prac-assessment-report_en.pdf. Accessed 13 Jan 2020.
4. de Bastos M, Stegeman BH, Rosendaal FR, Van Hylckama Vlieg A, Helmerhorst FM, Stijnen T, et al. Combined oral contraceptives: venous thrombosis. Cochrane Database Syst Rev. 2014;2014(3):CD010813. https://doi.org/10.1002/14651858.CD010813.pub2.
5. Douxfils J, Morimont L, Bouvy C. Oral contraceptives and venous thromboembolism: focus on testing that may enable prediction and assessment of the risk. Semin Thromb Hemost. 2020;46(8):872–86. https://doi.org/10.1055/s-0040-1714140.
6. Meade TW, Haines AP, North WRS, Chakrabarti R, Howarth DJ, Stirling Y. Haemostatic, lipid, and blood-pressure profiles of women on oral contraceptives containing 50 μg or 30 μg oestrogen. Lancet. 1977:948–51.
7. Bonnar J. Coagulation effects of oral contraception. Am J Obstet Gynecol. 1987;157(4 Pt 2):1042–8. https://doi.org/10.1016/s0002-9378(87)80129-1.
8. Sitruk-Ware R. New progestagens for contraceptive use. Hum Reprod Update. 2006;12(2):169–78. https://doi.org/10.1093/humupd/dmi046.
9. Sitruk-Ware R. Pharmacological profile of progestins. Maturitas. 2008;61(1–2):151–7. https://doi.org/10.1016/j.maturitas.2008.11.011.
10. Lete I, Chabbert-Buffet N, Jamin C, Lello S, Lobo P, Nappi RE, et al. Haemostatic and metabolic impact of estradiol pills and drospirenone-containing ethinylestradiol pills vs. levonorgestrel-containing ethinylestradiol pills: a literature review. Eur J Contracept Reprod Health Care. 2015;20(5):329–43. https://doi.org/10.3109/13625187.2015.1050091.
11. Didembourg M, Locquet M, Raskin L, Tchimchoua BT, Dogné J-M, Beaudart C, et al. Lower reporting of venous thromboembolisms events with natural estrogen-based COCs compared to ethinylestradiol containing pills: a disproportionality analysis of the Eudravigilance database. Contraception. 2024; https://doi.org/10.1016/j.contraception.2024.110727.
12. Douxfils J, Gaspard U, Taziaux M, Jost M, Bouvy C, Lobo RA, et al. Impact of estetrol (E4) on hemostasis, metabolism and bone turnover in postmenopausal women. Climacteric. 2023;26(1):55–63. https://doi.org/10.1080/13697137.2022.2139599.
13. Douxfils J, Klipping C, Duijkers I, Kinet V, Mawet M, Maillard C, et al. Evaluation of the effect of a new oral contraceptive containing estetrol and drospirenone on hemostasis parameters. Contraception. 2020;102(6):396–402. https://doi.org/10.1016/j.contraception.2020.08.015.
14. Douxfils J, Raskin L, Didembourg M, Donis N, Dogne JM, Morimont L, et al. Are natural estrogens used in contraception at lower risk of venous thromboembolism than synthetic ones? A systematic literature review and meta-analysis. Front Endocrinol (Lausanne). 2024;15:1428597. https://doi.org/10.3389/fendo.2024.1428597.
15. Morimont L, Didembourg M, Bouvy C, Jost M, Taziaux M, Oligschlager Y, et al. Low thrombin generation in postmenopausal women using estetrol. Climacteric. 2024;27(2):193–201. https://doi.org/10.1080/13697137.2023.2292066.
16. Morimont L, Jost M, Gaspard U, Foidart JM, Dogne JM, Douxfils J. Low thrombin generation in users of a contraceptive containing Estetrol and Drospirenone. J Clin Endocrinol Metab. 2022;108(1):135–43. https://doi.org/10.1210/clinem/dgac511.
17. Klipping C, Duijkers I, Parke S, Mellinger U, Serrani M, Junge W. Hemostatic effects of a novel estradiol-based oral contraceptive: an open-label, randomized, crossover study of estradiol

valerate/dienogest versus ethinylestradiol/levonorgestrel. Drugs R&D. 2011;11(2):159–70. https://doi.org/10.2165/11591200-000000000-00000.

18. Agren UM, Anttila M, Maenpaa-Liukko K, Rantala ML, Rautiainen H, Sommer WF, et al. Effects of a monophasic combined oral contraceptive containing nomegestrol acetate and 17beta-oestradiol compared with one containing levonorgestrel and ethinylestradiol on haemostasis, lipids and carbohydrate metabolism. Eur J Contracept Reprod Health Care. 2011;16(6):444–57. https://doi.org/10.3109/13625187.2011.604450.
19. Haverinen AH, Luiro KM, Szanto T, Kangasniemi MH, Hiltunen L, Sainio S, et al. Combined oral contraceptives containing estradiol valerate vs ethinylestradiol on coagulation: a randomized clinical trial. Acta Obstet Gynecol Scand. 2022;101(10):1102–11. https://doi.org/10.1111/aogs.14428.
20. Tchaikovski SN, Thomassen MC, Costa SD, Bremme K, Rosing J. Changes in haemostatic parameters during the menstrual cycle and subsequent use of drospirenone-containing oral contraceptives. Thromb Res. 2014;134(5):1032–7. https://doi.org/10.1016/j.thromres.2014.09.008.
21. Tchaikovski SN, van Vliet HA, Thomassen MC, Bertina RM, Rosendaal FR, Sandset PM, et al. Effect of oral contraceptives on thrombin generation measured via calibrated automated thrombography. Thromb Haemost. 2007;98(6):1350–6. https://doi.org/10.1160/th07-07-0439.
22. Kuhl H. Pharmacology of estrogens and progestogens: influence of different routes of administration. Climacteric. 2005;8(Suppl 1):3–63. https://doi.org/10.1080/13697130500148875.
23. Gaussem P, Alhenc-Gelas M, Thomas JL, Bachelot-Loza C, Remones V, Ali FD, et al. Haemostatic effects of a new combined oral contraceptive, nomegestrol acetate/17beta-estradiol, compared with those of levonorgestrel/ethinyl estradiol. A double-blind, randomised study. Thromb Haemost. 2011;105(3):560–7. https://doi.org/10.1160/TH10-05-0327.
24. Junge W, Mellinger U, Parke S, Serrani M. Metabolic and haemostatic effects of estradiol valerate/dienogest, a novel oral contraceptive: a randomized, open-label, single-centre study. Clin Drug Investig. 2011;31(8):573–84. https://doi.org/10.2165/11590220-000000000-00000.
25. Kluft C, Zimmerman Y, Mawet M, Klipping C, Duijkers IJM, Neuteboom J, et al. Reduced hemostatic effects with drospirenone-based oral contraceptives containing estetrol vs. ethinyl estradiol. Contraception. 2017;95(2):140–7. https://doi.org/10.1016/j.contraception.2016.08.018.
26. Douxfils J, Morimont L, Delvigne AS, Devel P, Masereel B, Haguet H, et al. Validation and standardization of the ETP-based activated protein C resistance test for the clinical investigation of steroid contraceptives in women: an unmet clinical and regulatory need. Clinical Chemistry and Laboratory Medicine (CCLM). 2020;58(2):294–305. https://doi.org/10.1515/cclm-2019-0471.
27. Evrard J, Morimont L, Didembourg M, Haguet H, Siriez R, Dogne JM, et al. Assessment of acquired activated protein C resistance with the FibWave and comparison with the ETP-based APC resistance. Int J Lab Hematol. 2021;43(4):802–12. https://doi.org/10.1111/ijlh.13427.
28. Morimont L, Dogne JM, Douxfils J. Letter to the Editors-in-Chief in response to the article of Abou-Ismail, et al. entitled "Estrogen and thrombosis: A bench to bedside review" (Thrombosis Research 192 (2020) 40–51). Thromb Res. 2020;193:221–3. https://doi.org/10.1016/j.thromres.2020.08.006.
29. Nicolaes GA, Thomassen MC, Tans G, Rosing J, Hemker HC. Effect of activated protein C on thrombin generation and on the thrombin potential in plasma of normal and APC-resistant individuals. Blood Coagul Fibrinolysis. 1997;8(1):28–38. https://doi.org/10.1097/00001721-199701000-00006.
30. Rosing J, Middeldorp S, Curvers J, Christella M, Thomassen LG, Nicolaes GA, et al. Low-dose oral contraceptives and acquired resistance to activated protein C: a randomised cross-over study. Lancet. 1999;354(9195):2036–40. https://doi.org/10.1016/s0140-6736(99)06092-4.

31. Middeldorp S, Meijers JC, van den Ende AE, van Enk A, Bouma BN, Tans G, et al. Effects on coagulation of levonorgestrel- and desogestrel-containing low dose oral contraceptives: a cross-over study. Thromb Haemost. 2000;84(1):4–8.
32. Raps M, Rosendaal F, Ballieux B, Rosing J, Thomassen S, Helmerhorst F, et al. Resistance to APC and SHBG levels during use of a four-phasic oral contraceptive containing dienogest and estradiol valerate: a randomized controlled trial. J Thrombosis Haemostasis. 2013;11(5):855–61. https://doi.org/10.1111/jth.12172.
33. Mannucci PM, Franchini M. Classic thrombophilic gene variants. Thromb Haemost. 2015;114(5):885–9. https://doi.org/10.1160/TH15-02-0141.
34. Hotoleanu C. Genetic risk factors in venous thromboembolism. Adv Exp Med Biol. 2017;906:253–72. https://doi.org/10.1007/5584_2016_120.
35. Douxfils J, Bouvy C, Morimont L. Evaluation of activated protein C resistance using thrombin generation test. Methods Mol Biol. 2023;2663:211–24. https://doi.org/10.1007/978-1-0716-3175-1_12.
36. Morimont L, Creinin MD, Gaspard U, Foidart JM, Douxfils J. Hormonal therapies and venous thrombosis: estrogen matters! Res Pract Thromb Haemost. 2023;7(1):100021. https://doi.org/10.1016/j.rpth.2022.100021.
37. de Visser MC, van Hylckama Vlieg A, Tans G, Rosing J, Dahm AE, Sandset PM, et al. Determinants of the APTT- and ETP-based APC sensitivity tests. J Thrombosis Haemostasis. 2005;3(7):1488–94. https://doi.org/10.1111/j.1538-7836.2005.01430.x.
38. Kobayashi T, Hirayama M, Nogami M, Meguro K, Iiduka M, Foidart JM, et al. Impact of Estetrol combined with Drospirenone on blood coagulation and fibrinolysis in patients with endometriosis: a multicenter, randomized, open-label, active-controlled, parallel-group study. Clin Appl Thromb Hemost. 2024;30:10760296241286514. https://doi.org/10.1177/10760296241286514.
39. Gerard C, Arnal JF, Jost M, Douxfils J, Lenfant F, Fontaine C, et al. Profile of estetrol, a promising native estrogen for oral contraception and the relief of climacteric symptoms of menopause. Expert Rev Clin Pharmacol. 2022;15(2):121–37. https://doi.org/10.1080/17512433.2022.2054413.
40. Bagot CN, Marsh MS, Whitehead M, Sherwood R, Roberts L, Patel RK, et al. The effect of estrone on thrombin generation may explain the different thrombotic risk between oral and transdermal hormone replacement therapy. J Thrombosis Haemostasis. 2010;8(8):1736–44. https://doi.org/10.1111/j.1538-7836.2010.03953.x.
41. Douxfils J, Morimont L, Creinin MD, Gaspard U, Foidart JM. Hormonal therapies and venous thrombosis: considerations for prevention and management-a reappraisal. Res Pract Thromb Haemost. 2023;7(4):100155. https://doi.org/10.1016/j.rpth.2023.100155.
42. Douxfils J, Morimont L, Gaspard U, Utian WH, Foidart JM. Estetrol is not a SERM but a NEST and has a specific safety profile on coagulation. Thromb Res. 2023;232:148–50. https://doi.org/10.1016/j.thromres.2022.09.007.
43. Foidart JM, Simon K, Utian WH, Mauvais-Jarvis F, Douxfils J, Dixon G, et al. Estetrol is safe and well tolerated during treatment of hospitalized men and women with moderate COVID-19 in a randomized, double-blind study. J Clin Med. 2023;12(12):3928. https://doi.org/10.3390/jcm12123928.
44. Morimont L, Donis N, Bouvy C, Mullier F, Dogne JM, Douxfils J. Laboratory testing for the evaluation of phenotypic activated protein C resistance. Semin Thromb Hemost. 2022;48(6):680–9. https://doi.org/10.1055/s-0042-1753511.
45. Reda S, Morimont L, Douxfils J, Ruhl H. Can we measure the individual Prothrombotic or Prohemorrhagic tendency by global coagulation tests? Hamostaseologie. 2020;40(3):364–78. https://doi.org/10.1055/a-1153-5824.
46. Food and Drug Administration: Combined Hormonal Contraceptives (CHCs) and the Risk of Cardiovascular Disease Endpoints – CHC-CVD final report 111022v2. 2011. https://www.fda.gov/media/82335/download. Accessed 26 Dec 2019.

47. Lidegaard O, Skovlund CW, Nielsen LH. FC3–19 Thrombotic diseases in users of estradiol/dienogest oral contraceptives: a historical national follow-up study 2009–2011. Eur J Contracept Reprod Health Care. 2013;18:S75.
48. Dinger J, Do Minh T, Heinemann K. Impact of estrogen type on cardiovascular safety of combined oral contraceptives. Contraception. 2016;94(4):328–39. https://doi.org/10.1016/j.contraception.2016.06.010.
49. Reed S, Koro C, DiBello J, Becker K, Bauerfeind A, Franke C, et al. Prospective controlled cohort study on the safety of a monophasic oral contraceptive containing nomegestrol acetate (2.5mg) and 17beta-oestradiol (1.5mg) (PRO-E2 study): risk of venous and arterial thromboembolism. Eur J Contracept Reprod Health Care. 2021;26(6):439–46. https://doi.org/10.1080/13625187.2021.1987410.
50. Schink T, Princk C, Braitmaier M, Haug U. Use of combined oral contraceptives and risk of venous thromboembolism in young women: a nested case-control analysis using German claims data. BJOG. 2022;129(13):2107–16. https://doi.org/10.1111/1471-0528.17268.
51. Heikinheimo O, Toffol E, Partonen T, But A, Latvala A, Haukka J. Systemic hormonal contraception and risk of venous thromboembolism. Acta Obstet Gynecol Scand. 2022;101(8):846–55. https://doi.org/10.1111/aogs.14384.
52. Bauerfeind A, von Stockum S, Boehnke T, Heinemann K. Venous thromboembolic risk of estradiol Valerate-Dienogest compared with Ethinyl estradiol-Levonorgestrel combined oral contraceptives. Obstet Gynecol. 2024;143(3):431–4. https://doi.org/10.1097/AOG.0000000000005509.
53. Vinogradova Y, Coupland C, Hippisley-Cox J. Use of combined oral contraceptives and risk of venous thromboembolism: nested case-control studies using the QResearch and CPRD databases. BMJ. 2015;350(may26 13):h2135. https://doi.org/10.1136/bmj.h2135.
54. Kiri VA. A pathway to improved prospective observational post-authorization safety studies. Drug Saf. 2012;35(9):711–24. https://doi.org/10.1007/BF03261968.
55. European Medicines Agency: Guideline on good pharmacovigilance practices (GVP) — Module VIII—Post-authorisation safety studies (Rev 3) — EMA/813938/2011 Rev 3*. 2017. https://www.ema.europa.eu/en/documents/scientific-guideline/guideline-good-pharmacovigilance-practices-gvp-module-viii-post-authorisation-safety-studies-rev-3_en.pdf. Accessed 3 Oct 2024.
56. Klipping C, Duijkers I, Mawet M, Maillard C, Bastidas A, Jost M, et al. Endocrine and metabolic effects of an oral contraceptive containing estetrol and drospirenone. Contraception. 2021;103(4):213–21. https://doi.org/10.1016/j.contraception.2021.01.001.
57. Gemzell-Danielsson K, Apter D, Zatik J, Weyers S, Piltonen T, Suturina L, et al. Estetrol-Drospirenone combination oral contraceptive: a clinical study of contraceptive efficacy, bleeding pattern and safety in Europe and Russia. BJOG. 2022;129(1):63–71. https://doi.org/10.1111/1471-0528.16840.
58. Creinin MD, Westhoff CL, Bouchard C, Chen MJ, Jensen JT, Kaunitz AM, et al. Estetrol-drospirenone combination oral contraceptive: North American phase 3 efficacy and safety results. Contraception. 2021;104(3):222–8. https://doi.org/10.1016/j.contraception.2021.05.002.
59. Chen MJ, Jensen JT, Kaunitz AM, Achilles SL, Zatik J, Weyers S, et al. Tolerability and safety of the estetrol/drospirenone combined oral contraceptive: pooled analysis of two multicenter, open-label phase 3 trials. Contraception. 2022;116:44–50. https://doi.org/10.1016/j.contraception.2022.10.004.
60. European Medicines Agency: Guideline on the use of statistical signal detection methods in the Eudravigilance Data Analysis System. 2007. https://www.ema.europa.eu/en/documents/regulatory-procedural-guideline/draft-guideline-use-statistical-signal-detection-methods-eudravigilance-data-analysis-system_en.pdf. Accessed 1 May 2024.
61. Creinin MD, Douxfils J, Beaudart C, Foidart J-M. Errors in the use of the FAERS database to assess the safety of Yasmin. Eur J Obstet Gynecol Reprod Biol. 2024; https://doi.org/10.1016/j.ejogrb.2024.10.053.

62. Skouby SO, Sidelmann JJ. Impact of progestogens on hemostasis. Horm Mol Biol Clin Investig. 2018;37(2) https://doi.org/10.1515/hmbci-2018-0041.
63. Regidor PA, Colli E, Schindler AE. Drospirenone as estrogen-free pill and hemostasis: coagulatory study results comparing a novel 4 mg formulation in a 24 + 4 cycle with desogestrel 75 mug per day. Gynecol Endocrinol. 2016;32(9):749–51. https://doi.org/10.3109/09513590.2016.1161743.
64. Lidegaard O, Nielsen LH, Skovlund CW, Skjeldestad FE, Lokkegaard E. Risk of venous thromboembolism from use of oral contraceptives containing different progestogens and oestrogen doses: Danish cohort study, 2001-9. BMJ. 2011;343:d6423. https://doi.org/10.1136/bmj.d6423.
65. Callegari LS, Zhao X, Schwarz EB, Rosenfeld E, Mor MK, Borrero S. Racial/ethnic differences in contraceptive preferences, beliefs, and self-efficacy among women veterans. Am J Obstet Gynecol. 2017;216(5):504.e1–e10. https://doi.org/10.1016/j.ajog.2016.12.178.
66. Fiebig DG, Knox S, Viney R, Haas M, Street DJ. Preferences for new and existing contraceptive products. Health Econ. 2011;20(Suppl 1):35–52. https://doi.org/10.1002/hec.1686.
67. Weisberg E, Bateson D, Knox S, Haas M, Viney R, Street D, et al. Do women and providers value the same features of contraceptive products? Results of a best-worst stated preference experiment. Eur J Contracept Reprod Health Care. 2013;18(3):181–90. https://doi.org/10.3109/13625187.2013.777830.
68. Cardona C, Sarnak D, Gemmill A, Gichangi P, Thiongo M, Anglewicz P. Are contraceptive method preferences stable? Measuring change in the preferred method among Kenyan women. Stud Fam Plan. 2024;55(3):193–214. https://doi.org/10.1111/sifp.12271.
69. Masini I, Frisch E, Andary R, McCallum E, Steller J, Patel J. Contraceptive-Induced Amenorrhea: Perceptions among a reproductive-age urban Southern California population. Contraception. 2023;127 https://doi.org/10.1016/j.contraception.2023.110229.
70. Dam A, Yeh PT, Burke AE, Kennedy CE. Contraceptive values and preferences of pregnant women, postpartum women, women seeking emergency contraceptives, and women seeking abortion services: a systematic review. Contraception. 2022;111:39–47. https://doi.org/10.1016/j.contraception.2021.10.007.
71. Hugon-Rodin J, Horellou MH, Conard J, Gompel A, Plu-Bureau G. Type of combined contraceptives, factor V Leiden mutation and risk of venous thromboembolism. Thromb Haemost. 2018;118(5):922–8. https://doi.org/10.1055/s-0038-1641152.
72. Khialani D, le Cessie S, Lijfering WM, Cannegieter SC, Rosendaal FR, van Hylckama Vlieg A. The joint effect of genetic risk factors and different types of combined oral contraceptives on venous thrombosis risk. Br J Haematol. 2020;191(1):90–7. https://doi.org/10.1111/bjh.16666.
73. Morimont L, Didembourg M, Haguet H, Modaffari E, Tillier M, Bouvy C, et al. Interlaboratory variability of activated protein C resistance using the ETP-based APC resistance assay. Res Pract Thromb Haemost. 2021;5(7):e12612. https://doi.org/10.1002/rth2.12612.
74. Morimont L. Hormone-induced coagulopathy – evaluation of the prothrombotic state using a global coagulation assay. Department of Pharmacy. Presses universitaires de Namur & Laure MORIMONT: University of Namur; 2023.
75. Meade TW, Haines AP, North WR, Chakrabarti R, Howarth DJ, Stirling Y. Haemostatic, lipid, and blood-pressure profiles of women on oral contraceptives containing 50 microgram or 30 microgram oestrogen. Lancet. 1977;2(8045):948–51. https://doi.org/10.1016/s0140-6736(77)90888-1.
76. Task Force on Oral Contraceptive. A multicentre study of coagulation and haemostatic variables during oral contraception: variations with four formulations. BJOG Int J Obstet Gynaecol. 2005;98(11):1117–28. https://doi.org/10.1111/j.1471-0528.1991.tb15364.x.
77. Melis GB, Fruzzetti F, Nicoletti I, Ricci C, Lammers P, Atsma WJ, et al. A comparative study on the effects of a monophasic pill containing desogestrel plus 20 ug ethinylestradiol, a triphasic combination containing levonorgestrel and a monophasic combination containing gestodene on coagulatory factors. Contraception. 1991;43:23–31.

78. Quehenberger P, Kapiotis S, Partan C, Schneider B, Wenzel R, Gaiger A, et al. Studies on oral contraceptive-induced changes in blood coagulation and fibrinolysis and the estrogen effect on endothelial cells. Ann Hematol. 1993;67(1):33–6. https://doi.org/10.1007/BF01709663.
79. Basdevant A, Conard J, Pelissier C, Guyene TT, Lapousterle C, Mayer M, et al. Hemostatic and metabolic effects of lowering the ethinyl-estradiol dose from 30 mcg to 20 mcg in oral contraceptives containing desogestrel. Contraception. 1993;48(3):193–204. https://doi.org/10.1016/0010-7824(93)90141-s.
80. Cachrimanidou AC, Hellberg D, Nilsson S, von Schoulz B, Crona N, Siegbahn A. Hemostasis profile and lipid metabolism with long-interval use of a desogestrel-containing oral contraceptive. Contraception. 1994;50(2):153–65. https://doi.org/10.1016/0010-7824(94)90051-5.
81. Norris LA, Bonnar J. The effect of oestrogen dose and progestogen type on haemostatic changes in women taking low dose oral contraceptives. Br J Obstet Gynaecol. 1996;103(3):261–7. https://doi.org/10.1111/j.1471-0528.1996.tb09716.x.
82. Oral C, Hemostasis Study G. The effects of seven monophasic oral contraceptive regimens on hemostatic variables: conclusions from a large randomized multicenter study. Contraception. 2003;67(3):173–85. https://doi.org/10.1016/s0010-7824(02)00476-6.
83. Endrikat J, Klipping C, Gerlinger C, Ruebig A, Schimdt W, Holler T, et al. A double-blind comparative study of the effects of a 23-day oral contraceptive regimen with 20 ug ethinyl estradiol and 75 ug gestodene and a 21-day regimen with 30 ug ethinyl estradiol and 75 ug gestodene on hemostatic variables, lipids, and carbohydrate metabolism. Contraception. 2001;64:235–41.
84. Alhenc-Gelas M, Plu-Bureau G, Guillonneau S, Kirzin JM, Aiach M, Ochat N, et al. Impact of progestagens on activated protein C (APC) resistance among users of oral contraceptives. J Thrombosis Haemostasis. 2004;2(9):1594–600. https://doi.org/10.1111/j.1538-7836.2004.00894.x.
85. Jespersen J, Endrikat J, Dusterberg B, Schmidt W, Gerlinger C, Wessel J, et al. A 1-year study to compare the hemostatic effects of oral contraceptive containing 20 microg of ethinylestradiol and 100 microg of levonorgestrel with 30 microg of ethinylestradiol and 100 microg of levonorgestrel. Contraception. 2005;72(2):98–104. https://doi.org/10.1016/j.contraception.2005.01.006.
86. Klipping C, Marr J. Effects of two combined oral contraceptives containing ethinyl estradiol 20 microg combined with either drospirenone or desogestrel on lipids, hemostatic parameters and carbohydrate metabolism. Contraception. 2005;71(6):409–16. https://doi.org/10.1016/j.contraception.2004.12.005.
87. Kluft C, Endrikat J, Mulder SM, Gerlinger C, Heithecker R. A prospective study on the effects on hemostasis of two oral contraceptives containing drospirenone in combination with either 30 or 20 microg ethinyl estradiol and a reference containing desogestrel and 30 microg ethinyl estradiol. Contraception. 2006;73(4):336–43. https://doi.org/10.1016/j.contraception.2005.09.015.
88. Oslakovic S, Zadro R. Comparison of the impact of four generations of progestins on hemostatic variables. Clin Appl Thrombosis/Hemostasis. 2014;20(4):448–55. https://doi.org/10.1177/1076029612463426.
89. Nappi RE, Paoletti AM, Volpe A, Chiovato L, Howard B, Weiss H, et al. Multinational, multicentre, randomised, open-label study evaluating the impact of a 91-day extended regimen combined oral contraceptive, compared with two 28-day traditional combined oral contraceptives, on haemostatic parameters in healthy women. Eur J Contracept Reprod Health Care. 2014;19(4):285–94. https://doi.org/10.3109/13625187.2014.918596.
90. Kemmeren JM, Algra A, Meijers JC, Bouma BN, Grobbee DE. Effects of second and third generation oral contraceptives and their respective progestagens on the coagulation system in the absence or presence of the factor V Leiden mutation. Thromb Haemost. 2002;87(2):199–205.
91. Winkler UH, Howie H, Buhler K, Korver T, Geurts TB, Coelingh Bennink HJ. A randomized controlled double-blind study of the effects on hemostasis of two progestogen-only

pills containing 75 microgram desogestrel or 30 microgram levonorgestrel. Contraception. 1998;57(6):385–92. https://doi.org/10.1016/s0010-7824(98)00045-6.
92. Oral Contraceptive and Hemostasis Study Group. An open label, randomized study to evaluate the effects of seven monophasic oral contraceptive regimens on hemostatic variables. Outline of the protocol. Oral Contraceptive and Hemostasis Study Group. Contraception. 1999;59(6):345–55. https://doi.org/10.1016/s0010-7824(99)00044-x.
93. Archer D, Mammen E, Grubb G. The effects of a low-dose monophasic preparation of levonorgestrel and ethinyl estradiol on coagulation and other hemostatic factor. Am J Obstet Gynecol. 1999;181:63–6.
94. Blanco-Molina MA, Lozano M, Cano A, Cristobal I, Pallardo LP, Lete I. Progestin-only contraception and venous thromboembolism. Thromb Res. 2012;129(5):e257–62. https://doi.org/10.1016/j.thromres.2012.02.042.
95. Ferreira AC, Montes MB, Franceschini SA, Toloi MR. Effects of two oral contraceptives, containing 30 or 20 microg of ethinyl estradiol in combination with gestodene, on blood coagulation and fibrinolysis in Brazilian women. Int J Fertil Womens Med. 2001;46(5):265–70.
96. van Hylckama Vlieg A, van der Linden IK, Bertina RM, Rosendaal FR. High levels of factor IX increase the risk of venous thrombosis. Blood. 2000;95(12):3678–82.
97. Adam A, Albert A, Boulanger J, Genot D, Demoulin A, Damas J. Influence of oral contraceptives and pregnancy on constituents of the kallikrein-kininogen system in plasma. Clin Chem. 1985;31(9):1533–6.
98. Jespersen J, Kluft C. Increased euglobulin fibrinolytic potential in women on oral contraceptives low in oestrogen–levels of extrinsic and intrinsic plasminogen activators, prekallikrein, factor XII, and C1-inactivator. Thromb Haemost. 1985;54(2):454–9.
99. Hoem NO, Johannesen S, Hauge G, Rud AC, Sandem S, Briseid K. Contact activation factors in plasma from women using oral contraceptives–increased levels of factor XII, kinin-free high molecular weight kininogen and acetone-activated kallikrein. Thromb Res. 1991;64(4):427–34. https://doi.org/10.1016/0049-3848(91)90343-u.
100. Winkler UH, Schindler AE, Endrikat J, Dusterberg B. A comparative study of the effects of the hemostatic system of two monophasic gestodene oral contraceptives containing 20 micrograms and 30 micrograms ethinylestradiol. Contraception. 1996;53(2):75–84. https://doi.org/10.1016/0010-7824(95)00271-5.
101. Fruzzetti F, Genazzani AR, Ricci C, De Negri F, Bersi C, Carmassi F. A 12-month clinical investigation with a 24-day regimen containing 15 ug ethinylestradiol plus 60 ug gestodene with respect to hemostasis and cycle control. Contraception. 2001;63:303–7.
102. Jespersen J, Petersen KR, Skouby SO. Effects of newer oral contraceptives on the inhibition of coagulation and fibrinolysis in relation to dosage and type of steroid. Am J Obstet Gynecol. 1990;163(1 Pt 2):396–403. https://doi.org/10.1016/0002-9378(90)90590-4.
103. Aldrighi JM, De Campos LS, Eluf Gebara OC, Petta CA, Bahamondes L. Effect of a combined oral contraceptive containing 20 microg ethinyl estradiol and 75 microg gestodene on hemostatic parameters. Gynecol Endocrinol. 2006;22(1):1–4. https://doi.org/10.1080/09513590500430328.
104. van Vliet HA, Bertina RM, Dahm AE, Rosendaal FR, Rosing J, Sandset PM, et al. Different effects of oral contraceptives containing different progestogens on protein S and tissue factor pathway inhibitor. J Thrombosis Haemostasis. 2008;6(2):346–51. https://doi.org/10.1111/j.1538-7836.2008.02863.x.
105. Raps M, Helmerhorst FM, Fleischer K, Dahm AE, Rosendaal FR, Rosing J, et al. The effect of different hormonal contraceptives on plasma levels of free protein S and free TFPI. Thromb Haemost. 2013;109(4):606–13. https://doi.org/10.1160/TH12-10-0771.
106. Henkens CM, Bom VJ, Seinen AJ, van der Meer J. Sensitivity to activated protein C; influence of oral contraceptives and sex. Thromb Haemost. 1995;73(3):402–4.
107. Kamphuisen PW, Rosendaal FR, Eikenboom JC, Bos R, Bertina RM. Factor V antigen levels and venous thrombosis: risk profile, interaction with factor V Leiden, and relation with

factor VIII antigen levels. Arterioscler Thromb Vasc Biol. 2000;20(5):1382–6. https://doi.org/10.1161/01.atv.20.5.1382.
108. Raps M, Helmerhorst F, Fleischer K, Thomassen S, Rosendaal F, Rosing J, et al. Sex hormone-binding globulin as a marker for the thrombotic risk of hormonal contraceptives. J Thrombosis Haemostasis. 2012;10(6):992–7. https://doi.org/10.1111/j.1538-7836.2012.04720.x.
109. Meijers JC, Middeldorp S, Tekelenburg W, van den Ende AE, Tans G, Prins MH, et al. Increased fibrinolytic activity during use of oral contraceptives is counteracted by an enhanced factor XI-independent down regulation of fibrinolysis: a randomized cross-over study of two low-dose oral contraceptives. Thromb Haemost. 2000;84(1):9–14.
110. Peters K, Gordon N, Ricciotti N, Hsieh J, Howard B, Weiss H. Hemostatic effects of two desogestrel-containing combined oral contraceptive regimens: a multinational, multicenter, randomized, open-label study. Clin Exp Obstet Gynecol. 2016;43(3):334–40.
111. Heit JA, Kobbervig CE, James AH, Petterson TM, Bailey KR, Melton LJ III. Trends in the incidence of venous thromboembolism during pregnancy or postpartum: a 30-years-based study. Ann Intern Med. 2005;143:697–706.
112. European Medicines Agency: Combined hormonal contraceptive (CHC)—chiormadinone acetate/ethinylestradiol Slightly increased risk of venous thromboembolism in women using chlormadinone acetate and ethinylestradiol containing combined hormonal contraceptives. 2024. https://www.aifa.gov.it/documents/20142/2254729/2024.03.22_NII_clormardinone-acetato-etinilestradiolo_EN.pdf. Accessed 6 Nov 2024.
113. Dinger JC, Bardenheuer K, Assmann A. International active surveillance study of women taking oral contraceptives (INAS-OC study). BMC Med Res Methodol. 2009;9(1):77. https://doi.org/10.1186/1471-2288-9-77.

Chapter 12
Effects of Combined Hormonal Contraception (CHC) on Bone and Collagen

Mark P. Brincat and Joel Pollacco

12.1 Introduction

Since its inception in the 1960s, the combined oral contraceptive (COC) pill and its subsequent derivative formulations such as the combined contraceptive vaginal ring (CCVR) and the combined contraceptive patch (CCP) have been used by millions of women worldwide [1–8]. Combined hormonal contraception (CHC) has been largely effective at avoiding unplanned pregnancies and is used to this effect, especially by women of young age, particularly in women requiring long-term commitment to arduous jobs such as military service women [9–11]. The COCP is increasingly being also used for its added non-contraceptive health benefits such as reduced menstrual bleeding and pain [7, 12]. This is especially true for young women engaging in strenuous physical activity on a daily basis such as athletes [3, 7, 11, 13, 14].

Bone is metabolically active tissue made of composite material. It is composed of structural proteins such as the collagens that impart it with its tensile strength and mineral content such as calcium phosphate and hydroxyapatite that confer it with compressive strength [4]. Different types of collagen are also found in other connective tissues such as muscle and skin. Bone [15–18] and muscle [18, 19] are all sensitive to estrogen meaning that combined hormonal contraception can exert either a

M. P. Brincat (✉)
Department of Obstetrics and Gynaecology, Faculty of Medicine and Surgery, University of Malta, Msida, Malta

Barts School of Medicine and Dentistry, Queen Mary University of London, Malta Campus, Gozo, Malta

J. Pollacco
Department of Obstetrics and Gynaecology, Faculty of Medicine and Surgery, University of Malta, Msida, Malta

A. R. Genazzani et al. (eds.), *Ethical, Efficacy and Safety Issues in Contraception*, Reproductive Medicine for Clinicians 4,
https://doi.org/10.1007/978-3-032-07322-8_12

beneficial or a harmful effect on these organs. This chapter aims to review the current state of evidence on the effects of combined hormonal contraception on bone and muscle.

12.2 CHC and Bone

12.2.1 An Overview of Bone Structure

Bone is a composite living tissue made up of organic matrix, an inorganic substance, as well as bone cells. The inorganic substance, which constitutes up to 70% of bone composition, consists of mineral material in the form of phosphates and hydroxyapatites, whereas the organic matrix is made up of complex protein structures such as collagen. Type I collagen makes up 90% of the organic matrix with the remaining 10% consisting of non-collagenous proteins such as glycosaminoglycans [4, 5].

The cellular component of bone is made up of three distinct types of cells, osteoblasts, osteocytes, and osteoclasts. The osteoblasts are the cells responsible for bone formation, whereas osteoclasts are responsible for resorption. Osteocytes are mature osteoblasts. In mature adult life, the bone responds to mechanical stresses, by undergoing bone formation in one part and bone resorption in another, such that the extent and magnitude of bone formation and resorption equal each other, not to result in net loss of bone content. This is called bone remodelling [3, 4, 20, 21]. In young adolescent women, there is more osteoblastic activity than osteoclastic activity as these patients are still in the process of accruing their peak bone mass (PBM). This is called bone modelling [21].

12.2.2 The Interplay of Female Sex Steroid Hormones with Bone

The exact mechanism by which estrogen exerts its action still has not yet been fully elucidated. Estrogen has a direct action on bone tissue by upregulating bone formation through the stimulation of osteoblastogenesis, while decreasing bone resorption by inducing osteoclast apoptosis [4, 22]. The increase in osteoblastogenesis and decrease in osteoclastolysis are partly achieved through modulation of the cytokine environment, leading to reduced NF-kB activity, inhibition of production of pro-osteoclastic cytokines such as IL-6 and IL-7, blocking of the RANK-L ligand activation of the osteoclasts, as well as TGF-ß signaling upregulation [4, 22–24]. Progesterone seems to exert its action on bone by its varying interplay on the glucocorticoid, androgen, or mineralocorticoid receptors [4].

12.2.3 Estrogen and Osteoporosis

The accrual of PBM is highly important as it prevents the development of osteoporotic disease later in life [15, 24–29]. This is partly achieved by the presence of endogenous estrogens in eumenorrheic post-menarchal females. Conversely, the risk of osteoporosis can be increased in older peri-menopausal females, as a result of low endogenous estrogens, at this life cycle stage [24].

12.2.4 Outcomes of Studies Evaluating Effect of CHC on Bone

One of the most readily available objective ways of quantifying bone mineralization is through bone densitometry. Derangements in bone metabolic activity such as the altered remodelling states associated with the lack or presence of estrogen is best characterized by bone histomorphometric studies [11]. However, in the absence of practicality to perform such tests, the acceptable alternative would be to use serum metabolites of markers of bone formation and resorption. These are termed bone turnover markers. The most commonly used bone-turnover markers are the carboxyterminal cross-linking telo-peptide of type I collagen (ß-CTX) as the marker of bone formation and procollagen type I N propeptide (PINP) as the bone formation marker [30]. These same bone turnover markers are indeed those that are recommended for use in clinical studies by the International Osteoporosis Foundation (IOF) and the International Federation of Clinical Chemistry (IFCC) [31]. They also advise to collect PINP samples during the early follicular phase as PINP levels tend to be falsely higher in the luteal phase [32], even though Martin et al. [30] did not find any significant differences in variations of the same bone turnover markers along different phases of the menstrual cycle.

12.2.5 The Effect of CHC on Bone in Young Females

There is still ongoing controversy with regard to the effect of CHCs on bone mineral density (BMD) as well as bone turnover markers (BTMs) with some studies showing no effect, while others showing either a negative or a positive effect. Lopez et al. [33] performed a systematic review to evaluate the effect of steroid hormonal contraceptives on the risk of bone fractures as well as measures of BMD or BTMs. In their systematic review, they analyze a total of 11 randomized controlled trials (RCTs) comparing CHCs and conclude that COCs do not seem to negatively affect bone density. However, there was huge heterogeneity in methodology of the trials included in the systematic review as well as in outcome reporting such as to preclude any meta-analysis.

This is in contrast to a previous systematic review by Liu and Lebrun [3], which reported a fair evidence for a positive effect of OCs on BMD in oligo/amenorrheic premenopausal women, supported by 7 out of 10 studies, followed by limited evidence of a positive effect of CHC on BMD in anorexic pre-menopausal women and healthy pre-menopausal women. In contrast with Lopez et al. [33], Liu and Lebrun include observational studies in addition to RCTs, therefore any conclusions reached could have been affected by the biases inherent to an observational study design.

There is an increasing drive for pharmaceutical companies to introduce ultra-low dose estrogen-containing COCs into the market [34] because of the increased benefits in terms of decreased risk of venous thrombo-embolism (VTE) [35] as well as the decreased risk of consequences of hepatic stimulation such as increased triglycerides. The combined oral contraceptive pill works by inhibiting the hypothalamo-pituitary-ovarian (HPO) axis, hence suppressing endogenous estrogen production [28, 36]. The consequent lack of estrogen in these patients might be detrimental especially in young women, who have not yet reached their PBM, resulting in increased bone resorption and subsequently decreased bone density [1, 26].

Out of the 13 RCTs, included in the systematic review by Lopez et al. [33], only 2 actually compared just differing doses of ethinylestradiol on BMD and BTM changes. Paoletti et al. [37] found a statistically significant decrease in urinary pyridinoline (PYR) and deoxypyridinoline (D-PYR), from 6 to 12 months in women taking both the 20 μg ethinylestradiol pill and those taking the 30-μg ethinylestradiol pill compared to baseline and controls, indicating decreased bone resorption with COC consumption. There were no significant differences between the two COC groups. Gargano et al. [29] perform a similar study to Paoletti et al., but use 3 mg drospirenone (DRSP) as the progestogenic component of the COC instead of 75 μg gestodene and they also include lumbar spine bone mineral density as an outcome in addition to 3 monthly BTM measurements. They report statistically significant evidence of decreased bone resorption from the sixth month onward for each treatment group compared to baseline and controls. There were no significant changes in bone density measurements in either treatment or control groups. The results obtained in both Gargano and Lopez could have been influenced by the fact that the participants included in the studies most likely had already achieved their peak bone mass, while the progestogenic component of the COC could have confounded the estrogenic effect on bone metabolism [29, 37].

There were two similar studies performed by Nappi et al. [34, 36] that confirmed the same results obtained by Gargano et al. However, one study [36] compared two COC regimens with differing doses of both ethinylestradiol (EE) and gestodene and the other study [34] compared two 30-μg ethinylestradiol pills with a different type of progestogen.

Conversely, no changes to bone density measurements were achieved in a 3-year double-blind randomized controlled study by Endrikat et al., [38], in which participants were randomized to treatment groups of 20 μg EE/100 μg levonorgestrel (LNG) or 30 μg EE/150 μg LNG. However, no significant findings could have been the result of direct comparison between the treatment groups as there was no reference control group in this study.

In a three-arm parallel design RCT study performed by Gersten et al. [39], 12- to 18-year-old adolescents were randomized to a 91-day extended regimen of levonorgestrel/ethinylestradiol or 28-day cyclical cycles of levonorgestrel/ethinylestradiol. Results showed no statistically significant differences between the extended regimens and controls; however, the cyclical regimen users had statistically significant smaller increases in BMD than controls, suggesting increased resorption, resulting in more difficulty to achieve their PBM. Rad et al. [40] also compare the effect of a continuous versus a cyclic regimen on BTMs but unlike, Gersten et al. find no significant difference. This could be because of the small numbers of recruited study participants as well as the large age range of 18–49, as opposed to Gersten et al., which recruit a study population < 20 years of age.

In Cibula et al. [41], the age group of the recruited study participants like Gersten et al. is limited to the under 20 and their study also reveals a negative bone density effect on the participants' bone densities. They do a crossover study in which study participants are randomized to a treatment group of 30 μg EE/75 μg gestodene and another group of 15 μg EE/60 μg gestodene, followed by switching treatment at 9 months, followed by another 9 months of treatment. Their findings confer impaired increased BMD in the 15 μg ethinylestradiol group as compared to the 30 μg one, suggesting impairment to attain peak bone density with the ultra-low dose estrogen COCs. Unfortunately, having the two COC regimens with a different dose progestogen hampers interpretation of the result, as to whether this is attributable to the different dose of estrogen or progestogen. A systematic review reporting on the effect of COCs on a number of health determinants including BMD in females under 18 years of age concluded that it is still unclear as to whether COCs have a negative impact on BMD [42]. This could be partly attributed to differences in design and observation of the individual studies showing minimal increase in BMD for the COC users [42].

Sørdal et al. [43] also report no significant differences in bone density outcomes between the treatment groups. However, this study is a two-arm comparison between completely different monophasic oral contraceptive regimens with a 24/4 regimen of COC of 2.5 mg nomogestrel/1.5 mg estradiol and a 21/7 day regimen of 150 mg levonorgestrel/30 mg ethinylestradiol as comparator. Gai et al. [7] report no statistically significant results and use a three-arm parallel comparison study design between two treatment groups and a control. However, they change both the type of progestogen in the COC and the ethinylestradiol dose, making interpretation of the results difficult as to whether those should be attributed to the former or the latter.

Hartard et al. [44] also recruit a relatively young age group of study participants (18–24 years of age); however, they use a three-arm parallel RCT design to compare the effect of two different COC regimens containing different progestogens on bone mineral density. In their conclusions, they remark that the vertebral BMD loss witnessed in the treatment group of the desogestrel-containing COC could be due to the weaker androgenic activity of desogestrel as opposed to levonorgestrel. In Berenson et al. [45], two COC regimens were compared as comparators together with a control group not on any hormonal contraception to a group of women on depot medroxyprogesterone acetate injection. In this study, users of COCs sustained a gain in lumbar spine BMD as opposed to DMPA users and controls.

The results obtained from the RCTs recruiting an adolescent population less than 20 years of age [39, 41, 44] seem to be consistent with a non-randomized study by Biason et al. [26] as well as a number of observational studies. Biason et al. [26] report a statistically significant decreased bone mineral content (BMC) acquisition in adolescent COC users as opposed to non-COC users after 1 year of follow-up. Polatti et al. [46] recruited 100 women assigned to a group receiving a monophasic oral contraceptive pill containing 20 µg ethinylestradiol and another 100 women not on any hormonal treatment as controls and followed these up for 5 years. The control group had a statistically significant increase in BMD at 5 years of follow-up compared to that of the COC group, showing that the COC most likely impaired adequate accrual of PBM in these adolescents. Similar results were also reported in another observational study by Shoepe et al. [27], in which non-COC users had 1.0%–2.6% greater BMD at the spine, 0.8%–1.8% greater BMD at the hip, and 1.1% greater whole body BMD, compared to COC users with an EE-containing COC varying between 20 and 35 µg. The study followed a relatively young population of 18–25 years and with a mean use of contraception of 3.3 years and yielded statistically significant results with a p-value <0.01, suggesting that low-dose estradiol COCs could play a role in preventing development of PBM in these adolescents. Almstedt et al. [2] find statistically significant decrease in BMD measurements at the lateral spine following the 12-month period in COC users as opposed to controls. However, these could be spurious findings resulting from the low participant numbers and the observational nature of the study. Conversely, four observational studies report a decrease in COC users of both bone formation BTMs and resorption BTMs, rendering interpretation of these findings somewhat confusing [5, 25, 47, 48].

12.2.6 Other CHC Formulations and BMD

One RCT evaluated urinary PYR and urinary D-PYR as markers of bone resorption in the CCVR users, CCP users, and controls [49] and found out that the CCVR and CCP reduced these bone resorption markers in a statistically significant manner compared to baseline and controls, implying a beneficial effect of these formulations on bone health.

12.2.7 The Effect of CHC on Bone in Peri-menopausal Females

In older women, contraception is mostly limited to the peri-menopausal age. Hence, there have been few studies that actually studied the influence of oral contraception on BMD and BTMs in such an aging population. Unlike in younger females, most of the studies seem to be at consensus that CHC tends to have a positive impact on bone health [3, 50, 51]. Liu and Lebrun [3] report good evidence being supported by 8 out of 11 studies, implying a positive effect of CHC on BMD in peri-menopausal females. These findings are further supported by a study by Gambacciani et al. [50], where spine BMD was increased at 12-month and 24 month follow-up periods, compared to age-matched peri-menopausal females that were eumenorrheic on no treatment or oligomenorrheic and on calcium supplements. A retrospective case–control study by Dombrowski et al. [51] is also in keeping with these findings. In this study, a cohort of 12,970 women having a mean age of 37.8 years was examined and those not having sustained bone fractures were found to be more likely to have been on oral contraception, suggesting that oral contraception has an important role in decreasing the age-related bone mass decline and hence preventing osteoporotic fractures.

All these findings seem to be consistent with a larger body of evidence that shows that the estrogen in HRT tends to have a beneficial effect in improving bone density of the lumbar spine and femoral neck in post-menopausal women [52–54] and reduction in cortical bone loss in post-menopausal females tends to be estrogen-dose-dependent [55]. There is also a witnessed improvement in the health of other connective tissues with HRT administration [56, 57], in particular prevention of decrease in inter-vertebral disc heights [58] and thinning of the carotid artery wall [59].

12.3 The Effect of CHC on Muscular Collagen

There is a paucity of studies on the effects of CHC on muscular collagen and these same studies are also contradictory. Chidi-Ogolu and Baar [19] suggest that estrogen exposure increases the muscle's sensitivity to anabolic stimulation. Thompson et al. [60] compared a low androgenicity COC and a high androgenicity COC's effects on a number of physical exercises. They found that a high androgenicity COC was associated with better isokinetic knee flexion at $240°s^{-1}$ in the late hormone phase compared to the earlier phase, while a low androgenicity COC reduced the time for counter-movement jump in the late hormone phase, implying the androgenic role of the progestogen component in the COC in actually improving physical activity performance. In stark contrast to these findings, Sung et al. [12] do not find any statistically significant changes in the muscle strength, muscle thickness, type I to type II muscle fibre ratio, muscle fibre thickness, and nuclear to fibre ratio following 12 weeks of strength training in COC users as opposed to controls, and muscular collagen synthesis rate was found to be reduced in COC users as opposed to controls in another study [18].

12.4 Conclusion

The effect of CHC on BMD, BTMs, and muscular collagen is still not clear from the published studies so far. There is a large amount of methodological heterogeneity, among the performed studies, with studies differing in terms of the types, doses of the estrogen and progestogen, as well as the formulation and regimes of the contraceptives. More often than not, there were studies, which altered more than one variable at a time between intervention and comparator COC regimens, such as changing both the estrogen and the progestogen component dose. These studies were fraught with difficulty in interpreting whether any observed differences are due to the change in estrogen or progestogen dose.

A number of studies performed in adolescents seem to suggest that the modern ultra-low dose COCs containing less than 20 μg ethinylestradiol may be associated with decreased rate of BMD increase in these adolescents, hence preventing them from reaching their PBM. This is particularly true in studies, where these patients were followed up for more than 2 years. Moreover, there is a paucity of studies that shows whether such decreased BMD at follow-up recovers after stopping COCs. More adequately powered studies are needed to further investigate low-dose estrogen-containing contraceptive pills with higher dose estrogen ones in an adolescent population less than 20 years of age, with follow-up rates of more than 2 years.

Declarations

Competing Interests The author(s) has no competing interests to declare that are relevant to the content of this manuscript.

Ethics Approval The author(s) declares that this manuscript does not include primary research with human participants.

The author(s) declares that this manuscript does not include primary studies involving animals.

References

1. Trémollieres F. Impact of oral contraceptive on bone metabolism. Best Pract Res Clin Endocrinol Metab. 2013;27(1):47–53.
2. Almstedt HC, Cook MM, Bramble LF, Dabir DV, LaBrie JW. Oral contraceptive use, bone mineral density, and bone turnover markers over 12 months in college-aged females. J Bone Miner Metab. 2020;38(4):544–54.

3. Liu SL, Lebrun CM. Effect of oral contraceptives and hormone replacement therapy on bone mineral density in premenopausal and perimenopausal women: a systematic review. Br J Sports Med. 2006;40(1):11–24.
4. Ampatzis C, Zervoudis S, Iatrakis G, Mastorakos G. Effect of Oral contraceptives on Bone mineral density. Acta Endocrinol (Buchar). 2022;18(3):355–60.
5. Wreje U, Brynhildsen J, Aberg H, Byström B, Hammar M, von Schoultz B. Collagen metabolism markers as a reflection of bone and soft tissue turnover during the menstrual cycle and oral contraceptive use. Contraception. 2000;61(4):265–70.
6. Pollacco J, Brincat M. An overview of current contraceptive modalities and historical perspectives: a review. GREM Gynecol Reproduct Endocrinol Metab. 2024;5-1/2024:021–6.
7. Gai L, Jia Y, Zhang M, Gai P, Wang S, Shi H, et al. Effect of two kinds of different combined oral contraceptives use on bone mineral density in adolescent women. Contraception. 2012;86(4):332–6.
8. Allaway HCM, Misra M, Southmayd EA, Stone MS, Weaver CM, Petkus DL, et al. Are the effects of Oral and vaginal contraceptives on bone formation in young women mediated via the growth hormone-IGF-I Axis? Front Endocrinol (Lausanne). 2020;11:334.
9. O'Leary TJ, Wardle S, Rawcliffe A, Chapman S, Mole J, Greeves J. Understanding the musculoskeletal injury risk of women in combat: the effect of infantry training and sex on musculoskeletal injury incidence during British Army basic training. BMJ Mil Health. 2023;169(1):57–61.
10. Double RL, Wardle S, O'Leary T, Weaden N, Bailey G, Greeves J. Hormonal contraceptive prescriptions in the UK armed forces. BMJ Mil Health. 2023;169(1):23–6.
11. Myers SJ, Knight RL, Wardle SL, Waldock KA, O'Leary TJ, Jones RK, et al. Effect of menstrual cycle and hormonal contraception on musculoskeletal health and performance: protocol for a prospective cohort design and cross-sectional comparison. JMIR Res Protoc. 2024;13:e50542.
12. Sung ES, Han A, Hinrichs T, Vorgerd M, Platen P. Effects of oral contraceptive use on muscle strength, muscle thickness, and fiber size and composition in young women undergoing 12 weeks of strength training: a cohort study. BMC Womens Health. 2022;22(1):150.
13. Seidman L, Seidman DS, Constantini NW. Hormonal contraception for female athletes presents special needs and concerns. Eur J Contracept Reprod Health Care. 2024;29(1):8–14.
14. Martin D, Sale C, Cooper SB, Elliott-Sale KJ. Period prevalence and perceived side effects of hormonal contraceptive use and the menstrual cycle in elite athletes. Int J Sports Physiol Perform. 2018;13(7):926–32.
15. Balasch J. Sex steroids and bone: current perspectives. Hum Reprod Update. 2003;9(3):207–22.
16. Eriksen EF, Colvard DS, Berg NJ, Graham ML, Mann KG, Spelsberg TC, et al. Evidence of estrogen receptors in Normal human osteoblast-like cells. Science. 1988;241(4861):84–6.
17. Oursler MJ, Osdoby P, Pyfferoen J, Riggs BL, Spelsberg TC. Avian osteoclasts as estrogen target cells. Proc Natl Acad Sci. 1991;88(15):6613–7.
18. Hansen M, Miller BF, Holm L, Doessing S, Petersen SG, Skovgaard D, et al. Effect of administration of oral contraceptives in vivo on collagen synthesis in tendon and muscle connective tissue in young women. J Appl Physiol (1985). 2009;106(4):1435–43.
19. Chidi-Ogbolu N, Baar K. Effect of estrogen on musculoskeletal performance and injury risk. Front Physiol. 2019;9:1834.
20. Seibel MJ. The use of molecular markers of bone turnover in the management of patients with metastatic bone disease. Clin Endocrinol. 2008;68(6):839–49.
21. Callegari ET, Garland SM, Gorelik A, Chiang CY, Wark JD. Bone turnover marker determinants in young women: results from the safe-D study. Ann Clin Biochem. 2018;55(3):328–40.
22. Riggs BL. The mechanisms of estrogen regulation of bone resorption. J Clin Invest. 2000;106(10):1203–4.
23. Manolagas SC. Birth and death of bone cells: basic regulatory mechanisms and implications for the pathogenesis and treatment of osteoporosis. Endocr Rev. 2000;21(2):115–37.
24. Hadji P, Colli E, Regidor PA. Bone health in estrogen-free contraception. Osteoporos Int. 2019;30(12):2391–400.

25. Garnero P, Sornay-Rendu E, Delmas PD. Decreased bone turnover in oral contraceptive users. Bone. 1995;16(5):499–503.
26. Biason TP, Goldberg TB, Kurokawa CS, Moretto MR, Teixeira AS, Nunes HR. Low-dose combined oral contraceptive use is associated with lower bone mineral content variation in adolescents over a 1-year period. BMC Endocr Disord. 2015;15:15.
27. Almstedt Shoepe H, Snow CM. Oral contraceptive use in young women is associated with lower bone mineral density than that of controls. Osteoporos Int. 2005;16:1538–44.
28. Ziglar S, Hunter TS. The effect of hormonal oral contraception on acquisition of peak bone mineral density of adolescents and young women. J Pharm Pract. 2012;25(3):331–40.
29. Gargano V, Massaro M, Morra I, Formisano C, Di Carlo C, Nappi C. Effects of two low-dose combined oral contraceptives containing drospirenone on bone turnover and bone mineral density in young fertile women: a prospective controlled randomized study. Contraception. 2008;78(1):10–5.
30. Martin D, Cooper SB, Tang JCY, Fraser WD, Sale C, Elliott-Sale KJ. Bone metabolic marker concentrations across the menstrual cycle and phases of combined oral contraceptive use. Bone. 2021;145:115864.
31. Vasikaran S, Eastell R, Bruyere O, Foldes A, Garnero P, Griesmacher A, et al. Markers of bone turnover for the prediction of fracture risk and monitoring of osteoporosis treatment: a need for international reference standards. Osteoporos Int. 2011;22:391–420.
32. Szulc P, Naylor K, Hoyle N, Eastell R, Leary E, Project NBHABTM. Use of CTX-I and PINP as bone turnover markers: National Bone Health Alliance recommendations to standardize sample handling and patient preparation to reduce pre-analytical variability. Osteoporos Int. 2017;28:2541–56.
33. Lopez LM, Grimes DA, Schulz KF, Curtis KM, Chen M. Steroidal contraceptives: effect on bone fractures in women. Cochrane Database Syst Rev. 2014;6
34. Nappi C, Sardo ADS, Greco E, Tommaselli GA, Giordano E, Guida M. Effects of an oral contraceptive containing drospirenone on bone turnover and bone mineral density. Obstet Gynecol. 2005;105(1):53–60.
35. Cromer BA, Bonny AE, Stager M, Lazebnik R, Rome E, Ziegler J, et al. Bone mineral density in adolescent females using injectable or oral contraceptives: a 24-month prospective study. Fertil Steril. 2008;90(6):2060–7.
36. Nappi C, Sardo ADS, Acunzo G, Bifulco G, Tommaselli G, Guida M, et al. Effects of a low-dose and ultra-low-dose combined oral contraceptive use on bone turnover and bone mineral density in young fertile women: a prospective controlled randomized study. Contraception. 2003;67(5):355–9.
37. Paoletti AM, Orrù M, Floris S, Mannias M, Vacca AMB, Ajossa S, et al. Evidence that treatment with monophasic oral contraceptive formulations containing ethinylestradiol plus gestodene reduces bone resorption in young women. Contraception. 2000;61(4):259–63.
38. Endrikat J, Mih E, Düsterberg B, Land K, Gerlinger C, Schmidt W, et al. A 3-year double-blind, randomized, controlled study on the influence of two oral contraceptives containing either 20 μg or 30 μg ethinylestradiol in combination with levonorgestrel on bone mineral density. Contraception. 2004;69(3):179–87.
39. Gersten J, Hsieh J, Weiss H, Ricciotti NA. Effect of extended 30 μg ethinyl estradiol with continuous low-dose ethinyl estradiol and cyclic 20 μg ethinyl estradiol oral contraception on adolescent bone density: a randomized trial. J Pediatr Adolesc Gynecol. 2016;29(6):635–42.
40. Rad M, Kluft C, de Kam ML, Meijer P, Cohen AF, Grubb GS, et al. Metabolic profile of a continuous versus a cyclic low-dose combined oral contraceptive after one year of use. Eur J Contracept Reprod Health Care. 2011;16(2):85–94.
41. Cibula D, Skrenkova J, Hill M, Stepan JJ. Low-dose estrogen combined oral contraceptives may negatively influence physiological bone mineral density acquisition during adolescence. Eur J Endocrinol. 2012;166(6):1003–11.

42. Warholm L, Petersen KR, Ravn P. Combined oral contraceptives' influence on weight, body composition, height, and bone mineral density in girls younger than 18 years: a systematic review. Eur J Contracept Reprod Health Care. 2012;17(4):245–53.
43. Sørdal T, Grob P, Verhoeven C. Effects on bone mineral density of a monophasic combined oral contraceptive containing nomegestrol acetate/17β-estradiol in comparison to levonorgestrel/ethinylestradiol. Acta Obstet Gynecol Scand. 2012;91(11):1279–85.
44. Hartard M, Kleinmond C, Luppa P, Zelger O, Egger K, Wiseman M, et al. Comparison of the skeletal effects of the progestogens desogestrel and levonorgestrel in oral contraceptive preparations in young women: controlled, open, partly randomized investigation over 13 cycles. Contraception. 2006;74(5):367–75.
45. Berenson AB, Radecki CM, Grady JJ, Rickert VI, Thomas A. A prospective, controlled study of the effects of hormonal contraception on bone mineral density. Obstet Gynecol. 2001;98(4):576–82.
46. Polatti F, Perotti F, Filippa N, Gallina D, Nappi RE. Bone mass and long-term monophasic oral contraceptive treatment in young women. Contraception. 1995;51(4):221–4.
47. de Papp AE, Bone HG, Caulfield MP, Kagan R, Buinewicz A, Chen E, et al. A cross-sectional study of bone turnover markers in healthy premenopausal women. Bone. 2007;40(5):1222–30.
48. Ott SM, Scholes D, LaCroix AZ, Ichikawa LE, Yoshida CK, Barlow WE. Effects of contraceptive use on bone biochemical markers in young women. J Clin Endocrinol Metab. 2001;86(1):179–85.
49. Massaro M, Di Carlo C, Gargano V, Formisano C, Bifulco G, Nappi C. Effects of the contraceptive patch and the vaginal ring on bone metabolism and bone mineral density: a prospective, controlled, randomized study. Contraception. 2010;81(3):209–14.
50. Gambacciani M, Cappagli B, Lazzarini V, Ciaponi M, Fruzzetti F, Genazzani AR. Longitudinal evaluation of perimenopausal bone loss: effects of different low dose oral contraceptive preparations on bone mineral density. Maturitas. 2006;54(2):176–80.
51. Dombrowski S, Jacob L, Hadji P, Kostev K. Oral contraceptive use and fracture risk-a retrospective study of 12,970 women in the UK. Osteoporos Int. 2017;28(8):2349–55.
52. Stevenson JC, Cust MP, Gangar KF, Hillard TC, Lees B, Whitehead MI. Effects of transdermal versus oral hormone replacement therapy on bone density in spine and proximal femur in postmenopausal women. Lancet. 1990;336(8710):265–9.
53. Lees B, Stevenson JC. The prevention of osteoporosis using sequential low-dose hormone replacement therapy with estradiol-17 beta and dydrogesterone. Osteoporos Int. 2001;12(4):251–8.
54. Hillard TC, Whitcroft SJ, Marsh MS, Ellerington MC, Lees B, Whitehead MI, et al. Long-term effects of transdermal and oral hormone replacement therapy on postmenopausal bone loss. Osteoporos Int. 1994;4(6):341–8.
55. Horsman A, Jones M, Francis R, Nordin C. The effect of estrogen dose on postmenopausal bone loss. N Engl J Med. 1983;309(23):1405–7.
56. Brincat M, Galea R, Baron YM, Xuereb A. Changes in bone collagen markers and in bone density in hormone treated and untreated postmenopausal women. Maturitas. 1997;27(2):171–7.
57. Brincat M, Moniz CF, Studd JW, Darby AJ, Magos A, Cooper D. Sex hormones and skin collagen content in postmenopausal women. Br Med J (Clin Res Ed). 1983;287(6402):1337–8.
58. Stevenson T, Brincat M, Pollacco J, Stevenson J. Effect of hormone replacement therapy on intervertebral disc height. Climacteric. 2023;26(2):110–3.
59. Muscat Baron Y, Brincat M, Galea R. Carotid artery wall thickness in women treated with hormone replacement therapy. Maturitas. 1997;27(1):47–53.
60. Thompson BM, Drover KB, Stellmaker RJ, Sculley DV, Janse de Jonge XAK. The effect of the menstrual cycle and oral contraceptive cycle on muscle performance and perceptual measures. Int J Environ Res Public Health. 2021;18(20)

Chapter 13
Hormonal Treatment for Endometriosis, Adenomyosis, and Fibromatosis

Claudia Silvestri, Alice Baronti, Giovanni Ferraro, Francesca Papini, Vito Cela, Andrea Giannini, Tommaso Simoncini, and Stefano Luisi

13.1 Introduction

Endometriosis, adenomyosis, and fibromatosis are gynecological disorders characterized by abnormal tissue growth and associated symptoms such as pain and abnormal bleeding. Understanding the pathophysiology of these conditions is crucial for effective management. Hormonal treatments play a significant role in controlling symptoms and disease progression. This text will explore the pathophysiological mechanisms, clinical manifestations, and hormonal treatment options for each condition.

13.1.1 Endometriosis: Pathophysiology and Clinical Manifestations

Endometriosis is a chronic condition where endometrial tissue, which normally lines the inside of the uterus, grows outside the uterine cavity. This ectopic endometrial tissue responds to hormonal changes of the menstrual cycle, leading to inflammation, pain, and the formation of adhesions and scar tissue. Common sites of endometriosis include the ovaries, fallopian tubes, and the pelvic lining [1, 2].

Clinically, endometriosis presents with dysmenorrhea, non-menstrual pelvic pain, dyspareunia, and infertility. The severity of symptoms does not always

C. Silvestri · A. Baronti · G. Ferraro · F. Papini · V. Cela · A. Giannini · T. Simoncini
S. Luisi (✉)
Obstetrics & Gynecology, Department of Clinical and Experimental Medicine, University of Pisa, Pisa, Italy
e-mail: andrea.giannini@unipi.it; tommaso.simoncini@unipi.it; stefano.luisi@unipi.it

A. R. Genazzani et al. (eds.), *Ethical, Efficacy and Safety Issues in Contraception*, Reproductive Medicine for Clinicians 4,
https://doi.org/10.1007/978-3-032-07322-8_13

correlate with the extent of the disease. Other symptoms may include heavy menstrual bleeding, bowel and bladder dysfunction, and fatigue. These symptoms can significantly impact the quality of life and daily functioning of affected women [3].

The exact cause of endometriosis is not fully understood, but several theories have been proposed. The most widely accepted theory is retrograde menstruation, where menstrual blood flows backward through the fallopian tubes into the pelvic cavity, allowing endometrial cells to implant and grow outside the uterus. Other theories include genetic predisposition, immune system dysfunction, and coelomic metaplasia, where cells lining the pelvic organs transform into endometrial-like cells [1].

13.1.1.1 Hormonal Treatment

Hormonal treatments aim to reduce or eliminate hormonal fluctuations to alleviate symptoms and slow disease progression. These treatments can include oral contraceptives, progestins, GnRH analogues, and other hormone-modulating agents.

Oral Contraceptive Pills (OCPs) Continuous or extended-cycle OCPs are commonly used to manage endometriosis. These pills work by suppressing ovulation and reducing menstrual flow, which can prevent endometriosis-associated dysmenorrhea [4]. However, OCPs may not be effective for non-menstrual pelvic pain or dyspareunia [5]. Extended-cycle OCPs can reduce the frequency of menstruation, thereby minimizing the cyclical hormonal changes that exacerbate endometriosis symptoms. Studies have shown that women taking continuous OCPs experience significant relief from dysmenorrhea and other cyclic pain symptoms. The benefits of OCPs include their ease of use, relatively low cost, and safety profile. However, some women may experience side effects such as nausea, breast tenderness, and mood changes.

Dienogest Dienogest is a progestin that has shown success in controlling disease progression, particularly in ovarian endometriomas. Studies have demonstrated that dienogest can reduce the size of endometriomas and provide symptomatic relief, even after recurrence [6–9]. Dienogest works by creating a hormonal environment that is less conducive to endometrial growth. It reduces estrogen levels while maintaining sufficient progesterone to prevent breakthrough bleeding. Clinical trials have shown that dienogest significantly reduces endometriosis-associated pelvic pain, improves quality of life, and decreases the size of endometriotic lesions [6]. Long-term use of dienogest is well-tolerated, with a low incidence of adverse effects such as weight gain and mood changes [9].

Levonorgestrel-Releasing Intrauterine System (LNG-IUS) The LNG-IUS is an effective treatment for endometriosis, especially for women who also require contraception. This device releases levonorgestrel locally within the uterus, reducing menstrual blood loss, pain, and the size of endometriotic lesions [10]. The LNG-IUS has been shown to improve endometriosis-associated symptoms and quality of life in women who prefer a long-term, reversible contraceptive option. The device can remain in place for up to five years and is associated with fewer systemic side effects compared to oral hormonal treatments.

13.1.2 Adenomyosis: Pathophysiology and Clinical Manifestations

Adenomyosis is a myometrial lesion characterized by the presence of endometrial glands and stroma located randomly and deeply within the myometrium [11].

According to the most widely accepted theory about adenomyosis' pathogenesis, it originates from the basal layer of the endometrium that invaginates between smooth muscle cell bundles or along lymphatic vessels deeply into the myometrium [12].

Looking at the state-of-the-art literature, current evidence demonstrate genetics as a driver through alterations in gene functions managing steroid hormone function, extracellular cell matrix dysregulation, angiogenesis, tissue injury and repair, and inflammatory mediators [13]. The resulting ectopic presence of endometrial tissue with its glands and stroma seems to affect normal contractile function and peristalsis of uterine smooth muscle, causing the typical symptoms of this disease [14].

The main clinical manifestations in women who suffer from adenomyosis are pelvic pain, dyspareunia, dysmenorrhea [11], heavy menstrual bleeding, infertility, and miscarriage [15]. Adenomyosis has frequently been associated with endometriosis and can also coexist with the presence of leiomyomas or congenital uterine anomalies [16–19].

13.1.2.1 Hormonal Treatment

As far as adenomyosis therapy, there are no established guidelines and this disease presents significant challenges in treatment but various hormonal treatments are being used off-label to manage adenomyosis as a hormone-dependent inflammatory condition [19].

GnRH Agonists GnRH agonists are a second-line treatment in symptomatic adenomyosis. They have an initial stimulatory effect, but with a continuous prolonged treatment a central downregulation with a deep suppression of gonadotropin secretion is induced. This inhibition of the hypothalamo-pituitary-ovarian axis suppresses ovarian function and induces profound hypo-estrogenism which can lead to side effects such as severe vaso-motor symptoms or bone loss but we have lack of information on what add-back therapy should be used in these cases [20].

Levonorgestrel-Releasing Intrauterine System (LNG-IUS) LNG-IUS is an efficient way to treat menorrhagia associated with adenomyosis for two different actions of this device: the former is the deciduation and subsequent marked hypotrophy of ectopic endometrium [21] and the latter is a direct effect of progestin on foci of adenomyosis [22, 23]; the reduction of menstrual flow is significant notwithstanding a high incidence of spotting and oligomenorrhea which are well-tolerated by patients [21].

Furthermore, LNG-IUS is effective in alleviating dysmenorrhea associated with adenomyosis with little effect on ovarian function and uterus volume can reduce in 6 months after insertion and later [24].

Etonogestrel Implant Etonogestrel implants are effective in reducing pelvic pain and menstrual flow of adenomyosis or endometriosis. In some patients, vaginal bleeding, amenorrhea, weight gain, and acne occurred as side effects [25].

Norethindrone (NETA) The use of NETA in adenomyosis is effective in relieving menorrhagia and pain. Like other progestins, is known to cause breakthrough bleeding. The regime "three weeks on, one week off" aims to minimize the side effect of breakthrough bleeding since it causes incomplete suppression of the hypothalamic-pituitary-ovarian axis, perhaps causing less of a hypoestrogenic effect. Other less frequent symptoms are changes in menstrual flow, amenorrhea, changes in cervical secretions, erosion, edema, weight gain or loss, cholestatic jaundice, allergic rash with or without pruritus, melasma or chloasma, and mental depression [26].

Dienogest (DNG) DNG is a progestational 19-norsteroid derivative, a synthetic oral progestin with highly selective binding to progestin receptors. Its mechanism of action consists in antiovulatory and mild hypoestrogenic effects, and antiproliferative activity in human endometrial cells. Thanks to its hormonal profile, DNG is used as a treatment for painful symptoms of endometriosis without causing any severe hypoestrogenic adverse effects and it is expected to be an effective treatment for painful symptoms associated with adenomyosis. The DNG improves pain in patients with adenomyosis who wish fertility preservation, at various ages despite a high incidence of irregular genital bleeding [27].

Combined Oral Contraceptives (COCs) COCs act by the reduction or elimination of ovarian activity and a total progestogenic antiproliferation, at best resulting in amenorrhea [28].

COCs are used for adenomyosis management to decrease the menstrual flow, in particular when given continuously, and a pseudogestational status which causes decidualization and atrophy of the endometrium [29]. The resulting amenorrhea can be an advantage for patients with dysmenorrhea and menorrhagia. The best choice for adenomyosis-related pain seems to be monophasic, low-dose COCs with a continuous administration, which show safety, good efficacy as far as high tolerability and low costs. As for side effects, many women report irregular bleedings and COCs have been often associated with an increased risk of venous thrombosis, thus are not suggested in patients with other risk factors such as thrombophilia or hypertension [29].

13.1.3 Fibromatosis: Pathophysiology and Clinical Manifestations

Fibromatosis, or desmoid tumors, are benign fibroblastic neoplasms that can occur in any musculoaponeurotic structure of the body, including the uterus. Uterine fibromatosis, also known as uterine fibroids or leiomyomas, are the most common benign tumors in women of reproductive age. These tumors are composed of smooth muscle cells and fibrous connective tissue and they can occur in different size and number.

The pathogenesis of fibromatosis involves genetic, hormonal, and environmental factors. Estrogen and progesterone are believed to play a crucial role in the development and growth of fibroids, as these tumors often become smaller after menopause when hormone levels decline [30].

Clinically, uterine fibromatosis can present with a variety of symptoms, including heavy menstrual bleeding, pelvic pressure or pain, frequent urination, constipation, and reproductive issues such as infertility and recurrent pregnancy loss. The severity of symptoms depends on the size, number, and location of the fibroids. Large fibroids can cause significant distortion of the uterine cavity and adjacent pelvic organs [30, 31].

13.1.3.1 Hormonal Treatment

Hormonal treatments for fibromatosis aim to reduce the size of the fibroids and alleviate associated symptoms. These treatments include GnRH antagonists, combination therapies, and progestin-releasing intrauterine devices.

GnRH Antagonists GnRH antagonists are a valid option for the medical treatment of fibromatosis. These drugs work by directly inhibiting the release of gonadotropins, leading to a rapid decline in estrogen and progesterone levels. Clinical studies have demonstrated that GnRH antagonists can reduce fibroid volume by 30%–50% within 4–8 weeks, providing significant symptom relief [32]. However, similar to GnRH analogues, long-term use of GnRH antagonists can lead to hypoestrogenic side effects such as hot flashes, bone loss, and vaginal dryness. Add-back therapy is often recommended to minimize these side effects.

Relugolix Combination Therapy For women of reproductive age with moderate to severe symptomatic fibromatosis, relugolix combination therapy is indicated.

This therapy involves the use of relugolix, a GnRH antagonist, in combination with low doses of estrogen and progestin. This combination helps to maintain a favorable benefit/risk profile by reducing bleeding and pelvic discomfort while preventing the hypoestrogenic side effects associated with GnRH antagonist monotherapy. Clinical trials have shown that relugolix combination therapy significantly improves symptoms and quality of life in women with fibromatosis [33].

13.2 Conclusion

Hormonal treatments play a crucial role in managing endometriosis, adenomyosis, and fibromatosis by alleviating symptoms and controlling disease progression. Understanding the pathophysiological mechanisms and clinical manifestations of these conditions is essential for selecting the most appropriate treatment options. Continuous or extended-cycle OCPs, dienogest, GnRH analogues, LNG-IUS, and GnRH antagonists are among the effective hormonal treatments available. Each treatment has its benefits and potential side effects, and the choice of therapy should be individualized based on the patient's symptoms, preferences, and overall health.

Declarations

Competing Interests The author(s) has no competing interests to declare that are relevant to the content of this manuscript.

Ethics Approval The author(s) declares that this manuscript does not include primary research with human participants.

The author(s) declares that this manuscript does not include primary studies involving animals.

References

1. Burney RO, Giudice LC. Pathogenesis and pathophysiology of endometriosis. Fertil Steril. 2012;98:511–9.
2. Bulun SE. Endometriosis. N Engl J Med. 2009;360:268–79.
3. Taylor HS, Giudice LC, Lessey BA, et al. Treatment of endometriosis-associated pain with Elagolix, an Oral GnRH antagonist. N Engl J Med. 2017;377:28–40.
4. Edelman A, Micks E, Gallo MF, Jensen JT, Grimes DA. Continuous or extended cycle vs. cyclic use of combined hormonal contraceptives for contraception. Cochrane Database Syst Rev. 2014;2014(7):CD004695.
5. Brown J, Farquhar C. Endometriosis: an overview of Cochrane reviews. Cochrane Database Syst Rev. 2014;2014(3):CD009590.
6. Harada T, Momoeda M, Taketani Y, et al. Dienogest is as effective as intranasal buserelin acetate for the relief of pain symptoms associated with endometriosis–a randomized, double-blind, multicenter, controlled trial. Fertil Steril. 2009;91:675–81.

7. Petraglia F, Hornung D, Seitz C, et al. Reduced pelvic pain in women with endometriosis: efficacy of long-term dienogest treatment. Arch Gynecol Obstet. 2012;285:167–73.
8. Strowitzki T, Faustmann T, Gerlinger C, Schumacher U, Ahlers C, Seitz C. Safety and tolerability of dienogest in endometriosis: pooled analysis from the European clinical study program. Int J Women's Health. 2015;7:393–401.
9. Lee JH, Song JY, Yi KW, et al. Effectiveness of Dienogest for treatment of recurrent endometriosis: multicenter data. Reprod Sci. 2018;25:1515–22.
10. Lethaby A, Hussain M, Rishworth JR, Rees MC. Progesterone or progestogen-releasing intrauterine systems for heavy menstrual bleeding. Cochrane Database Syst Rev. 2015;4:CD002126.
11. Taran FA, Wallwiener M, Kabashi D, et al. Clinical characteristics indicating adenomyosis at the time of hysterectomy: a retrospective study in 291 patients. Arch Gynecol Obstet. 2012;285:1571–6.
12. Benagiano G, Habiba M, Brosens I. The pathophysiology of uterine adenomyosis: an update. Fertil Steril. 2012;98:572–9.
13. Zhai J, Vannuccini S, Petraglia F, Giudice LC. Adenomyosis: mechanisms and pathogenesis. Semin Reprod Med. 2020;38:129–43.
14. Antero MF, Ayhan A, Segars J, Shih IM. Pathology and pathogenesis of Adenomyosis. Semin Reprod Med. 2020;38:108–18.
15. Vannuccini S, Tosti C, Carmona F, et al. Pathogenesis of adenomyosis: an update on molecular mechanisms. Reprod Biomed Online. 2017;35:592–601.
16. Koninckx PR, Ussia A, Zupi E, Gomel V. Association of Endometriosis and Adenomyosis: vast literature but scant conclusive data. J Minim Invasive Gynecol. 2018;25:745–8.
17. Dababou S, Garzon S, Laganà AS, et al. Linzagolix: a new GnRH-antagonist under investigation for the treatment of endometriosis and uterine myomas. Expert Opin Investig Drugs. 2021;30:903–11.
18. Feghali E, Etrusco A, Haydamous J, et al. Concurrent diagnosis of Adenomyosis and congenital uterine anomalies: a review. J Pers Med. 2023;13:716.
19. Etrusco A, Barra F, Chiantera V, et al. Current medical therapy for Adenomyosis: from bench to bedside. Drugs. 2023;83:1595–611.
20. Streuli I, Dubuisson J, Santulli P, de Ziegler D, Batteux F, Chapron C. An update on the pharmacological management of adenomyosis. Expert Opin Pharmacother. 2014;15:2347–60.
21. Fedele L, Bianchi S, Raffaelli R, Portuese A, Dorta M. Treatment of adenomyosis-associated menorrhagia with a levonorgestrel-releasing intrauterine device. Fertil Steril. 1997;68:426–9.
22. van der Walt LA, Sanfilippo JS, Siegel JE, Wittliff JL. Estrogen and progestin receptors in human uterus: reference ranges of clinical conditions. Clin Physiol Biochem. 1986;4:217–28.
23. Azziz R. Adenomyosis in pregnancy. A review. J Reprod Med. 1986;31:224–7.
24. Ji F, Yang XH, Ai Xing Zi AL, Ha Ni Ke Zi TX, He Y, Ding Y. Role of levonorgestrel-releasing intrauterine system in dysmenorrhea due to adenomyosis and the influence on ovarian function. Clin Exp Obstet Gynecol. 2014;41:677–80.
25. Niu X, Luo Q, Wang C, Zhu L, Huang L. Effects of Etonogestrel implants on pelvic pain and menstrual flow in women suffering from adenomyosis or endometriosis: results from a prospective, observational study. Medicine (Baltimore). 2021;100:e24597.
26. Muneyyirci-Delale O, Chandrareddy A, Mankame S, Osei-Tutu N, Gizycki H. Norethindrone acetate in the medical management of adenomyosis. Pharmaceuticals (Basel). 2012;5:1120–7.
27. Osuga Y, Fujimoto-Okabe H, Hagino A. Evaluation of the efficacy and safety of dienogest in the treatment of painful symptoms in patients with adenomyosis: a randomized, double-blind, multicenter, placebo-controlled study. Fertil Steril. 2017;108:673–8.
28. Schindler AE. Non-contraceptive use of hormonal contraceptives. Gynecol Endocrinol. 2008;24:235–6.
29. Pontis A, D'Alterio MN, Pirarba S, de Angelis C, Tinelli R, Angioni S. Adenomyosis: a systematic review of medical treatment. Gynecol Endocrinol. 2016;32:696–700.
30. Lumsden MA, Hamoodi I, Gupta J, Hickey M. Fibroids: diagnosis and management. BMJ. 2015;351:h4887.

31. Donnez J, Dolmans MM. Uterine fibroid management: from the present to the future. Hum Reprod Update. 2016;22:665–86.
32. Rackow BW, Arici A. Options for medical treatment of myomas. Obstet Gynecol Clin N Am. 2006;33:97–113.
33. Friedman AJ, Lobel SM, Rein MS, Barbieri RL. Efficacy and safety considerations in women with uterine leiomyomas treated with gonadotropin-releasing hormone agonists: the estrogen threshold hypothesis. Am J Obstet Gynecol. 1990;163:1114–9.

Part V
Combined Hormonal Contraception Effects on Polycystic Ovary, Breast, Breast Cancer and Other Cancer Patients

Chapter 14
Metabolic Effects of Combined Hormonal Contraception and Its Use in Polycystic Ovary Syndrome

David Vasquez Awad

14.1 Introduction

PCOS is a set of signs and symptoms that have been recognized since the eighteenth century, associated with irregular menstrual cycles, obesity, hirsutism, and obesity. In 1935, Stein and Leventhal unified this syndrome linked to anovulation and that is why it is also known as Stein Leventhal syndrome and recently, androgenic ovary syndrome [1, 2].

All diagnostic criteria proposed to date require that other causes of anovulation and other causes of hyperandrogenism be ruled out. PCOS is the most common endocrine disorder in women of reproductive age and is the cause of around 80% of hirsutism [1]. The clinical spectrum of PCOS is broad and depends on variables such as age, developmental stage, genetics, racial, and environmental factors.

Several professional organizations have proposed diagnostic criteria for PCOS. In 2003, the "Rotterdam Criteria" were proposed with the presence of two of three features needed to establish the diagnosis of PCOS: oligo-amenorrhea or amenorrhea, clinical or biochemical evidence of hyperandrogenism, and polycystic ovaries on ultrasound, ruling out other causes of anovulation and hyperandrogenism [3]. This definition implies the existence of four phenotypes: phenotype 1, which encompasses the three criteria; phenotype 2, in which oligo-or anovulation and clinical or biochemical hyperandrogenism occur; phenotype 3, in which clinical or biochemical hyperandrogenism and polycystic ovaries occur; and phenotype 4, whose features are anovulation and polycystic ovaries. In 2009, the Androgen Excess and Polycystic Ovary Syndrome Society proposed that the presence of hyperandrogenism (clinical or biochemical), accompanied by ovulatory dysfunction, polycystic ovaries, or both (only three) as essential criteria for establishing the

D. Vasquez Awad (✉)
National Academy of Medicine, Bogotá, Colombia

A. R. Genazzani et al. (eds.), *Ethical, Efficacy and Safety Issues in Contraception*, Reproductive Medicine for Clinicians 4,
https://doi.org/10.1007/978-3-032-07322-8_14

diagnosis of PCOS), excluding other causes of anovulation and hyperandrogenism [4, 5]. The clinical and metabolic implications of PCOS, as well as the prognosis, may differ according to the phenotype.

14.2 Pathophysiology

Regarding its pathophysiology, the average production of androgens and estrogens is increased in PCOS. There is an increase in the values of testosterone, androstenedione, and 17α- hydroxyprogesterone. These substances have ovarian origin and depend on the luteinizing hormone (LH). Dehydroepiandrosterone (DHEA) and DHEA sulfate have adrenal origin. There is an increase in estrone concentrations (peripheral conversion), which causes obesity typical of the syndrome to generate peripheral conversion of estrone to estradiol in the fatty tissue. A fundamental role is played by the altered role of gonadotropin-releasing factor (GnRH), which increases the pulse frequency, generating the release of GnRH and thus altering the LH/FSH relationship. The latter leads to increased conversion to androgens in theca cells, an increase in the number of small preantral and antral follicles. The alteration of the LH/FSH relationship with a reduction in FSH and aromatase then prevents the growth and subsequent rupture of the follicles, which generates chronic anovulation. The extended ovarian stroma increases the production of androgens that cannot be aromatized to estrogens and, likewise, there is inhibition of sex hormone–binding globulin (SHBG) which increases the concentration of free androgens [2, 5].

From a metabolic point of view, most patients will present with insulin resistance which leads to compensatory hyperinsulinemia by the beta cells of the pancreas. Hyperinsulinism generates some of the characteristics of POS: [1] it decreases the synthesis of SHBG; [2] it decreases hepatic synthesis of insulin-like growth factor–binding protein 1 (IGF BP-1); [3] insulin, acting synergistically with LH, increases ovarian synthesis of androgens; [4] hyperinsulinemia stops follicular maturation and contributes to the sensitization of the pituitary gland to GnRH, increasing the release of LH; [5] at the endometrial level, insulin favors the synthesis of estrone and endometrial hyperplasia [5].

In patients with PCOS, an increase in proinflammatory adipocytokines, a procoagulant state, and markers of endothelial dysfunction are observed, as occurs in patients with metabolic syndrome. As in this syndrome, women with PCOS have an increase in total cholesterol, LDL cholesterol and triglycerides, and a reduction in HDL2 and apolipoprotein A-I [6].

Hyperandrogenism increases visceral fat and perpetuates insulin resistance, which contributes to an increase in androgens both systemically and locally, and in the portal system increases visceral fat. Obese women with PCOS are at increased risk of developing metabolic syndrome with impaired glucose tolerance and type 2 diabetes mellitus, and experience twice as many cardiovascular risk factors.

However, there is little direct evidence of increased or premature morbidity and mortality from cardiovascular events in patients with PCOS [2, 6].

There are genes that regulate the secretion, action of gonadotropins, folliculogenesis, insulin secretion, weight and energy regulation, and the biosynthesis and action of androgens. DENND1A and THADA states have been identified [7].

14.3 Diagnosis

The diagnosis is clinical, paraclinical, and ultrasound. Symptoms include oligomenorrhea, weight gain, hirsutism, and acne. Signs include overweight and obesity, acne, and signs of hyperandrogenism or insulin resistance. Complementary paraclinical tests include glycemia, insulin, glycosylated hemoglobin, lipid profile, free and total testosterone, and in some cases androstenedione and DHEA sulfate. Other laboratory tests may be necessary to establish a differential diagnosis [2, 7].

14.4 Treatment

As a systemic disease, PCOS must be managed by a multidisciplinary team and on an individual basis. The first line of treatment includes lifestyle modification with appropriate diet and exercise; carbohydrate intolerance is indicated. Cyclic progestins prevent endometrial hyperplasia and depot progestins can be used as contraception as well as progestin-releasing intrauterine devices. Infertility requires study and management with ovulation inducers as the first line, particularly aromatase inhibitors, and subsequent management should be given in specialized fertility clinics. Spironolactone, finasteride, and GnRH analogues can be used as antiandrogens. Skin management is carried out by dermatology.

Eventually can be important the assessment and follow up by Psychiatrist and Psychologist.

14.5 Contraceptive Use in Patients with PCOS

COs are first-line tools in women with PCOS to control hirsutism, acne, and irregular cycles. Combined COs (estrogens progestins) are superior to progestin-only COs as well as injectable ones. COs have non-contraceptive contraceptive benefits and the physician treating PCOS should be familiar with their management. The estrogenic component of CO increases the synthesis of SHBG which reduces biologically active free androgens and thus the bioavailability for the peripheral conversion of testosterone to dihydrotestosterone mediated by 5-alpha reductase [2].

On the other hand, progestins contribute to the negative feedback on LH which leads to the stimulation of theca cells for the synthesis of androgens. Some progestins, commonly called antiandrogens, exert competitive inhibition at the androgen receptor. Finally, by counteracting the permanent effect of estrogens on the endometrium, progestins prevent endometrial hyperplasia. In adolescence, control of the menstrual cycle and the clinical manifestations of hyperandrogenism are priorities, with CO being the first-line treatment [8, 9].

All COs studied are useful regardless of the type of progestins they contain. Some progestins such as levonorgestrel and norethindrone have androgenic effects and others are considered antiandrogenic. Among the latter, in decreasing order of anti-androgenicity, we have cyproterone, dienogest, drospirenone, trimegestone, levonorgestrel, and chlormadinone. In clinical practice, these latter progestins are used more as a component of OCs for PCOS. Given that the management of PCOS is multidisciplinary, it is worth noting that CO is only one of the tools for its treatment and is aimed at the management of irregular cycles, acne, and hirsutism as well as the prevention of endometrial hyperplasia. In women without a desire for fertility, CO is a very appropriate therapy since it would also cover this indication [10].

The metabolic management of PCOS is more about lifestyle habits, low-calorie diet, exercise, metformin, inositol, and the prevention of cardiovascular alterations typical of the increased risk that comes with the increased risk of metabolic syndrome. No increase in cardiovascular morbidity has been demonstrated in patients with PCOS who consume CO; What's more, most of the information favors the use of CO. Although no significant reduction in waist circumference or waist–hip ratio is observed, a significant increase in HDL cholesterol and SHBG levels is observed. The area under the glucose curve is reduced in CO users; Additionally, the area under the insulin curve is not altered in CO users. However, in patients with PCOS and morbid obesity, impaired glucose tolerance is observed with the use of CO [2, 11].

A systematic review and meta-analysis of prospective cohort studies and controlled clinical trials evaluated the effect of combined hormonal contraceptives on markers of insulin resistance and dyslipidemia in patients with POS. The review included 35 studies with 42 cohorts, using ethinyl estradiol with different progestins. It was found that no significant changes occurred in fasting blood glucose and insulin, total cholesterol, LDL cholesterol, and HOMA-IR. There was an increase in HDL cholesterol and triglycerides without clinical significance. The increase in triglycerides is because of the estrogenic component of CO but is below the risk level for generating pancreatitis [12].

Finally, in relation to the effect of CO on chronic inflammation mediators in women with PCOS, a meta-analysis found that most preparations increase C-reactive protein and produce a non-significant increase in homocysteine levels and a decrease in inhibitor 1, CO plasminogen activator containing desogestrel, norgestimate, and drospirenone [12].

14.6 Conclusion

The treatment of PCOS must be multidisciplinary since its pathophysiology and clinical symptoms involve different organs and systems. Treatment includes lifestyle changes, a low-calorie diet, exercise, and the use of metformin, inositol, and other anti-obesity drugs as well as antiandrogens.

The use of CO in PCOS is more aimed at controlling the cycle and symptoms of hyperandrogenism and preventing endometrial hyperplasia. The metabolic impact in favor or against CO in PCOS has yet to be elucidated, but its contraceptive and non-contraceptive benefits make it a fundamental tool in the management of these patients.

Declarations

Competing Interests The author(s) has no competing interests to declare that are relevant to the content of this manuscript.

Ethics Approval The author(s) declares that this manuscript does not include primary research with human participants.

The author(s) declares that this manuscript does not include primary studies involving animals.

References

1. Martin KA, Anderson RR, Chang RH, Ehrman DA, Lobo RA, Murad MH, et al. Evaluation and treatment of hirsutism in premenopausal women: an Endocrine Society clinical practice guideline. J Clin Endocrinol Metab. 2018;103(4):1233–57. https://doi.org/10.1210/jc.2018-00241.
2. Ruiz A. Anticoncepción hormonal y su uso en Ovario Androgénico-Síndrome de Ovarios poliquísticos. En: Vásquez Awad D, Palacios S, Anticoncepción hormonal, Ed. Kimpres, 2020. p. 375–393.
3. Rotterdam ESHRE/ASRM-Sponsored PCOS Consensus Workshop Group. Revised 2003 consensus on diagnostic and long-term health risks related to polycystic ovary syndrome. Fertil Steril. 2004;81(1):19–25. https://doi.org/10.1016/j.fertnstert.2003.10.0004.
4. Azziz R, Carmina E, Dewailly D, Diamanti-Kandarakis E, Escobar-Morreale HF, Futterweit W, et al. The androgen excess and PCOS society criteria for the polycystic ovary syndrome: the complete task force report. Fertil Steril. 2009;91(2):456–88.
5. Ehrmann DA, Barnes RB, Rosenfield RL. Polycystic ovary syndrome as a form of functional ovarian hyperandrogenism due to dysregulation of androgen secretion. Endocr Rev. 1995;16:322–53.
6. Diamanti-Kandarakis E, Dunaif A. Insulin resistance and the polycystic ovary syndrome revisited: an update on mechanisms and implications. Endocr Rev. 2012;33:981–1030.
7. Dumesic DA, Oberfield SE, StenerVictorin E, Marshall JC, Laven JS, Legro RS. Scientific statement on the diagnostic criteria, epidemiology, pathophysiology, and molecular genetics of polycystic ovary syndrome. Endocr Rev. 2015;36:487–525.
8. Legro RS, Arslanian SA, Ehrmann DA, et al. Diagnosis and treatment of polycystic ovary syndrome: an Endocrine Society clinical practice guideline. J Clin Endocrinol Metab. 2013;98:4565–92.

9. Teede HJ, Misso ML, Deeks AA, et al. Assessment and management of polycystic ovary syndrome: summary of an evidence-based guideline. Med J Aust. 2011;195:S65–112.
10. Fauser BC, Tarlatzis BC, Rebar RW, et al. Consensus on women's health aspects of polycystic ovary syndrome (PCOS): the Amsterdam ESHRE/ASRM-sponsored 3rd PCOS Consensus Workshop Group. Fertil Steril. 2012;97(1):28–38.e25.
11. Conway G, Dewailly D, Diamanti, Kandarakis E, et al. The polycystic ovary syndrome: a position statement from the European Society of Endocrinology. Eur J Endocrinol. 2014;171:1–29.
12. Halperin IJ, Kumar SS, Stroup DF, Laredo SE. The association between the oral contraceptive pill and insulin resistance, dysglycemia and dyslipidemia in women with polycystic ovary syndrome: a systematic review and meta-analysis of observational studies. Hum Reprod. 2022;26:191–201.

Chapter 15
Combined Oral Contraception, Benign Breast Diseases, and Breast Cancer

Anne Gompel

15.1 Introduction

Hormonal contraception concerns a large proportion of young women. Across the world, in 2019, according to INED [1], 922 million women or their partners were contraceptive users. Hormonal contraception encompasses the combined pill and oral progestin and is used by 16% of women, and progestin by injections or implants concerns 10% of women [1]. Combined oral contraception (COC) is the first contraception used in Western, and Northern Europe, Northern Africa, Northern and South America, and Oceania [2].

15.1.1 Benign Breast Diseases (BBDs) and Contraception

15.1.1.1 BBD Consists of Fibroadenoma (FA), Adenoma Phyllodes, and Fibrocystic Disease (FCD)

FA are benign, not associated with an increased risk of breast cancer, and occur in young women. There is usually no indication to perform a surgical treatment. Phyllodes may have the potential for recurrence and are classified as benign, borderline, or malignant [3] and the recommended treatment is surgical ablation [3]. Usually, the diagnosis is suspected in a rapidly growing FA, and the size is larger than the usual FA. They contain estradiol and/or progesterone receptors as FA [3].

A. Gompel (✉)
Université Paris Cité, Department of Gynecology, Paris, France
e-mail: anne.gompel@parisdescartes.fr

A. R. Genazzani et al. (eds.), *Ethical, Efficacy and Safety Issues in Contraception*, Reproductive Medicine for Clinicians 4,
https://doi.org/10.1007/978-3-032-07322-8_15

Multiple FA is a condition where at least three FAs are in the breast. The diagnosis for benignity and follow-up is not always easy. They represent about 10%–15% of the patients with FA. Some studies suggested an increased risk of breast cancer in this context.

FCD can variably contain different histopathologic characteristics. It can vary from simple cysts, due to some degree of fibrosis in the stroma, a consequence of the edema at the end of the menstrual cycle, this edema regressing is replaced by fibrosis which can wrap and tighten the ducts, producing cysts. The lining epithelium may remain unicellular or proliferation can be associated. Proliferation may concern ducts or lobules and can consist of simple proliferative disease or proliferation with atypia. Mastalgia is associated with the swelling of the breast at the end of the menstrual cycle. It is always present in the context of FCD and can be extremely severe.

These different lesions are associated with different levels of risk of breast cancer. Studies showed that FCD without proliferative disease is associated with a mild increase in breast cancer, with a RR: 1.27 (1.15–1.41), FCD with a proliferative disease without atypia, a RR: 1.88 (1.66–2.12) and FCD with a proliferative disease with atypia, a RR: 4.24 (3.26–5.41) [4]. Having had biopsies showing several foci with proliferative disease is associated with an even higher RR of breast cancer [5]. Atypical hyperplasia of the ducts was associated with a greater risk than having an atypical lobular hyperplasia [5].

15.1.2 Contraception and Incidence of BBD

Several studies have shown since the first generation of COC that women users had a lower incidence of FA and FCD [6–10]. This protective effect was increased with a longer duration of use. Some studies suggested that this protective effect was only observed for COC use before the first full-term pregnancy [8, 10]. In a more recent study, which included 61,617 women from a screening program in Sweden, aged 40–69 years, current and long ($\geq$8 years) COC use was associated with a reduced risk of fibroadenoma, HR = 0.65 (0.47–0.90), in premenopausal women [11]. COC did not influence the other types of BBD. It is to be noted that the diagnosis, in this retrospective cohort, was made in the context of screening mammograms and not in the context of a clinical consultation for a lump or mastalgia, which could have introduced a bias for the accuracy of diagnosis and its clinical relevance.

15.1.3 Which Contraception in Women with BBD?

No specific studies have looked at the effect of initiating a COC after diagnosing FA. In practice, follow-up of the FA can be recommended: if its size increases during the COC, or if it is painful, a shift to a progestin contraception or a lower dose

COC can be proposed. No recommendations exist about this question. The natural history of FA is to stabilize or decrease in size with time. A biopsy can be indicated to eliminate a carcinoma or a phyllode if the lump is growing.

The main clinical symptom of FCD is mastalgia which can be extremely disabling and thus needs to be treated. Several randomized studies have demonstrated the efficacy of antigonadotropic progestins in the treatment of FCD and the control of mastalgia. At the longer term, these treatments help to decrease the size of the cysts [12–14]. COC can help to reduce mastalgia in some patients with FCD but not in all. In case of persistent mild mastalgia, percutaneous progesterone can be associated with COC, daily applied on the breast, but it will not always be sufficient. In case of persistent mastalgia and growing cysts, an antigonadotropic progestin could be much more efficient. Long-term duration mastalgia has been associated with an increased risk of breast cancer [15]. Whereas in a series of French women with BBD, followed up in two clinical departments, women who have used norsteroids (predominantly lynestrenol at 10 mg) had a lower risk of breast cancer than non-users [16]. The trend of the decrease in the risk was associated with increased duration of use. The addition of percutaneous progesterone did not alter the protective effect of progestin [17]. The progestin used were either norsteroids at 10 mg/day or pregnane/norpregnane derivatives as chlormadinone acetate or nomegestrol acetate, respectively at 10 or 5 mg/day, 20/27 days [16, 18]. At the doses used, these progestins have a contraceptive efficacy.

In women with multiple adenomas, a progestin treatment had also a beneficial effect on the size of the FAs [19].

In women with a diagnosis of atypical hyperplasia, which is a precancerous lesion that carries a high probability of getting invasive cancer in the next 25 years, it is not certain that COC can be prescribed safely. As the next paragraph will show, the usual opinion is that COC may have a promoter effect on occult cancer or precancerous lesions such as hyperplasia with atypia, explaining the mild increased risk of breast cancer in users, a risk which decreases progressively after stopping. However, no data are available on that topic except an old study that did not observe an increase in the risk of breast cancer, in women with proliferative disease, with COC [20].

15.2 Hormonal Contraception and the Risk of Breast Cancer (Table 15.1)

15.2.1 COC

There have been many publications addressing the risk of breast cancer and COC [21–26] (Table 15.1). In the meta-analysis from the Collaborative Group on Hormonal Factors in Breast Cancer [21] which pooled data from 54 studies, the risk of breast cancer was increased in current users: RR = 1.24 (1.15–1.33), and

Table 15.1 Contraception and risk of breast cancer

Study	Design	Cases (N)	Controls (N)/ Population	Risk	Comments
Torres-de la Roche et al. 2023	Meta-analysis	44,295	2,275,304	OR = 1.33 (1.19–1.49)	Substantial Heterogeneity in the studies, I2 value of `182%.
Collaborative group of hormonal factors in breast cancer 1995	Meta-analysis			RR = 1.24 (1.15–1.33) Disappeared in 10 years	
UK Fitzpatrick et al. 2023	Case-control	9498	18,171	OR = 1.33[1.26–1.41] ORa = 1.25 [1.18–1.33] Risk decreased progressively after cessation	Cases had more recent birth Some factors of adjustment are missing: family history, age at FFTP, BBD, PA
USA Nurses' health study II Burchardt 2021	Prospective cohort	5799	113,187	>5 years: HR: 1.56 (1.23–1.99) <5 years HR: 1.19 (0.95–1.49) Risk stop after 5/10 years	Many factors of adjustment
Swedish Niemeyer Hultstrand 2023	Prospective cohort	3842	1,500,000	IRR: 1.03 (0.91–1.16) First 5 years of use: IRR: 1.39 (1.14–1.69) Disappeared in 5 years	Adjustments: parity, age at first birth, smoking, BMI, infertility, polycystic ovarian syndrome, endometriosis

progressively disappeared 10 or more years after stopping COC. The latest meta-analysis reported an increased risk, pooling studies between 2017 and 2021, of HR = 1.33 (1.19–1.49) in ever-users and suggested that the risk was persistent after the end of use [22]. However, the authors pointed out the important heterogeneity among the studies which does not allow to firmly accept the evidence.

Several important studies have been published since this meta-analysis.

A Swedish nationwide prospective cohort study included 1.5 million women, 15–35 years old, and did not find any increase in the risk of breast cancer, IRR 1.03 (0.91–1.16) [26]. However, during the first 5 years of use, there was a significant increase in the risk (IRR 1.39 (1.14–1.69)) which was not any more apparent after 5 years. This strongly suggests an effect on preexisting lesions, because of the short duration of COC use and the cancer. The risk was significantly increased in the years after interrupting COC (<5 years; IRR 1.66 (1.45–1.90) and 5–10 years after stopping COC (IRR 1.22 (1.08–1.38)) [26].

In a case–control study of breast cancer, using a computerized UK primary care database, an increased risk was observed. The non-adjusted OR was OR = 1.33 (1.26–1.41) for breast cancer in women aged <50 years who used a COC [24]. After adjusting on time since the last birth, number of recorded births, BMI, and alcohol intake (but were missing important factors, such as age at first pregnancy and family history of breast cancer as well as history of BBD, physical activity), the OR was ORa = 1.25 (1.18–1.35) [24]. The ORs declined over time since the last use. It is important to note, however, that the mean use of any hormonal contraceptives was between 2.8 and 3.7 years. So, what is apparent here, is the consequence of a rapid promoter effect likely on occult cancers. The authors also calculated the number of excess cases of breast cancer attributable to COC from their case–control study: according to age, the attributable number of cases is different since the number of breast cancer cases is low before the age of 35 years: for use at ages 16–20 years, this number could be about 8 per 100,000 users (an increase in incidence from 0.084% to 0.093%); for use at ages 25–29, about 61 per 100,000 users (from 0.50% to 0.57%); and for use at ages 35–39, about 265 per 100,000 users (from 2.0% to 2.2%) [24].

In another study, from the Nurses' cohort, the factors for adjustment were far more complete, including age, calendar period, age of menarche, BMI at age 18 years, diagnosis of BBD, family history of breast cancer, breastfeeding duration index, alcohol consumption, physical activity, screening mammography in the last 2 years, variation of weight since age 18 years, and birth index [23]. The results showed an HRa = 1.31 (1.09–1.58) for COC current users, the risk increased with duration of use and decreased after stopping: no associations were observed after 5 years of cessation, and duration of use was not associated with breast cancer risk in past OC users. They looked at the effect of COC composition, and COC containing norgestrel appears to be at higher risk as in the study from a Danish register [25]. The excess number of cases attributable to COC in the Nurses' study, corresponded to 4 excess cases per 100,000 person-years among past users and 36 excess cases per 100,000 person-years among current users. For the users of COC containing norgestrel, the numbers were 6 excess cases per 100,000 person-years for past users and 96 excess cases per 100,000 person-years for current users [23].
This is compared to the rate of breast cancer during pregnancy, which is estimated to be about 1/3000 pregnancies, or for the WHO to 10% of breast cancer in women <40 years.

15.2.2 *Progestin Contraceptives and the Risk of Breast Cancer*

15.2.2.1 Oral and Injectable Progestin Contraceptives

The UK database previously cited also performed a meta-analysis on progestin contraceptives, including the most recent studies and their own data, and reported an increased risk for all progestin contraceptives [24]. The ORs were similar to COC for oral progestin (OR = 1.35 (1.26–1.47) and ORa = 1.26 (1.16–1.37)), for injectable progestin (OR = 1.30 (1.12–1.50) and ORa = 1.25 (1.07–1.45)). A potential bias is that women who have used progestin contraception may have different risk factors for breast cancer than women who used COC and as well women who did not use any hormonal contraception.

In the Swedish study [26], progestin contraception was associated with an increased risk of IRR = 1.32 (1.20–1.45), adjusted for age at the start of each exposure, level of education, place of birth, age at first full-term pregnancy, number of children, having received ovulation stimulating treatment and any diagnosis of infertility, polycystic ovarian syndrome, or endometriosis, or an IRR = 1.26 (1.12–1.42) adjusted on the same factors+ BMI and smoking. All types of progestin-only contraception were associated with a significant increase in the risk, with the exception of MPA injectable. Similar to COC, the risk decreased after cessation of the contraceptives.

15.2.2.2 IUD Containing Norgestrel (IUS)

The risk associated with IUS was also calculated in the meta-analysis from the UK and found to be OR = 1.21 (1.14–1.28) [24]. In the Swedish study, the IRR = 1.21 (1.01–1.33) [26]. The authors pointed out that they could not differentiate the use in premenopausal or postmenopausal women, which could have caused a bias; as we said above, the risk factors for adjustment were not complete in these studies. In a previous meta-analysis, the results suggested that the risk of breast cancer was increased in women over 50 years/postmenopausal [27].

15.2.3 Conclusions

From all these data, it is suggested that COC and, to the same extent, progestin contraception exert a promoter effect, in the short term, on pre-existing lesions in the breast and by this effect, increase the risk of breast cancer. This effect is more clinically relevant after the age of 35 years.

This suggests contraindicating COC and progestin contraception as the first line in women over that age if they have important risk factors for breast cancer. However, the benefits of ovarian, colorectal, and endometrial cancers of the hormonal contraceptive have to be balanced by the increased risk of breast cancer. The specific case of carriers of BRCA variants will be discussed in the next paragraph.

15.3 Hormonal Contraception in Women Carriers of BRCA Pathogenic Variants

Several meta-analyses have looked at the risk of breast cancer in women carriers of BRCA pathogenic variants (PV). The last one [28] analyzed separately studies reporting the level of risk as HR and studies reporting as OR. The analysis included 7525 patients in the studies who reported on the HR and 9106 patients in the ORs studies. The results were not similar since in the case of HR, it was reported as increased, but not for the OR. Concerning the studies which reported a hazard ratio, the value was, HR: 1.55 (1.36–1.76), and for the studies which reported an odd ratio, OR = 1.06 (0.90–1.25). The level of risk was higher for BRCA2 than BRCA1 carriers. The ER+ breast cancer is the most frequent in the context of BRCA2, whereas triple-negative breast cancers occur more frequently in BRCA1 carriers. For BRCA1 carriers, the HR = 1.44 (1.16–1.78), and for BRCA2, the HR = 1.73 (1.13–2.30). For the OR, no increase was seen either for BRCA1 or BRCA2 carriers.

Another meta-analysis [29] also reported an increased risk of breast cancer, but which was significant only after 5 years of use. The risk of breast cancer for carriers of BRCA1 PV was: OR/RR/HR = 1.24 (1.09–1.41) and BRCA2: OR/RR/HR = 1.40 (1.10–1.78). For use above 5 years, in BRCA1 carriers, OR/RR/HR = 1.40 (1.26–1.57), and in BRCA2 carriers OR/RR/HR = 1.49 (1.15–1.93).

Both meta-analyses reported a significant decrease in the risk of ovarian cancer, HR = 0.62 (0.52–0.74) and OR = 0.49 (0.38–0.63) in the first meta-analysis [28] and for BRCA1 carriers, HR = 0.51 (0.41–0.64) and for BRCA2 HR = 0.57 (0.41–0.80) [29].

Tubal ligation was associated with a lower risk of ovarian cancer at least in the study from Antonionou et al., which calculated the HR = 0.44 (0.26–0.74), but not in the three other studies calculating an OR = 0.74 (0.53–1.03).

These results open the discussion of which contraception to be used in BRCA carriers. Avoiding using COC will contribute to preventing a certain proportion of breast cancers. However, the protective effect on ovarian cancer and endometrial cancer will be lost. Whereas breast cancer can be detected using screening [30], this is not the case for ovarian cancer. There is also the question of the validity of interpreting MRI under a combined pill. No study has examined this question but it was reported a background parenchymal enhancement in some women using an IUS, as during the menstrual cycle in the luteal phase [31]. It is also to take into account that a prophylactic oophorectomy is recommended in BRCA1 carriers at an age of 35–40 years and 40–45 years in BRCA2 carriers. However, this is not always accepted or respected. In a recent publication, about 60% of the BRCA carriers had performed an oophorectomy and thus about 40% did not [32]. This suggests that there could be a benefit of using COC for women who are reluctant to perform at a young age the oophorectomy.

15.4 Contraception in Women with a History of Breast Cancer

There are only two studies which had looked at the risk of recurrence in women survivors of breast cancer and have used an IUS.

The first one of low power is a case–control study which has included 199 women with breast cancer some of whom used the IUS [33]. Seventy-nine women used it after the diagnosis and 120 controls did not. There was no difference in the recurrence in both groups: HRa = 1.86 (0.86–4.00). However, among 38 women who kept the IUS after the diagnosis, the risk of recurrence appeared to be higher: HR = 3.39 (1.01–11.35) [33].

A Cochrane review was conducted to analyze the preventive effect on endometrial diseases (polyps and hyperplasia) of an IUS in women using tamoxifen (24–60 months) [34]. In this study, not designed to look at the effect of IUS on the prognosis of breast cancer patients, the recurrence and deaths from breast cancer were analyzed. The recurrence was not increased, but with large confidence intervals: OR = 1.74 (0.64–4.74), and based on 11 recurrences with IUS versus 7 for the controls and 8 deaths in each group.

15.5 Conclusions

Data remain scarce and guidelines suggest avoiding any hormonal contraception including the IUS in women survivors of breast cancer [35]. However, some of these can have benign uterine diseases associated with bleeding. Then the balance risk-benefit of using the IUS appears positive and after a discussion with the oncologist, according to the personal history of the patient, most of the experts consider that in case of gynecological indication (bleeding), IUS can be used with a stringent follow-up.

The first choice for most patients should be a Copper IUD.

A barrier method can be also proposed if a previous use was efficient in a given woman. Just to be mentioned, MPA and megestrol acetate are used at high doses in metastatic breast cancer patients. They cannot be recommended because of side effects in other women, but in case of oncologic indications, they have a contraceptive effect.

Emergency contraception can be used in all cases.

It is important to highlight that several studies have reported a lack of contraception in women survivors of breast cancer, with a proportion of women from 20% to 80% missing any method of contraception in this context, where pregnancy needs to be programmed for the less [36].

Declarations

Competing Interests The author(s) has no competing interests to declare that are relevant to the content of this manuscript.

Ethics Approval The author(s) declares that this manuscript does not include primary research with human participants.

The author(s) declares that this manuscript does not include primary studies involving animals.

References

1. Ined – Institut national d'études démographiques [Internet]. [cité 28 mars 2024]. What are the most widely used contraceptive methods across the world? – the issue today – demographic fact sheets. Disponible sur: https://www.ined.fr/en/everything_about_population/demographic-facts-sheets/faq/most-widely-used-contraceptive-methods-world/
2. Division UP. Contraceptive use by method 2019: data booklet [Internet]. UN; 2019 [cité 28 mars 2024]. Disponible sur: https://digitallibrary.un.org/record/3849735
3. Tan BY, Acs G, Apple SK, Badve S, Bleiweiss IJ, Brogi E, et al. Phyllodes tumours of the breast: a consensus review. Histopathology. 2016;68(1):5–21.
4. Hartmann LC, Sellers TA, Frost MH, Lingle WL, Degnim AC, Ghosh K, et al. Benign breast disease and the risk of breast cancer. N Engl J Med. 2005;353(3):229–37.
5. Degnim AC, Dupont WD, Radisky DC, Vierkant RA, Frank RD, Frost MH, et al. Extent of atypical hyperplasia stratifies breast cancer risk in 2 independent cohorts of women. Cancer. 2016;122(19):2971–8.
6. Brinton LA, Vessey MP, Flavel R, Yeates D. Risk factors for benign breast disease. Am J Epidemiol mars. 1981;113(3):203–14.
7. Vessey M, Yeates D. Oral contraceptives and benign breast disease: an update of findings in a large cohort study. Contraception. 2007;76(6):418–24.
8. Charreau I, Plu-Bureau G, Bachelot A, Contesso G, Guinebretiére JM, Lê MG. Oral contraceptive use and risk of benign breast disease in a French case-control study of young women. Eur J Cancer Prev. 1993;2(2):147–54.
9. Sitruk-Ware R, Thalabard JC, Benotmane A, Mauvais-Jarvis P. Risk factors for breast fibroadenoma in young women. Contraception. 1989;40(3):251–68.
10. Rohan TE, Miller AB. A cohort study of oral contraceptive use and risk of benign breast disease. Int J Cancer. 1999;82(2):191–6.
11. Johansson A, Christakou AE, Iftimi A, Eriksson M, Tapia J, Skoog L, et al. Characterization of benign breast diseases and association with age, hormonal factors, and family history of breast cancer among women in Sweden. JAMA Netw Open. 2021;4(6):e2114716.
12. Uzan S, Denis C, Pomi V, Varin C. Double-blind trial of promegestone (R 5020) and lynestrenol in the treatment of benign breast disease. Eur J Obstet Gynecol Reprod Biol. 1992;43(3):219–27.
13. Schindler AE. Dydrogesterone and other progestins in benign breast disease: an overview. Arch Gynecol Obstet févr. 2011;283(2):369–71.
14. Winkler UH, Schindler AE, Brinkmann US, Ebert C, Oberhoff C. Cyclic progestin therapy for the management of mastopathy and mastodynia. Gynecol Endocrinol déc. 2001;15(Suppl 6):37–43.
15. Plu-Bureau G, Lê MG, Sitruk-Ware R, Thalabard JC. Cyclical mastalgia and breast cancer risk: results of a French cohort study. Cancer Epidemiol Biomarkers Prev juin. 2006;15(6):1229–31.
16. Plu-Bureau G, Lê MG, Sitruk-Ware R, Thalabard JC, Mauvais-Jarvis P. Progestogen use and decreased risk of breast cancer in a cohort study of premenopausal women with benign breast disease. Br J Cancer. 1994;70(2):270–7.

17. Plu-Bureau G, Lê MG, Thalabard JC, Sitruk-Ware R, Mauvais-Jarvis P. Percutaneous progesterone use and risk of breast cancer: results from a French cohort study of premenopausal women with benign breast disease. Cancer Detect Prev. 1999;23(4):290–6.
18. Peters F. Multicentre study of gestrinone in cyclical breast pain. Lancet. 1992;339(8787):205–8.
19. Grouthier V, Chakhtoura Z, Tejedor I, Badachi Y, Goffin V, Touraine P. Positive association between progestins and the evolution of multiple fibroadenomas in 72 women. Endocr Connect juin. 2020;9(6):570–7.
20. Dupont WD, Page DL, Rogers LW, Parl FF. Influence of exogenous estrogens, proliferative breast disease, and other variables on breast cancer risk. Cancer. 1989;63(5):948–57.
21. Collaborative Group on Hormonal Factors in Breast Cancer. Breast cancer and hormonal contraceptives: collaborative reanalysis of individual data on 53 297 women with breast cancer and 100 239 women without breast cancer from 54 epidemiological studies. Lancet. 1996;347(9017):1713–27.
22. Torres-de la Roche LA, Acevedo-Mesa A, Lizarazo IL, Devassy R, Becker S, Krentel H, et al. Hormonal contraception and the risk of breast cancer in women of reproductive age: a meta-analysis. Cancers (Basel). 2023;15(23):5624.
23. Burchardt NA, Eliassen AH, Shafrir AL, Rosner B, Tamimi RM, Kaaks R, et al. Oral contraceptive use by formulation and breast cancer risk by subtype in the nurses' health study II: a prospective cohort study. Am J Obstet Gynecol. 2022;226(6):821.e1–821.e26.
24. Fitzpatrick D, Pirie K, Reeves G, Green J, Beral V. Combined and progestagen-only hormonal contraceptives and breast cancer risk: a UK nested case-control study and meta-analysis. PLoS Med. 2023;20(3):e1004188.
25. Mørch LS, Skovlund CW, Hannaford PC, Iversen L, Fielding S, Lidegaard Ø. Contemporary hormonal contraception and the risk of breast cancer. N Engl J Med. 2017;377(23):2228–39.
26. Niemeyer Hultstrand J, Gemzell-Danielsson K, Kallner HK, Lindman H, Wikman P, Sundström-Poromaa I. Hormonal contraception and risk of breast cancer and breast cancer in situ among Swedish women 15-34 years of age: a nationwide register-based study. Lancet Reg Health Eur. 2022;21:100470.
27. Conz L, Mota BS, Bahamondes L, Teixeira Dória M, Françoise Mauricette Derchain S, Rieira R, et al. Levonorgestrel-releasing intrauterine system and breast cancer risk: a systematic review and meta-analysis. Acta Obstet Gynecol Scand. 2020;99(8):970–82.
28. van Bommel MHD, IntHout J, Veldmate G, Kets CM, de Hullu JA, van Altena AM, et al. Contraceptives and cancer risks in BRCA1/2 pathogenic variant carriers: a systematic review and meta-analysis. Hum Reprod Update. 2023;29(2):197–217.
29. Park J, Huang D, Chang YJ, Lim MC, Myung SK. Oral contraceptives and risk of breast cancer and ovarian cancer in women with a BRCA1 or BRCA2 mutation: a meta-analysis of observational studies. Carcinogenesis. 2022;43(3):231–42.
30. Lubinski J, Kotsopoulos J, Moller P, Pal T, Eisen A, Peck L, et al. MRI surveillance and breast cancer mortality in women with BRCA1 and BRCA2 sequence variations. JAMA Oncol. 2024;10(4):493–9.
31. Huck LC, Truhn D, Wilpert C, Zanderigo E, Raaff V, Dethlefsen E, et al. Background parenchymal enhancement in contrast-enhanced MR imaging suggests systemic effects of intrauterine contraceptive devices. Eur Radiol. 2022;32(11):7430–8.
32. Metcalfe K, Eisen A, Senter L, Armel S, Bordeleau L, Meschino WS, et al. International trends in the uptake of cancer risk reduction strategies in women with a BRCA1 or BRCA2 mutation. Br J Cancer. 2019;121(1):15–21.
33. Trinh XB, Tjalma WAA, Makar AP, Buytaert G, Weyler J, van Dam PA. Use of the levonorgestrel-releasing intrauterine system in breast cancer patients. Fertil Steril. 2008;90(1):17–22.
34. Dominick S, Hickey M, Chin J, Su HI. Levonorgestrel intrauterine system for endometrial protection in women with breast cancer on adjuvant tamoxifen. Cochrane Database Syst Rev. 2015;12:CD007245.

35. WHO. World Health Organization. Medical eligibility criteria for contraceptive use.
36. Sebbag C, Rousset-Jablonski C, Coussy F, Ray-Coquard I, Garin C, Evrevin C, et al. Contraception in breast cancer survivors from the FEERIC case-control study (performed on behalf of the Seintinelles research network). Breast. 2023;67:62–70.

Chapter 16
Hormonal Contraception and Cancer

Giovanni Grandi, Lia Feliciello, Lorenzo Aguzzoli, and Antonio La Marca

16.1 Introduction

Hormonal contraception (HC), which includes methods such as oral contraceptive pills, vaginal rings, patches, injections, implants and levonorgestrel-releasing intrauterine systems (LNG-IUS), is commonly used for family planning during reproductive life. Containing steroid hormones, both estrogens and progestins, it has been extensively studied for its potential link to cancer risk, uncovering a complex relationship between hormonal exposure and cancer development. The connection between HC and cancer risk is multifaceted and varies depending on factors such as the type of cancer, the length of HC use, and other individual characteristics such as age, body mass index, family history, genetic predisposition, lifestyle choices, smoking, and human papilloma virus (HPV) status [1].

Moreover, the research concerning the relationship between cancer risk and HC use is complicated by a number of other factors: the peak incidence of the majority of cancers at an older age with a long interval from last or first HC use, the use of multiple hormonal formulations during the women's life, the existence of many confounding factors, some of which may be directly related to contraceptive use (number of pregnancies, length of breast-feeding, age of first pregnancy, the number

G. Grandi (✉) · L. Feliciello · A. La Marca
Department of Medical and Surgical Sciences for Mother, Child and Adult, University of Modena and Reggio Emilia, Azienda Ospedaliero-Universitaria di Modena, Modena, Italy
e-mail: giovanni.grandi@unimore.it; antonio.lamarca@unimore.it

L. Aguzzoli
Santa Maria Hospital, Reggio Emilia, Italy

University of Modena and Reggio Emilia, Reggio Emilia, Italy
e-mail: lorenzo.aguzzoli@ausl.re.it

A. R. Genazzani et al. (eds.), *Ethical, Efficacy and Safety Issues in Contraception*, Reproductive Medicine for Clinicians 4,
https://doi.org/10.1007/978-3-032-07322-8_16

of sexual partners, the use of barrier contraceptives, etc.), and different composition of HC formulations used.

In summary, HC use can both increase and decrease the risk of various cancers, depending on the specific type of cancer and individual factors. This chapter is finalized to describe the most important associations described in the literature between HC use and cancer incidence, with the exclusion of the relationship with the most common cancer diagnosed in women such as breast cancer [2].

16.2 Ovarian Cancer

All studies about the relationship between HC use and ovarian cancer (OC) have clearly and constantly demonstrated that the use of combined oral contraceptives (COCs) significantly reduces the risk of OC: the degree of risk reduction correlating positively with the duration of use (more than 50% of reduction for 15 years of use). The first meta-analysis published by Beral et al. involving 45 epidemiological studies indicated that women who used COCs experienced a substantial decrease in OC risk with protective effects persisting for decades after cessation, being more evident for perimenopausal COC use [3]: studies concerning borderline and not epithelial cancers found the same decreasing trend. The reduction of the risk involves all the histotypes of OC with the exclusion of mucinous OC: this is similar of what happens after tubal ligation (due to the retrograde menstruation inhibition effect). In women with a high risk of OC (up to 40% lifetime), COCs can exert a similar protective effect, and their use should be recommended (such as *BRCA* mutation carriers and Lynch syndrome) [4, 5]. The benefit risk ratio is particularly evident in women at the highest risk for OC, such as *BRCA 1* mutation carriers.

The protective effects of COCs use against OC are further supported by biological mechanisms that may involve alterations in hormone metabolism and reduced exposure to estradiol (E2), which is implicated in ovarian carcinogenesis [6]. Additionally, the role of inflammation and its interaction with hormonal factors in the etiology of OC has been suggested, indicating a complex interplay between HC use and cancer risk [7, 8]. The development of OC is a consequence of repeated microtrauma of the ovarian surface epithelium during ovulation. However, not only "incessant ovulation inhibition" is included in this mechanism. Indeed, also progestin-only contraceptive (POCs) methods, including progestin-only pills, injections such as depot-medroxyprogesterone acetate (DMPA), and implants, have also been associated with reduced OC risk but by a lesser degree in comparison to combined formulations. This would suggest that the protective mechanism could be dependent also on gonadotropin levels, particularly follicle-stimulating hormone

(FSH), which differ between CHCs and POCs users. The three "actors" involved in the pathogenesis of serous, endometrioid, and clear-cell OC have been described in the retrograde menstruation, the ovulation (germinative epithelium of the ovary), and the fimbriae [9]: HC probably acts on both the inhibition of ovulation and reduction of retrograde menstruation, with no activity on the fimbriae. Moreover, the use of LNG-IUS has been linked to a decreased risk of OC, although the underlying biological mechanisms remain less clear, probably linked to a similar reduction of retrograde menstruation [7–9]. The use of HCs is generally contraindicated in survivors of stromal OC, in particular granulosa cells histotype [2].

- *Risk reduction*: HC use, especially of COCs, has been associated with a significant reduction in the risk of OC and borderline tumors. This protection is for all histotypes of OC, with the exclusion of mucinous one. This protective effect is lighter with the use of POCs.
- *Protective effect*: The protective effect appears to increase with the duration of use, is highest for the perimenopausal use and may persist for decades after cessation of HC use.
- *Mechanism*: The reduction in risk is thought to be related to the suppression of ovulation, reducing the number of times the ovarian epithelium is exposed to the damaging effects of incessant ovulations, but probably dependent on the reduction of retrograde menstruation too.

16.3 Endometrial Cancer

Numerous studies have examined the role of HC in modulating endometrial cancer (EC) risk. Research consistently shows that the use of HC is associated with a reduced risk of EC, with protective effects lasting for years after discontinuation of the contraceptive method. Even in women younger than 40, the use of CHCs decreases the risk of EC. The protective mechanism is the regulation of the endometrial lining: progestin induces secretory changes in the endometrial tissue, counteracting the proliferative action of estrogens [10]. Also the use of the LNG-IUS, especially in high dose 52 mg LNG-IUSs, may actually reduce the risk of EC, and this effect is thought to be due to the local progestin released by the device, in this way by maintaining a thinner endometrium; the LNG-IUS may prevent the development of precancerous conditions (hyperplasia with atypia, endometrial intraepithelial neoplasia, EIN) and reduce the likelihood of EC [11]. Even the use of copper IUD was associated with a protective action against EC due to its inflammatory effect on the endometrium and the stabilization of the endometrium-suppressor oncogenic PTEN [12].

The endometrium differs from the breast. Proliferation in the endometrium is seen in the follicular phase (with over 80% of the endometrial cells proliferating) (E2 dominated), while proliferation in the breast is seen typically in the luteal phase (with, however, only 10% of the epithelial breast cells proliferating) (progesterone dominated).

- *Risk reduction*: Similarly to OC, the use of CHC was always associated with a reduced risk for EC. Similarly, the use of LNG-IUS but also of copper IUD was associated with a similar reduced risk for EC.
- *Protective effect*: The protective effect can last for many years after stopping the HC, and the risk reduction is more significant with longer durations of use.
- *Mechanism*: This protective effect is likely due to the progestin component of the contraceptives, which counteracts the proliferative effects of estrogens on the endometrial lining, and it is probably more evident in the progestin dominant modern CHC formulations in comparison to the older ones.

16.4 Cervical Cancer

The use of HCs, especially when used for more than 5 years, has been associated with a modest increase in the risk of cervical cancer (CC), although the overall risk remains relatively low [13]. The proposed mechanism is that steroids of contraceptives can affect the immune system, reducing the body's ability to eliminate human papilloma virus (HPV) infection: a chronic or persistent infection with high-risk strains of HPV can increase the likelihood of developing precancerous lesions or, in more severe cases, invasive cancer.

There is limited specific data regarding adenocarcinoma histotype risk and contraception. Long-term use of COCs may increase the incidence of both types of CC [14]. While some studies suggest that the copper IUD may offer protection against cervical intraepithelial neoplasia (CIN) and invasive cervical cancer, other research has indicated a slight increase in the risk of CIN with the use of both copper IUDs and LNG-IUS [15].

CC is caused by HPV infection, and HPV exposure is not independent of HCs use. Women who use HCs are more likely to be exposed to genital HPV than those who use barrier contraceptive methods or who do not have sexual intercourses. Finally, the impact of primary (nonvalent vaccination) and secondary (population screening) prevention measures should be considered in this complex relationship.

In the next research, it will be helpful to understand how the effect of HC on vaginal microbiome, in particular in combined ones (with the increase in lactobacillus species), could have a protective role in HPV possible transformation of the uterine cervix.

- *Increased risk*: Long-term use of HC, especially for 5 years or more, has been associated with an increased risk of CC, particularly in women infected with HPV.
- *Risk postdiscontinuation*: The risk diminishes gradually after discontinuation and may return to baseline levels 10 years after stopping use.
- *Mechanism*: The increase in risk might be due to hormonal changes affecting the cervix, potentially making it more susceptible to HPV infection and progression to invasive cancer.

16.5 Colorectal Cancer

COCs might offer some protection against colorectal cancer (CRC), especially for women who have used them long term. This potential benefit is believed to be associated with the antiinflammatory and cell-regulating properties of estrogens, which could play a role in preventing the formation of tumor cells lifelong. The precise mechanisms are still not fully understood, but estrogens appear to influence the activity of certain genes that control cell growth and apoptosis (programmed cell death), potentially reducing the risk of abnormal cell proliferation that can lead to cancer. Moreover, HCs may have an impact on the gut microbiome or regulate immune system responses, which could provide additional protection against CRC [16].

For these reasons, CHC use is not contraindicated following CRC treatment. In the case of Lynch syndrome, antigonadotropic contraceptives might be advantageous, as they reduce the risk of both OC, EC, and CRC [17].

- *Risk reduction*: Some evidence suggests that CHC use may reduce the risk of colorectal cancer, the most frequent neoplasm in nonsmokers of both sexes combined in Western countries.
- *Potential mechanism*: The proposed mechanism involves the influence of estrogens on bile acids, insulin sensitivity, and inflammation, all of which are factors in CRC development and last during menopause for postmenopausal hormone therapy (HT) (Fig. 16.1).

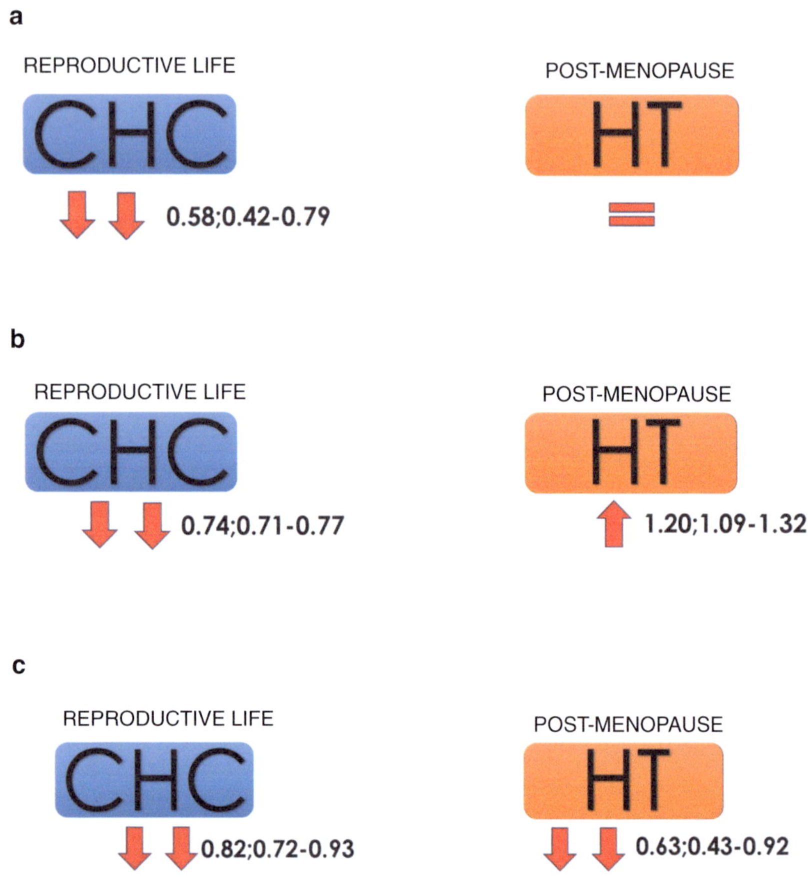

Fig. 16.1 Hormonal therapies and cancer risk in the lifetime. CHC, combined hormonal contraceptives; HT, postmenopausal hormone therapy. Relative risks (RR) with 95% confidence intervals are reported. (**a**) Lifetime hormonal therapies and endometrial cancer risk: partially concordant. (**b**) Lifetime hormonal therapies and ovarian cancer risk: completely discordant ("the effect of ovulation"). (**c**) Lifetime hormonal therapies and colorectal cancer risk: completely concordant ("the estrogenic effect")

16.6 Liver Cancer

The evidence is inconclusive to establish a relation between oral contraceptives and the risk of hepatocellular carcinoma [18, 19].

There is no evidence to suggest that HC use should be avoided in the cancer survivors if liver function is normal or in the absence of liver transplantation. If liver function is impaired, nonhormonal contraceptives should be considered as the first option. In the case of liver transplantation, CHC and the copper IUD are not recommended due to the use of immunosuppressive drugs [2].

16.7 Pancreatic Cancer

No data in the literature establish a link between HC therapy and pancreatic cancer (PC). A meta analysis of observational studies by Tang et al. found no significant association between the use of HC and PC [20] and also other researchers failed to find that the use of exogenous hormones, such as estrogens and progestins, was associated with an increased risk of PC; however, a slight increase in risk is seen if the use of such therapy is prolonged for more than 10 years.

16.8 Thyroid Cancer

According to the data available in the literature, there is no evidence of a connection between the use of HC use and the risk of thyroid cancer: in a prospective study, Braganza et al. found no direct link between HC or postmenopausal HT and cancer risk [21]. However, other research suggests that the use of exogenous steroids may be associated with an increased risk of TC after menopause.

Nonhormonal contraception should be the preferred option for women who have had thyroid cancer. While HC is not explicitly contraindicated, it should be used with caution [2].

There is generally limited research on contraceptive use among survivors of non-gynecological endocrine cancers. Women in this group need accurate information and access to safe and effective contraception that does not interfere with their condition. Most experts agree that the copper IUD is the safest and most effective contraceptive method, including for emergency contraception. It rarely leads to infections and can be safely used by immune-compromised women [22].

16.9 Hematological Cancers

Hematological cancers are not influenced by gonadal steroids, and the use of HC is not involved in their development, progression, or recurrence rate. The only potential exception appears to be follicular lymphoma, as its incidence seems to be positively associated with gonadal steroids [23]. On the other hand, there are some growing evidence that COC use can reduce the risk of hematological cancers at all, according to the Royal College of General Practitioners study [24]. Since there is no available data on the impact of COC on possible recurrence, it is considered cautious to avoid using COCs in survivors of follicular lymphoma. International guidelines do not impose any restrictions on the use of contraception, whether during or after treatment for a hematological malignancy [25].

In individuals with chronic diseases, the choice of contraceptive method is influenced by the risks of infection, thrombosis, bleeding, and anemia, as well as the stage and symptoms of the disease. For patients with pancytopenia, extended-cycle COCs are preferred to minimize bleeding risks, which are higher with IUDs, progestogen-only pills, and subdermal implants. The LNG-IUS high dose 52 mg has a lower bleeding. IUDs are generally contraindicated in pancytopenia due to infection risks. COCs are not recommended for women with thrombophilia or increased blood viscosity. For patients with Hodgkin's lymphoma, which increases the risk of thrombosis and may involve jaundice or cholestasis, HC is typically avoided. However, research suggests that COCs do not raise the risk of breast cancer in these patients. Safer alternatives include natural methods and condoms [26]. Conditions like Waldenström's macroglobulinemia, plasma cell neoplasms, and polycythemia vera, which increase thrombosis risk, also warrant avoiding COCs, though other contraceptive methods are acceptable. For follicular lymphoma, COCs are not recommended, particularly after treatment. In aggressive NK cell leukemia, where anemia, thrombocytopenia, and liver issues are common, contraception is contraindicated, except for natural methods and condoms [2].

16.10 Other Cancers

Adrenocortical carcinoma is a very rare tumor, associated with hormone secretion (cortisol, aldosterone, testosterone, or estrogens). It may occur in children and adults. Due to the low frequency of these neoplasms, there are few specific published findings related to contraceptive use and the risk for these cancers.

Meningiomas are neoplasms of the membranes covering the brain and spinal cord. Meningiomas show an evident female predominance (a female-to-male ratio of 2.5:1), especially in women of reproductive age [27]: the size of meningiomas increases during pregnancy and decreases after delivery. Furthermore, a hormonal modulation, probably due to high doses of progesterone stimulation, has always been proposed. How the risk of meningioma could change from "progestin-only therapy" (especially with progesterone derivatives such as cyproterone acetate, chlormadinone acetate, or nomegestrol acetate) to "combined therapy" has not been fully understood: central estrogen modulation of risk could be very important and a real game changer in the cause–event hormonal effect, as we do not know any POP containing these specific progestins in the market or in the experimental phase for contraceptive purposes. In fact, a recent meta-analysis including 13 studies (1,948,360 participants) reporting on the association between OC use and the risk of meningioma did not find evidence of any significant association between OC use and meningioma risk in female patients (relative risk = 0.99; 95% CI = 0.87–1.13), while showing a 30% reduction of glioma occurrence (RR 0.7; 95% CI, 0.6–0.81) [28].

16.11 Net Cancer Effect

In the view of the individual user of HC is very important the net cancer effect, putting all the oncological risk/benefits together. Considering all the possible cancers as a whole, the use of COCs was associated to a—24% reduced risk of main gynecological cancers (incidence rate ratio 95%; confidence interval 0.76; 0.63–0.91) and a neutral effect on cancers at all (0.96; 0.90–1.03) [24]. This net cancer protective effect was confirmed also from United States independent data (0.97; 0.95–0.99) [29].

16.12 Conclusions

Communicating cancer risk information is a crucial part of contraceptive counselling. Reliable epidemiological assessment of any association of hormone therapy use with cancer requires large numbers and careful controls of all potential sources of appreciable bias. It is also important a life-time approach, so it is very important to consider how the use of different hormonal formulations as HC during reproductive life and HT in postmenopause can affect the risk of cancer occurrence: this is clearly reported in Fig. 16.1, in particular for endometrial, ovarian, and colorectal cancer.

CHCs use has always shown a significant protective effect on the risk of ovarian cancer, especially for the use during the perimenopausal period. Similarly, the risk of endometrial cancer is reduced by about 50% in ever users of CHCs, a benefit which is greater with increasing duration of use. A positive association has been found between increased risk of uterine cervical cancer and long-term CHCs use, but this risk is influenced by different HPV exposures in users and nonusers of HC and it will be affected by actual primary prevention policies (vaccination). Colorectal cancer is the most frequent neoplasm in nonsmokers of both sexes combined in Western countries and CHCs use seems to reduce its risk (as postmenopausal hormone therapy does). Confirmed data derived from independent international trials state that the risk of any cancers as a whole does not appear to be increased in CHCs users, while that of gynecological ones seems even reduced. The effect of progestin-only methods has not been studied that much: however, the protective effects appear to be more limited than the combined ones on some organs (i.e., ovaries, colon-rectum).

Unfortunately we do not have any data about different estrogens (E2, ethinyl-estradiol or estetrol) or different progestins activity on the modulation of oncological risk, with the exclusion of breast tissue in which the use of natural estrogens or progestins derived from progesterone seems to have preclinical and clinical evidence of higher safety in comparison with other available compounds [30, 31]: it will be the goal of the future research to identify some possible differences in this crucial association (natural vs. synthetic steroids).

Declarations

Competing Interests The author(s) has no competing interests to declare that are relevant to the content of this manuscript.

Ethics Approval The author(s) declares that this manuscript does not include primary research with human participants.

The author(s) declares that this manuscript does not include primary studies involving animals.

References

1. Gompel A, Ramirez I, Bitzer J, European Society of Contraception Expert Group on Hormonal Contraception. Contraception in cancer survivors – an expert review. Part I. Breast and gynaecological cancers. Eur J Contracept Reprod Health Care. 2019;24(3):167–74.
2. Cagnacci A, Ramirez I, Bitzer J, Gompel A. Contraception in cancer survivors – an expert review. Part II. Skin, gastrointestinal, haematological and endocrine cancers. Eur J Contracept Reprod Health Care. 2019;24(4):299–304.
3. Collaborative Group on Epidemiological Studies of Ovarian Cancer, Beral V, Doll R, Hermon C, Peto R, Reeves G. Ovarian cancer and oral contraceptives: collaborative reanalysis of data from 45 epidemiological studies including 23,257 women with ovarian cancer and 87,303 controls. Lancet. 2008;371(9609):303–14.
4. Iodice S, Barile M, Rotmensz N, Feroce I, Bonanni B, Radice P, et al. Oral contraceptive use and breast or ovarian cancer risk in BRCA1/2 carriers: a meta-analysis. Eur J Cancer. 2010;46(12):2275–84.
5. Grandi G, Sammarini M, Del Savio MC, Toss A, Facchinetti F. Combined hormonal contraceptives in BRCA gene mutation carriers: why not? Eur J Contracept Reprod Health Care. 2019;24(6):417–9.
6. Michels KA, Pfeiffer RM, Brinton LA, Trabert B. Modification of the associations between duration of oral contraceptive use and ovarian, endometrial, breast, and colorectal cancers. JAMA Oncol. 2018;4(4):516–21.
7. Iversen L, Fielding S, Lidegaard Ø, Mørch LS, Skovlund CW, Hannaford PC. Association between contemporary hormonal contraception and ovarian cancer in women of reproductive age in Denmark: prospective, nationwide cohort study. BMJ. 2018;362:k3609. https://doi.org/10.1136/bmj.k3609.
8. Phung MT, Lee AW, Wu AH, Berchuck A, Cho KR, Cramer DW, et al. Depot-medroxyprogesterone acetate use is associated with decreased risk of ovarian cancer: the mounting evidence of a protective role of progestins. Cancer Epidemiol Biomarkers Prev. 2021;30(5):927–35.
9. Grandi G, Toss A, Cortesi L, Botticelli L, Volpe A, Cagnacci A. The association between endometriomas and ovarian cancer: preventive effect of inhibiting ovulation and menstruation during reproductive life. Biomed Res Int. 2015;2015:751571.
10. Zapata LB, Whiteman MK, Marchbanks PA, Curtis KM. Intrauterine device use among women with ovarian cancer: a systematic review. Contraception. 2010;82(1):38–40.
11. Dashti SG, Chau R, Ouakrim DA, Buchanan DD, Clendenning M, Young JP, et al. Female hormonal factors and the risk of endometrial cancer in lynch syndrome. JAMA. 2015;314(1):61–71.
12. Lin MC, Burkholder KA, Viswanathan AN, Neuberg D, Mutter GL. Involution of latent endometrial precancers by hormonal and nonhormonal mechanisms. Cancer. 2009;115(10):2111–8.
13. International Collaboration of Epidemiological Studies of Cervical Cancer, Appleby P, Beral V, Berrington de González A, Colin D, Franceschi S, et al. Cervical cancer and hormonal contraceptives: collaborative reanalysis of individual data for 16,573 women with cervical

cancer and 35,509 women without cervical cancer from 24 epidemiological studies. Lancet. 2007;370(9599):1609–21.
14. Moodley M, Moodley J, Chetty R, Herrington CS. The role of steroid contraceptive hormones in the pathogenesis of invasive cervical cancer: a review. Int J Gynecol Cancer. 2003;13(2):103–10.
15. Averbach S, Silverberg MJ, Leyden W, Smith-McCune K, Raine-Bennett T, Sawaya GF. Recent intrauterine device use and the risk of precancerous cervical lesions and cervical cancer. Contraception. 2018:S0010-7824(18)30144–6. https://doi.org/10.1016/j.contraception.2018.04.008.
16. Bosetti C, Bravi F, Negri E, La Vecchia C. OC and colorectal cancer risk: a systematic review and meta-analysis. Hum Reprod Update. 2009;15:489–98.
17. Barra F, Perrone U, Ferrero S, Bogliolo S, Ottonello S, Gustavino C, Iasci A, Grandi G, Pulliero A, Centurioni MG, Izzotti A. Perception about benefits and risks related to combined hormonal contraceptives use in women with Lynch syndrome. Ann Med. 2024;56(1):2370568
18. Cibula D, Gompel A, Mueck AO, La Vecchia C, Hannaford PC, Skouby SO, et al. Hormonal contraception and risk of cancer. Hum Reprod Update. 2010;16(6):631–50.
19. Maheshwari S, Sarraj A, Kramer J, El-Serag HB. Oral contraception and the risk of hepatocellular carcinoma. J Hepatol. 2007;47(4):506–13.
20. Tang B, Lv J, Li Y, Yuan S, Wang Z, He S. Relationship between female hormonal and menstrual factors and pancreatic cancer: a meta-analysis of observational studies. Medicine (Baltimore). 2015;94(7):e177.
21. Braganza MZ, Berrington de González A, Schonfeld SJ, Wentzensen N, Brenner AV, Kitahara CM. Benign breast and gynecologic conditions, reproductive and hormonal factors, and risk of thyroid cancer. Cancer Prev Res (Phila). 2014;7(4):418–25.
22. Rzepka J, Malmur M, Zalewski K, Gózdz S, Bidziński M. Contraception for cancer survivors. Ginekol Pol. 2013;84(11):955–8.
23. Kane EV, Roman E, Becker N, Bernstein L, Boffetta P, Bracci PM, et al. Menstrual and reproductive factors, and hormonal contraception use: associations with non-Hodgkin lymphoma in a pooled analysis of InterLymph case-control studies. Ann Oncol. 2012;23(9):2362–74.
24. Iversen L, Sivasubramaniam S, Lee AJ, Fielding S, Hannaford PC. Lifetime cancer risk and combined oral contraceptives: the Royal College of General Practitioners' Oral Contraception Study. Am J Obstet Gynecol. 2017;216(6):580.e1–9.
25. Roman E, Smith A, Appleton S, Crouch S, Kelly R, Kinsey S, et al. Myeloid malignancies in the real-world: occurrence, progression and survival in the UK's population-based Haematological Malignancy Research Network 2004-15. Cancer Epidemiol. 2016;42:186–98.
26. De Bruin ML, Sparidans J, van't Veer MB, Noordijk EM, Louwman MWJ, Zijlstra JM, et al. Breast cancer risk in female survivors of Hodgkin's lymphoma: lower risk after smaller radiation volumes. J Clin Oncol. 2009;27(26):4239–46.
27. Grandi G, Marani G, Facchinetti F, Bahamondes L. We don't have elements to scare women who use oral contraceptives based on nomegestrol or chlormadinone about the risk of meningioma. Let's be careful and honest! Eur J Contracept Reprod Health Care. 2022;27(5):355–6.
28. Yang X, Liu F, Zheng J, Cheng W, Zhao C, Di J. Relationship between oral contraceptives and the risk of gliomas and meningiomas: a dose-response meta-analysis and systematic review. World Neurosurg. 2021;147:e148–62.
29. Michels KA, Brinton LA, Pfeiffer RM, Trabert B. Oral contraceptive use and risks of cancer in the NIH-AARP diet and health study. Am J Epidemiol. 2018;187(8):1630–41.
30. Grandi G, Toss A, Cagnacci A, Marcheselli L, Pavesi S, Facchinetti F, Cascinu S, Cortesi L. Combined hormonal contraceptive use and risk of breast cancer in a population of women with a family history. Clin Breast Cancer. 2018;18(1):e15–24.
31. Fruzzetti F, Fidecicchi T, Gambacciani M. Oestrogens in oral contraception: considerations for tailoring prescription to women's needs. Eur J Contracept Reprod Health Care. 2024;29(3):93–102.

Part VI
Progestin Only Contraception

Chapter 17
Progestin-Only Pills

Santiago Palacios

17.1 Introduction

Progestin-only pills (POPs) are a hormonal contraceptive method that contains exclusively progestins, without estrogens. These formulations have been designed to prevent pregnancy by inhibiting ovulation, modifying cervical mucus, and altering the endometrium, thereby hindering the implantation of a fertilized ovum [1]. Unlike combined oral contraceptives, POPs are particularly useful for women who cannot utilize estrogens, such as those who are breastfeeding or have a history of venous thrombosis [2].

The significance of POPs lies in their capacity to provide an effective and safe contraceptive option for a wide range of women. In many clinical contexts, women with contraindications to combined methods find in POPs a viable alternative, thereby allowing for greater personalization of contraceptive care [3]. Furthermore, the increase in acceptance and use of POPs reflects the need for more flexible and accessible contraceptive options in a world that values family planning and women's empowerment.

The objectives of this chapter are to explore in depth the characteristics, efficacy, and safety of progestin-only pills, as well as their place in modern clinical practice. Current formulations, the evolution of progestins used, and future directions in the research and development of hormonal contraceptive methods will also be addressed.

S. Palacios (✉)
Palacios Clinics, Madrid, Spain
e-mail: spalacios@clinicapalacios.com

A. R. Genazzani et al. (eds.), *Ethical, Efficacy and Safety Issues in Contraception*, Reproductive Medicine for Clinicians 4,
https://doi.org/10.1007/978-3-032-07322-8_17

17.2 History and Development

The history of progestin-only pills (POPs) is embedded within the broader context of the evolution of hormonal contraceptive methods. The introduction of the combined oral contraceptive pill in the 1960s marked a significant milestone in contraception, but it also highlighted the need for safe options for women who could not use estrogens. Consequently, in 1970, the first progestin-only pill, known as the "mini-pill," was launched, containing norethisterone. This method provided an alternative for those with medical contraindications [4].

Throughout the 1980s and 1990s, the development of new formulations of POPs focused on improving efficacy and reducing side effects. The introduction of more potent progestins, such as desogestrel in 1999 and drospirenone in 2000, represented a significant advancement. These progestins not only demonstrated enhanced efficacy in suppressing ovulation but also exhibited a more favorable side effect profile, which facilitated their acceptance in clinical practice [5].

Over the decades, the use of POPs has increased, particularly in contexts where combined pills are not suitable. The World Health Organization (WHO) has promoted POPs as a reliable option, especially for breastfeeding women or those with health conditions that contraindicate the use of estrogens [5]. As research in hormonal contraception advances, POPs continue to evolve, with recent studies investigating new progestins and formulations that could further enhance their efficacy and safety.

In summary, the evolution of POPs has been marked by the necessity for safe and effective contraceptive options for a diverse range of women. Their development has responded to changes in the understanding of reproductive health and individual needs, solidifying their role as a cornerstone of modern contraception.

17.3 Mechanism of Action

Progestin-only pills (POPs) operate through several mechanisms that contribute to their efficacy in preventing pregnancy. These mechanisms include the inhibition of ovulation, changes in cervical mucus, and effects on the endometrium.

17.3.1 Inhibition of Ovulation

The primary mechanism of action of POPs is the inhibition of ovulation. The administration of progestins suppresses the release of luteinizing hormone (LH) through negative feedback on the pituitary gland. The reduction in LH levels prevents the maturation and release of the ovum from the ovary. Although some formulations of POPs may not consistently suppress ovulation in all women, recent studies have demonstrated that progestins such as desogestrel and drospirenone are highly effective in inhibiting ovulation in the majority of users, thereby providing a reliable contraceptive method [6].

17.3.2 Changes in Cervical Mucus

Another fundamental mechanism is the alteration of the characteristics of cervical mucus. Progestins cause an increase in the viscosity of cervical mucus, which hinders the passage of sperm through the cervical canal. This change acts not only as a physical barrier but may also affect the ability of sperm to survive in the female reproductive tract [7, 8]. The efficacy of this mechanism is particularly relevant in clinical practice, as it provides an additional layer of protection against pregnancy.

17.3.3 Effects on the Endometrium

Finally, POPs also induce changes in the endometrium, which are essential for preventing the implantation of a fertilized ovum. Exposure to progestins causes the endometrium to transform into a secretory phase, making the environment less receptive to implantation. This modification includes reduced vascularization and alteration of endometrial secretions, which can hinder the nesting of the blastocyst [9]. These effects are crucial for the overall efficacy of POPs as contraceptive methods.

In conclusion, the mechanism of action of progestin-only pills combines the inhibition of ovulation, changes in cervical mucus, and modification of the endometrium. These multiple approaches ensure a high efficacy in preventing pregnancy, supporting their use as a safe and reliable contraceptive option.

17.4 Progestogens Used in POPs

17.4.1 Brief History of Progestogens

The first generations of progestogens in progestogen-only pills (POPs) included compounds like norethisterone and medroxyprogesterone. Introduced in the 1950s and 1960s, these progestogens were selected for their ovulation-inhibiting capacity and resistance to oral metabolism. Norethisterone was the first widely used synthetic progestogen, with early studies confirming ovulation inhibition in over 95% of cycles. However, these compounds displayed side effects such as fluid retention and mood changes due to their androgenic properties [10].

Levonorgestrel, a second-generation progestogen introduced in the 1970s, represented an improvement in terms of efficacy and side effect profile. Compared with norethisterone and medroxyprogesterone, levonorgestrel presented fewer side effects related to fluid retention and a lower incidence of mood changes [11]. Controlled studies showed ovulation inhibition close to 99% under ideal conditions; however, its androgenic activity led to side effects such as acne and hirsutism in some women.

17.4.2 Commentary on Modern Progestogens

With the development of third- and fourth-generation progestogens, such as desogestrel and drospirenone, the goal was to enhance safety, tolerability, and reduce adverse effects.

Desogestrel

(a) Efficacy and side effect profile: In phase III studies, desogestrel has demonstrated high efficacy in ovulation inhibition, with prevention rates exceeding 99% in perfect use and efficacy around 97% under typical conditions [12, 13]. Desogestrel's ovulation inhibition is robust, even with slightly inconsistent dosing, which is advantageous in clinical practice. In terms of side effects, studies reported lower incidences of androgenic effects such as acne and weight gain compared with older progestogens. However, irregular bleeding remains a commonly reported side effect, although it is not associated with serious adverse events [12, 13].

(b) Advantages compared with other progestogens: The high affinity of desogestrel for progesterone receptors allows for robust ovulation inhibition with less variability in efficacy compared with levonorgestrel. Additionally, its low androgenic profile improves tolerability in women who have experienced adverse effects with earlier progestogens [14].

Drospirenone

(a) Antimineralocorticoid properties: Drospirenone, a fourth-generation progestogen, is characterized by its antimineralocorticoid properties, which provide additional benefits regarding fluid retention and premenstrual symptom management. In phase III studies, these properties showed benefits in terms of reducing edema and symptoms like bloating and discomfort, especially compared with desogestrel and levonorgestrel [15, 16].

(b) Clinical uses and safety profile: Drospirenone has demonstrated contraceptive efficacy comparable to other progestogens, inhibiting ovulation in over 99% of cycles when taken correctly. Furthermore, phase III clinical trials highlighted a favorable cardiovascular safety profile, as low doses do not significantly increase the risk of thrombotic events. Its low androgenic activity also reduces the incidence of acne and adverse metabolic effects, making it particularly suitable for women prone to fluid retention or premenstrual mood changes [17, 18].

Other Progestogens Used in POPs

Other progestogens such as gestodene and norgestrel have been explored to a lesser extent in POPs. Gestodene, a third-generation progestogen, has shown strong contraceptive efficacy in smaller studies, with low androgenic activity, reducing side effects like acne. In contrast, norgestrel has been less popular due to its higher androgenic profile, which may increase the likelihood of mood changes and weight gain [19].

17.5 Efficacy of Drospirenone and Desogestrel in POPs

17.5.1 Pregnancy Prevention Rate

Both drospirenone and desogestrel are highly effective in progestogen-only pills (POPs), with studies reporting high efficacy in preventing pregnancy. For drospirenone, clinical trials indicate a typical-use efficacy rate of approximately 91–94%, with perfect-use efficacy approaching 99% when taken consistently [17, 18]. Its primary mechanism is ovulation inhibition, achieved through its strong affinity for progesterone receptors, effectively suppressing ovulation in over 99% of cycles under optimal adherence conditions [20]. Desogestrel, in comparison, exhibits similar effectiveness. Typical-use efficacy is reported around 93–95%, with perfect-use rates close to 99%, largely due to its ability to inhibit ovulation consistently [14]. This strong suppression of ovulation in both drospirenone and desogestrel makes them competitive with combined oral contraceptives (COCs), although without the cardiovascular risks associated with estrogen.

17.5.2 Factors Affecting Efficacy

Efficacy for both drospirenone and desogestrel POPs is highly dependent on adherence, as they must be taken at approximately the same time each day. Drospirenone has a relatively shorter half-life, meaning that missed or delayed doses can reduce plasma concentrations, potentially allowing follicular development and ovulation, thus impacting effectiveness [21]. Gastrointestinal disturbances, such as vomiting or diarrhea, can also impair drug absorption, further impacting efficacy. Desogestrel, with its slightly longer half-life, offers marginally more flexibility; however, consistent adherence remains essential to maintain its effectiveness [22]. The absence of estrogen in both types of POPs eliminates the dual suppression of ovulation present in COCs, increasing reliance on adherence to maintain contraceptive effectiveness.

17.5.3 Comparison with Combined Oral Contraceptives and Other Contraceptive Methods

In terms of efficacy, drospirenone and desogestrel POPs are slightly less effective than COCs in typical-use scenarios, though comparable under perfect use. COCs, which combine estrogen and progestogen, have typical-use effectiveness rates around 94–97% because of the dual suppression of ovulation. For women unable to use estrogen, drospirenone and desogestrel POPs provide a viable and effective alternative, offering similar contraceptive benefits without the added cardiovascular risks associated with estrogen [23]. When compared with long-acting reversible contraceptives (LARCs), such as intrauterine devices (IUDs) or implants, both drospirenone and desogestrel POPs are less effective due to LARCs' minimal reliance on user adherence. However, their oral administration and noninvasiveness make them an attractive option for women preferring a daily method. Drospirenone, in particular, offers additional benefits for women experiencing premenstrual symptoms, thanks to its antimineralocorticoid effects, while desogestrel may offer a slight advantage in terms of flexibility due to its pharmacokinetic profile [24].

17.6 Indications and Benefits of POPs

17.6.1 Groups of Women Who Benefit from POPs (Table 17.1)

Progestogen-only pills (POPs), including drospirenone and desogestrel formulations, are particularly advantageous for specific groups of women. Breastfeeding women represent a primary population who benefit from POPs, as they do not interfere with lactation or alter milk composition. POPs are a safe contraceptive option postpartum, as they do not contain estrogens, which can reduce milk production. Studies show that desogestrel and drospirenone POPs have no adverse effects on breastfeeding duration or infant growth, positioning them as a preferred choice for lactating mothers who require contraception [2, 6, 24].

Another group that benefits from POPs is women with contraindications to estrogens. Women with a history of cardiovascular disease, hypertension, or a predisposition to thromboembolic disorders should avoid estrogen-containing contraceptives due to their increased risk of cardiovascular events. For these women, POPs offer an effective alternative that circumvents estrogen-related risks while maintaining a high degree of contraceptive efficacy [6]. Furthermore, women with migraine, particularly those with aura, often face restrictions on estrogen-containing methods, making POPs a safer choice [6].

Table 17.1 Indications for the use of POPs

Indication	Description
Breastfeeding women	Safe for lactating women, as they do not affect milk production
Women with contraindications to estrogen	Ideal for those with conditions like thromboembolic disorders, migraines with aura, or certain cancers
Women with a history of thrombosis	Provides a lower risk for thromboembolic events compared to estrogen-containing contraceptives
Women experiencing side effects from estrogen	Suitable for women who have had adverse reactions to combined hormonal contraceptives
Women desiring a flexible contraceptive method	Offers daily dosing without the need for estrogen, which is often easier for some women to manage
Women with heavy menstrual bleeding	Can help manage menstrual cycles and reduce heavy bleeding
Women with specific health conditions	Effective for women with conditions like polycystic ovary syndrome (PCOS) or endometriosis, where estrogen may exacerbate symptoms

17.6.2 Advantages of POPs over Other Methods

POPs present notable advantages over combined oral contraceptives (COCs) and other contraceptive methods, particularly due to the absence of estrogens. Without the associated risks of estrogen, such as increased blood pressure and thromboembolic events, POPs offer a safer profile, especially for women at elevated cardiovascular risk. In comparative studies, women on POPs report fewer estrogen-related side effects, such as breast tenderness, nausea, and migraines, thereby enhancing their acceptability and adherence [24, 25].

Moreover, POPs offer greater flexibility in administration, particularly with newer formulations. Desogestrel has a slightly longer half-life compared to traditional progestins, providing a broader dosing window and enhancing user adherence. Similarly, drospirenone POPs, despite their shorter half-life, provide consistent ovulation suppression when taken as directed, though adherence remains essential. This flexibility makes POPs suitable for women with varying schedules or those seeking an alternative to more rigidly timed contraceptive methods. Additionally, the option to stop and start POPs with a quick return to fertility makes them a versatile choice compared to long-acting methods like IUDs or implants, which require medical removal [24, 25].

17.7 Side Effects and Risks of Drospirenone and Desogestrel POPs

17.7.1 Common Side Effects (Table 17.2)

Both drospirenone and desogestrel POPs share several common side effects, primarily due to their progestogenic activity. Menstrual irregularities, such as breakthrough bleeding, are frequently reported, especially in the first few months of use, with desogestrel exhibiting a slightly higher incidence of irregular bleeding than drospirenone [26]. Some users also report mild mood changes, headaches, and breast tenderness. However, drospirenone has unique antimineralocorticoid properties, which can alleviate bloating and fluid retention, offering an advantage over desogestrel for users sensitive to these symptoms [17].

17.7.2 Rare Side Effects and Health Concerns

Serious side effects associated with both drospirenone and desogestrel are rare, but certain health concerns remain. Progestogen-only pills in general have a minimal risk profile compared to estrogen-containing contraceptives, particularly in terms of

Table 17.2 Common and rare side effects of POPs

Side effect category	Specific side effects	Notes
Common side effects	Irregular bleeding or spotting	May improve after a few months of use
Nausea	Generally mild	Can often be managed with timing of doses
Headaches	May occur more frequently in women with a history of migraines	
Breast tenderness	Can fluctuate, less with drospirenone	Often resolves over time
Mood changes	Some women may experience anxiety or depression	
Weight gain	Variable, less with drospirenone	Some users report changes in weight
Rare side effects	Deep vein thrombosis (DVT)	Very low risk compared to combined hormonal contraceptives
Pulmonary embolism	Risk associated with underlying conditions	
Hypertension	Can occur, less with drospirenone	Monitoring may be necessary for women with a history of high blood pressure
Impact on bone density	Long-term use may affect bone health	Monitoring may be necessary

thromboembolic events. However, some studies have suggested that high doses of desogestrel might slightly increase the risk of breast tenderness and acne due to its androgenic activity, although the risk remains low overall [27]. Drospirenone's antimineralocorticoid effect, though beneficial in reducing bloating, has raised concerns about potential hyperkalemia in users with kidney or adrenal conditions. Yet, studies report that the risk of significant hyperkalemia is negligible for most healthy women, making drospirenone generally safe [28].

17.7.3 Comparison of Side Effects with Other Contraceptive Methods

Compared to combined oral contraceptives (COCs), both drospirenone and desogestrel POPs generally exhibit a lower risk of side effects linked to estrogen, such as nausea, increased blood pressure, and risk of thromboembolism. COCs tend to cause more breast tenderness and mood swings due to the combined estrogen-progestogen effect, making POPs a preferable option for women sensitive to estrogen or at increased cardiovascular risk [23, 28]. While desogestrel has a slight androgenic effect, leading to occasional reports of acne and weight changes, drospirenone's antimineralocorticoid properties often reduce bloating and weight gain associated with fluid retention, offering a side-effect profile similar to COCs that contain drospirenone [17, 18].

Long-acting reversible contraceptives (LARCs) like IUDs and implants offer fewer daily side effects due to their steady hormone release, but may initially cause heavier bleeding or cramping, particularly with copper IUDs. POPs, by contrast, provide a more flexible, user-controlled option with reversible effects and a quick return to fertility upon discontinuation, making them attractive for women seeking a noninvasive, short-term contraceptive [24].

17.8 Practical Considerations for Using POPs

17.8.1 Administration and Compliance

Both drospirenone and desogestrel POPs require daily intake at the same time each day to maintain their efficacy. However, drospirenone offers greater flexibility regarding missed pills compared to desogestrel. With drospirenone, a missed dose can be taken within 24 h without significantly impacting its contraceptive effectiveness, whereas desogestrel must be taken within a narrower 12-h window, making it less forgiving of delayed doses [29, 30]. This added flexibility with drospirenone can improve adherence, especially for users with unpredictable schedules, reducing the likelihood of contraceptive failure due to missed doses.

17.8.2 Tips for Effective Use

To maximize effectiveness, users should incorporate daily reminders or use electronic alerts to ensure timely intake. For women who do miss a dose, following specific instructions is essential: for drospirenone, the missed pill can be taken within a day without additional contraception; with desogestrel, if more than 12 h have passed, a backup method, such as condoms, should be used for the next 2 days [29, 30]. POP users should also avoid any drugs that may interact with these contraceptives, such as certain antiepileptic medications, which may lower efficacy.

17.9 Future Directions and Recent Studies in POPs

17.9.1 Innovations in POP Formulations

Recent advancements in progestogen-only pill (POP) formulations aim to enhance efficacy, safety, and user compliance. Innovations include the development of extended-release formulations that allow for less frequent dosing, thereby improving adherence among women with busy lifestyles. For example, researchers are exploring the use of biodegradable implants that release progestogens steadily over extended periods, potentially reducing the daily burden of oral contraceptives while maintaining high contraceptive efficacy [31]. Furthermore, advances in delivery methods, such as transdermal patches and vaginal rings that deliver progestogens, are under investigation, which may offer alternatives to traditional oral administration and cater to varying patient preferences.

17.9.2 Ongoing Research on Efficacy and Safety

Current studies continue to evaluate the efficacy and safety profiles of both drospirenone and desogestrel in diverse populations. Research is focusing on the long-term effects of POPs on reproductive health, particularly concerning bone density and cardiovascular health. For instance, a multi-centre trial is examining the impact of drospirenone on bone mineral density in young women using POPs over extended periods [32]. Additionally, studies are assessing the potential for progestogen-only contraceptives to reduce menstrual-related disorders, thereby broadening their appeal beyond mere contraception [26]. Ongoing research is also investigating the interaction of POPs with other medications and their impact on efficacy, particularly in women with comorbidities.

17.9.3 *Perspectives on Hormonal Contraception in Reproductive Health*

The landscape of hormonal contraception is evolving, with a growing emphasis on personalization in reproductive health. The integration of patient-centered approaches in contraceptive counseling allows for tailored contraceptive choices that consider individual health profiles, lifestyle, and preferences [33]. Future directions in hormonal contraception, particularly with POPs, include the exploration of how genetic factors may influence individual responses to progestogens, potentially leading to more effective personalized contraceptive regimens. Furthermore, increasing awareness of the need for accessible contraception options among underserved populations will drive future research and policy initiatives aimed at improving reproductive health outcomes globally [34].

In conclusion, the future of progestogen-only contraceptives looks promising, with ongoing research and innovations expected to enhance their role in reproductive health. As the scientific community continues to uncover the benefits and risks of POPs, these contraceptives will likely become even more integral to women's health strategies worldwide.

Declarations

Competing Interests The author(s) has no competing interests to declare that are relevant to the content of this manuscript.

Ethics Approval The author(s) declares that this manuscript does not include primary research with human participants.

The author(s) declares that this manuscript does not include primary studies involving animals.

References

1. Teal S, Edelman A. Contraception selection, effectiveness, and adverse effects: a review. JAMA. 2021;326(24):2507–18. https://doi.org/10.1001/jama.2021.21392. PMID: 34962522.
2. Kubba A, Gemzell-Danielsson K, Palacios S, Wiegratz I, Grandi G, Colli E, Regidor PA. The drospirenone (DRSP)-only pill: clinical implications in the daily use. Eur J Contracept Reprod Health Care. 2023;28(1):36–43. https://doi.org/10.1080/13625187.2022.2164186.
3. Festin MPR. Overview of modern contraception. Best Pract Res Clin Obstet Gynaecol. 2020;66:4–14. https://doi.org/10.1016/j.bpobgyn.2020.03.004. Epub 2020 Mar 13. PMID: 32291177.
4. Graham S, Fraser IS. The progestogen-only mini-pill. Contraception. 1982;26(4):373–88. https://doi.org/10.1016/0010-7824(82)90104-4. PMID: 6759029.
5. Liu S, Kciuk O, Frank M, Tyson N. Progestins of today and tomorrow. Curr Opin Obstet Gynecol. 2022;34(6):344–50. https://doi.org/10.1097/GCO.0000000000000819. Epub 2022 Aug 19. PMID: 36036464.
6. Gaffield ML, Kiarie J. WHO medical eligibility criteria update. Contraception. 2016;94(3):193–4. https://doi.org/10.1016/j.contraception.2016.07.001. PMID: 27503261.

7. Zuniga C, Blanchard K, Harper CC, Wollum A, Key K, Henderson JT. Effectiveness and efficacy rates of progestin-only pills: a comprehensive literature review. Contraception. 2023;119:109925. https://doi.org/10.1016/j.contraception.2022.109925. Epub 2022 Dec 17. PMID: 36535414.
8. Kumar TC, Shah RS, Chitlange SM, Hazari KT, Gopalkrishnan K, Vadigoppula AD, Vernekar VJ, Borkar DM, Puri CP. Effects of intranasal administration of norethisterone on folliculogenesis, cervical mucus, vaginal cytology, endometrial morphology and reproductive-endocrine profile in women. Contraception. 1991;44(3):245–67. https://doi.org/10.1016/0010-7824(91)90016-9. PMID: 1764942.
9. Rivera R, Yacobson I, Grimes D. The mechanism of action of hormonal contraceptives and intrauterine contraceptive devices. Am J Obstet Gynecol. 1999;181(5 Pt 1):1263–9. https://doi.org/10.1016/s0002-9378(99)70120-1. PMID: 10561657.
10. Huvinen E, Holopainen E, Heikinheimo O. Norethisterone and its acetate – what's so special about them? BMJ Sex Reprod Health. 2021;47(2):102–9. https://doi.org/10.1136/bmjsrh-2020-200619. Epub 2020 May 12. PMID: 32398290.
11. Sapapsap B, Leelakanok N, Boonpattharatthiti K, Siritientong T, Methaneethorn J. A systematic review and meta-analysis of the prevalence and association between levonorgestrel and ectopic pregnancy. Expert Opin Drug Saf. 2023;22(10):929–41. https://doi.org/10.1080/14740338.2023.2247965. Epub 2023 Aug 17. PMID: 37577925.
12. Rice CF, Killick SR, Dieben T, Bennink HC. A comparison of the inhibition of ovulation achieved by desogestrel 75 mg and levonorgestrel 30 mg daily. Hum Reprod. 1999;14:982–5.
13. Rice C, Killick S, Hickling D, Bennink HC. Ovarian activity and vaginal bleeding patterns with a desogestrel-only preparation at three different doses. Hum Reprod. 1996;11:737–40.
14. Stone SC. Desogestrel. Clin Obstet Gynecol. 1995;38(4):821–8. https://doi.org/10.1097/00003081-199538040-00017. PMID: 8616978.
15. Regidor PA, Mueller A, Mayr M. Pharmacological and metabolic effects of drospirenone as a progestin-only pill compared to combined formulations with estrogen. Womens Health (Lond). 2023;19:17455057221147388. https://doi.org/10.1177/17455057221147388. PMID: 36744531; PMCID: PMC9905034.
16. Rapkin AJ, Winer SA. Drospirenone: a novel progestin. Expert Opin Pharmacother. 2007;8(7):989–99. Review.
17. Archer DF, Ahrendt HJ, Drouin D. Drospirenone-only oral contraceptive: results from a multicenter noncomparative trial of efficacy, safety and tolerability. Contraception. 2015;92(5):439–44. https://doi.org/10.1016/j.contraception.2015.07.014. Epub 2015 Jul 29.
18. Palacios S, Colli E, Regidor PA. Multicenter, phase III trials on the contraceptive efficacy, tolerability and safety of a new drospirenone only pill. Acta Obstet Gynecol Scand. 2019;98(12):1549–57. https://doi.org/10.1111/aogs.13688.
19. Kaplan B. Desogestrel, norgestimate, and gestodene: the newer progestins. Ann Pharmacother. 1995;29(7–8):736–42. https://doi.org/10.1177/106002809502907-817. PMID: 8520092.
20. Duijkers IJ, Heger-Mahn D, Drouin D, Skouby S. A randomized study comparing the effect on ovarian activity of a progestin-only pill (POP) containing desogestrel and a new POP containing drospirenone in a 24/4 regimen. Eur J Contracept Reprod Health Care. 2015;20:419–27.
21. Chiara Del Savio M, De Fata R, Facchinetti F, Grandi G. Drospirenone 4 mg-only pill (DOP) in 24+4 regimen: a new option for oral contraception. Expert Rev Clin Pharmacol. 2020;13(7):685–94. https://doi.org/10.1080/17512433.2020.1783247. Epub 2020 Jun 22. PMID: 32538188.
22. Faculty of Family Planning & Reproductive Health Care, Clinical Effectiveness Unit. Desogestrel-only pill (Cerazette). J Fam Plann Reprod Health Care. 2003;29(3):162–4. https://doi.org/10.1783/147118903101197593. PMID: 12885316.
23. Palacios S, Colli E, Regidor PA. Efficacy and cardiovascular safety of the new estrogen-free contraceptive pill containing 4 mg drospirenone alone in a 24/4 regime. BMC Womens Health. 2020;20(1):218. https://doi.org/10.1186/s12905-020-01080-9. PMID: 33008401; PMCID: PMC7530969.

24. Regidor PA. The clinical relevance of progestins in hormonal contraception: present status and future developments. Oncotarget. 2018;9:34628–38.
25. de Melo NR. Estrogen-free oral hormonal contraception: benefits of the progestin-only pill. Womens Health (Lond). 2010;6(5):721–35. https://doi.org/10.2217/whe.10.36.
26. Palacios S, Colli E, Regidor PA. A multicenter, double-blind, randomized trial on the bleeding profile of a drospirenone-only pill 4 mg over nine cycles in comparison with desogestrel 0.075 mg. Arch Gynecol Obstet. 2019;300(6):1805–12.
27. McClamrock HD, Adashi EY. Pharmacokinetics of desogestrel. Am J Obstet Gynecol. 1993;168(3 Pt 2):1021–8. https://doi.org/10.1016/0002-9378(93)90332-d. PMID: 8447355.
28. Krattenmacher R. Drospirenone: pharmacology and pharmacokinetics of a unique progestin. Contraception. 2000;62:29–38.
29. Rosenberg MJ, Burnhill MS, Waugh MS, Grimes DA, Hillard PJ. Compliance and oral contraceptives: a review. Contraception. 1995;52(3):137–41. Review.
30. Duijkers IJM, Heger-Mahn D, Drouin D, Colli E, Skouby S. Maintenance of ovulation inhibition with a new progestin-only pill containing drospirenone after scheduled 24-h delays in pill intake. Contraception. 2016;93(4):303–9. https://doi.org/10.1016/j.contraception.2015.12.007. Epub 2015 Dec 17.
31. Gilbert AL, Hoffman BL. Contraceptive technology: present and future. Obstet Gynecol Clin N Am. 2021;48(4):723–35. https://doi.org/10.1016/j.ogc.2021.07.001. PMID: 3475629.
32. Hadji P, Colli E, Regidor PA. Bone health in estrogen-free contraception. Osteoporos Int. 2019;30(12):2391–400. https://doi.org/10.1007/s00198-019-05103-6. Epub 2019 Aug 24. Erratum in: Osteoporos Int. 2020;31(7):1399. doi: 10.1007/s00198-020-05426-9. PMID: 31446440; PMCID: PMC7203087.
33. Schivone GB, Glish LL. Contraceptive counseling for continuation and satisfaction. Curr Opin Obstet Gynecol. 2017;29(6):443–8. https://doi.org/10.1097/GCO.0000000000000408. PMID: 28938374.
34. Lo Faro V, Johansson T, Johansson Å. The risk of venous thromboembolism in oral contraceptive users: the role of genetic factors-a prospective cohort study of 240,000 women in the UK Biobank. Am J Obstet Gynecol. 2024;230(3):360.e1–360.e13. https://doi.org/10.1016/j.ajog.2023.09.012. Epub 2023 Sept 19. PMID: 37734636.

Chapter 18
Intrauterine Devices: Efficacy and Risks: Insights from the Real-World Evidence

Oskari Heikinheimo

18.1 Introduction

With more than 160 million users globally, contraception by means of intrauterine contraceptive device (IUD) is one of the most commonly used reversible contraceptive methods worldwide. There is considerable geographical variation in the use of IUD. According to United Nations statistics from 2019, IUDs are used a lot in Southeastern Asia (e.g., in North Korea, Uzbekistan, Turkmenistan, and China) with approximately 24% rate of overall use among fertile-aged women. In Europe, IUDs are used frequently in eastern and northern countries (approximately 8%) with top figure of 18% in Moldova. Also, the Baltic states and Nordic countries all have high use of IUD. Lower rates of IUD use (approximately 4%) have been reported in southern European countries [28].

The contraceptive efficacy of contraceptive methods is expressed as Pearl index (PI), i.e., the number of contraceptive failures (i.e., pregnancies) during the first year of use in 100 fertile-aged women. Classical comparison of PIs during perfect and typical use of different contraceptive methods has been presented by James Trussell [27]. Contraception by means of IUD is very effective with PI values of 0.2 and 0.6 during perfect, and 0.3 and 0.8 during typical, use of LNG-IUD and Cu-IUD, respectively.

The rationale for IUD use is evident. High contraceptive efficacy in all women, long duration of action, safety, several associated health benefits (especially LNG-IUD), and minimal need of routine follow-up are clear benefits of intrauterine contraception [6].

O. Heikinheimo (✉)
Department of Obstetrics and Gynecology, University of Helsinki and Helsinki University Hospital, Helsinki, Finland
e-mail: oskari.heikinheimo@helsinki.fi

A. R. Genazzani et al. (eds.), *Ethical, Efficacy and Safety Issues in Contraception*, Reproductive Medicine for Clinicians 4,
https://doi.org/10.1007/978-3-032-07322-8_18

The present review focuses on the efficacy and safety especially of hormone (i.e., levonorgestrel) releasing IUD. Specifically, results of the first large-scale clinical trials evaluating LNG-IUD versus Cu-IUD performed already in the 1980s, and those of recent real-world data and epidemiological studies are discussed and compared.

18.2 Contraceptive Efficacy

Before its first market approval in Finland in 1990, the clinical performance of LNG-IUD was studied in several international multicenter studies [1, 23].

Contraceptive efficacy, expulsion, discontinuation, and side effects of LNG-IUD (releasing 20 μg of LNG/d) versus Nova-T Cu-IUD (copper surface area of 200 mm^2) were studied in a randomized clinical trial (RCT) performed in the Nordic countries and Hungary by Andersson et al. [1]. The study enrolled women aged 18–38 years with proven fertility (i.e., history of at least one pregnancy) between 1982 and 1984; the follow-up was 5 years. With more than 2750 participants, the study accumulated approximately 14.000 women-years (WY) of follow-up. Similarly, a multinational RCT by Sivin et al. [23] compared the contraceptive efficacy of LNG-IUD versus copper T 380Ag IUD during 5-year follow-up among 2245 fertile women aged 18–38 years. The PIs during the first year of use were 0.1 for LNG-IUD and 0.9 for Cu-IUD in the study by Andersson et al. [1], and 0.2 and 0.3 by Sivin et al. [23]. The 5-year cumulative pregnancy rates of 0.5% and 1.1% were reported for the LNG-IUD, and 5.9% and 1.4% for Cu-IUD [1, 23].

Contraceptive efficacy, reported as cumulative annual pregnancy rates in LNG- and Cu-IUD users by Andersson et al. [1], is shown in Fig. 18.1. In addition, the cumulative 5-year pregnancy rates in different age groups are depicted in Fig. 18.2 (panel on the left). With 5-year cumulative pregnancy rate of approximately ≤4%, both types of IUDs were very effective, yet the LNG-IUD was more effective.

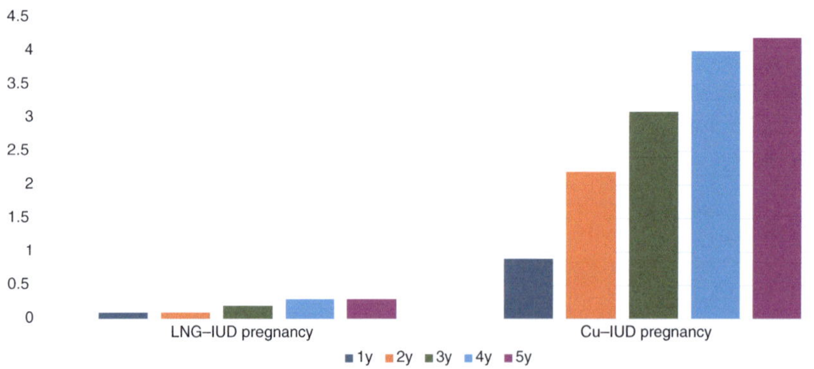

Fig. 18.1 Five-year cumulative rate (%) of pregnancy in LNG-IUD versus Cu-IUD users [1]

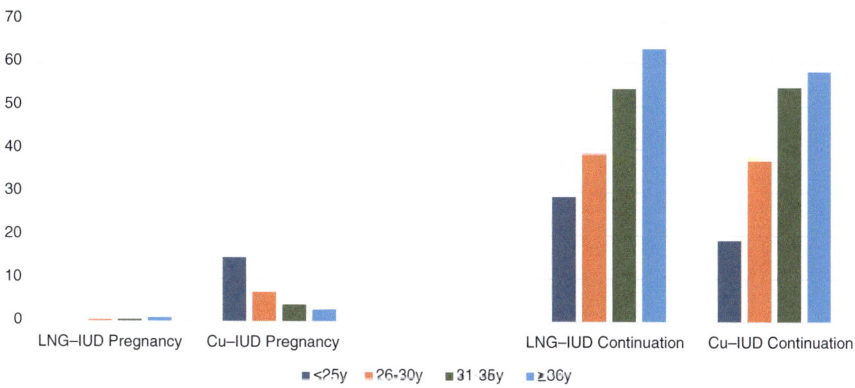

Fig. 18.2 Five-year cumulative rate (%) of pregnancy and continuation of LNG-IUD versus Cu-IUD user in different age groups [1]

Moreover, the LNG-IUD was similarly effective in all age categories, whereas the efficacy of Cu-IUD was lower among younger age cohorts with 5-year cumulative pregnancy rate of 14.9% among women ≤25 years of age and 6.9% those between 26 and 30 years [1].

Contraceptive efficacy of IUDs has been recently revisited in large European Active Surveillance Study for Intrauterine Devices (EURAS-IUD) trial, a prospective noninterference study performed in six European countries [11]. The study enrolled nearly 61,500 women aged between 18 and 50 years, who received an IUD between 2006 and 12. Approximately two-thirds (67%) of the women received the LNG52mg-IUD and 28% received various brands of Cu-IUDs. The follow-up was 1 year. A PI of 0.06 was found for LNG-IUD and 0.52 for Cu-IUD. Similarly, as in the early study by Andersson et al. [1], the contraceptive efficacy of Cu-IUDs was somewhat reduced among the youngest age cohort (PI 1.4 in women aged 18–29) compared to that seen (PI 0.57) among 30–39-year-olds [11].

The value of the high contraceptive efficacy of long-acting reversible contraceptives (i.e., IUDs and contraceptive implants [LARC]) is highlighted especially in highly fertile women, such as young women or those after induced abortion. The CHOICE study performed in St Louis area of the United States assessed the effects of free-of-charge LARC provision on the rate of unintended pregnancy especially among teenagers [22]. Approximately 37% of the study participants chose an IUD. Free-of-charge LARC provision was associated with significantly decreased rate of teenage pregnancy and abortion. Moreover, this effect was similar in all age groups [22]. Similarly, in a study performed in the City of Vantaa in Finland, provision of free-of-charge LARC decreased significantly the rate of induced abortion among women younger than 25 years of age, but not among older women [9].

Postabortal IUD contraception has been shown to decrease the need of subsequent induced abortion by approximately two-thirds in several cohort studies [10]. In a randomized clinical trial, rapid postabortal provision of IUD by the clinic responsible for abortion care, compared with initiating oral contraceptives and

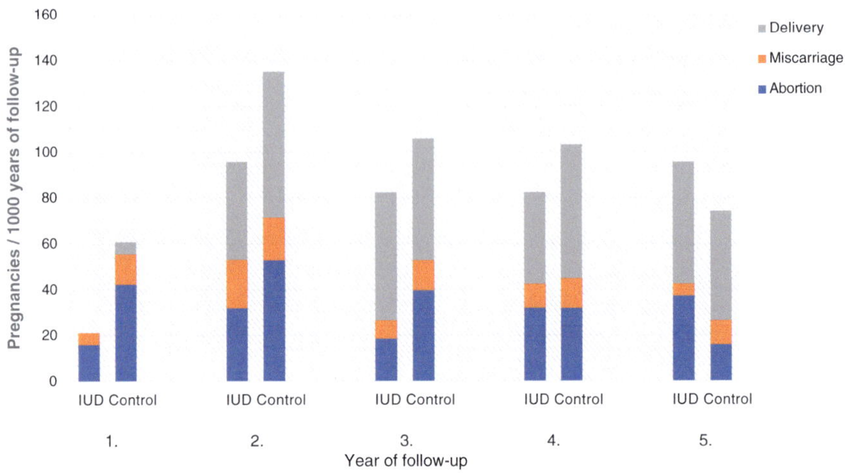

Fig. 18.3 Pregnancy outcomes following routine early provision of IUD after first-trimester induced abortion during 5-year follow-up [19]

directing women to primary healthcare for IUD provision, significantly reduced the need of another abortion during the 5-year follow-up [18]. This decline was significant during the first 2 years of the follow-up. However, the rates of delivery or miscarriage were not significantly affected by the intervention (Fig. 18.3) [19].

18.3 IUD Discontinuation

Continuation rates and reasons for discontinuation were studied already in the first prospective clinical trials comparing LNG-IUD and Cu-IUD [1, 23]. In brief, the first-year continuation rates of IUDs have been high, with approximately 80% of all study participants. The 5-year continuation rates of LNG-IUD and Cu-IUD use were 47% and 45% in the study by Andersson et al. [1] and 33% and 41% by Sivin et al. [23]. Continuation rates of both LNG-IUD and Cu-IUD were higher in older age cohorts (Fig. 18.2, panel on the left) [1]. The main reasons for discontinuation were bleeding problems (approximately 11–16%), planning pregnancy (11–12%), other medical reasons (6–8%), and pain (4%) in both studies. Discontinuation of LNG-IUD use for hormonal reasons (i.e., oily skin, acne) and amenorrhea was more common than that of Cu-IUD in both studies [1, 23].

The real-life discontinuation of any contraceptive method, including that of IUD, is difficult to study reliably. However, 2-year discontinuation rates of different LARC-methods were studied in a recent Finnish retrospective cohort study [21]. The study utilized a combination of different Finnish national registers to monitor the IUD discontinuations among women receiving their first LARC method free-of-charge in the City of Vantaa in the Helsinki metropolitan area. The 2-year cumulative rate of LNG-IUD discontinuation (24.2/100 WY [95% CI 21.7–26.9]) was significantly lower than that of Cu-IUD (37.8/100 [31.0–45.8]). Similarly, as reported by Andersson et al. [1], IUD discontinuation was higher among young women (aged <30 vs. ≥30–44 years), those who had given birth during previous year and those who spoke other than national language [21].

Thus the 2-year discontinuation rates of IUD contraception in this recent real-life study [21] are surprisingly similar to those reported in a RCT performed some 40 years ago by Andersson et al. [1] (i.e., 34.4 for LNG-IUD and 29.3 for Cu-IUD). The only difference was higher rate of LNG-IUD discontinuation in the early studies [1, 23].

Concerning the main reasons for IUD discontinuations, bleeding problems were the dominant reason in both the old RCTs and the new real-life studies [1, 21, 23]. Amenorrhea was a common reason for discontinuation in the old trials. However, it may be speculated that as absence of bleeding during LNG-IUD use was a new concept in the 1980s, it also resulted in discontinuations in these first trials.

18.4 Risks Associated with Intrauterine Contraception

18.4.1 Uterine Perforation

Risk of uterine perforation is a unique complication associated with IUD contraception. The incidence and risk factors of uterine perforation have been studied recently prospectively in the EURAS-IUD study [11], and in a registry-based APEX-IUD [20] and Finnish studies [13]. The risk of perforation was small in all studies irrespective of the study design. The highest rate of perforation (1.1 for Cu-IUD and 1.4 for LNG-IUD/1000 insertions) was seen in the prospective EURAS-IUD study, whereas a rate of 0.4/1000 was reported in a registry-based study from Finland [13]. Importantly, the risk of perforation did not differ between LNG-IUD and Cu-IUD [11].

Similar risk factors for uterine perforation have emerged in different study settings. Insertion during postpartum period to lactating woman increased the risk of IUD perforation up to six- to sevenfold in the EURAS-IUD and APEX-IUD studies [11, 20]. Nevertheless, IUD perforation continues to be rare event, and more than 99% of IUD insertions do not result in perforation even if performed in lactating women.

Clinical symptoms and sequela of uterine perforation have been studied systematically in a registry-based study by Kaislasuo et al. [14] and prospectively in the EURAS-IUD study. In both of these studies, the majority of cases of uterine perforation presented with rather minimal symptoms.

In case series of 75 patients identified via Finnish hospital registry, approximately 70% of the patients had only mild symptoms (such as mild abdominal pain and/or bleeding), and 30% of the cases were asymptomatic and perforation was diagnosed incidentally due to, e.g., missing stings or unplanned pregnancy [14]. Similarly, among the 81 uterine perforations recorded in the EURAS-IUD study, no serious medical sequelae or organ injuries were reported [11]. Abdominally placed IUDs are typically removed laparoscopically. However, the necessity of the surgical removal may also be questioned in cases of asymptomatic patients.

18.5 IUD Expulsion

Unnoticed expulsion—a typical complication of IUD contraception—is not risky per se, but exposes the woman to the risks of unplanned pregnancy. The randomized trial comparing LNG-IUD and Cu-IUD by Andersson et al. [1] reported 5-year cumulative expulsion rate of approximately 5% for both devices, whereas higher expulsion rates (i.e., 11.8% for LNG-IUD and 7.4% for Cu-IUD) were reported by Sivin et al. [23].

The rate and risk factors of IUD expulsion have recently been studied in two large studies from Europe and North America. Besides contraceptive efficacy of IUDs, EURAS-IUD study assessed the risk of ectopic pregnancy and uterine perforation in EU area [11]. The Association of Perforation and Expulsion of Intrauterine Devices (APEX-IUD) study performed in California and Washington states used Kaiser Permanente healthcare data of more than 326,000 women aged ≤50 years receiving an IUD between 2001 and 2018 [7].

The APEX-IUD study characterized the risk factors of IUD expulsion. In adjusted analyses, current or past heavy menstrual bleeding, overweight and obesity, age below 25 years, and parity of ≥4 emerged as significant risk factors for IUD expulsion [2].

The adjusted hazard ratios (95Cis) of IUD expulsion and perforation according to postpartum timing, breastfeeding status, HMB status and IUD type reported in the APEX-IUD study are shown in Table 18.1.

18.6 Ectopic Pregnancy

The association of intrauterine contraception and the risk of ectopic pregnancy (EP) is often confusing. It is important to note that the incidence of all pregnancies—including EPs—is decreased during IUD use. However, in rare cases of pregnancy during IUD use, the proportion of EPs of all pregnancies is increased in women using IUD compared to women not using IUD.

Concerning the efficacy of different types of IUDs in reducing the risk of EP, the EURAS-IUD reported an EP incidence rate of 0.02/100 WY (95%CI 0.01–0.03) for LNG52mg-IUD and 0.08/100 WY (0.04–0.13) for Cu-IUD [11].

The protective effect of contraceptive use, including IUD use on the risk of EP, was highlighted in a recent Swedish national registry-based study on the risk of EP

Table 18.1 Hazard ratios (adjusted HR [95%CI]) of IUD perforation and expulsion by different risk factors [7]

	Perforation	Expulsion
Postpartum timing (vs. interval insertion)		
0 to 3 days	2.73 (1.33–5.63)	5.34 (4.47–6.39)
4 days to ≤6 weeks	6.71 (4.80–9.38)	1.22 (1.05–1.41)
>6 to ≤14 weeks	4.64 (3.48–6.18)	1.06 (0.95–1.18)
>14 to ≤52 weeks	2.93 (2.15–4.00)	1.43 (1.29–1.60)
Breastfeeding (vs. not breastfeeding)	1.37 (1.12–1.66)	0.71 (0.64–0.78)
Heavy menstrual bleeding (vs. no recorded HMB)	1.53 (1.10–2.13)	2.84 (2.66–3.03)
IUD type (LNG-IUD vs. Cu-IUD)	1.49 (1.25–1.78)	0.69 (0.65–0.73)

Table 18.2 Incidence rates of ectopic pregnancy (EP) according to method of hormonal contraception (HC) [15]

Type of HC	EP incidence rate/1000 WY (95% CI)
Any contraceptive	0.28 (0.26–0.29)
LNG 13.5mg IUD	2.76 (2.26–3.35)
LNG 52mg IUD	0.30 (0.28–0.33)
Combined HC (vaginal)	0.26 (0.20–0.34)
Combined HC (patch)	0.49 (0.30–0.75)
Combined HC (oral)	0.20 (0.19–0.22)
Etonogestrel implant	0.31 (0.26–0.37)
Progestin-only pill (medium dose)	0.24 (0.21–0.27)
Progestin-only pill (low dose)	0.81 (0.70–0.93)
DMPA injection	0.06 (0.04–0.10)

among women using versus not using hormonal contraception [15]. The study included all Swedish women (nearly 1.7 million) purchasing hormonal contraception and subsequent diagnosis of EP during 2005–16 (n = 1915). The study found that the overall incidence of EP in women using hormonal contraception was lower than the national incidence (0.28 vs. 0.83/1000 women years). The reduced incidence of EP was especially clear among women using all types of combined hormonal contraception, medium-dosed progestin-only pills, etonogestrel-releasing implants, and LNG52mg-IUD [15]. However, an increased risk of EP was seen among women using the low-dose LNG13.5mg-IUD [15] (Table 18.2).

A subsequent Swedish retrospective cohort study compared the risk of EP during the use of differentially dosed LNG-IUDs (i.e., 13.5, 19.5, and 52 mg). The study identified altogether 2252 women diagnosed with EP in the Stockholm County, of whom 105 were using a known type of LNG-IUD at the time of diagnosis. However, the Pearl index for EP was significantly higher among users of the

LNG13.5mg-IUD (0.136 [95%CI 0.11–0.18]) and LNG19.5mg-IUD (0.037 [0.02–0.07]) compared to the LNG52mg-IUD (0.009 [0.006–0.01]). The relative risk of being diagnosed with EP was 14.49 (9.0–23.3) during LNG13.5mg-IUD use and 4.44 (1.6–12.0) during LNG19.5mg-IUD use compared to that of LNG52mg-IUD [5].

Thus, even though the overall risk of EP is low with any of type of LNG-IUDs used, a high-dosed LNG-IUD should be considered for patients with risk factors of EP (such as history of EP) [15].

18.7 Risk of Gynecological Cancer

The overall effect of intrauterine contraception—including various types of IUDs—on the risk of cervical cancer has been summarized in a systematic review and meta-analysis [4]. Based on analysis of 16 studies, the meta-analysis concluded that women using IUD experience approximately 30% reduced risk (i.e., OR 0.64 [95%CI 0.53–0.77]) of cervical cancer. The biological explanation of this reduced risk remains uncertain, but may be related to low level inflammatory reaction in the endocervical canal and/or cervical manipulation associated with IUD use [4].

Similarly, a recent expert review on IUD use and the risk of endometrial, cervical, and ovarian cancer summarized that the risk of gynecological cancers is decreased in association with IUD use [16]. In the studies included, the risk of endometrial cancer associated with IUD use varied from 0.4 to 0.81 (OR or RR), and that of cervical cancer from 0.38 to 0.64 [16]. Less consistent effects were seen concerning IUD use on the risk of ovarian cancer, with OR/RR figures varying from 0.53 to 1.76. Low-grade uterine inflammatory reaction associated with all IUDs and strong local progestogenic effects of LNG-IUD on the endometrium are likely to explain significantly the reduced risk of gynecological cancer associated with IUD use.

As the mechanisms of action of Cu-IUD and LNG-IUD differ, their effect(s) on the risk of especially hormone-dependent cancers are likely to differ. The risk of breast cancer during LNG-IUD use has been studied recently in several epidemiological studies both in the Nordic countries and in the United Kingdom. Table 18.3 summarizes the effects of LNG-IUD use on the risk of breast and other gynecological cancers in fertile-aged women reported in these studies. A clear pattern emerges—most of these studies have observed a slightly increased risk of breast cancer, whereas the risk of endometrial cancer and that of ovarian cancer has decreased significantly in all these studies.

Even though LNG-IUD exerts its contraceptive effects mainly via its local effects on cervical mucus and endometrium, minute amounts of circulating levonorgestrel are present and likely to have an effect on breast epithelium. It may thus be speculated that the effects of LNG-IUD on the breast are similar to those seen during the use of continuous combined hormone replacement therapy [3]. However, the epidemiological studies on the risk of breast cancer associated with LNG-IUD use have

Table 18.3 Recent epidemiological studies on LNG-IUD use and associated risk of gynecological cancer in fertile-aged women (HR/OR/SIR [95% CI])

Ref	Study country and subjects	Study design	Breast cancer	Endometrial cancer	Ovarian cancer	Cervical cancer
Soini et al. [24]	Finland, women aged 30–49 years with heavy menstrual bleeding	Retrospective cohort		SIR 0.50 (0.35–0.70)		
Soini et al. [25, 26]	Finland, women aged 30–49 years with heavy menstrual bleeding	Retrospective cohort	*Ductal ca* SIR 1.20 (1.14–1.25) *Lobular ca* SIR 1.33 (1.20–1.46)		SIR 0.59 (0.47–0.73)	
Iversen et al. [12]	Denmark, women 15–49 years	Retrospective cohort		HR 0.58 (0.36–0.95)		
Fitzpatrick et al. [8]	UK, women aged <50 years	Nested case-control	OR 1.32 (1.17–1.49)			
Mørch et al. [30]	Denmark, women 15–49 years	Retrospective cohort	HR 1.4 (1.2–1.5)			
Yi et al. [29]	Sweden, women 18–50 years	Retrospective cohort	HR 1.13 (1.10–1.17)	HR 0.67 (0.56–0.80)	HR 0.86 (0.75–0.99)	HR 0.91 (0.84–0.99)

covered time periods when only the LNG52mg-IUD has been available on the market. As the LNG52mg-IUD is also used for the treatment of heavy menstrual bleeding, it is plausible that some of the risk factors of HMB explain also in part the increased risk of breast cancer. Moreover, whether this risk differs during use of the newer, low-dose LNG-IUDs remain to be seen.

In brief, LNG-IUD use has been reported to have dual effects on the risk of different gynecological cancers. However, no studies have assessed the possible effect of LNG-IUD contraception on the overall risk of cancer-related death.

18.8 Summary and Conclusions

1. Intrauterine contraception by means of LNG- or Cu-IUDs is very effective [1]. In clinical and real-world studies, LNG-IUD is somewhat more effective than Cu-IUD [1, 11]. Similarly, the continuation rates of IUD use are high [1, 21]. The contraceptive benefits of IUDs are important in all, and especially in highly fertile young women [19].

2. Intrauterine contraception is also very safe. IUD-specific risks of perforation are rare event (1/1000) and rarely dangerous [14, 20]. Expulsion predisposing to unplanned pregnancy is seen with an overall rate of approximately 5%/5-years in both prospective clinical trials and in RWD. Several risk factors of both perforation and expulsion are known [7].
3. Intrauterine contraception has very few health risks. LNG-IUD use is associated with slight increase in breast cancer [8, 17, 29], and Cu-IUD can increase uterine bleeding and menstrual pain [1].
4. Intrauterine contraception has several health benefits. IUD use is associated with reduced risk of cervical cancer [4]. Use of LNG-IUD is associated with decreases in uterine bleeding and dysmenorrhea, increased B-Hb and body iron stores [1], and decreased risk of uterine and ovarian cancer [12, 29].

Declarations

Competing Interests The author(s) has no competing interests to declare that are relevant to the content of this manuscript.

Ethics Approval The author(s) declares that this manuscript does not include primary research with human participants.

The author(s) declares that this manuscript does not include primary studies involving animals.

References

1. Andersson K, Odlind V, Rybo G. Levonorgestrel-releasing and copper-releasing (Nova T) IUDs during five years of use: a randomized comparative trial. Contraception. 1994;49(1):56–72. https://doi.org/10.1016/0010-7824(94)90109-0. PMID: 8137626.
2. Anthony MS, Zhou X, Schoendorf J, Reed SD, Getahun D, Armstrong MA, Gatz J, Peipert JF, Raine-Bennett T, Fassett MJ, Saltus CW, Ritchey ME, Ichikawa L, Shi JM, Alabaster A, Wahdan Y, Wang J, Xie F, Merchant M, Hunter S, Chiu VY, Postlethwaite D, Rothman KJ, Im TM, Chillemi G, Takhar HS, Asiimwe A, Pisa F. Demographic, reproductive, and medical risk factors for intrauterine device expulsion. Obstet Gynecol. 2022;140(6):1017–30. https://doi.org/10.1097/AOG.0000000000005000. Epub 2022 Nov 2. PMID: 36357958; PMCID: PMC9665953.
3. Collaborative Group on Hormonal Factors in Breast Cancer. Type and timing of menopausal hormone therapy and breast cancer risk: individual participant meta-analysis of the worldwide epidemiological evidence. Lancet. 2019;394(10204):1159–68. https://doi.org/10.1016/S0140-6736(19)31709-X. Epub 2019 Aug 29. PMID: 31474332; PMCID: PMC6891893.
4. Cortessis VK, Barrett M, Brown Wade N, Enebish T, Perrigo JL, Tobin J, Zhong C, Zink J, Isiaka V, Muderspach LI, Natavio M, McKean-Cowdin R. Intrauterine device use and cervical cancer risk: a systematic review and meta-analysis. Obstet Gynecol. 2017;130(6):1226–36. https://doi.org/10.1097/AOG.0000000000002307. PMID: 29112647.
5. Elgemark K, Graner S, McTaggart J, Ramirez Löfström J, Sörensen D, Envall N, Kopp Kallner H. The 13.5-mg, 19.5-mg, and 52-mg levonorgestrel-releasing intrauterine systems and risk of ectopic pregnancy. Obstet Gynecol. 2022;140(2):227–33. https://doi.org/10.1097/AOG.0000000000004846. Epub 2022 Jul 6. PMID: 35852273.

6. Faculty of Sexual & Reproductive Healthcare Guideline. Intrauterine contraception. BMJ Sex Reprod Health. 2023;49:1–142. Available at https://srh.bmj.com/content/49/Suppl_1/1.
7. Fassett MJ, Reed SD, Rothman KJ, Pisa F, Schoendorf J, Wahdan Y, Peipert JF, Gatz J, Ritchey ME, Armstrong MA, Raine-Bennett T, Postlethwaite D, Getahun D, Shi JM, Xie F, Chiu VY, Im TM, Takhar HS, Wang J, Anthony MS. Risks of uterine perforation and expulsion associated with intrauterine devices. Obstet Gynecol. 2023;142(3):641–51. https://doi.org/10.1097/AOG.0000000000005299. Epub 2023 Aug 3. PMID: 37535968; PMCID: PMC10424817.
8. Fitzpatrick D, Pirie K, Reeves G, Green J, Beral V. Combined and progestogen-only hormonal contraceptives and breast cancer risk: a UK nested case-control study and meta-analysis. PLoS Med. 2023;20(3):e1004188. https://doi.org/10.1371/journal.pmed.1004188. PMID: 36943819; PMCID: PMC10030023.
9. Gyllenberg F, Juselius M, Gissler M, Heikinheimo O. Long-acting reversible contraception free of charge, method initiation, and abortion rates in Finland. Am J Public Health. 2018;108(4):538–43. https://doi.org/10.2105/AJPH.2017.304280. Epub 2018 Feb 22. PMID: 29470111; PMCID: PMC5844404.
10. Heikinheimo O, Suhonen S. Contraception after induced abortion and childbirth. In: Meriggiola MC, Gemzell-Danielsson K, editors. Female and male contraception. Springer Nature Switzerland AG; 2021. p. 229–42.
11. Heinemann K, Reed S, Moehner S, Minh TD. Comparative contraceptive effectiveness of levonorgestrel-releasing and copper intrauterine devices: the European Active Surveillance Study for Intrauterine Devices. Contraception. 2015;91(4):280–3. https://doi.org/10.1016/j.contraception.2015.01.011. Epub 2015 Jan 16. PMID: 25601350.
12. Iversen L, Fielding S, Lidegaard Ø, Hannaford PC. Contemporary hormonal contraception and risk of endometrial cancer in women younger than age 50: a retrospective cohort study of Danish women. Contraception. 2020;102(3):152–8. https://doi.org/10.1016/j.contraception.2020.06.008. Epub 2020 Jun 25. PMID: 32592798.
13. Kaislasuo J, Suhonen S, Gissler M, Lähteenmäki P, Heikinheimo O. Intrauterine contraception: incidence and factors associated with uterine perforation—a population-based study. Hum Reprod. 2012;27(9):2658–63. https://doi.org/10.1093/humrep/des246. Epub 2012 July 3. PMID: 22763376.
14. Kaislasuo J, Suhonen S, Gissler M, Lähteenmäki P, Heikinheimo O. Uterine perforation caused by intrauterine devices: clinical course and treatment. Hum Reprod. 2013;28(6):1546–51. https://doi.org/10.1093/humrep/det074. Epub 2013 Mar 22. PMID: 23526304.
15. Kopp-Kallner H, Linder M, Cesta CE, Segovia Chacón S, Kieler H, Graner S. Method of hormonal contraception and protective effects against ectopic pregnancy. Obstet Gynecol. 2022;139(5):764–70. https://doi.org/10.1097/AOG.0000000000004726. Epub 2022 Apr 5. PMID: 35576335; PMCID: PMC9015020.
16. Minalt N, Caldwell A, Yedlicka GM, Joseph S, Robertson SE, Landrum LM, Peipert JF. Association between intrauterine device use and endometrial, cervical, and ovarian cancer: an expert review. Am J Obstet Gynecol. 2023;229(2):93–100. https://doi.org/10.1016/j.ajog.2023.03.039. Epub 2023 Mar 29. PMID: 37001577.
17. Mørch LS, Skovlund CW, Hannaford PC, Iversen L, Fielding S, Lidegaard Ø. Contemporary hormonal contraception and the risk of breast cancer. N Engl J Med. 2017;377(23):2228–39. https://doi.org/10.1056/NEJMoa1700732. PMID: 29211679.
18. Mørch LS, Meaidi A, Corn G, Hargreave M, Wessel Skovlund C. Breast Cancer in Users of Levonorgestrel-Releasing Intrauterine Systems. JAMA. 2024 Nov 12;332(18):1578–1580. https://doi.org/10.1001/jama.2024.18575. PMID: 39412770; PMCID: PMC11558473
19. Pohjoranta E, Suhonen S, Gissler M, Ikonen P, Mentula M, Heikinheimo O. Early provision of intrauterine contraception as part of abortion care-5-year results of a randomised controlled trial. Hum Reprod. 2020;35(4):796–804. https://doi.org/10.1093/humrep/deaa031. PMID: 32266392.
20. Pohjoranta E, Suhonen S, Mentula M, Gissler M, Heikinheimo O. Pregnancy outcomes following routine early provision of intrauterine device after first-trimester induced abortion –

a secondary analysis of a randomized controlled trial with a 5-year follow up. Acta Obstet Gynecol Scand. 2024;103(2):342–50. https://doi.org/10.1111/aogs.14724. Epub ahead of print. PMID: 37983839.
21. Reed SD, Zhou X, Ichikawa L, Gatz JL, Peipert JF, Armstrong MA, Raine-Bennett T, Getahun D, Fassett MJ, Postlethwaite DA, Shi JM, Asiimwe A, Pisa F, Schoendorf J, Saltus CW, Anthony MS, APEX-IUD Study Team. Intrauterine device-related uterine perforation incidence and risk (APEX-IUD): a large multisite cohort study. Lancet. 2022;399(10341):2103–12. https://doi.org/10.1016/S0140-6736(22)00015-0. Erratum in: Lancet. 2022;400(10354):732. PMID: 35658995.
22. Saloranta TH, Gyllenberg FK, But A, Gissler M, Laine MK, Heikinheimo O. Free-of-charge long-acting reversible contraception: two-year discontinuation, its risk factors, and reasons. Am J Obstet Gynecol. 2020;223(6):886.e1–886.e17. https://doi.org/10.1016/j.ajog.2020.06.023. Epub 2020 Jun 17. PMID: 32562657.
23. Secura GM, Madden T, McNicholas C, Mullersman J, Buckel CM, Zhao Q, Peipert JF. Provision of no-cost, long-acting contraception and teenage pregnancy. N Engl J Med. 2014;371(14):1316–23. https://doi.org/10.1056/NEJMoa1400506.
24. Sivin I, el Mahgoub S, McCarthy T, Mishell DR Jr, Shoupe D, Alvarez F, Brache V, Jimenez E, Diaz J, Faundes A, et al. Long-term contraception with the levonorgestrel 20 mcg/day (LNg 20) and the copper T 380Ag intrauterine devices: a five-year randomized study. Contraception. 1990;42(4):361–78. https://doi.org/10.1016/0010-7824(90)90046-x. Erratum in: Contraception. 1991;43(1):100. PMID: 2124179.
25. Soini T, Hurskainen R, Grénman S, Mäenpää J, Paavonen J, Pukkala E. Cancer risk in women using the levonorgestrel-releasing intrauterine system in Finland. Obstet Gynecol. 2014;124(2 Pt 1):292–9. https://doi.org/10.1097/AOG.0000000000000356. PMID: 25004338.
26. Soini T, Hurskainen R, Grénman S, Mäenpää J, Paavonen J, Pukkala E. Impact of levonorgestrel-releasing intrauterine system use on the cancer risk of the ovary and fallopian tube. Acta Oncol. 2016a;55(11):1281–4. https://doi.org/10.1080/0284186X.2016.1175660. Epub 2016 May 5. PMID: 27148621.
27. Soini T, Hurskainen R, Grénman S, Mäenpää J, Paavonen J, Joensuu H, Pukkala E. Levonorgestrel-releasing intrauterine system and the risk of breast cancer: a nationwide cohort study. Acta Oncol. 2016b;55(2):188–92. https://doi.org/10.3109/0284186X.2015.1062538. Epub 2015 Aug 4. PMID: 26243443.
28. Trussell J. Contraceptive failure in the United States. Contraception. 2011;83(5):397–404. https://doi.org/10.1016/j.contraception.2011.01.021. Epub 2011 Mar 12. PMID: 21477680; PMCID: PMC3638209.
29. United Nations. World contraceptive use. 2024. Available at: https://www.un.org/development/desa/pd/data/world-contraceptive-use.
30. Yi H, Zhang N, Huang J, Zheng Y, Hong QH, Sundquist J, Sundquist K, Zheng X, Ji J. Association of levonorgestrel-releasing intrauterine device with gynecologic and breast cancers: a national cohort study in Sweden. Am J Obstet Gynecol. 2024;231(4):450.e1–450.e12. https://doi.org/10.1016/j.ajog.2024.05.011. Epub 2024 May 15. PMID: 38759709.

Chapter 19
Contraceptive Implants and Injectables

Luis Bahamondes, Cassia T. Juliato, and M. Valeria Bahamondes

19.1 Subdermal Contraceptive Implants

More than 700 million women worldwide use modern contraceptives [1, 2], including long-acting reversible contraceptives (LARCs) and injectables. These methods are associated with substantial reductions in the high rates of unplanned pregnancies and associated health issues, particularly in low- and middle-income countries and settings. The use of modern contraceptives is an important tool in women's empowerment, providing access to better education and employment opportunities and contributing to economic and social development [3, 4].

19.1.1 Types of Progestin-Containing Subdermal Contraceptive Implants

Contraceptive implants are progestogen-only methods that do not contain oestrogen [5]. There are two widely used contraceptive implants approved by health authorities: the etonogestrel-releasing (ENG) implant and the levonorgestrel (LNG) implant. The ENG implant contains 68 mg of 3-keto-desogestrel (the active metabolite of ENG) in a single preloaded silicone rod measuring 4 cm in length and 2 mm

L. Bahamondes (✉) · C. T. Juliato
Department of Obstetrics and Gynaecology, University of Campinas Faculty of Medical Sciences (UNICAMP), Campinas, SP, Brazil
e-mail: bahamond@caism.unicamp.br

M. V. Bahamondes
Independent consultant, Austin, TX, USA

A. R. Genazzani et al. (eds.), *Ethical, Efficacy and Safety Issues in Contraception*, Reproductive Medicine for Clinicians 4,
https://doi.org/10.1007/978-3-032-07322-8_19

in diameter. It is approved by different health authorities for use for up to 3 years [6]. The LNG implant consists of two silicone rods, each measuring 2.5 × 43 mm and containing 75 mg of LNG in a polymer matrix, and it is approved by different health authorities for use up to 5 years.

Both implants have the same mechanisms of action: anovulation, thickening of cervical mucus, and endometrial suppression [7]. The contraceptive actions of both implants begin 8 h after placement. The clearance of both ENG and LNG is rapid, and the serum levels are almost undetectable 1 week after implant removal [8]. Although both the LNG and ENG implants inhibit ovulation, some ovarian follicular activity persists [9]. The suppression of ovulation after ENG implant placement occurs within 24 h, and the peak serum level is reached on day 4 after placement. In contrast, the maximum serum concentration of LNG is achieved 24–72 h after placement, and it then falls very slowly over 3–7 years.

19.1.2 Contraceptive Efficacy and Safety

LNG and ENG implants are among the most effective contraceptives worldwide. There is no difference between typical and perfect use with LARC methods, including implants, because these contraceptives do not rely on user action. Consequently, their efficacy remains consistent and is not influenced by user characteristics such as parity or age [10, 11]. The World Health Organization (WHO) conducted a multicentre randomised study and found that the cumulative pregnancy rate of both the ENG and LNG implants up to the first 3 years was 0.4 per 100 woman-years (W-Ys), which was significantly lower than that of short-acting contraceptive methods [12]. Additionally, this low pregnancy rate was maintained for up to 5 years after placement of both implants, including when the ENG implant was tested for extended use for up to 5 years [6].

In a pooled analysis of 11 clinical trials with 1,755 W-Ys of exposure among ENG implant users, the contraceptive failure rate was 0.34 (95% confidence interval [CI], 0.13–0.74) [13]. When providing guidance to users and potential users, it is important to explain that the possibility of becoming pregnant is 4 in 1000 users. Additionally, other studies showed that being overweight (≥70 kg at admission) did not significantly increase the risk of contraceptive failure after ENG implant placement. Furthermore, only one pregnancy was reported (0.8 per 100 W-Ys; 95% CI, 1.0–5.3) among LNG implant users weighing ≥70 kg [6, 14]. The contraceptive failure rate among users of both types of implants is extremely low, making it difficult to identify failures in women with different body mass indexes. It has been observed that the ENG plasma concentration is inversely related to body weight, and in obese women (body mass index of ≥41 kg/m^2), the ENG concentration can be nearly 48% lower than that in women of normal weight [15, 16].

The use of contraceptive implants is safe for most women. One concern is the impact of implant use on bone mineral density because contraceptive implants contain only progestin. Few studies have focused on this issue. One study assessed bone mineral density at the distal and ultra-distal radius of the non-dominant forearm at baseline and at 18 and 36 months after either ENG or LNG implant placement in 111 women [17]. No differences were observed in the bone mineral density of users of either implant at 36 months after device placement at the ultra-distal radius, which is the portion containing more trabecular bone.

Implants induce endometrial changes, mainly atrophic endometrium with dilated, thin-walled vessels. Vessel dilation causes abnormal bleeding patterns in some women [18]. This bothersome bleeding can result in premature discontinuation of implant use or affect women's quality of life. Thus, it is important to alert potential users of such complications before placement [19, 20].

In a United States (US)-based study involving 825 ENG implant recipients who were aged 13.5–32.5 years and followed up for 3 years, researchers identified factors associated with bothersome uterine bleeding and the impact of these factors on implant discontinuation [21]. Among the 27% of women who reported bothersome uterine bleeding, it was more commonly associated with previous experience of irregular menses (odds ratio, 1.36; 95% CI, 1.11–1.68) and irregular and infrequent menses (odds ratio, 1.41; 95% CI, 1.07–1.86). The authors found that participants who received medical treatment including non-specified hormonal medications, 45 (33%) nonsteroidal anti-inflammatory drugs, and 11 (8%) both agents for management of bleeding had a higher rate of implant discontinuation at 1 year (hazard ratio, 1.98; 95% CI, 1.39–2.81). Nevertheless, 50% of subjects were still using the implant by 3 years after placement.

In the above-mentioned WHO trial [12], the rates of bleeding disturbances that resulted in discontinuation of ENG and LNG implant use were 16.7 per 100 W-Ys (95% CI, 14.4–19.3) and 12.5 per 100 W-Y (95% CI, 10.5–14.9), respectively. Furthermore, the US-based CHOICE study showed an ENG implant discontinuation rate of 44% at 3 years, and almost half of users reported bothersome abnormal uterine bleeding as the reason for discontinuation [22]. However, almost 50% of ENG implant users reported amenorrhoea or infrequent bleeding [23]. Women with normal uterine bleeding during the first few months of use tended to continue these patterns over the next 2 years [16]. The proposed treatments for women with bothersome bleeding are continuous and cyclic combined oestrogen–progestin oral contraceptives (COCs), progestin-only pills, tranexamic acid, non-steroidal anti-inflammatory drugs, ulipristal acetate, and tamoxifen [24]. Although all these treatments successfully control bleeding, abnormal bleeding recurs after treatment in many women.

The relatively low adoption of implants is associated with several barriers, one of which is the need for more than one visit to perform the placement. Other advantages of single-visit placement are that it allows for immediate initiation of contraceptive protection, reduces costs, and minimizes the possibility that women might not return for placement. Our group evaluated 590 single-visit ENG implant placements and found one pregnancy in a woman in whom the placement was performed within days 1–5 of menstrual cycle [25]. In a US-based study, the authors reported practice characteristics associated with single-visit placement of LARCs. They found that single-visit placement was highest for those who self-paid and those seen by an obstetrician–gynaecologist [26].

Contraindications for use of contraceptive implants include severe decompensated liver disease, hepatocellular adenoma, malignant liver tumours, and breast cancer [27]. A recent meta-analysis provided evidence that use of progestin-only contraceptives is associated with a slight increase in breast cancer risk [28]. The relative risk of current or recent use of contraceptive implants was slightly increased 1.28 (95% CI, 1.08–1.51; heterogeneity χ^2_3, 7.3; $p = 0.06$).

There have been concerns regarding the safety of using some contraceptives, including implants, in areas with a high prevalence of HIV infection because their use may increase a women's susceptibility to HIV acquisition. A randomised multicentre study conducted by the WHO in 12 settings in Sub-Saharan African countries compared intramuscular depot medroxyprogesterone acetate (DMPA-IM), a copper intrauterine device (IUD), and an LNG implant among 7,829 women [29]. The authors reported no significant differences in HIV risk among the three contraceptives evaluated, providing reassurance regarding the safety and effectiveness of all methods.

Progestin implants have a lesser metabolic impact than COCs, and their influence on haemostasis, blood pressure, lipids, liver and renal function, carbohydrates, and insulin release are also considered to be minimal. However, there is no information regarding users with elevated risks of cardiovascular disease and diabetes [30].

19.1.3 Postpartum and Post-abortion Placement and Use of Implants During Breastfeeding

ENG and LNG implants should be offered to women during the immediate postpartum and post-abortion periods. This is important because many women do not return for another visit 6–8 weeks postpartum. Thus, immediate postpartum or post-abortion implant placement prevents unplanned pregnancies. Both the ENG and LNG implants do not affect breastfeeding or cause infant weight gain. A Brazil-based study evaluated patient acceptance of the ENG implant in the immediate postpartum period among adolescents and young adults. After 1 year of follow-up, the continuation rate was 87.5%, and 90.0% of women reported that they were satisfied with the method [31, 32]. Regarding post-abortion implant placement, the American College of Obstetricians and Gynaecologists reported that women are satisfied with the convenience of receiving the contraceptive method of their choice immediately after an abortion [33, 34].

19.1.4 Return of Fertility After Implant Removal

Among women who do not use any type of contraceptive, the possibility of becoming pregnant after 1 year of sexual intercourse is almost 82% [35], and the pregnancy rate depends on the age of the woman [36, 37]. One study showed that after removal of both ENG and LNG implants, the return of fertility was high, ranging from 76.5% to 85.6% [38], which are expected rates [39]. It is important to communicate to users that implant use does not impair future fertility because some women believe that using contraceptives can induce infertility. One study showed that 20–40% of participants agreed or strongly agreed with this misconception [40].

19.1.5 Drug Interactions

Implants have several drug–drug interactions that can either reduce their contraceptive effectiveness or affect the effectiveness of other drugs. The first-line treatment for severe nodular acne and treatment-resistant acne is isotretinoin, which is a potent teratogen [41, 42]. In one study, the ENG concentration remained at >90 pg/mL during isotretinoin therapy without changes from baseline [43]. In addition, topiramate, a first-line treatment for migraine prophylaxis [44], is often used by women of reproductive age. Many of these women need effective contraception because topiramate is potentially teratogenic [45]. In one study, the baseline serum ENG concentration, as well as that measured at different times during the use of topiramate for migraines (100 mg/day) and epilepsy (400 mg/day), was reduced by concomitant topiramate use. The ENG concentrations fell below the levels needed for ovulatory suppression, potentially resulting in contraceptive failure [46].

Rifampin is a commonly prescribed antibiotic for tuberculosis [47]. The pharmacokinetic and pharmacodynamic effects of a short course of rifampin (600 mg daily for 2 weeks) on serum ENG concentrations were evaluated in women who had used the ENG implant for 12–32 months [48]. The study showed significant decreases in serum ENG concentrations from baseline (median, 164.0 pg/mL [range, 94.4–265.0 pg/mL]) compared to the post-treatment period (median, 47.8 pg/mL [range, 24.7–82.8 pg/mL]) ($p < 0.001$). This study indicates that concomitant use of rifampin during ENG implant use significantly decreases the serum ENG concentrations and increases the risk of ovulation [48].

A major concern is the potential for drug interactions when using concomitant antiretroviral therapy (ART) in women with HIV infection. One study assessed the pharmacokinetics of ENG and LNG implants in users of either rilpivirine- or darunavir-based ART over 48 weeks post-implant placement compared with control women without HIV [49]. The main results showed that at week 24, both the ENG and LNG concentrations were similar between the rilpivirine and control groups; however, progestin exposure was higher in the darunavir group than in the control group, with similar results at week 48. The authors concluded that both implants are appropriate contraceptive options for women on either rilpivirine- or darunavir/ritonavir-based ART. Another study focused on the interaction between the ENG implant and two ART regimens (one containing efavirenz and the other containing ritonavir-boosted lopinavir) in HIV-positive women [50]. The authors found a reduction in the bioavailability of ENG associated with the efavirenz-based highly active ART regimen (decreases of 63.4%, 53.7%, and 70.0% in the area under the curve, maximum concentration, and minimum concentration of ENG, respectively), but not in the lopinavir/ritonavir-based highly active ART regimen. They concluded that the administration of efavirenz as ART decreased the bioavailability of ENG.

A pharmacokinetics study involving double-dose LNG implants (300 mg LNG) among 27 young women on ART with 600 mg efavirenz showed that the double dose was not effective in overcoming the drug–drug interaction with efavirenz, leading to ovulatory activity [51]. A similar study involving double-dose ENG implants in users of efavirenz-based ART [52] showed two (2%) ovulations over 108 women-months in 2 of 36 participants in the double implant group, resulting in a 97.7% reduction of the possibility of ovulation in the double implant group over 48 weeks [52].

19.1.6 Non-contraceptive Benefits

The efficacy of an ENG implant versus the LNG 52-mg IUD in controlling endometriosis-associated pelvic pain was reported up to 6 months after device placement [53]. The study assessed daily scores of noncyclic pelvic pain, dysmenorrhoea, daily bleeding patterns from a menstrual calendar, and health-related quality of life (QoL) using the Endometriosis Health Profile-30 questionnaire. Both the ENG implant and the hormonal IUD significantly improved endometriosis-associated pelvic pain, dysmenorrhoea, and health-related QoL in all domains. The most common bleeding patterns at 180 days of follow-up among ENG implant users were amenorrhoea and infrequent bleeding. Additionally, an ancillary study correlated endometriosis-associated pain with serum levels of ENG, CA-125, and soluble CD23 for up to 2 years after either implant or IUD placement. The main results showed that users of the ENG implant had reduced serum levels of soluble CD23 and CA-125 by 24 months after either implant or IUD placement; however, there was no correlation between pain scores and ENG serum levels [54].

Additionally, the ENG implant was used off-label for pain control in women with adenomyosis. A systematic review showed a significant reduction in pelvic pain and dysmenorrhoea when comparing baseline levels to those post-placement (ranging from 12 to 36 months), as well as an increase in haemoglobin levels after ENG implant placement [55]. We suggest that more studies are necessary to confirm the potential value of both the ENG and LNG implants in women with endometriosis and adenomyosis.

Additionally, it has been reported that use of the ENG implant is associated with a reduced risk of ovarian and endometrial cancer, possibly due to the anovulation induced by the implant (OR = 0.30; 95% CI 0.12–0.73; $p = 0.008$) [14]. However, further studies are needed to confirm these findings.

19.1.7 Extended Use

Health authorities in all the countries in which the ENG implant was commercialized approved the use of the ENG implant for up to 3 years after placement. Nevertheless, after the WHO completed a randomised comparison trial with ENG and LNG implants, it was decided to extend the use of the ENG implant up to 5 years because the pharmacokinetics data indicated high levels of ENG beyond the approved duration. A total of 390 women accepted the extended use [6]. No pregnancies were reported among the >200 women who accepted the extended use up to 5 years, and the overall 5-year cumulative pregnancy rate was of 0.6 per 100 W-Ys (95% CI, 0.2–1.8). Although few adolescents were enrolled, which was a limitation, the study provided evidence about the high contraceptive effectiveness beyond the approved 3 years. A US-based study also confirmed the effectiveness of the ENG implant beyond 3 years [56].

19.1.8 Training and Complications at Placement Time

Any implant programme must include proper training in placement and removal, not only with models but also with actual users or potential users, even though the learning curve is simple. Lack of training is associated with myths and poor knowledge, which can affect women's choices. Our group assessed the impact of training healthcare providers (HCPs) on the ENG implant using both models and real women [57]. We observed that after training, 78.2% of the HCPs began offering and inserting up to five implants per month, and 17.6% inserted six to ten per month.

A study conducted in Spain examined the impact of a structured ENG implant training programme on HCPs (gynaecologists, general practitioners, and midwives). There was an increase in inclusion of the implant in contraceptive guidance in the post-training period, and almost 50% of the HCPs became competent in insertion and removal. We consider that theoretical training alone is not adequate; practical training should be compulsory for HCPs involved in implant provision [58].

Contraceptive implants are associated with several complications, mainly migration due to incorrect placement procedures, which is mainly associated with the ENG implant. Although extremely rare (1 in 100,000), there have been reports of implants migrating into pulmonary arteries, and a review of the literature on this topic was recently published [59]. However, the more common complication is non-palpable implants found below the muscle fascia, which can be easily detected by ultrasonography [60, 61].

In 2019, a publication described the anatomical assessment of the medial upper arm and potential sites for ENG implant placement [62]. The study involved the dissection of 40 female cadaveric arms and reported that at 3–5 cm posterior to the sulcus, there are no major neurovascular structures. It was also noted that if a woman maintains elbow flexion with her hand underneath her head, the ulnar nerve is displaced anteriorly toward the sulcus. The authors recommended placing the ENG implant at that location to avoid injury associated with improper deep insertion and further migration. Although the authors only recommended this insertion location for the ENG implant, it is also appropriate for the LNG implant.

19.2 Injectable Contraceptives

19.2.1 Types of Injectable Contraceptives

Injectable contraceptive methods are popular worldwide, particularly in sub-Saharan Africa. Although they are not classified as LARCs like IUDs and implants, their lack of a daily administration requirement promotes continued use. Injectable contraceptives are divided into combined oestrogen–progestin injectable contraceptives (CICs) and progestin-only injectables, such as depot medroxyprogesterone acetate (DMPA), administered by either an IM or subcutaneous (SC) route, and norethisterone enanthate (NET-EN), also administered IM. DMPA is the most widely used injectable method and the fourth most prevalent contraceptive globally, with 42 million women of reproductive age using it in more than 130 countries [63]. DMPA is a progestin-only injectable contraceptive and has been available from various manufacturers for more than 40 years. It is approved by health authorities in more than 179 countries, and it is administered via IM injection in the upper arm or buttock.

Traditionally, DMPA is administered at a dosage of 150 mg IM every 3 months (13 weeks), is completely reversible, and has a 4-week grace period for users unable to return for injections on their scheduled date. However, the 104-mg subcutaneous (SC) dosage, which allows for self-administration, is an appealing alternative in many countries because it enhances contraceptive access, continuation, and autonomy [64]. DMPA-SC in the prefilled Uniject injection system is known in many countries as Sayana®Press (Pfizer, New York, NY), and it is approved by health authorities in nearly 60 countries. Studies have shown that women can learn to successfully self-administer injectable contraceptives [65]. A recent meta-analysis of three randomized controlled trials showed significantly higher 1-year continuation rates among women who self-administered DMPA-SC than among those who returned to an HCP for injections [66].

NET-EN was introduced to the market in 1957 as the first progestogen-only injectable contraceptive, preceding the introduction of DMPA. It is administered intramuscularly (IM) at a dose of 200 mg every 2 months and is approved by health authorities in more than 60 countries. After IM administration, NET-EN (as a pro-drug of norethisterone) is rapidly converted into norethisterone by esterases, and this drug exhibits weak androgenic and estrogenic activity [67]. Following an IM injection of 200 mg NETE, the mean maximum concentration of ethinyl-oestradiol (oEE) was 32% compared to combined oral contraceptives (COCs) with 30 μg of oEE [68], indicating that the exposure to oEE is significantly lower than with COCs. The metabolism of norethisterone can be affected by finasteride and dutasteride, as these drugs inhibit 5α-reductase, which plays an important role in its metabolism. Additionally, rifampicin and bosentan are CYP3A4 inducers, and their concurrent administration with NET-EN can affect norethisterone levels by 42% and 23%, respectively. Carbamazepine and St. John's wort may also accelerate norethisterone clearance [69].

Both forms of DMPA, as well as NET-EN and CIC injections, suppress ovulation and have a secondary mechanism of thickening cervical mucus or thinning the endometrium. All injectable contraceptives are on the WHO list of essential medicines. The DMPA SC form is equally effective with a 30% lower dose, regardless of body weight [66]. It has been suggested that race, ethnicity, or BMI does not affect the efficacy of the DMPA-SC formulation [70]. The administration of DMPA-SC is considered equivalent to DMPA-IM; however, the SC form may offer some advantages due to its lower dose and potential for self-injection, which is common in many settings, particularly in sub-Saharan countries [71].

Regarding CICs, there are two available on the market. One contains medroxyprogesterone acetate (MPA) 25 mg and oestradiol cypionate 5 mg, commonly branded as Cyclofem. The other contains norethisterone enanthate (50 mg) and oestradiol valerate (5 mg), commonly branded as Mesygina. Even though they are approved by health authorities in many countries, their uptake and use are limited, primarily because they require monthly injections.

19.2.2 Efficacy

The contraceptive efficacy of DMPA is similarly high between the IM and SC routes, with a typical-use failure rate of 6.0 per 100 W-Ys in the first year and a cumulative rate of only 0.7 per 100 W-Ys over 3 years [11, 72]. The contraceptive efficacy is high and comparable to long-acting reversible contraceptives and female surgical contraception, ranging from 0.0 to 1.1 per 100 W-Ys [73, 74]. The efficacy of the two brands commercialized worldwide is similar. The typical-use failure rate of NET-EN is 2.0 per 100 woman-years (W-Ys) in the first year.

19.2.3 Return of Fertility

One concern with the use of DMPA is the delay in the return of fertility after discontinuation. It has been described that the time to conception after the last injection of DMPA is almost 10 months, which could be problematic for women who stop using it with the intention of becoming pregnant in a short time [75]. An Australian-based large trial reported that the median delay in the return of fertility was 9.2 months [76].

Regarding CIC, the return of fertility was assessed among women who used the CIC containing medroxyprogesterone acetate (MPA) 25 mg and oestradiol cypionate 5 mg in Brazil, Chile, Colombia, and Peru. The authors followed 70 women after discontinuation of the contraceptive and found that the return to fertility rate was 1.4 per 100 women at the end of the first month and 82.9 per 100 women at 1 year. More than 50% were pregnant within 6 months [35]. However, within the first month after discontinuation, the pregnancy rate was extremely low, indicating a small delay in the return of fertility.

The return of ovulation (not fertility) was studied when SC DMPA (Sayana Press; 104 mg/0.65 mL MPA in the Uniject device) was administered every 4 months for 1 year instead of every 3 months. Serum progesterone was used as a surrogate endpoint for ovulation and was monitored in weeks 38–42 and 46–50 after the final (third) injection [77]. The main results indicated that 10 out of 19 women (53%; 95% CI: 29–76) ovulated within 50 weeks of their last injection, and the median time from the last injection to first ovulation was 1.1 months shorter (13.1 vs. 14.2 months) when injections were given every 4 months for 1 year.

19.2.4 Safety and Comorbidities

Progestin-only injectables are suitable for most conditions, with the only absolute contraindications being hormone-dependent cancers such as breast cancer and women with liver disease. Neither DMPA-SC nor DMPA-IM or NET-EN increases blood pressure or the risk of adverse cardiovascular events, making them suitable for women with hypertension or cardiovascular diseases. Due to the low levels of oEE produced after the IM administration of one ampoule of NET-EN there is no increased risk of venous thromboembolism or hepatic adenoma [68]. The primary adverse effect and most frequent reason for discontinuation of progestin-only injectables is the development of menstrual bleeding changes, which are more common than in users of combined methods [78]. Unscheduled and unpredictable bleeding is prevalent during the first year of use but tends to decrease thereafter. The proportion of women who develop amenorrhoea increases over time (40–50% after 1 year and 80% after 5 years of DMPA use) [79]. In addition, other side effects among users of DMPA and NET-EN like breast tenderness, headaches, abnormal uterine bleeding have been reported. Weight gain is another side effect associated with DMPA use. Although numerous studies have explored this topic, a systematic review of 16 studies revealed no significant weight differences between methods, with most studies reporting weight gain of approximately 2 kg (4.4 pounds) over 6–12 months of use [80].

Concerns regarding the use of DMPA and the risk of acquiring HIV have been raised. A study involving 7,800 HIV-seronegative women in high-risk areas showed no difference in HIV acquisition rates among users of DMPA, the copper IUD, or the LNG implant after 18 months [29]. Additionally, a 2020 systematic review of 36 studies showed no significant differences in HIV risk among users of DMPA-IM, the LNG implant, or the copper IUD [81].

Another concern is the impact of DMPA (although not for NET-EN users) on bone metabolism and decreased bone mass. The pathophysiology involves the suppression of gonadotropin secretion, reducing ovarian production of oestradiol. Under hypo-oestrogenic conditions, bone resorption exceeds bone formation, resulting in decreased bone mass [82]. However, several studies have indicated that this bone mass decline reverses after discontinuation of DMPA. The best available data suggest that DMPA use does not reduce peak bone mass or increase the risk of osteoporotic fractures later in life in women at average risk of osteoporosis [83].

Concerns have also been raised about the potential development of diabetes mellitus in DMPA users. However, a study involving 240 women (White, African American, and Hispanic) showed only mild increases in fasting insulin and glucose levels (3 mg/dL and 4 units, respectively, over baseline values) in some participants, and these changes were not likely to be clinically significant [84].

Considering the two CICs, the discontinuation rates due to amenorrhea, spotting, and menstrual irregularity were significantly lower compared to NET-EN. However, higher rates of discontinuation due to gastrointestinal disturbances were reported with CICs compared to NET-EN [85].

19.2.5 Non-contraceptive Benefits and Side Effects

Various non-contraceptive benefits are associated with DMPA use, such as decreased menstrual flow, reduced pain secondary to endometriosis, and endometrial protection in women with polycystic ovarian syndrome. Additionally, DMPA reduces the number of sickle cell crises in women with sickle cell disease [86].

As previously mentioned, the main adverse effect of progestin-only injectables is the development of menstrual bleeding changes, which can be unexpected and unpredictable. The two most commonly available forms of CICs are medroxyprogesterone acetate (MPA)/oestradiol cypionate and NET-EN/oestradiol valerate. CICs, which contain both oestrogen and progestin, tend to cause fewer menstrual changes than progestin-only methods [87, 88]. Adding oestrogen to long-acting progestin builds up the endometrium, thus regulating bleeding patterns and resulting in more regular bleeding cycles than obtained with injectable progestin-only methods [88]. When women use COCs cyclically, bleeding occurs upon oestrogen withdrawal, mimicking a typical menstrual period. Given monthly, CICs allow serum oestrogen levels to fall similarly, resulting in withdrawal bleeding [89].

A systematic review showed that compared with DMPA users, women using a CIC with DMPA 25 mg plus oestradiol cypionate 5 mg experienced less amenorrhoea and fewer discontinuations due to amenorrhoea or menstrual changes. CIC users had more regular (cyclical) bleeding and fewer instances of infrequent bleeding than DMPA users. However, CIC users had higher discontinuation rates due to events such as headaches than did DMPA users [87]. Nevertheless, CICs are an appealing contraceptive option because of their high effectiveness (<1 per 100 W-Ys), reversibility, and the lack of a need for daily administration or coital-related actions.

Studies comparing the two combinations showed that NET-EN 50 mg plus oestradiol valerate 5 mg resulted in a lower overall rate of early discontinuation and a lower discontinuation due to amenorrhoea or prolonged bleeding compared with DMPA 25 mg plus oestradiol cypionate 5 mg. The NET-EN plus oestradiol valerate group also experienced more regular (cyclical) bleeding and fewer prolonged bleeding episodes than the DMPA plus oestradiol cypionate group. The groups did not differ in the rates of amenorrhoea, although the statistical significance of almost all these findings depended on one trial conducted in China [90].

19.2.6 Extended Use

There are no major studies regarding the extended use of DMPA, whether via IM or SC routes, NET-EN, or CICs. However, a new initiative organized by Family Health International 360 studied the performance of Sayana® Press when used every 4 months instead of 3. With this strategy, women could benefit from longer pregnancy prevention, fewer visits to healthcare facilities, lower costs for public services and out-of-pocket expenses for users, and lower plasma levels of MPA. The study was conducted with 710 women at risk of pregnancy in Brazil, Chile, and the Dominican Republic. Participants were randomized to receive injections in the abdomen or thigh, and 40 women received injections in the back of the upper arm for comparative pharmacokinetic analyses. No pregnancies (Pearl Index of 0.00; 95% CI 0.00–0.59) were observed during the trial among 629.3 woman-years (W-Ys) of follow-up. However, MPA serum concentrations were higher when the injection was administered in the abdomen compared to the thigh and arm [91]. Regarding the acceptability of this injection schedule, 1 year after study initiation, 90% of participants were satisfied with Sayana® Press, and 75% reported that they preferred using the contraceptive every 4 months. Participants liked the amenorrhea induced by the contraceptive but disliked the bleeding disturbances [92].

19.3 Conclusions

Both ENG and LNG implants and injectables are highly effective and safe contraceptives. Both implants, as members of the LARC 'family,' contribute to reductions in the global maternal mortality ratio and unplanned pregnancy rate, which remain high mainly in low- and middle-income countries and settings. Both implants provide similarly high contraceptive effectiveness (4 per 1,000 W-Ys), which approaches the efficacy of permanent contraception, and injectables also provide high contraceptive effectiveness. They are extremely safe contraceptives with few contraindications because they are progestin-only methods. They can be used by women with hypertension, diabetes, and current or past venous thromboembolism as well as by nulligravidas, by adolescents, and during the postpartum and post-abortion periods. Notably, their use may induce profound endometrial atrophy, which can induce bothersome bleeding; this is the main cause of discontinuation. Injectable contraceptives offer high effectiveness and high continuation rates. Cultural acceptance of the resulting menstrual patterns varies among women, highlighting the importance of regional considerations when choosing the most appropriate contraceptive methods.

In Boxes 19.1 and 19.2, we present a summary of the principal characteristics of the current contraceptive implants available on the market and the injectables contraceptives.

Box 19.1 Main characteristics of the currently available contraceptive implants

Characteristics	Etonogestrel (ENG) implant	Levonorgestrel (LNG) implant
Brand name, active ingredients, and main characteristics	Implanon NXT, one rod with 68 mg of 3-keto-desogestrel (the active metabolite of ENG. Preloaded in an inserter with the trocar	Jadelle, two rods with containing 75 mg of LNG each rod. The trocar is separate from the implants
Temporal changes in the active pharmaceutical ingredients in blood after placement	After placement, steroid serum concentrations are detected to levels associated with ovulation inhibition within 8 h. If placement occurs within the first 5 days of the menstrual cycle, the contraceptive effect is almost immediate	After placement, steroid serum concentrations are detected to levels associated with ovulation inhibition within 8 h. If placement occurs within the first 5 days of the menstrual cycle, the contraceptive effect is almost immediate
Approved life-span use	Three years	Five years
Effectiveness	0.4/100 women-years up to 3 years after device placement	0.4/100 women-years up to 5 years after device placement
Complexity of placement and removal	Easy and quick insertion (< than 1 min) and removal procedure (< than 4 min)	Easy and quick insertion (< than 2 min) and removal procedure (< than 6 min)

(continued)

Box 19.1 (continued)

Characteristics	Etonogestrel (ENG) implant	Levonorgestrel (LNG) implant
Return to fertility	Rapid return of fertility after removal	Rapid return of fertility after removal
Contraindications	Abnormal uterine bleeding without diagnosis, decompensated cirrhosis, hepatocellular adenoma, or malignant hepatoma, systemic lupus erythematosus with positive (or unknown) antiphospholipid antibodies; ischemic heart disease or stroke while using an implant; current or history of breast cancer	Abnormal uterine bleeding without diagnosis, decompensated cirrhosis, hepatocellular adenoma, or malignant hepatoma, systemic lupus erythematosus with positive (or unknown) antiphospholipid antibodies; ischemic heart disease or stroke while using an implant; current or history of breast cancer
Major side effects	Bothersome uterine bleeding, acne	Bothersome uterine bleeding, acne
Non-contraceptive benefits	Improved visual analogue scale pain scores for cyclic pelvic pain and dysmenorrhea in women with endometriosis. Reduction of the risk of ovarian cancer, probably due to suppression of ovulation. Reduce acne	Reduction of the risk of ovarian cancer, probably due to suppression of ovulation
Post-partum and post-abortion use	It is safe	It is safe
Temporal changes in the active pharmaceutical ingredients in blood after removal	After removal, plasma steroid levels fall rapidly, being below the threshold for detection by the assay (20 pg/mL) within about 4 days	After removal, plasma steroid levels fall rapidly, being below the threshold for detection by the assay (20 pg/mL) within about 4 days
Advantages of use	A very safe method of contraception. Anemia, hypertension, gallbladder disease, diabetes, pelvic inflammatory disease, thromboembolic events, cardiovascular events, and neoplastic diseases are similar to those in women not using implants. Excellent option for women who do not like daily, weekly, monthly contraceptive care. Reduces the risk of ectopic pregnancy; however, if a pregnancy does occur, ectopic pregnancy must be ruled out because the risk of tubal implantation	A very safe method of contraception. Anemia, hypertension, gallbladder disease, diabetes, pelvic inflammatory disease, thromboembolic events, cardiovascular events, and neoplastic diseases are similar to those in women not using implants. Excellent option for women who do not like daily, weekly, monthly contraceptive care. Reduces the risk of ectopic pregnancy; however, if a pregnancy does occur, ectopic pregnancy must be ruled out because the risk of tubal implantation

Box 19.1 (continued)

Characteristics	Etonogestrel (ENG) implant	Levonorgestrel (LNG) implant
Disadvantages of use	Bleeding patterns can range from amenorrhoea to frequent and prolonged bleeding. Irregular and unpredictable bleeding are the major disadvantages. Weight gain is a common reason for discontinuation; however, weight gain is under debate. It could provoke breast tenderness, emotional lability/mood changes, headache	Bleeding patterns can range from amenorrhoea to frequent and prolonged bleeding. Irregular and unpredictable bleeding are the major disadvantages. Weight gain is a common reason for discontinuation; however, weight gain is under debate. It could provoke breast tenderness, emotional lability/mood changes, headache
Recommended follow-up procedures after placement	After insertion, there is no need for attention by either the user or the provider until time of removal	After insertion, there is no need for attention by either the user or the provider until time of removal

Box 19.2 Main characteristics of the currently available injectable contraceptives

Characteristics	Depot medroxyprogesterone acetate (DMPA)	Norethisterone-Enanthate (NET-EN)	Combined injectables
Brand name, active ingredients, and main characteristics	Depo-provera (150 mg of medroxyprogesterone acetate) and Sayana Press (104 mg of medroxyprogesterone acetate)	Noretisterat (200 mg of norethisterone enanthate)	Cyclofem (medroxyprogesterone acetate 25 mg and oestradiol cypionate 5 mg) Mesygina (norethisterone enanthate 50 mg and oestradiol valerate 5 mg)
Temporal changes in the active pharmaceutical ingredients in blood after placement	If injection occurs within the first 5 days of the menstrual cycle, the contraceptive effect is almost immediate. If administered after the first 5 days of a menstrual cycle, it takes 3 days to become effective	If injection occurs within the first 5 days of the menstrual cycle, the contraceptive effect is almost immediate. If administered after the first 5 days of a menstrual cycle, it takes 3 days to become effective	If injection occurs within the first 5 days of the menstrual cycle, the contraceptive effect is almost immediate
Approved life-span use	Three months	Two months	One month
Effectiveness	6/100 women-years	2/100 women-years	0.4/100 women-years
Complexity of administration	IM injection. For Sayana Press could be self-injected	IM injection	IM injection

(continued)

Box 19.2 (continued)

Characteristics	Depot medroxyprogesterone acetate (DMPA)	Norethisterone-Enanthate (NET-EN)	Combined injectables
Return to fertility	Some delay in the return of fertility after last injection	Rapid return of fertility after last injection	Rapid return of fertility after last injection
Contraindications	Abnormal uterine bleeding without diagnosis, decompensated cirrhosis, hepatocellular adenoma, or malignant hepatoma, systemic lupus erythematosus with positive (or unknown) antiphospholipid antibodies; ischemic heart disease or stroke while using an implant; current or history of breast cancer	Abnormal uterine bleeding without diagnosis, decompensated cirrhosis, hepatocellular adenoma, or malignant hepatoma, systemic lupus erythematosus with positive (or unknown) antiphospholipid antibodies; ischemic heart disease or stroke while using an implant; current or history of breast cancer	Oestrogen-responsive tumours of the breast or genital tract. Current or individual history of cardiovascular disease, current liver disease or liver tumours, and over age 40 if a smoker. Unexplained abnormal vaginal bleeding
Major side effects	Bothersome uterine bleeding, breast tenderness, headache, weight gain, dizziness	Bothersome uterine bleeding, breast tenderness, headache, weight gain, dizziness	Bothersome uterine bleeding, breast tenderness, headache, weight gain, dizziness
Non-contraceptive benefits	Improved visual analogue scale pain scores for cyclic pelvic pain and dysmenorrhoea in women with endometriosis. Protection against endometrial cancer and uterine fibroids. Reduced sickle cell crises in women with sickle cell anaemia side effects Reduction of the risk of ovarian cancer, probably due to suppression of ovulation	Reduction of the risk of ovarian cancer, probably due to suppression of ovulation	None

(continued)

Box 19.2 (continued)

Characteristics	Depot medroxyprogesterone acetate (DMPA)	Norethisterone-Enanthate (NET-EN)	Combined injectables
Post-partum and post-abortion use	It is safe	It is safe	It is safe only 6-weeks after delivery or 2 weeks after medical termination
Temporal changes in the active pharmaceutical ingredients in blood after removal	After removal, plasma steroid levels fall rapidly, being below the threshold for detection by the assay (20 pg/mL) within about 4 days	After removal, plasma steroid levels fall rapidly, being below the threshold for detection by the assay (20 pg/mL) within about 4 days	Not available
Advantages of use	Highly safe. Decreased risk of iron-deficiency anaemia. Could be administered at post-partum including among breastfeeding women, starting 6 weeks postpartum	Highly safe. Decreased risk of iron-deficiency anaemia. Could be administered at post-partum including among breastfeeding women, starting 6 weeks postpartum	Highly safe. Could be administered at post-partum including among breastfeeding women, starting 6 weeks postpartum
Disadvantages of use	Bleeding patterns can range from amenorrhoea to frequent and prolonged bleeding. Irregular and unpredictable bleeding are the major disadvantages. Weight gain is a common reason for discontinuation; however, it is under debate. Delayed return to fertility and bone mineral density loss are under debate	Bleeding patterns can range from amenorrhoea to frequent and prolonged bleeding. Irregular and unpredictable bleeding are the major disadvantages	The administration must be performed every 30 days
Recommended follow-up procedures after injection	After injection, there is no need for attention by either the user or the provider until time of new injection	After injection, there is no need for attention by either the user or the provider until time of new injection	After injection, there is no need for attention by either the user or the provider until time of new injection

Declarations

Competing Interests The author(s) has no competing interests to declare that are relevant to the content of this manuscript.

Ethics Approval The author(s) declares that this manuscript does not include primary research with human participants.

The author(s) declares that this manuscript does not include primary studies involving animals.

References

1. UN, Department of Economic and Social Affairs, Population Division. World family planning highlights – 2017 (ST/ESA/SER.A/414). 2017. Available at: https://www.un.org/en/development/desa/population/publications/pdf/family/WFP2017_Highlights.pdf. Accessed 23 Apr 2024.
2. Bahamondes L, Villaroel C, Guzmánn NF, Oizerovich S, Velazquez-Ramirez N, Monteiro I. The use of long-acting reversible contraceptives in Latin America and the Caribbean: current landscape and recommendations. Hum Reprod Open. 2018;1:hox030. https://doi.org/10.1093/hropen/hox030. eCollection 2018
3. Gigante DP, de França G, De Lucia RE, Lima NP, Dos Santos Motta JV, Gonçalves H, et al. Adolescent parenthood associated with adverse socio-economic outcomes at age 30 years in women and men of the Pelotas, Brazil: 1982 Birth Cohort Study. BJOG. 2019;126(3):360–7. https://doi.org/10.1111/1471-0528.15428.
4. Darroch J, Sully E, Biddlecom A. Adding it up: investing in contraception and maternal and newborn health. New York, NY: Guttmacher Institute; 2017.
5. Le J, Tsourounis C. Implanon: a critical review. Ann Pharmacother. 2001;35:329–36. https://doi.org/10.1345/aph.10149.
6. Ali M, Akin A, Bahamondes L, Brache V, Habib N, Landoulsi S, et al. Extended use up to 5 years of the etonogestrel-releasing subdermal contraceptive implant: comparison to levonorgestrel-releasing subdermal implant. Hum Reprod. 2016;31:2491–8. https://doi.org/10.1093/humrep/dew222.
7. Brache V, Faundes A, Johansson E, Alvarez F. Anovulation, inadequate luteal phase and poor sperm penetration in cervical mucus during prolonged use of Norplant implants. Contraception. 1985;31:261–73. https://doi.org/10.1016/0010-7824(85)90096-4.
8. Makarainen L, van Veek A, Tuomivaara L, Asplund B, Coelingh-Bennink H. Ovarian function during the use of a single contraceptive implant: Implanon compared with Norplant. Fertil Steril. 1998;69:714–21. https://doi.org/10.1016/s0015-0282(98)00015-6.
9. Blumenthal PD, Gemzell-Danielsson K, Marintcheva-Petrova M. Tolerability and clinical safety of Implanon. Eur J Contracept Reprod Health Care. 2008;13(Suppl 1):29–36. https://doi.org/10.1080/13625180801960012.
10. Grimes D. Forgettable contraception. Contraception. 2009;80:497–9. https://doi.org/10.1016/j.contraception.2009.06.005.
11. Winner B, Peipert JF, Zhao Q, Buckel C, Madden T, Allsworth JE, et al. Effectiveness of long-acting reversible contraception. N Engl J Med. 2012;366:1998–2007. https://doi.org/10.1056/NEJMoa1110855.
12. Bahamondes L, Brache V, Meirik O, Ali M, Habib N, Landoulsi S. A 3-year multicentre randomized controlled trial of etonogestrel- and levonorgestrel-releasing contraceptive implants, with non-randomized matched copper-intrauterine device controls. Hum Reprod. 2015;30:2527–38. https://doi.org/10.1093/humrep/dev221.

13. Darney P, Patel A, Rosen K, Shapiro LS, Kaunitz AM. Safety and efficacy of a single-rod etonogestrel implant (Implanon): results from 11 international clinical trials. Fertil Steril. 2009;91:1646–53. https://doi.org/10.1016/j.fertnstert.2008.02.140.
14. McNicholas C, Maddipati R, Zhao Q, Swor E, Peipert JF. Use of the etonogestrel implant and levonorgestrel intrauterine device beyond the U.S. Food and Drug Administration-approved duration. Obstet Gynecol. 2015;125:599–604. https://doi.org/10.1097/AOG.0000000000000690.
15. Mornar S, Chandra A, Mistretta S, Neustadt A, Martinez G, Gilliam M. Pharmacokinetics of the etonogestrel contraceptive implant in obese women. Am J Obstet Gynecol. 2012;207(110):e1–6. https://doi.org/10.1016/j.ajog.2012.05.002.
16. Morrell KM, Cremers S, Westhoff C, Davis AR. Etonogestrel levels in normal- weight, overweight and obese women after 1 year or more of contraceptive implant use. Contraception. 2016;93:263–5. https://doi.org/10.1016/j.contraception.2015.11.005.
17. Monteiro-Dantas C, Espejo-Arce X, Lui-Filho JF, Fernandes AM, Monteiro I, Bahamondes L. A three-year longitudinal evaluation of the forearm bone density of users of etonogestrel- and levonorgestrel-releasing contraceptive implants. Reprod Health. 2007;4:11. https://doi.org/10.1186/1742-4755-4-11.
18. Dinh A, Sriprasert I, Williams AR, Archer DF. A review of the endometrial histologic effects of progestins and progesterone receptor modulators in reproductive age women. Contraception. 2015;91:360–7. https://doi.org/10.1016/j.contraception.2015.01.008.
19. Mansour D, Fraser IS, Edelman A, Vieira CS, Kaunitz AM, Korver T, et al. Can initial vaginal bleeding patterns in etonogestrel implant users predict subsequent bleeding in the first 2 years of use? Contraception. 2019;100:264–8. https://doi.org/10.1016/j.contraception.2019.05.017.
20. Peterson AM, Brown A, Savage A, Dempsey A. Prevalence of early discontinuation and associated factors among a retrospective cohort of etonogestrel contraceptive implant users. Eur J Contracept Reprod Health Care. 2019;24:475–9. https://doi.org/10.1080/13625187.2019.1666361.
21. Milliren CE, DiVasta AD, Edwards AJ, Maslyanskaya S, Borzutzky C, Pitts S. Contraceptive implant-associated bleeding in adolescent/young adult clinical practice: associated factors, management, and rates of discontinuation. J Adolesc Health. 2023;72:583–90. https://doi.org/10.1016/j.jadohealth.2022.11.007.
22. Diedrich JT, Zhao Q, Madden T, Secura GM, Peipert JF. Three-year continuation of reversible contraception. Am J Obstet Gynecol. 2015;213(662):e1–8. https://doi.org/10.1016/j.ajog.2015.08.001.
23. Mansour D, Korver T, Marintcheva-Petrova M, Fraser IS. The effects of Implanon on menstrual bleeding patterns. Eur J Contracept Reprod Health Care. 2008;13:13–28. https://doi.org/10.1080/13625180801959931.
24. Henkel A, Goldthwaite LM. Management of bothersome bleeding associated with progestin-based long-acting reversible contraception: a review. Curr Opin Obstet Gynecol. 2020;32:408–15. https://doi.org/10.1097/GCO.0000000000000664.
25. Manhiça SI, Bahamondes L, Laporte M, Anjos F, Viscola M, Garcia E, et al. Single-visit long-acting reversible contraception provision and pregnancy rates within 3 months. Int J Gynaecol Obstet. 2023;161:1028–32. https://doi.org/10.1002/ijgo.14630.
26. Stuart GS, Yates L, Crump J, Allison BA, Navarro AL, Tadikonda A, et al. Single-visit insertion of long-acting reversible contraception in a single health system. Contraception. 2023;123:110009. https://doi.org/10.1016/j.contraception.2023.110009.
27. Curtis KM, Tepper NK, Jatlaoui TC, et al. U.S. Medical eligibility criteria for contraceptive use. MMWR Recomm Rep. 2016;65:1–103. https://doi.org/10.15585/mmwr.rr6503a1.
28. Fitzpatrick D, Pirie K, Reeves G, Green J, Beral V. Combined and progestagen-only hormonal contraceptives and breast cancer risk: a UK nested case–control study and meta-analysis. PLoS Med. 2023;20:e1004188. https://doi.org/10.1371/journal.pmed.1004188.
29. Evidence for Contraceptive Options and HIV Outcomes (ECHO) Trial Consortium. HIV incidence among women using intramuscular depot medroxyprogesterone acetate, a copper

intrauterine device, or a levonorgestrel implant for contraception: a randomised, multicentre, open-label trial. Lancet. 2019;394:303–13. https://doi.org/10.1016/S0140-6736(19)31288-7.
30. Dorflinger LJ. Metabolic effects of implantable steroid contraceptives for women. Contraception. 2002;65:47–62. https://doi.org/10.1016/s0010-7824(01)00290-6.
31. Braga GC, Ferriolli E, Quintana SM, Ferriani RA, Pfrimer K, Vieira CS. Immediate postpartum initiation of etonogestrel -releasing implant: a randomized controlled trial on breastfeeding impact. Contraception. 2015;92:536–42. https://doi.org/10.1016/j.contraception.2015.07.009.
32. Barbieri MM, Herculano TB, Dantas Silva A, Bahamondes L, Juliato CRT, Surita FG. Acceptability of ENG-releasing subdermal implants among postpartum Brazilian young women during the COVID-19 pandemic. Int J Gynaecol Obstet. 2021;154:106–12. https://doi.org/10.1002/ijgo.13663.
33. American College of Obstetricians and Gynecologists. Access to postabortion contraception. ACOG Committee Opinion no. 833. Obstet Gynecol. 2021;138:e91–5.
34. Makins A, Cameron S. Post pregnancy contraception. Best Pract Res Clin Obstet Gynaecol. 2020;66:41–54. https://doi.org/10.1016/j.bpobgyn.2020.01.004.
35. Bahamondes L, Lavin P, Ojeda G, et al. Return of fertility after discontinuation of the once-a-month injectable contraceptive Cyclofem. Contraception. 1997;55:307–10. https://doi.org/10.1016/s0010-7824(97)00034-6.
36. Schwartz D, Mayaux MJ. Female fecundity as a function of age: results of artificial insemination in 2193 nulliparous women with azoospermic husbands. Federation CECOS. N Engl J Med. 1982;306:404–6. https://doi.org/10.1056/NEJM198202183060706.
37. Bongaarts J. Infertility after age 30: A false alarm. Fam Plann Perspect. 1982;14:75–8.
38. Damtie Y, Kefale B, Arefaynie M, Yalet M, Adane B. Fertility return after hormonal contraceptive discontinuation and associated factors among women attended Family Guidance Association of Ethiopia Dessie model clinic, Northeast Ethiopia: a cross-sectional study. PLoS One. 2023;18:e0287440. https://doi.org/10.1371/journal.pone.0287440.
39. Mansour D, Gemzell-Danielsson K, Inki P, Jensen JT. Fertility after discontinuation of contraception: a comprehensive review of the literature. Contraception. 2011;84:465–77. https://doi.org/10.1016/j.contraception.2011.04.002.
40. Bell SO, Karp C, Moreau C, PMA Principal Investigators Group, Gemmill A. "If I use family planning, I may have trouble getting pregnant next time I want to": a multicountry survey-based exploration of perceived contraceptive-induced fertility impairment and its relationship to contraceptive behaviors. Contraception X. 2023;5:100093. https://doi.org/10.1016/j.conx.2023.100093.
41. Zaenglein AL, Pathy AL, Schlosser BJ, et al. Guidelines of care for the management of acne vulgaris. J Am Acad Dermatol. 2016;74:945–73.e33. https://doi.org/10.1016/j.jaad.2015.12.037.
42. Mitchell AA, Van Bennekom CM, Louik C. A pregnancy-prevention program in women of childbearing age receiving isotretinoin. N Engl J Med. 1995;333:101–6. https://doi.org/10.1056/NEJM199507133330206.
43. Lazorwitz A, Seale R, Davis A, Guiahi M. A pilot study on the effect of isotretinoin on serum etonogestrel concentrations in contraceptive implant users. Contraception. 2020;102:58–60. https://doi.org/10.1016/j.contraception.2020.04.011.
44. Kouremenos E, Arvaniti C, Constantinidis TS, Giannouli E, Fakas N, Kalamatas T, et al. Consensus of the Hellenic Headache Society on the diagnosis and treatment of migraine. J Headache Pain. 2019;20:113. https://doi.org/10.1186/s10194-019-1060-6.
45. World Health Organization. Medical eligibility criteria for contraceptive use. Geneva; 2015.
46. Lazorwitz A, Pena M, Sheeder J, Teal S. Effect of topiramate on serum etonogestrel concentrations among contraceptive implant users. Obstet Gynecol. 2022;139:579–87. https://doi.org/10.1097/AOG.0000000000004697.
47. Centers for Disease Control and Prevention. Treatment regimens for Latent TB Infection (LTBI); 2020. Available at: https://www.cdc.gov/tb/topic/treatment/ltbi.htm. Accessed on 1 May 2024.

48. Lazorwitz A, Sheeder J, Teal S. The effect of rifampin on serum etonogestrel concentrations and biomarkers of ovulation among contraceptive implant users: a pharmacokinetic and pharmacodynamic study. Contraception. 2023;123:110035. https://doi.org/10.1016/j.contraception.2023.110035.
49. Nakalema S, Chappell CA, Pham M, Byakika P, Kaboggoza J, Walimbwa SI, et al. Pharmacokinetics of levonorgestrel and etonogestrel contraceptive implants over 48 weeks with rilpivirine- or darunavir-based antiretroviral therapy. J Antimicrob Chemother. 2022;77:3144–52. https://doi.org/10.1093/jac/dkac296.
50. Vieira CS, Bahamondes MV, de Souza RM, Brito MB, Rocha TR, Amaral E, et al. Effect of antiretroviral therapy including lopinavir/ritonavir or efavirenz on etonogestrel-releasing implant pharmacokinetics in HIV-positive women. J Acquir Immune Defic Syndr. 2014;66:378–85. https://doi.org/10.1097/QAI.0000000000000189.
51. Cirrincione LR, Nakalema S, Chappell CA, Byakika-Kibwika P, Kyohairwe I, Winchester L, et al. Effect of double-dose levonorgestrel subdermal implant in women taking efavirenz-based antiretroviral therapy: the DoubLNG pharmacokinetic study. Contraception. 2023;122:109975. https://doi.org/10.1016/j.contraception.2023.109975.
52. Chappell CA, Lamorde M, Nakalema S, Kyohairwe I, Byakika-Kibwika P, Meyn LA, et al. A randomized trial of double vs single-dose etonogestrel implant to overcome the interaction with efavirenz-based antiretroviral therapy. Am J Obstet Gynecol. 2024;S0002-9378(24):00424–1. https://doi.org/10.1016/j.ajog.2024.03.001.
53. Carvalho N, Margatho D, Cursino K, Benetti-Pinto CL, Bahamondes L. Control of endometriosis-associated pain with etonogestrel-releasing contraceptive implant and 52-mg levonorgestrel-releasing intrauterine system: randomized clinical trial. Fertil Steril. 2018;110:1129–36. https://doi.org/10.1016/j.fertnstert.2018.07.003.
54. Margatho D, Carvalho NM, Bahamondes L. Endometriosis-associated pain scores and biomarkers in users of the etonogestrel-releasing subdermal implant or the 52-mg levonorgestrel-releasing intrauterine system for up to 24 months. Eur J Contracept Reprod Health Care. 2020;25:133–40. https://doi.org/10.1080/13625187.2020.1725461.
55. Chene G, Baffet H, Cerruto E, Nohuz E, Agostini A. The role of progestin subdermal implant in the management of adenomyosis: a systematic review. Eur J Contracept Reprod Health Care. 2024;29:61–8. https://doi.org/10.1080/13625187.2024.2314298.
56. Xia YY, Gronwald J, Karlan B, et al. Contraceptive use and the risk of ovarian cancer among women with a BRCA1 or BRCA2 mutation. Gynecol Oncol. 2022;164:514–21. https://doi.org/10.1016/j.ygyno.2022.01.014.
57. De Nadai MN, Vieira CS, Monteiro I, et al. Practical training of health care providers in insertion of contraceptive implants: findings from two Brazilian centres. Eur J Contracept Reprod Health Care. 2021;26(6):499–502. https://doi.org/10.1080/13625187.2021.1942448.
58. Leon-Larios F, Llamazares MJA, Reisen HM, Ribes IP, Novoa MR, Lahoz-Pascual I. Impact of the hands-on clinical training program for subdermic implant on contraceptive counseling and users' choice in Spain: a 6-month follow-up study. Contraception. 2024;132:110372. https://doi.org/10.1016/j.contraception.2024.110372.
59. Grange R, Magand N, Grand N, Leroy S, Corsini T, Azarnoush K, et al. Endovascular retrieval of a migrated contraceptive implant into the pulmonary artery: case report and review of literature. CVIR Endovascular. 2024;7:35. https://doi.org/10.1186/s42155-024-00450-w.
60. Abubeker FA, Tufa TH, Tolu LB, Sium AF, Grentzer JM, Welderufael MB, et al. Localization and removal of nonpalpable contraceptive implants: experience from a teaching hospital in Ethiopia: a case series. Int J Gynecol Obstet. 2024;164:1125–31. https://doi.org/10.1002/ijgo.15166.
61. Ruelle Y, Haghighi S, Gui O. Effects of a short training workshop on the insertion/removal of intrauterine devices and contraceptive implants by general practice residents and their supervisors in France. Contraception. 2023;127:110117. https://doi.org/10.1016/j.contraception.2023.110117.

62. Iwanaga J, Fox MC, Rekers H, Schwartz L, Tubbs RS. Neurovascular anatomy of the adult female medial arm in relationship to potential sites for insertion of the etonogestrel contraceptive implant. Contraception. 2019;100:26–30. https://doi.org/10.1016/j.contraception.2019.02.007.
63. World Health Organization. Family planning: a global handbook for providers. 2018. Available from: https://www.who.int/publications/i/item/family-planning%2D%2D-a-global-handbook-for-providers.
64. Dragoman MV, Gaffield ME. The safety of subcutaneously administered depot medroxyprogesterone acetate (104mg/0.65mL): a systematic review. Contraception. 2016;94:202–15. https://doi.org/10.1016/j.contraception.2016.02.003.
65. Bahamondes L, Marchi NM, Nakagava HM, et al. Self-administration with UniJect of the once-a-month injectable contraceptive Cyclofem. Contraception. 1997;56:301–4. https://doi.org/10.1016/s0010-7824(97)00162-5.
66. Nabhan A, Elshafeey F, Mehrain LM, Kabra R, Elshabrawy A. Self-administered subcutaneous medroxyprogesterone acetate for improving contraceptive outcomes: a systematic review and meta-analysis. BMC Womens Health. 2021;9(21):359. https://doi.org/10.1186/s12905-021-01495-y.
67. Hapgood JP, Koubovec D, Louw A, Africander D. Not all progestins are the same: implications for usage. Trends Pharmacol Sci. 2004;25:554–7. https://doi.org/10.1016/j.tips.2004.09.005.
68. Friedrich C, Berse M, Klein S, Rohde B, Höchel J. In vivo formation of ethinylestradiol after intramuscular administration of Norethisterone Enantate. J Clin Pharmacol. 2018;58:781–9. https://doi.org/10.1002/jcph.1079.
69. Korhonen T, Turpeinen M, Tolonen A, Laine K, Pelkonen O. Identification of the human cytochrome P450 enzymes involved in the in vitro biotransformation of lynestrenol and norethindrone. J Steroid Biochem Mol Biol. 2008;110:56–66. https://doi.org/10.1016/j.jsbmb.2007.09.025.
70. Toh YC, Jain J, Rahnny MH, Bode FR, Ross D. Suppression of ovulation by a new subcutaneous depot medroxyprogesterone acetate (104 mg/0.65 mL) contraceptive formulation in Asian women. Clin Ther. 2004;26:1845–54. https://doi.org/10.1016/j.clinthera.2004.11.013.
71. Kaunitz AM, Darney PD, Ross D, Wolter KD, Speroff L. Subcutaneous DMPA vs. intramuscular DMPA: a 2-year randomized study of contraceptive efficacy and bone mineral density. Contraception. 2009;80:7–7. https://doi.org/10.1016/j.contraception.2009.02.005.
72. Jain J, Jakimiuk AJ, Bode FR, Ross D, Kaunitz AM. Contraceptive efficacy and safety of DMPA-SC. Contraception. 2004;70:269–75. https://doi.org/10.1016/j.contraception.2004.06.011.
73. Garza-Flores J, Morales del Olmo A, Fuziwara JL, et al. Introduction of cyclofem® once-a-month injectable contraceptive in Mexico. Contraception. 1998;58:7–12. https://doi.org/10.1016/s0010-7824(98)00062-6.
74. Hall P, Bahamondes L, Diaz J, Petta C. Introductory study of the once-a-month, injectable contraceptive Cyclofem in Brazil, Chile, Colombia, and Peru. Contraception. 1997;56:353–9. https://doi.org/10.1016/s0010-7824(97)00185-6.
75. Kaunitz AM. Injectable contraception. New and existing options. Obstet Gynecol Clin North Am. 2000;27:741–80. https://doi.org/10.1016/s0889-8545(05)70171-6.
76. Fraser IS, Dennerstein GJ. Depo-Provera use in an Australian metropolitan practice. Med J Aust. 1994;160:553–6.
77. Taylor DJ, Deese J, Bahamondes L, et al. Return to ovulation after Sayana Press is injected every 4 months for one year: empirical and pharmacokinetic/pharmacodynamic modeling results. Contracept X. 2022;4:100080. https://doi.org/10.1016/j.conx.2022.100080.
78. Bachmann G, Korner P. Bleeding patterns associated with non-oral hormonal contraceptives: a review of the literature. Contraception. 2009;79:247–58. https://doi.org/10.1016/j.contraception.2008.10.012.
79. Hubacher D, Lopez L, Steiner MJ, Dorflinger L. Menstrual pattern changes from levonorgestrel subdermal implants and DMPA: systematic review and evidence-based comparisons. Contraception. 2009;80:113–8. https://doi.org/10.1016/j.contraception.2009.02.008.

80. Lopez LM, Ramesh S, Chen M, Edelman A, Otterness C, Trussell J, Helmerhorst FM. Progestin-only contraceptives: effects on weight. Cochrane Database Syst Rev. 2016;28:CD008815. https://doi.org/10.1002/14651858.CD008815.pub4.
81. Curtis KM, Hannaford PC, Rodriguez MI, Chipato T, Steyn PS, Kiarie JN. Hormonal contraception and HIV acquisition among women: an updated systematic review. BMJ Sex Reprod Health. 2020;46:8–16. https://doi.org/10.1136/bmjsrh-2019-200509.
82. Gbolade BA. Depo-Provera and bone density. J Fam Plann Reprod Health Care. 2002;28:7–11. https://doi.org/10.1783/147118902101195910.
83. Bertrand JT, Ross J, Sullivan TM, Hardee K, Shelton JD. Contraceptive method mix: updates and implications. Glob Health Sci Pract. 2020;8:666–79. https://doi.org/10.9745/GHSP-D-20-00229.
84. Berenson AB, van den Berg P, Williams KJ, Rahman M. Effect of injectable and oral contraceptives on glucose and insulin levels. Obstet Gynecol. 2011;117:41–7. https://doi.org/10.1097/AOG.0b013e318202ac23.
85. Newton JR, D'arcangues C, Hall PE. A review of "once-a-month" combined injectable contraceptives. J Obstet Gynaecol (Lahore). 1994;4(Suppl 1):S1–34. https://doi.org/10.3109/01443619409027641.
86. Gupta V, Chawla S, Goel PK. Injectable depot medroxy progesterone acetate: a safe contraceptive choice in public health system of India. Int J Prev Med. 2020;11:180. https://doi.org/10.4103/ijpvm.IJPVM_163_19. eCollection 2020
87. Gallo MF, Grimes DA, Lopez LM, Schulz KF, d'Arcangues C. Combination injectable contraceptives for contraception. Cochrane Database Syst Rev. 2013;3:CD004568.
88. Goldberg AB, Grimes DA. Injectable contraceptives. In: Hatcher RA, Trussell J, Nelson AL, Cates W, Stewart F, Kowal D, editors. Contraceptive technology. 19th ed. New York: Ardent Media, Inc.; 2007. p. 157–79.
89. Kaunitz AM, Arias R, McClung M. Bone density recovery after depot medroxyprogesterone acetate injectable contraception use. Contraception. 2008;77:67–76. https://doi.org/10.1016/j.contraception.2007.10.005.
90. Sang GW, Shao QX, Ge RS, Ge JL, Chen JK, Song S, Fang KJ, He ML, Luo SY, Chen SF, et al. A multicentred phase III comparative clinical trial of Mesigyna, Cyclofem and Injectable No. 1 given by intramuscular injection to Chinese women. II. The comparison of bleeding patterns. Contraception. 1995;51:185–92. https://doi.org/10.1016/0010-7824(95)00014-2.
91. Deese J, Brache V, Bahamondes L, et al. Contraceptive effectiveness, pharmacokinetics, and safety of Sayana® Press when injected every four months: a multicenter phase 3 trial. EClinicalMedicine. 2022;44:101273. https://doi.org/10.1016/j.eclinm.2022.101273. eCollection 2022
92. Burke HM, Packer C, Fuchs R, et al. Acceptability of the contraceptive Sayana®Press when injected every four months: results from a twelve-month trial in Brazil, Chile and the Dominican Republic. Contraception. 2022;113:95–100. https://doi.org/10.1016/j.contraception.2022.04.007.

Part VII
Other Aspects of Hormonal Contraception in Women and Men

Chapter 20
Quality of Life and Sexuality in Women Using Hormonal Contraceptives

Johannes Bitzer

20.1 Introduction

Millions of women use hormonal contraceptives to protect them against unwanted pregnancy. These methods are based on the interaction with the physiology of the menstrual cycle and the impact of these hormones on ovulation, the endometrium, and the cervical mucus. For decades, the knowledge about these methods has accumulated with respect to efficacy, effectiveness, and health risks, and based on this practice, guidelines have been issued. During the years, it has become evident that hormonal contraceptives can have a negative (side effects) and a positive effect (benefit) on different aspects of general health including physical, mental, and sexual health. The impact on the individual quality of life of the user as a subjective experience has important consequences regarding the decision to use hormonal contraceptives and the continuation or discontinuation of use which increases the risk of unwanted pregnancies [1].

In this chapter, a short overview regarding empirical studies about the impact of hormonal contraceptives on quality of life including sexual health will be given followed by a practical model how to include quality of life and sexual health into the contraceptive counseling and care.

J. Bitzer (✉)
Department of Obstetrics and Gynecology, University Hospital Basel, Basel, Switzerland
e-mail: Johannes.Bitzer@usb.ch

A. R. Genazzani et al. (eds.), *Ethical, Efficacy and Safety Issues in Contraception*, Reproductive Medicine for Clinicians 4,
https://doi.org/10.1007/978-3-032-07322-8_20

20.2 Quality of Life and Sexual Health in Users of Hormonal Contraception—Measurement and Empirical Findings

In 1993, WHO defined quality of life as "*individuals' perception of their position in life in the context of the culture and value systems in which they live in relation to their goals, standards, and concerns*" [2].

This definition includes the concept that quality of life is the result of a dynamic balance between a person's subjective needs and the degree to which these needs are fulfilled.

Later, QoL was stronger based on the biopsychosocial model and the WHOQOL-BREF included besides the general rating of three domains (physical health, psychological, social relationship), which should cover the main elements of wellbeing [3] (Fig. 20.1).

There are many questionnaires used to empirically study the impact of contraceptives on the quality of life including nonhormonal methods (Fig. 20.2). In a systematic review, the authors found that the most used was the Short Form-36 questionnaires, followed by the EQ-5FD. On the whole, 23 questionnaires were used across 78 studies [4].

Regarding measurement of sexual health in the context of contraception, again different tools were used: screening tool for FSD like the FSFI, a diagnostic tool for differentiation and quantification of sexual dysfunctions like the FSDR-R, tools for comparative studies like the CSFQ-F and short questionnaire like the Arizona Sexual Experience Scale (ASEX) or the Sexual Desire Inventory, a diagnostic tool for etiopathogenesis [5] (Fig. 20.3).

The different studies concerning QoL and sexual health using different measures and methodologies came to controversial results [4–6].

The observational studies investigating QoL and sexual health before and after use of hormonal contraceptives found no change, negative change, and positive change in variable percentages.

Comparing different contraceptive methods (hormonal, nonhormonal, etc.) in clinical trials resulted also in a large variety of results with contradictory outcomes.

There are several reasons explaining this lack of precision and the uncertainties.

- The outcomes (QoL and sexual health) are subjective patient-reported outcomes, which cannot be measured objectively like clinical or laboratory parameters but need standardized questionnaires.
- There is no single best questionnaire comparable to physical objective measurements like laboratory values, etc., making results difficult to compare or integrate.
- There are a large number of intervening variables between the contraceptive method and the QoL and sexual function increasing the risk of bias and confounders.

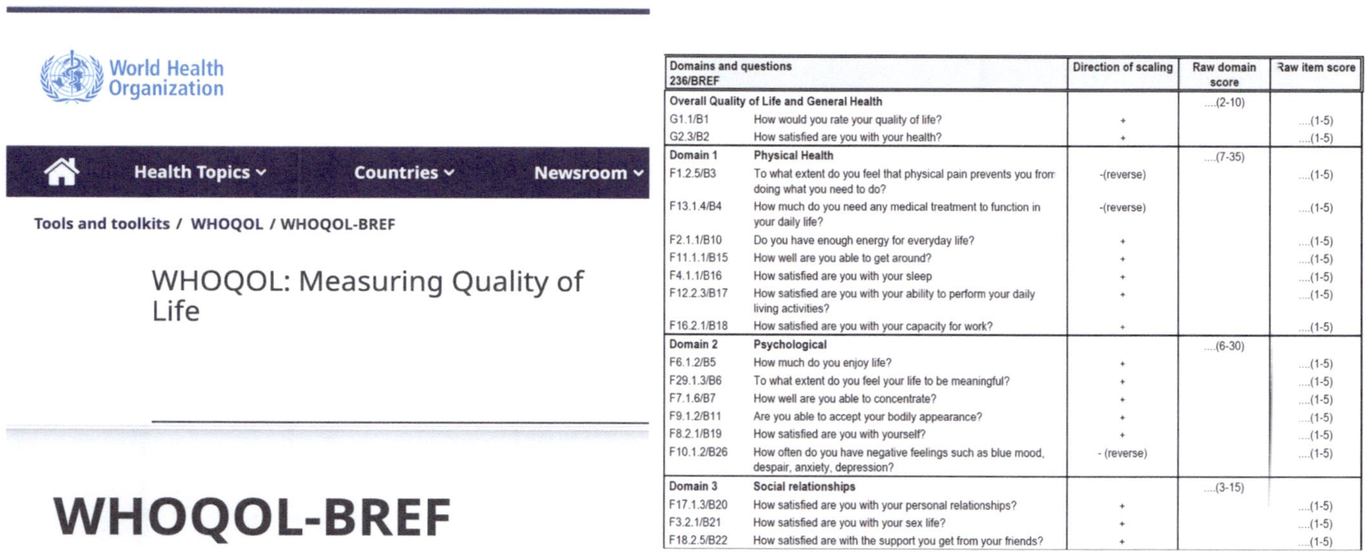

Domains and questions 236/BREF		Direction of scaling	Raw domain score	Raw item score
Overall Quality of Life and General Health			....(2-10)	
G1.1/B1	How would you rate your quality of life?	+		....(1-5)
G2.3/B2	How satisfied are you with your health?	+		....(1-5)
Domain 1	**Physical Health**		....(7-35)	
F1.2.5/B3	To what extent do you feel that physical pain prevents you from doing what you need to do?	-(reverse)		....(1-5)
F13.1.4/B4	How much do you need any medical treatment to function in your daily life?	-(reverse)		....(1-5)
F2.1.1/B10	Do you have enough energy for everyday life?	+		....(1-5)
F11.1.1/B15	How well are you able to get around?	+		....(1-5)
F4.1.1/B16	How satisfied are you with your sleep	+		....(1-5)
F12.2.3/B17	How satisfied are you with your ability to perform your daily living activities?	+		....(1-5)
F16.2.1/B18	How satisfied are you with your capacity for work?	+		....(1-5)
Domain 2	**Psychological**		....(6-30)	
F6.1.2/B5	How much do you enjoy life?	+		....(1-5)
F29.1.3/B6	To what extent do you feel your life to be meaningful?	+		....(1-5)
F7.1.6/B7	How well are you able to concentrate?	+		....(1-5)
F9.1.2/B11	Are you able to accept your bodily appearance?	+		....(1-5)
F8.2.1/B19	How satisfied are you with yourself?	+		....(1-5)
F10.1.2/B26	How often do you have negative feelings such as blue mood, despair, anxiety, depression?	- (reverse)		....(1-5)
Domain 3	**Social relationships**		....(3-15)	
F17.1.3/B20	How satisfied are you with your personal relationships?	+		....(1-5)
F3.2.1/B21	How satisfied are you with your sex life?	+		....(1-5)
F18.2.5/B22	How satisfied are with the support you get from your friends?	+		....(1-5)

Fig. 20.1 WHOQOL-BREF

MEASURING THE HEALTH-RELATED QUALITY OF LIFE OF WOMEN USING CONTRACEPTION: A SYSTEMATIC REVIEW AND ANALYSIS OF AVAILABLE TOOLS

Institute for Women's Health
Submitted as partial fulfilment of the requirements for the MSc in Reproductive Science and Women's Health, University College London

freq.	General	Freq.
	Short Form-36 Questionnaire	30
	EQ-5D	8
	Quality of Life and Satisfaction Questionnaire (Q-LESQ)	6
	Rand-36	5
	Short Personal Experience Questionnaire (SPEQ)	3
	Visual Analogue Scale (VAS)	3
	WHOQoL	3
	EQ-5D vas	2
	SF-12	2
	SF-36v2	2
	Women's Health Questionnaire	2
	Daily Record of Severity of Problems (DRSP)	1
	EORTC OLQ-C30	1
	EQ-5D-3L	1
	General Effect Study Medication Questionnaire (GESQ)	1
	General Health Questionnaire - 12	1
	HRQL (SF-8)	1
	HRQOL -4	1
	Short Form questionnaire-6 Dimensions (SF-6D)	1
	Sickness Impact Profile	1
	WHO-S	1
	WHOQoL-BREF	1
	Youth Quality of Life Instrument	1
		78

Fig. 20.2 Measuring health-related quality of life in women using contraception

Fig. 20.3 Measuring sexuality in the context of contraception

1. Screening tool for FSD	FSFI
2. Diagnostic tool for differentiation and quantification of FSD	FSDR-R
3. Tool for clinical relevant quantitative assessment of changes before/after treatment (RCT)	Changes in Sexual Functioning Questionnaire (CSFQ-F)
4. Diagnostic tool for FSD in specific clinical conditions	Arizona Sexual Experiences Scale© (ASEX) Five-item rating scale
5. Diagnostic tool for aetiopathogenesis	Sexual Desire Inventory© (SDI©)

20.3 The Variability of the Individual Biopsychosocial Impact of Hormonal Contraceptives on the Quality of Life and Sexuality of the Users

A major reason regarding the limitations of observational and clinical trials lies in the fact that contraception in general and hormonal contraceptives specifically can have a neutral, a negative, or a positive effect on QoL and sexual health depending on the response of the individual user.

There are five dimensions which interact with the profile of the user determining the subjective experience:

Separating Reproduction from Sexuality
Although being the rationale for contraception and *liberating sexual activity from the fear of pregnancy*, contraception can also be experienced on an emotional level as a *deprivation of a profound potency and profound sense of the sexual encounter* leading to insecurity, low mood, and dissatisfaction.

Impact on the Relationship
Contraception including hormonal contraception is experienced and practiced in the context of a relationship.

The perception can be positive as a *means of autonomy and self-determination* of the user. It can increase attractivity for the partner. But at the same *time*, *conflicts can arise*: Wish for a child in one partner, questions about shared responsibility for contraception, shared risk taking can *change the perception and make it more negative.*

Contraceptive Methods Have a Social Image Impacting the Experience of the Individual User
Contraception is a behavior which is embedded into a sociocultural and political context.

On one hand, hormonal contraception can be perceived as a big step forward regarding women's emancipation, as an efficient and safe protection. On the other hand, the history of the pill has shown that there are also risks, which depending on the media and the family culture may contribute to a negative image of "pills" being against nature, dangerous and imposed by "Big Pharma."

The Hormones Used in Hormonal Contraception Can Have Bidirectional Actions (Negative, Positive, Neutral) on the Physical and the Mental Level [6–8]
Estrogens have a positive action on the emotional regulation of the brain and on vaginal health.

Estrogens stabilize the endometrium improving tolerability.

On the other hand, estrogen preparations can indirectly have an antiandrogenic effect contributing to less desire or too much estrogen can contribute to heavy bleeding.

Progestogens can have a mood stabilizing effect on the brain in patients with PMS PMDD, and they counteract estrogen excess and reduce bleeding.

Some progestogens have a mood-lowering action depending on the interaction with the GABA receptor.

20.4 The Individualized Approach

Based on this biopsychosocial understanding of the complex interaction and the different ways hormonal contraceptives can have an impact on QoL and sexual Health, healthcare professionals need to integrate physical, mental, sexual, and social health of the individual patient into contraceptive counseling and care.

The biopsychosocial diagnostic assessment includes the following (Fig. 20.4).

Medical History and Examination

- The physical/medical history and examination focuses on risk factors for VTE, metabolic complications, malignancies to ensure safe prescribing using the medical eligibility criteria (WHO, FRSH).
- The assessment of quality of life and sexual health includes questions about physical symptoms like bleeding, pain, skin changes, etc.
- The mental health history explores mental health risk factors like PMS, PMDD, postpartum depression on one hand but also self-reported chronic stress and signs thereof like sleep problems.
- The sexual history includes questions not only about risks of sexually transmitted infections and how to protect oneself, but also questions about sexual activity, satisfaction with the sex life, problems with desire, arousal, sexual pain.

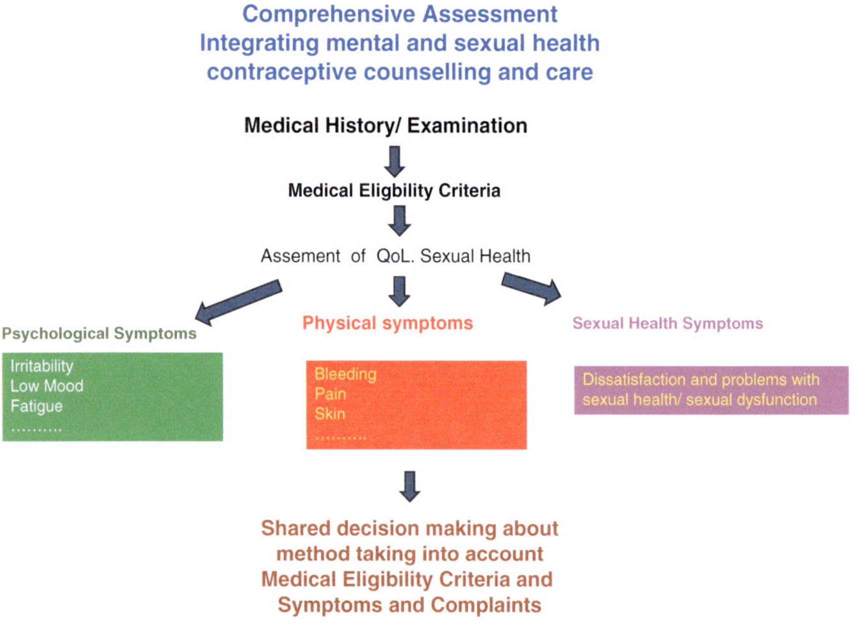

Fig. 20.4 Biopsychosocial assessment of the user's profile

Based on the individual profile, the HCP can help the patient to

- Find the method with the best safety profile using Medical Eligibility Criteria.
- Find the method with no negative or positive effects on mental and sexual health.

20.5 Comprehensive Care (Fig. 20.5)

If problems of mental health and/or sexuality are reported, the HCP should evaluate the severity and the individual distress.

Listening, providing information and basic counseling regarding stress, emotional, and sexual problems can be of great help and may be the first and only place and time for the patient to mention these problems to a healthcare professional.

Depending on the gravity and the wish of the patient, another consultation can be offered to address these issues in more detail and make eventually a referral to specialized treatments.

Regarding the choice of hormonal contraceptives and the follow-up of users, it is important to consider the possible effects of their use on QoL and sexual health depending on the type of the steroids, the dosages, combinations, and regimens [9]

- Estrogens especially applied in a continuous mode can exert a mood elevator effect in the brain and contribute to vulvovaginal health, thus having a positive effect in women with depressive mood and/or vulvovaginal atrophy accompanied by pain and arousal difficulties.

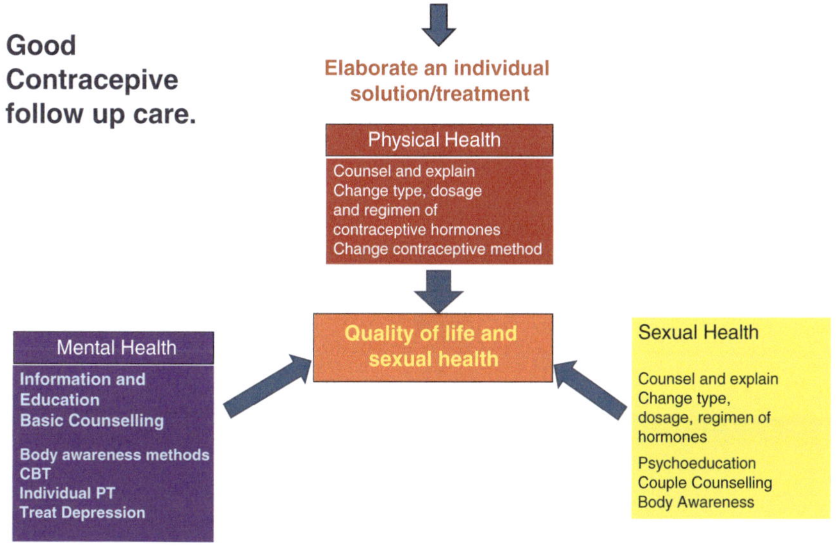

Fig. 20.5 Comprehensive follow-up care

- Some preparations with EE as component may lower free testosterone and contribute to preexisting low desire, and thus, the choice would be more among estradiol containing OCs eventually combined with an androgenic progestin.
- Regarding progestogen-only contraceptives due to the interaction with the GABA receptor, these preparations might exert a positive effect on irritability and anxious mood through their sedative effect but may have negative consequences on preexisting episodes of depressed mood or depression. It seems that androgenic progestins would have these effects more than nonandrogenic neutral progestins.
- Preexisting PMS PMDD seem to be effectively treated by drospirenone containing combined contraceptives and/or eventually drospirenone alone and/or long cycle regimen with different CHC.

20.6 Summary and Recommendations

- Quality of life and sexual health are important factors contributing to the satisfaction and continuation of users of hormonal contraception.
- Hormonal contraceptives can have a negative, neutral, or positive impact on the major elements of QoL and sexual health depending on the medical and psychosocial profile of the user.
- The choice of hormonal contraceptives and follow-up care should include assessment of mental and sexual health to detect major problems and provide supportive counseling.
- Depending on the individual mental or sexual health problem, professionals can help to find the hormonal contraceptive with the most likely positive effect on mental and sexual health.

Declarations

Competing Interests The author(s) has no competing interests to declare that are relevant to the content of this manuscript.

Ethics Approval The author(s) declares that this manuscript does not include primary research with human participants.

The author(s) declares that this manuscript does not include primary studies involving animals.

References

1. Sanders SA, Graham CA, Bass JL, Bancroft J. A prospective study of the effects of oral contraceptives on sexuality and wellbeing and their relationship to discontinuation. Contraception. 2001;64:51–8.
2. https://www.who.int/tools/whoqol

3. https://www.who.int/publications/i/item/WHO-HIS-HSI-Rev.2012.03
4. Giraldi A, Rellini A, Pfaus JG, Bitzer J. Questionnaires for assessment of female sexual dysfunction: a review and proposal for a standardized screener. J Sex Med. 2011;8:2681–706.
5. Davis A, Castano P. Oral contraceptives and libido in women. Annu Rev Sex Res. 2004;15:297–320.
6. Schaffir J. Hormonal contraception and sexual desire: a critical review. J Sex Marital Ther. 2006;32:305–14.
7. Genazzani AR, Monteleone M, Gambacciani M. Hormonal influence on the central nervous system. Maturitas. 2002;43(Suppl. 1):S11–7.
8. Lundin C, Danielsson KG, Bixo M, Moby L, Bengtsdotter H, Jawad I, et al. Combined oral contraceptive use is associated with both improvement and worsening of mood in the different phases of the treatment cycle-a double-blind, placebo-controlled randomized trial. Psychoneuroendocrinology. 2017;76:135–43.
9. Zethraeus N, Dreber A, Ranehill E, Blomberg L, Labrie F, von Schoultz B, et al. A first-choice combined oral contraceptive influences general well-being in healthy women: a double-blind, randomized, placebo-controlled trial. Fertil Steril. 2017;107:1238–45.

Chapter 21
Emergency Contraception

Kristina Gemzell-Danielsson, H. W. Raymond Li, and Sharon T. Cameron

21.1 Introduction

Emergency contraception (EC) refers to methods used to prevent pregnancy after unprotected intercourse or contraceptive failure. EC is an important option for reducing unintended pregnancies and is distinct from regular contraceptive methods in that it is used postcoitally. The most commonly used methods today are levonorgestrel (LNG), ulipristal acetate (UPA), and the copper intrauterine device (Cu-IUD). Each method has unique characteristics regarding efficacy, mechanism of action, and suitability for different situations.

21.2 Historical Background

The concept of postcoital contraception dates back to ancient times. Historical texts, such as those by Soranos of Ephesus in the second century AD, described rudimentary methods including vaginal washing, sneezing, and jumping, aimed at

K. Gemzell-Danielsson (✉)
Department of Women's and Children's Health, Division of Obstetrics and Gynaecology, Karolinska Institutet and Karolinska University Hospital, Stockholm, Sweden
e-mail: kristina.gemzell@ki.se

H. W. R. Li
Department of Obstetrics and Gynaecology, The University of Hong Kong, Queen Mary Hospital, Pok Fu Lam, Hong Kong

S. T. Cameron
Chalmers Sexual and Reproductive Health Centre, Edinburgh, UK

A. R. Genazzani et al. (eds.), *Ethical, Efficacy and Safety Issues in Contraception*, Reproductive Medicine for Clinicians 4,
https://doi.org/10.1007/978-3-032-07322-8_21

preventing sperm transport/function and hence preventing pregnancy after intercourse. However, modern EC only began to develop significantly in the latter half of the twentieth century. Early oral methods included high doses of ethinyl estradiol and levonorgestrel, known as the Yuzpe regimen, has largely been replaced by more effective and better-tolerated options like LNG and UPA.

21.3 Methods of Emergency Contraception

21.3.1 Levonorgestrel

Levonorgestrel is a synthetic progestogen initially developed to be administered as two 0.75 mg doses taken 12 h apart [1, 2], but later on, studies showed it was as effective as a single 1.5 mg dose [3]. It is most effective when taken within 24 h of unprotected intercourse, reducing the risk of pregnancy by 60–89% [4]. Its effectiveness decreases with time after intercourse, but with effects seen up to 96 h after intercourse. The regulatory approval is for use within 72 h.

21.3.2 Ulipristal Acetate

Ulipristal acetate is a selective progesterone receptor modulator. A single 30 mg dose of UPA can be taken up to 120 h (5 days) after unprotected intercourse, maintaining higher efficacy over a longer period compared to LNG. Studies have shown that UPA reduces the risk of pregnancy by approximately 85% when taken within 120 h of unprotected sex [5].

21.3.3 Cu-IUD

The Cu-IUD is the most effective form of emergency contraception, with an efficacy rate of almost 99% when inserted within 5 days of unprotected intercourse [4, 6, 7]. Additionally, it provides ongoing contraception for up to 10 years, making it a long-term solution as well as an emergency option. Despite its effectiveness, access to the Cu-IUD can be limited by the need for a trained healthcare provider to perform the insertion.

21.4 Mechanisms of Action

21.4.1 Inhibiting or Postponing Ovulation

The primary mechanism of action of LNG and UPA is the inhibition or delay of ovulation (Fig. 21.1). LNG prevents the LH surge necessary for ovulation if taken early enough in the menstrual cycle after selection of the dominant follicle. However, it does not prevent ovulation, and hence its efficacy is reduced, if taken when LH levels have already started to rise [8, 9]. UPA, on the other hand, remains effective

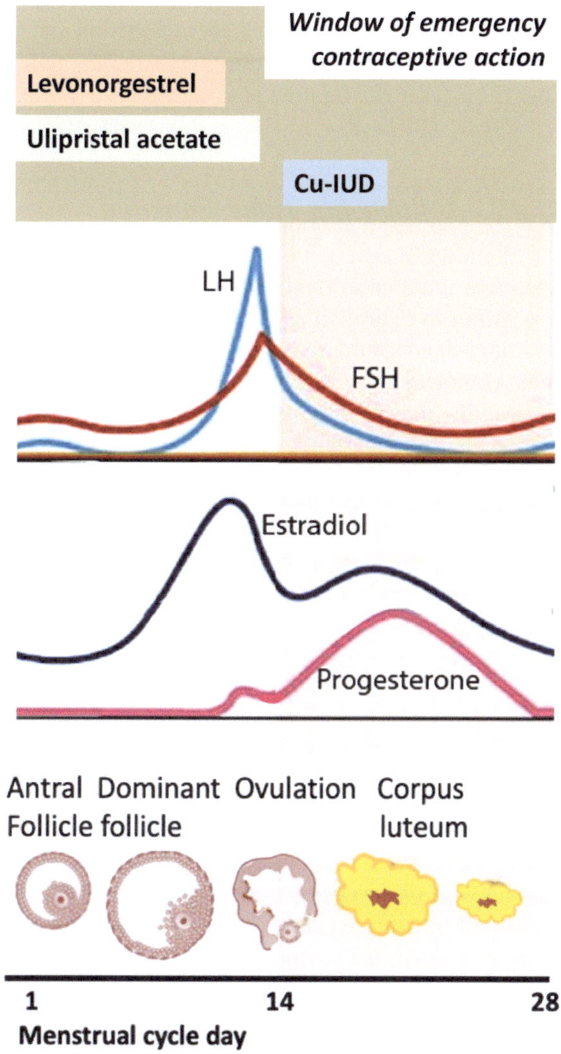

Fig. 21.1 Window of action of oral emergency contraceptive pills

even after the LH surge has begun, until its peak, thus providing a slightly broader window for intervention [10]. If taken after the LH peak, neither LNG nor UPA prevents ovulation.

21.4.2 Influencing Sperm Function and Fertilization

Studies suggested that LNG has no significant effect on sperm function or fertilization [11, 12], while UPA might inhibit the progesterone-induced acrosome reaction, hyperactivation, and intracellular calcium in human sperm [13]. The Cu-IUD has a toxic effect on sperm (and probably on the oocyte too) and may prevent fertilization [14]. The relevance of impaired sperm function and fertilization to EC of the latter is not certain as in most circumstances sperm could have reached the egg by the time EC is taken if ovulation has occurred.

21.4.3 Influencing Tubal Function

LNG was reported to inhibit muscular contractility of the fallopian tube [15] but was shown to reduce ciliary beating and muscular contractility only at suprapharmacological concentrations in another report [16]. The Cu-IUD may increase muscular contractility in the fallopian tube [17]. An increase or reduction in tubal contractility may result in asynchronized gametes or embryo transport, but whether or how much it contributes to a contraceptive effect is uncertain.

21.4.4 Inhibiting Implantation

While some in vitro studies demonstrated contrasting effects on certain histological and/or molecular changes in endometrial tissue after treatment with LNG and UPA, it is not known how these alterations affect implantation [18, 19]. The better approach to study implantation in vitro is by embryo-endometrial tissue coculture attachment assays. Attachment of human blastocysts or trophoblastic spheroids onto endometrial cells was shown not to be impaired by in vitro treatment with LNG and UPA at concentrations corresponding to pharmacological levels [20–22]. These findings were further supported by clinical trials which revealed that both LNG [23, 24] and UPA [25] were only effective as EC when administered before but not after ovulation. In summary, current evidence does not support any effect of LNG and UPA on endometrial receptivity or embryo implantation [9, 18, 19], which distinguishes them from abortifacients.

On the other hand, the Cu-IUD induces inflammatory reactions in the endometrium and may interfere with embryo implantation [14]. This extra window of action in the postfertilization phase may explain its superior efficacy for EC compared to oral LNG or UPA.

One important point to note is that all the mentioned EC methods including LNG, UPA, and Cu-IUD do not act by disrupting an already-implanted embryo and hence are not abortifacients. Hence, these methods should be used within 5 days of unprotected intercourse to ensure their effectiveness.

21.5 Contraindications and Side Effects

Both LNG and UPA have minimal contraindications. The main contraindication is known hypersensitivity to the drug. Cu-IUDs share the same contraindications as their use for regular contraception, such as active pelvic infection or uterine lesions that distort the cavity.

The most common side effects of EC drugs include headache, dysmenorrhea, and nausea. UPA may prolong the menstrual cycle by 1–2 days, whereas LNG may shorten it [2, 3, 5], but alterations in the next menstruation may vary among individual users. Neither method significantly affects the volume or duration of menstrual bleeding. Overall, the side effect profiles of LNG and UPA are similar, making both options generally well-tolerated.

21.6 Effectiveness and Repeat Use

The effectiveness of EC methods is difficult to quantify precisely due to ethical constraints on placebo-controlled trials. However, clinical studies and observational data indicate that UPA is generally more effective than LNG, and the Cu-IUD is the most effective overall [26]. The likelihood of pregnancy after unprotected intercourse depends on the timing within the menstrual cycle, with the highest risk occurring during the fertile window—the 5 days leading up to and including the day of ovulation.

EC methods can be used repeatedly as needed, but frequent use within a single menstrual cycle can lead to irregular bleeding patterns. If vomiting occurs within 3 h of taking an EC drug, a repeat dose is necessary. It is important to inform women that EC does not provide ongoing protection and that additional unprotected intercourse after taking EC can still result in pregnancy.

A Cochrane review reported that the risk of pregnancy is increased threefold among women who have further unprotected sex in the same menstrual cycle after using EC [26]. An effective method of contraception should therefore be started as soon as possible—known as "quick starting."

All hormonal methods of contraception can be started immediately after LNG. However, given that UPA is a progesterone receptor modulator, starting a progestogen-containing contraception at this time has been shown to affect the ability of UPA to delay ovulation [27]. It is, therefore, recommended to start an ongoing hormonal contraception, if desired, at least 5 days after UPA to avoid this risk.

Increasingly across Europe and many other parts of the world, women access EC directly from a pharmacist. A UK trial (Bridge-it trial) explored pharmacists providing a 3-month supply of the desogestrel progestogen-only pill to women as bridging contraception at the same time as LNG EC [28]. The rationale for the study was that this would give women 3 months of effective temporary contraception during which time they could get access to their preferred ongoing method with their usual contraception provider. The study reported that 4 months later the use of effective contraception was 20% greater among women receiving the progestogen-only pill intervention than controls receiving EC only ($P = 0.011$). The authors concluded that provision of a bridging supply of progestogen-only pill with EC from a pharmacist could offer the potential to prevent more unintended pregnancies for women after EC.

21.7 Impact on Pregnancy and Breastfeeding

EC drugs do not harm an existing pregnancy. Studies have shown that LNG does not affect pregnancy outcomes or harm children born after its use [29]. Although similar data for UPA is limited, clinical observations suggest it does not negatively impact pregnancy either. EC drugs can also be used during breastfeeding, making them a safe option for lactating women. As UPA is excreted in breast milk, breastfeeding is not recommended within 1 week of UPA intake, during which time breast milk can be expressed and discarded [30]. However, based on data on mifepristone use showing no harmful levels in breast milk and no negative impact on newborns, national guidelines allow breastfeeding following the use of UPA [31].

21.8 Drug Interactions

LNG and UPA are metabolized via the cytochrome P450 enzyme system, meaning that enzyme-inducing drugs (such as certain anticonvulsants and antibiotics) can reduce their effectiveness. UPA's effectiveness can also be affected by drugs that raise gastric pH. UPA binds to the progesterone receptor. Consequently, if a woman has taken a progestogen-containing product, UPA should not be used for the next 7 days based on a theoretical risk to reduce the receptor binding and thus effect of UPA. Conversely, after UPA use, progestogen-containing methods should not be started for the next 5 days based on the observation that this would attenuate the ability of UPA to delay ovulation and render it less effective as EC. This makes LNG a preferable option in cases where immediate initiation of hormonal contraception is required or in case of missed contraceptive pills.

21.9 Counseling and Education

Effective use of EC requires proper counseling and education. Women should be informed about the different options available, their mechanisms of action, side effects, and the appropriate timing for use. It is crucial to dispel myths and misconceptions about EC, such as the incorrect belief that EC pills can terminate an existing pregnancy or that they are effective beyond the specified window of use.

Healthcare providers should also educate women on the effectiveness of contraceptive methods. Usually, EC methods are seen as a backup option rather than a primary method of contraception. In case of the use of less effective contraceptive methods, EC pills could be kept at home to allow rapid use when needed. Additionally, discussions about the availability of the Cu-IUD and the need for a trained provider for its insertion should be included in counseling sessions.

21.10 Newer Potential Options

21.10.1 Levonorgestrel-Releasing Intrauterine Device

It has been postulated that the levonorgestrel IUD (LNG-IUD) might also be an effective IUD for EC given the effects of LNG on sperm transport, capacitation, the acrosome reaction, and fallopian tube transport. If effective, then this would increase the range of options available to women seeking EC and may be acceptable to those wishing to use LNG-IUD as an ongoing method of regular contraception. A Cochrane review examined the evidence from one randomized controlled study of women comparing the 52 mg LNG-IUD (n = 317) to the Cu-IUD (n = 321) for EC. The trial reported low pregnancy rates in both arms with only one pregnancy in the LNG-IUD arm and none in the CU-IUD [32]. The Cochrane review concluded that this did not provide definitive evidence on the effectiveness of LNG-IUD for EC and that more comparative studies are needed to see if the LNG-IUD is as effective as the Cu-IUD for EC [33].

Various prostaglandins play important roles in a number of reproductive processes including ovulation, gamete function, fertilization, and implantation. Cyclooxygenase inhibitors such as meloxicam and celecoxib that block prostaglandin synthesis have been explored for their effects on ovulation, either used alone or in combination with LNG or UPA [34, 35]. A recent randomized placebo-controlled trial demonstrated that coadministration of LNG 1.5 mg and piroxicam 40 mg resulted in significantly higher percentage of pregnancies prevented and lower pregnancy rate (0.2% versus 1.7%) compared with LNG 1.5 mg alone [36]. This is the first proof-of-concept study suggesting potential roles of a combination of a cyclooxygenase inhibitor and the current oral EC agents to achieve improved efficacy in pregnancy prevention.

21.11 Conclusion

Emergency contraception is a critical tool for preventing unintended pregnancies after unprotected intercourse. Among the available methods, the Cu-IUD is the most effective, while oral EC may be more convenient and allows over-the-counter provision and self-management. Understanding the mechanisms, effectiveness, and potential interactions of these methods is crucial for their optimal use and for advising patients appropriately. Ongoing studies will explore improved counseling models for start of regular contraceptive methods after the use of EC pills as well as EC regimens with improved efficacy. Development of an on-demand use of repeated doses of oral EC is also on the research agenda. Continued education and access to EC are essential components of reproductive healthcare, empowering women to make informed choices of birth control methods.

Declarations

Competing Interests The author(s) has no competing interests to declare that are relevant to the content of this manuscript.

Ethics Approval The author(s) declares that this manuscript does not include primary research with human participants.

The author(s) declares that this manuscript does not include primary studies involving animals.

References

1. Ho PC, Kwan MSW. A prospective randomized comparison of levonorgestrel with the Yuzpe regimen in post-coital contraception. Hum Reprod. 1993;8(3):389–92.
2. von Hertzen H, WHO Research Group on Post-ovulatory Methods of Fertility Regulation. Regulation randomised controlled trial of levonorgestrel versus the Yuzpe regimen of combined oral contraceptives for emergency contraception. Lancet. 1998;352:428–33.
3. von Hertzen H, Piaggio G, Ding J, Chen J, Song S, Bártfai G, Ng E, Gemzell-Danielsson K, Oyunbileg A, Wu S, Cheng W, Lüdicke F, Pretnar-Darovec A, Kirkman R, Mittal S, Khomassuridze A, Apter D, Peregoudov A, WHO Research Group on Post-ovulatory Methods of Fertility Regulation. Low dose mifepristone and two regimens of levonorgestrel for emergency contraception: a WHO multicentre randomised trial. Lancet. 2002;360(9348):1803–10.
4. Lalitkumar PG, Berger C, Gemzell-Danielsson K. Emergency contraception. Best Pract Res Clin Endocrinol Metab. 2013;27(1):91–101.
5. Glasier AF, Cameron ST, Fine PM, Logan SJ, Casale W, Van Horn J, Sogor L, Blithe DL, Scherrer B, Mathe H, Jaspart A, Ulmann A, Gainer E. Ulipristal acetate versus levonorgestrel for emergency contraception: a randomised non-inferiority trial and meta-analysis. Lancet. 2010;375(9714):555–62.
6. Gemzell-Danielsson K. Mechanism of action of emergency contraception. Contraception. 2010;82(5):404–9.
7. Envall N, Groes Kofoed N, Kopp-Kallner H. Use of effective contraception 6 months after emergency contraception with a copper intrauterine device or ulipristal acetate – a prospective observational cohort study. Acta Obstet Gynecol Scand. 2016;95(8):887–93.

8. Hapangama D, Glasier AF, Baird DT. The effects of peri-ovulatory administration of levonorgestrel on the menstrual cycle. Contraception. 2001;63(3):123–9.
9. Gemzell-Danielsson K, Marions L. Mechanisms of action of mifepristone and levonorgestrel when used for emergency contraception. Hum Reprod Update. 2004;10(4):341–8.
10. Brache V, Cochon L, Jesam C, Maldonado R, Salvatierra AM, Levy DP, Gainer E, Croxatto HB. Immediate pre-ovulatory administration of 30 mg ulipristal acetate significantly delays follicular rupture. Hum Reprod. 2010;25(9):2256–63.
11. Yeung WSB, Chiu PCN, Wang CH, Yao YQ, Ho PC. The effects of levonorgestrel on various sperm functions. Contraception. 2002;66(6):453–7.
12. Hermanny A, Bahamondes MV, Fazano F, Marchi NM, Ortiz ME, Genghini MHRR, Croxatto HB, Bahamondes L. In vitro assessment of some sperm function following exposure to levonorgestrel in human fallopian tubes. Reprod Biol Endocrinol. 2012;10:8.
13. Ko JK, Huang VW, Li RH, Yeung WS, Ho PC, Chiu PC. An in vitro study of the effect of mifepristone and ulipristal acetate on human sperm functions. Andrology. 2014;2(6):868–71. https://doi.org/10.1111/j.2047-2927.2014.00261.x
14. Ortiz ME, Croxatto HB. Copper-T intrauterine device and levonorgestrel intrauterine system: biological bases of their mechanism of action. Contraception. 2007;75(6 Suppl):S16–30.
15. Wanggren K, Stavreus-Evers A, Olsson C, Andersson E, Gemzell-Danielsson K. Regulation of muscular contraceptions in the human Fallopian tube through prostaglandins and progestogens. Hum Reprod. 2008;23(10):2359–68.
16. Li HWR, Liao SB, Yeung WSB, Wai Sum O, Ho PC. Mifepristone, but not levonorgestrel, has suppressive effect on tubal function at pharmacological dose which may contribute to emergency contraceptive action. Paper presented at: 47th Annual Meeting of the Society for the Study of Reproduction, Grand Rapids, MI, USA, 19–23 July 2014.
17. Lindblom B, Hamberger L. Copper and contractility of the human fallopian tube. Am J Obstet Gynecol. 1981;141(4):398–402.
18. Li HWR, Resche-Rigon M, Bagchi IC, Gemzell-Danielsson K, Glasier A. Does ulipristal acetate emergency contraception (ella®) interfere with implantation? Contraception. 2019;100(5):386–90.
19. Endler M, Li R, Gemzell Danielsson K. Effect of levonorgestrel emergency contraception on implantation and fertility: a review. Contraception. 2022;109:8–18.
20. Lalitkumar PG, Lalitkumar S, Meng CX, Stavreus-Evers A, Hambiliki F, Bentin-Ley U, Gemzell-Danielsson K. Mifepristone, but not levonorgestrel, inhibits human blastocyst attachment to an in vitro endometrial three-dimensional cell culture model. Hum Reprod. 2007;22(11):3031–7.
21. Berger C, Boggavarapu NR, Menezes J, Lalitkumar PGL, Gemzell-Danielsson K. Effects of ulipristal acetate on human embryo attachment and endometrial cell gene expression in an in vitro co-culture system. Hum Reprod. 2015;30:800–11.
22. Li HWR, Li YX, Li TT, Fan H, Ng EHY, Yeung WSB, Ho PC, Lee KF. Effect of ulipristal acetate and mifepristone at emergency contraception dose on the embryo-endometrial attachment using an in vitro human trophoblastic spheroid and endometrial cell co-culture model. Hum Reprod. 2017;32(12):2414–22.
23. Novikova N, Weisberg E, Stanczyk FZ, Croxatto HB, Fraser IS. Effectiveness of levonorgestrel emergency contraception given before or after ovulation – a pilot study. Contraception. 2007;75(2):112–8.
24. Noe G, Croxatto HB, Salvatierra AM, Reyes V, Villarroel C, Munoz C, Morales G, Retamales A. Contraceptive efficacy of emergency contraception with levonorgestrel given before or after ovulation. Contraception. 2010;81(5):414–20.
25. Li HWR, Lo SST, Ng EHY, Ho PC. Efficacy of ulipristal acetate for emergency contraception and its effect on the subsequent bleeding pattern when administered before or after ovulation. Hum Reprod. 2016;31(6):1200–7.
26. Shen J, Che Y, Showell E, Chen K, Cheng L. Interventions for emergency contraception. Cochrane Database Syst Rev. 2019;1(1):CD001324.

27. Brache V, Cochon L, Duijkers IJ, Levy DP, Kapp N, Monteil C, Abitbol JL, Klipping C. A prospective, randomized, pharmacodynamic study of quick-starting a desogestrel progestin-only pill following ulipristal acetate for emergency contraception. Hum Reprod. 2015;30(12):2785–93.
28. Cameron ST, Glasier A, McDaid L, Radley A, Baraitser P, Stephenson J, Gilson R, Battison C, Cowle K, Forrest M, Goulao B, Johnstone A, Morelli A, Patterson S, McDonald A, Vadiveloo T, Norrie J. Use of effective contraception following provision of the progestogen-only pill for women presenting to community pharmacies for emergency contraception (Bridge-It): a pragmatic cluster-randomised crossover trial. Lancet. 2020;396(10262):1585–94.
29. Meng CX, Gemzell-Danielsson K, Stephansson O, Kang JZ, Chen QF, Cheng LN. Emergency contraceptive use among 5677 abortion-seeking women in Shanghai, China. Hum Reprod. 2009;24(7):1612–8.
30. World Health Organization. Medical eligibility criteria for contraceptive use. 5th ed. WHO; 2015. http://apps.who.int.
31. Sääv I, Fiala C, Hämäläinen JM, Heikinheimo O, Gemzell-Danielsson K. Medical abortion in lactating women—low levels of mifepristone in breast milk. Acta Obstet Gynecol Scand. 2010;89(5):618–22.
32. Turok DK, Gero A, Simmons RG, Kaiser JE, Stoddard GJ, Sexsmith CD, Gawron LM, Sanders JN. Levonorgestrel vs copper intrauterine devices for emergency contraception. N Engl J Med. 2021;384(4):335–44.
33. Ramanadhan S, Goldstuck N, Henderson JT, Che Y, Cleland K, Dodge LE, Edelman A. Progestin intrauterine devices versus copper intrauterine devices for emergency contraception. Cochrane Database Syst Rev. 2023;2(2):CD013744.
34. Weiss EA, Gandhi M. Preferential cyclooxygenase 2 inhibitors as a nonhormonal method of emergency contraception: a look at the evidence. J Pharm Pract. 2016;29(2):160–4.
35. Cahill EP, Lerma K, Shaw KA, Blumenthal PD. Potential candidate for oral pericoital contraception: evaluating ulipristal acetate plus cyclo-oxygenase-2 inhibitor for ovulation disruption. BMJ Sex Reprod Health. 2022;48(3):217–21.
36. Li RHW, Lo SST, Gemzell-Danielsson K, Fong CHY, Ho PC, Ng EHY. Oral emergency contraception with levonorgestrel plus piroxicam: a randomised double-blind placebo-controlled trial. Lancet. 2023;402(10405):851–8.

Chapter 22
Reversible Male Contraception: New Technologies and Perspectives

Regine Sitruk-Ware

22.1 Introduction

The global unintended pregnancy rate is about 50% of all pregnancies worldwide [1, 2], and it is even higher among adolescents in the United States [3]. At present, the responsibility of preventing unintended pregnancies falls almost entirely on women. Contraceptive choices for men are limited and lacking, with condoms and withdrawal both subject to high failure rates, and vasectomy, which is meant to be a permanent method and therefore not easily or reliably reversible. The limited options leave men with insufficient choices to support their own reproductive health needs, while also preventing them from taking a more active role in contraceptive decision-making within relationships.

Even though there is a glaring unmet need for more methods of male contraception, support and funding for research and development has been significantly lacking. Only not-for-profit or government organizations conducted research in male contraception, and this field has struggled with little funding over the past decades.

22.2 Acceptability and Demand for Male Contraception

Would men use contraceptives if more choices were available? Multinational survey data suggest that between 29% and 71% of men across continents would use a male hormonal contraceptive [4] (Fig. 22.1). More recent market research from the Male

R. Sitruk-Ware (✉)
Center for Biomedical Research. Population Council, New York, NY, USA
e-mail: regine@popcouncil.org

A. R. Genazzani et al. (eds.), *Ethical, Efficacy and Safety Issues in Contraception*, Reproductive Medicine for Clinicians 4,
https://doi.org/10.1007/978-3-032-07322-8_22

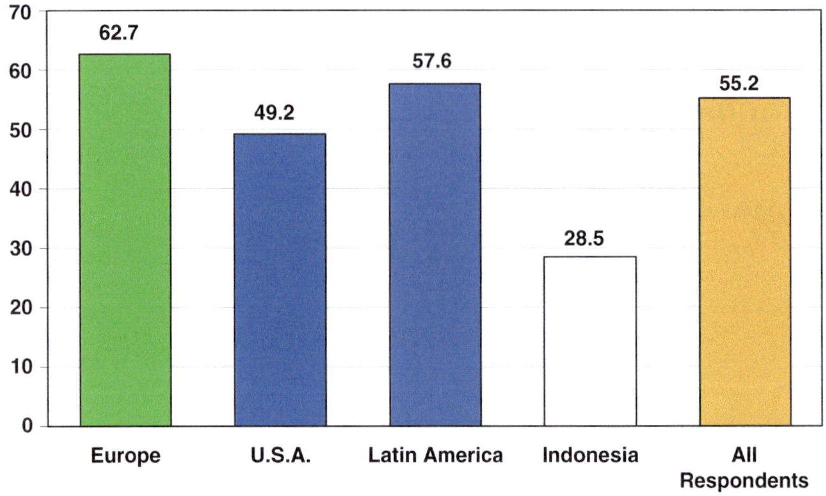

Fig. 22.1 Adapted from Heineman et al. 2005. In a Multinational Survey on Attitudes, Desires, and Acceptability of Male Fertility Control, 9345 men were interviewed in four continents. The percentage of men willing to use a male method if available is represented in this figure

Contraceptive Initiative indicates that 82% of US men ages 18–44 whose partners experienced an unplanned pregnancy in the past are interested in new methods of male contraception, with the majority saying they want to share contraceptive responsibility with their partner [5]. Importantly, another international study found that only 2% of women surveyed said they would not trust their partners to use a male hormonal contraception (MHC) [6]. These results were encouraging and indicated strong interest for male methods among both men and women.

Another recent multinational survey conducted by *Desireline*, and funded by the Bill & Melinda Gates Foundation, involved 19,000 adult men from eight different countries: Nigeria, Kenya, Cote d'Ivoire, Democratic Republic of the Congo, Vietnam, Bangladesh, India, and the United States [7]. That survey showed that men and their partners are strongly in favor of new forms of male contraception and that women trust their partners to use them responsibly. The study found that 78%–98% of men, depending on the country, would take a male contraceptive pill if available. The demand was high among men regardless of their relationship status. An important finding was that about half of the eligible men in the United States indicated they would try novel male contraceptives within 12 months of market introduction following the Dobbs decision that resulted in an abortion ban in several states [7]. Therefore, over the past two decades, there has been an increased interest in male contraception, and new advocacy groups as well as a few small industrial entities have emerged. However, more work is needed to substantiate these survey data with real-world experiences of men, and to educate men about contraceptive options.

22.3 Hormonal Methods of Male Contraception

Reversible MHC has been tested for around 50 years [8]. Various injections and implants have been tested in over 2,000 couples worldwide, together demonstrating reversibility [9] and around 95% effectiveness in preventing pregnancy, rates comparable to the female pill and better than condoms.

22.3.1 Mechanism of Action of Male Hormonal Contraception

MHC is based on the use of exogenously administered androgen alone or together with an antigonadotrophic agent, a gonadotrophin-releasing hormone (GnRH) analog or, usually, a progestin, to suppress secretion or action of GnRH in the hypothalamus and decrease the pituitary production of both gonadotropins, luteinizing hormone (LH) and follicle-stimulating hormone (FSH). The progestin ensures the suppression of the gonadotropins followed by a decrease in endogenous testosterone and sperm production. Hence, a supplemental androgen is required in order to maintain the normal male secondary characteristics. While many progestin and testosterone-containing products are approved by various regulatory agencies, none is approved for the indication of MHC. Most of the available progestins have long been approved and used for female contraception, and testosterone (T) formulations are widely approved for the treatment of hypogonadal men.

The pharmacological action by which the contraceptive effect is attained when using combined progestin and androgen is well known, via suppression of LH and FSH, resulting in suppression of sperm production as well as decreasing the intratesticular levels of testosterone.

The suppression of LH by the progestin or other antigonadotropin agent also reduces the intratesticular production of testosterone. Testosterone is required for maintaining the blood–testis barrier, completion of meiosis, Sertoli cell-spermatid adhesion, and spermiation [10, 11].

The suppression of FSH in addition to the deprivation of intratesticular testosterone induces marked suppression of spermatogenesis and sperm production without affecting the spermatogonial stem cells [11].

The expected efficacy of male hormonal contraception is demonstrated by the suppression of sperm concentration to very low levels (currently defined as ≤1 million/mL of ejaculate). This endpoint derives from the recommendations of the World Health Organization (WHO), demonstrating the correlation of this threshold and the prevention of pregnancy [12]. In that WHO study, no pregnancy occurred while the men were azoospermic. For men with sperm concentrations in the range of 0–3 million/mL, the pregnancy rate was 1.4 (95% CI 0.4–3.7) per 100 person-years [12]. The same threshold is now accepted and is recommended by expert groups reviewing the evidence [13, 14].

Based on published expert recommendations [13] and the WHO study [12] showing a correlation of sperm concentration with pregnancy occurrence, azoospermia or severe oligospermia such as a sperm concentration of ≤1 million/mL is proposed as a threshold to demonstrate the product's efficacy, and sufficient to allow clinical studies of pregnancy prevention in the female partner [12–14].

The suppression of the intratesticular levels of testosterone (ITT) maintains the suppression of spermatogenesis [15]. Coviello et al (2004) showed that a 6-month contraceptive treatment with exogenous T plus low-dose oral LNG resulted in a dramatic decrease in ITT by 98% as well as a 93% decrease in androgenic bioactivity. The exogenous administration of T did not increase the ITT levels and, therefore, is unable to restart sperm production [15].

It has been shown that suppression of serum LH correlates with suppression of spermatogenesis [16, 17]. In a study of combined progestin (NES) and androgen (T), in separate transdermal gels, the suppression of LH and FSH concentrations ≤ 1.0 IU/L after 4 weeks of therapy was highly associated with sperm concentrations ≤ 1 million/mL after 24 weeks of therapy [17]. Indeed, LH or FSH concentrations greater than 1 IU/L after 4 weeks of transdermal testosterone/Nestorone treatment had 97% sensitivity for predicting failure to suppress spermatogenesis after 24 weeks of treatment [18]. Thus, suppression of LH and FSH concentrations to ≤ 1.0 IU/L after 4 weeks of therapy would predict the likelihood of effectiveness of spermatogenic suppression in longer-term studies [18].

Hormonal methods must maintain relatively constant serum concentrations of androgen and progestin either from continuous release from an implant or injection, or daily administration in order to prevent rebound of sperm output and maintain the expected contraceptive efficacy.

The *Eunice Kennedy Shriver* National Institute of Child Health and Development (NICHD) and the Population Council, together with 15 centers across the globe, including sites in North and South America, Europe, and Africa, are currently finalizing a study in over 400 couples of a hormonal contraceptive gel that men apply to their shoulders once a day for about 18 months [18]. The investigators conducting this trial noted that men are interested and engaged in using these methods. The male study participants often expressed a desire to continue using the method for contraception after their time in the study ends, and their female partners are often disappointed to return to their previous methods.

The gel is applied on the skin of the shoulders and 10% of the applied dose is absorbed into the systemic circulation [19]. It delivers a very active progestin, Nestorone® (segesterone acetate) that blocks the sperm production and at the same time blocks the production of endogenous T, requiring the concomitant administration of exogenous T combined with the progestin in the same gel formulation (Fig. 22.2).

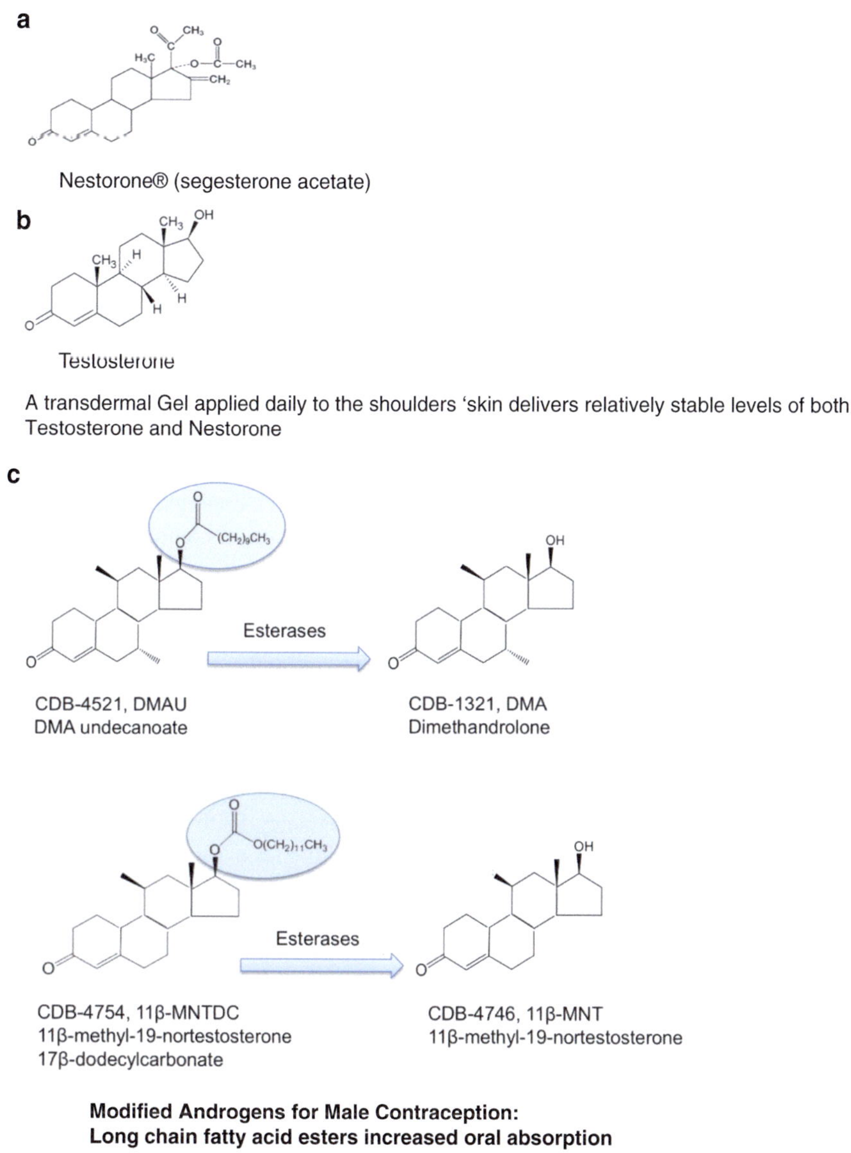

Fig. 22.2 (**a**) Nestorone® (segesterone acetate). (**b**) Testosterone. A transdermal gel applied daily to the shoulders' skin delivers relatively stable levels of both testosterone and Nestorone. (**c**) Modified androgens for male contraception: Long-chain fatty acid esters increased oral absorption

After about 12 weeks of treatment, or sometimes earlier, sperm production is fully suppressed, and the couple can use it as their sole method of contraception. When treatment is stopped, sperm production resumes to the normal range of sperm concentrations.

The transdermal gel is easy to apply but requires daily attention by the user, and precautions to avoid transfer of active ingredients to partners and children, as is currently recommended for marketed T gel products. Compliance with daily application is a major factor for ensuring efficacy, similar to other user-controlled methods in women.

22.3.2 Adverse Events Experience from Male Hormonal Contraception

A minority of men testing male hormonal contraceptives experience side effects that will be familiar to some women who have used hormonal contraceptives (e.g., weight gain, acne, and increase or decrease in libido, mood swings). Of interest, in a double-blind study of a combined progestin + androgen injection, Mommers et al. [20] demonstrated that about 10% of the placebo group also reported similar adverse events, indicating that the assessment of side effects should take in account background "noise" [20]. Nevertheless, men say they are willing to share the burden of side effects with women, and the concept of "shared risk" has been proposed to reframe the risk analysis in this situation. In this paradigm, men take on the risk of side effects from contraceptive use to protect their partners from the risk of undesirable effects of their contraceptive or unintended pregnancy. With a number of states in the United States, and countries now further limiting access to safe abortion, the risks for many women of an unplanned pregnancy have risen sharply, furthering the imperative to look at shared risk by a couple when assessing potential contraceptive side effects [21].

22.3.3 Modified Androgens (Fig. 22.2)

In order to combine both progestational and androgenic agents in one oral tablet, new molecules have been synthesized by the National Institute of Child Health and Human Development in order to develop an oral reversible male contraceptive pill [22]. Two novel androgens, dimethandrolone undecanoate (DMAU) and 11beta-methyl-19-nortestosterone-17beta-dodecylcarbonate (11β-MNTDC), both bind to androgen and progesterone receptors, and both have actions of androgens and progestins, with good oral bioavailability. These novel modified androgens are being developed as pills and injections for male contraception. Short-term 28-day completed studies confirmed that both DMAU and 11β-MNTDC were rapidly converted to their active derivatives. They suppress both LH and FSH while maintaining the male secondary sexual characteristics. Longer-term studies are underway to demonstrate suppression of spermatogenesis [23, 24].

22.4 Nonhormonal Male Contraceptives

Nonhormonal products are less advanced but show promise in laboratory testing [23, 24]. A prototype "reversible vasectomy" has been tested in India as Reversible Inhibitor of Sperm Under Guidance (RISUG), and now in the United States, named Plan A™. It entails an injected gel that forms a plug to prevent the passage of sperm. The plug can be broken down or degrades to allow for reversal. Another nonsurgical reversible vasectomy is under development with the injection of biodegradable gels (Adam™) that will ensure reversibility after 1 or 3 years of use.

Other approaches include the search for molecules that prevent sperm swimming (inhibition of sperm motility) or maturation and activation (inhibition of fertilization capacity). However, these new contraceptives are likely more than a decade away from introduction. They are described in recent reviews on the development of male nonhormonal contraception [23, 24].

One particular target is the sperm protein EPPIN, which is present on the surface of human spermatozoa. O'Rand et al. identified EP055 as a small organic compound that targets EPPIN on the surface of sperm and inhibits motility. EP055 has the potential to be a male contraceptive that would provide a reversible male method [25, 26].

Among other more advanced new methods, two approaches show promise for an oral nonhormonal contraceptive: antagonists to the retinoic acid receptor and inhibitors of adenylyl cyclase involved in sperm motility.

22.4.1 Retinoic Acid Receptor Antagonists or Synthesis Inhibitors

Mice with deletion of one of several of the retinoic acid receptors are sterile [27]. Retinoic acid receptor alpha activity is indispensable for the spermatogenic process, and, therefore, its antagonists have potential as male contraceptive agents.

Structure–activity studies have been conducted for the design of novel alpha-selective ligands [28]. A specific retinoic acid-alpha antagonist for male contraception, YCT-529, is currently being tested in a first-in-human clinical study, evaluating single ascending oral doses in healthy volunteers to establish the pharmacology and safety of this first potential oral nonhormonal male contraceptive [29] (NCT06094283).

22.4.2 *Soluble Adenylyl Cyclase*

Soluble adenylyl cyclase (sAC) is a unique enzyme required for sperm motility. Recently, a novel sAC inhibitor was shown to induce rapid, short-lived, reversible motility defects in sperm that prevented fertility in mice. Inhibition of sAC may have promise as an "on-demand" contraceptive for men [30].

22.5 Regulatory Challenges

In contrast to contraceptive products for women, there is no regulatory guidance for the development of male contraceptive products published by the Food and Drug Administration (FDA) or the European Medicines Agency (EMA).

Contraceptive products are used for prevention of a condition, unwanted pregnancy, in women. Guidelines are available for female hormonal contraception development [[31], 31]. In the absence of any guidelines for male contraceptive products, some relevant elements of the female guidance might also be applied to development programs in the male. Indeed, male contraception studies present a unique situation where the treatment is taken by the man and the clinical outcome of unwanted pregnancy is assessed in his female partner. Proper counseling for the couple about the possible risk of failure is needed, avoiding the risk of mistrust in the couple in case of failure, as well as providing information on options available in case of unscheduled pregnancy, according to the country's regulations. A surrogate marker of efficacy is measurable in the male, such as azoospermia for hormonal contraception. For nonhormonal methods acting on the sperm motility or function, the surrogate markers of efficacy remain to be defined.

22.6 Conclusions

Consensus recommendations from the research community have been published suggesting metrics for evaluating novel MHC and establishing effectiveness and safety standards, but whether these will be adopted by regulators is unknown [14]. Greater advocacy is needed to push the field forward and convince funders and the pharmaceutical industry that there is a demand for this technology.

The development of male contraceptives will not replace female contraceptives. Access to contraception and safe abortion are a fundamental human right for all people and a necessary component of public health. However, many men wish to share the burden of contraception with their partners; others want their own reproductive autonomy. Men are ready, but their contraceptive options are sparse.. Research must continue to develop effective, reversible options for men, to allow shared responsibility in the couple's fertility regulation as many men wish to take a more active role in family planning. Most research for male contraception has been funded through the public sector, but their funding capacity is limited. Given the high demand, it is time to encourage industry partners to engage in this field and speed up the development of new contraceptive choices for men.

Declarations

Competing Interests The author(s) has no competing interests to declare that are relevant to the content of this manuscript.

Ethics Approval The author(s) declares that this manuscript does not include primary research with human participants.

The author(s) declares that this manuscript does not include primary studies involving animals.

References

1. Guttmacher institute: unintended pregnancy in the United States: Fact Sheet March 2022. https://www.guttmacher.org/fact-sheet/induced-abortion-worldwide
2. Polls CB, Bradley SEK, Bankole A, Akinrinola TO, Croft TN, Singh S. Contraceptive failure rates in the developing world: an analysis of demographic and health survey data in 43 countries [Internet]. Guttmacher Institute; 2016. https://www.guttmacher.org/sites/default/files/report_pdf/contraceptive-failure-rates-in-developingworld_.pdf
3. Kantorová V, Wheldon MC, Dasgupta ANZ, Ueffing P, Castanheira HC. Contraceptive use and needs among adolescent women aged 15-19: Regional and global estimates and projections from 1990 to 2030 from a Bayesian hierarchical modelling study. PLoS One. 2021;16(3):e0247479.
4. Heinemann K, Saad F, Wiesemes M, White S, Heinemann L. Attitudes toward male fertility control: results of a multinational survey on four continents. Hum Reprod Oxf Engl. 2005 Feb;20(2):549–56.
5. Friedman M, Nickels L, Sokal D, Hamlin A King G, Levine D, Vahdat H, Shane K Interest among U.S. men for new male contraceptive options. https://www.malecontraceptive.org/uploads/1/3/1/9/131958006/mci_consumerresearchstudy.pdf. Male Contraceptive Initiative. Accessed 12 Aug 2023
6. Glasier A. Acceptability of contraception for men: a review. Contraception. 2010;82(5):453–6.
7. Kretchmer S. Desireline survey. https://www.malecontraceptive.org/uploads/1/3/1/9/131958006/reproductive_health_summit_male_ct_research_feb2023.pdf
8. Nieschlag E, Nieschlag S. Why we need more methods for male contraception. Andrology. 2023 Mar;11(3):421–4.
9. Liu PY, Swerdloff RS, Christenson PD, Handelsman DJ, Wang C. Rate, extent, and modifiers of spermatogenic recovery after hormonal male contraception: an integrated analysis. Lancet. 2006;367(9520):1412–20.
10. Smith LB, Walker WH. The regulation of spermatogenesis by androgens. Semin Cell Dev Biol. 2014;30:2–13.
11. McLachlan RI, O'Donnell L, Meachem SJ, Stanton PG, de Kretser David M, Pratis K, Robertson DM. Hormonal regulation of spermatogenesis in primates and man: insights for development of the male hormonal contraceptive. J Androl. 2002;23(2):149–62.
12. World Health Organization Task Force on the Regulation of Male Fertility. Contraceptive efficacy of testosterone-induced azoospermia and oligozoospermia in normal men. Fertil Steril. 1996;65(4):821–9.

13. Aaltonen P, Amory JK, Anderson RA, et al. 10th Summit Meeting consensus: recommendations for regulatory approval for hormonal male contraception. J Androl. 2007;28(3):362–3.
14. Wang C, Meriggiola MC, Amory JK, Barratt CLR, Behre HM, Bremner WJ, Ferlin A, Honig S, Kopa Z, Lo K, Nieschlag E, Page ST, Sandlow J, Sitruk-Ware R, Swerdloff RS, Wu FCW, Goulis DG. Practice and development of male contraception: European Academy of Andrology and American Society of Andrology guidelines. Andrology. 2023;12(7):1470–500.
15. Coviello AD, Bremner WJ, Matsumoto AM, Herbst KL, Amory JK, Anawalt BD, Yan X, Brown TR, Wright WW, Zirkin BR, Jarow JP. Intratesticular testosterone concentrations comparable with serum levels are not sufficient to maintain normal sperm production in men receiving a hormonal contraceptive regimen. J Androl. 2004;25(6):931–8.
16. Mahabadi V, Amory JK, Swerdloff RS, Bremner WJ, Page ST, Sitruk-Ware R, Christensen PD, Kumar N, Tsong YY, Blithe D, Wang C. Combined transdermal testosterone gel and the progestin nestorone suppresses serum gonadotropins in men. J Clin Endocrinol Metab. 2009;94(7):2313–20.
17. Ilani N, Roth MY, Amory JK, Swerdloff RS, Dart C, Page ST, Bremner WJ, Sitruk-Ware R, Kumar N, Blithe DL, Wang C. A new combination of testosterone and nestorone transdermal gels for male hormonal contraception. J Clin Endocrinol Metab. 2012;97(10):3476–86.
18. Amory JK, Blithe DL, Sitruk-Ware R, Swerdloff RS, Bremner WJ, Dart C, Liu PY, Thirumalai A, Nguyen BT, Anawalt BD, Lee MS, Page ST, Wang C. Design of an international male contraceptive efficacy trial using a self-administered daily transdermal gel containing testosterone and segesterone acetate (Nestorone). Contraception. 2023 Aug;124:110064.
19. Anawalt BD, Roth MY, Ceponis J, Surampudi V, Amory JK, Swerdloff RS, Liu PY, Dart C, Bremner WJ, Sitruk-Ware R, Kumar N, Blithe DL, Page ST, Wang C. Combined nestorone-testosterone gel suppresses serum gonadotropins to concentrations associated with effective hormonal contraception in men. Andrology. 2019;7(6):878–87.
20. Mommers E, Kersemaekers WM, Elliesen J, Kepers M, Apter D, Behre HM, Beynon J, Bouloux PM, Costantino A, Gerbershagen HP, Gronlund L, Heger-Mahn D, Huhtaniemi I, Koldewijn EL, Lange C, Lindenberg S, Meriggiola MC, Meuleman E, Mulders PF, Nieschlag E, Perheentupa A, Solomon A, Vaisala L, Wu FC, Zitzmann M. Male hormonal contraception: a double-blind, placebo-controlled study. J Clin Endocrinol Metab. 2008;93(7):2572–80.
21. Campelia GD, Adashi EY, Amory JK. Shared risk and shared responsibility: the ethics of male contraceptives. Andrology. 2024;12(7):1605–9. https://doi.org/10.1111/andr.13649. Epub ahead of print
22. Long JE, Lee MS, Blithe DL. Update on novel hormonal and nonhormonal male contraceptive development. J Clin Endocrinol Metab. 2021;106(6):e2381–92.
23. Yan W, Amory JK. Emerging approaches to male contraception. Andrology. 2024;115(6):1369–76. https://doi.org/10.1111/andr.13652. Epub ahead of print
24. Page ST, Amory JK. The world needs better male contraceptives: what is taking so long? FASEB J. 2022;36(12):e22658.
25. O'Rand MG, Hamil KG, Adevai T, Zelinski M. Inhibition of sperm motility in male macaques with EP055, a potential non-hormonal male contraceptive. PLoS One. 2018;13(4):e0195953.
26. Chung SS, Wolgemuth DJ. Role of retinoid signaling in the regulation of spermatogenesis. Cytogenet Genome Res. 2004;105(2-4):189–202.
27. Noman MAA, Kyzer JL, Chung SSW, Wolgemuth DJ, Georg GI. Retinoic acid receptor antagonists for male contraception: current status†. Biol Reprod. 2020;103(2):390–9.
28. A double-blind, placebo controlled, first in human study to evaluate safety, tolerability, pharmacokinetics, and pharmacodynamics of single ascending oral doses of YCT-529 https://clinicaltrials.gov/study/NCT06094283?term=NCT06094283&rank=1

29. Balbach M, Rossetti T, Ferreira J, Ghanem L, Ritagliati C, Myers RW, Huggins DJ, Steegborn C, Miranda IC, Meinke PT, Buck J, Levin LR. On-demand male contraception via acute inhibition of soluble adenylyl cyclase. Nat Commun. 2023;14(1):637.
30. Establishing effectiveness and safety for hormonal drug products intended to prevent pregnancy guidance for industry. https://www.fda.gov/regulatory-information/search-fda-guidance-documents/establishing-effectiveness-and-safety-hormonal-drug-products-intended-prevent-pregnancy-guidance
31. Clinical investigation of steroid contraceptives in women – scientific guideline. https://www.ema.europa.eu/en/clinical-investigation-steroid-contraceptives-women-scientific-guideline

Part VIII
Hormonal Contraception and Medical Benefits

Chapter 23
Uterine Bleeding and Hormonal Contraception

Cuauhtémoc Celis-González, Cecilia X. Flores Granados, and Juan Rivero Corona

23.1 Introduction

Abnormal uterine bleeding (AUB) is a highly prevalent condition, estimated to affect up to 30% of nonpregnant women of reproductive age. It significantly impacts quality of life—physically, socially, emotionally, sexually, and financially [1, 2]. It is also the leading cause of gynecological consultation among adolescents [3].

In 2007, the International Federation of Gynecology and Obstetrics (FIGO) published the first standardized program for the nomenclature and parameters of normal uterine bleeding (defined between the 5th and 95th percentiles based on large-scale epidemiological studies). This system was designed to reduce ambiguity in the assessment [4] of AUB during reproductive years.

Although AUB can be managed with certain nonhormonal medications, this chapter will focus primarily on treatment using hormonal contraceptives across different stages of a woman's life.

C. Celis-González (✉)
Latin American Federation of Obstetrics and Gynecology Societies (FLASOG), Mexico City, Mexico

C. X. Flores Granados
Department of Reproductive Biology, High-Specialty Medical Unit, Hospital of Gynecology and Obstetrics No. 3 "Dr. Víctor Manuel Espinosa de los Reyes Sánchez," National Medical Center "La Raza," Mexican Social Security Institute (IMSS), Mexico City, Mexico

J. R. Corona
Department of Gynecological Endoscopic Surgery, Hospital Juárez de México, Mexico City, Mexico

A. R. Genazzani et al. (eds.), *Ethical, Efficacy and Safety Issues in Contraception*, Reproductive Medicine for Clinicians 4,
https://doi.org/10.1007/978-3-032-07322-8_23

23.2 Definitions

23.2.1 Normal Menstrual Cycle

A cycle is considered normal when it lasts between 24 and 38 days, or more practically, 31 ± 7 days. The normal duration of menstruation is less than 8 days. Regarding cycle regularity, two age groups are defined: one includes women between 26 and 41 years old; the second group includes those aged 18–25 or 42–45. For the first group, regularity is defined by a variation of ≤7 days between the shortest and longest cycle over the last 6 months. For the second group, a variation of ≤9 days is considered normal [4, 5].

The definition of normal bleeding volume has changed. Previously, 5–80 ml was the range for normal bleeding. Recently, the National Institute for Health and Care Excellence (NICE) redefined it as *"excessive menstrual blood loss that interferes with a woman's physical, social, emotional, or occupational quality of life,"* categorizing it as heavy or abnormal bleeding (Table 23.1).

Table 23.1 Normal ranges of the menstrual cycle

Menstrual cycle	Type	Normal ranges
Frequency	Normal	24-38 days
Regularity cyclo by cycle 12 months	Regular	Variation ± 7 to 9 days
Duration	Normal	until 7 days
Volume monthly menstrual loss (ml)	Normal	5 - 80 ml Quality of life

AUB
Anything outside these limits

23.3 Abnormal Uterine Bleeding

Abnormal uterine bleeding (AUB) refers to bleeding from the uterus that deviates from the norm in terms of amount, duration, frequency, or regularity [4]. In non-pregnant, reproductive-age women, AUB is classified as either chronic or acute. Chronic AUB refers to bleeding that has been abnormal in frequency, duration, regularity, or volume for most of the past 6 months. Acute AUB refers to a heavy bleeding episode severe enough to require immediate medical intervention to minimize or prevent further blood [5] loss.

23.4 Heavy Menstrual Bleeding

Heavy menstrual bleeding (HMB) is defined as excessive menstrual blood loss that interferes with a woman's physical, social, emotional, or material quality of life. It may occur alone or along with other symptoms. HMB is one of the most common reasons for gynecological consultation, affecting approximately 30% of women globally during their reproductive years. It significantly affects daily activities, work productivity, and sexual health, and associated symptoms may also have clinical consequences on women's health [6].

23.5 Acute Uterine Bleeding

Acute uterine bleeding is defined as an episode of heavy bleeding that, in the opinion of the healthcare provider, is severe enough to warrant urgent intervention to prevent further blood loss. This may occur in the context of ongoing chronic AUB or without such a background history [7].

23.6 FIGO Classification: PALM–COEIN System

FIGO developed an effective mnemonic system to classify the potential causes of AUB in reproductive-age women. The *PALM–COEIN* system (illustrated in Fig. 23.1) classifies causes into structural and nonstructural categories.

- *PALM* (structural causes):
  - Polyp (P)
  - Adenomyosis (A)
  - Leiomyoma (L)
  - Malignancy and hyperplasia (M)
- *COEIN* (nonstructural causes):
  - Coagulopathy (C)
  - Ovulatory dysfunction (O)
  - Endometrial disorders (E)
  - Iatrogenic (I)
  - Not yet classified

Leiomyomas are further divided into those that include submucosal fibroids and those that do not affect the uterine cavity [8, 9].

It is worth noting that a more comprehensive description of ovulatory disorders has recently been published, allowing for a better understanding of these conditions.

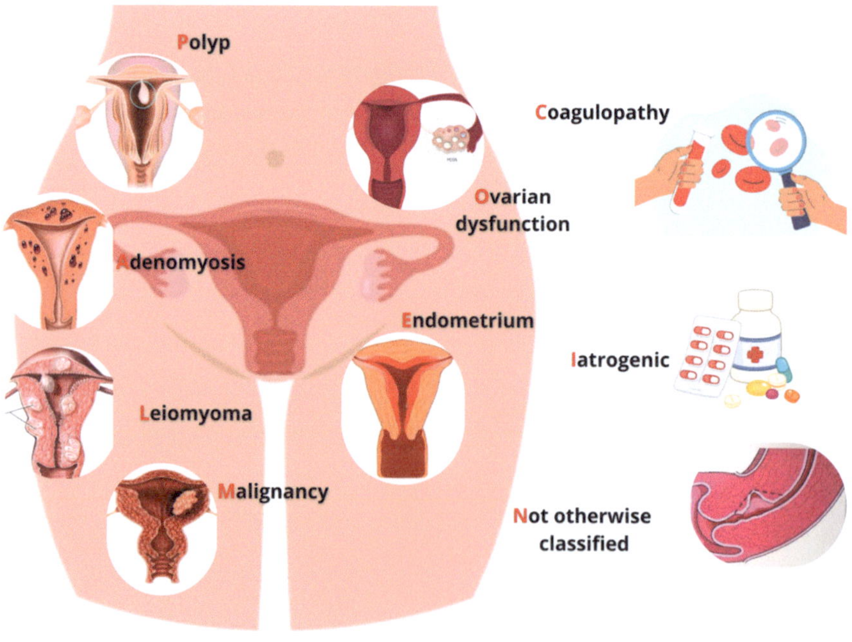

Fig. 23.1 FIGO system 2 provides a structured classification causes of AUB

In the current context, ovulatory disorders (AUB-O) encompass a variety of abnormalities in normal ovulatory function, ranging from irregular to infrequent or absent ovulation. To date, in the context of managing patients with abnormal uterine bleeding (AUB), the diagnosis of ovulatory disorders has primarily been based on a detailed menstrual history to meet the criteria established by the FIGO System 1 [10].

The new FIGO classification identifies four types of ovulatory disorders:

1. *Type I: Hypothalamic*
2. *Type II: Pituitary*
3. *Type III: Ovarian*
4. *Type IV: Polycystic ovary syndrome (PCOS)*

The acronym *HyPO-P* represents these categories where the "P" is separated from the other three categories, recognizing that it does not reside in a single anatomical location. The term "ovulatory disorder" is not synonymous with "anovulation"; instead, it refers to a spectrum from episodic to chronic [10] disorders.

The new system recognizes three basic strata once an ovulatory disorder is diagnosed. The first level involves categorization as follows: Type I: Hypothalamic; Type II: Pituitary; Type III: Ovarian; and Type IV: Polycystic ovary syndrome (PCOS). The second level requires assignment based on known or suspected anatomical knowledge [10] (Fig. 23.2).

The FIGO HyPO-P system for the classification of ovulatory disorders is presented for consideration as a global standard, designed to harmonize definitions and categories in a way that informs clinical care, facilitates the education of patients

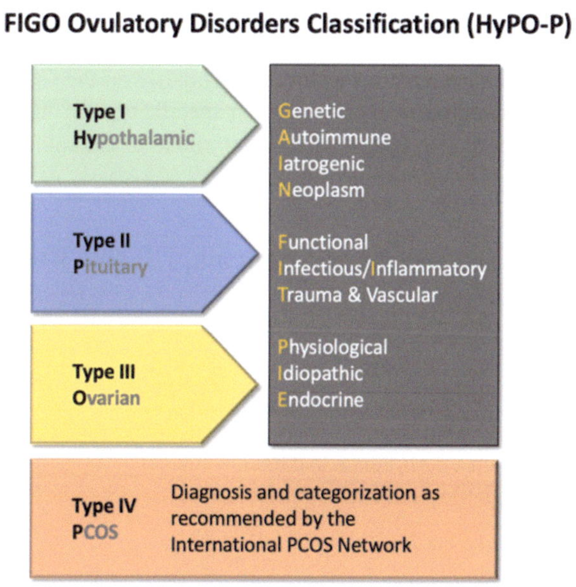

Fig. 23.2 Graphic representation of the ovulatory disorder classification system proposed by FIGO, taken from reference (10)

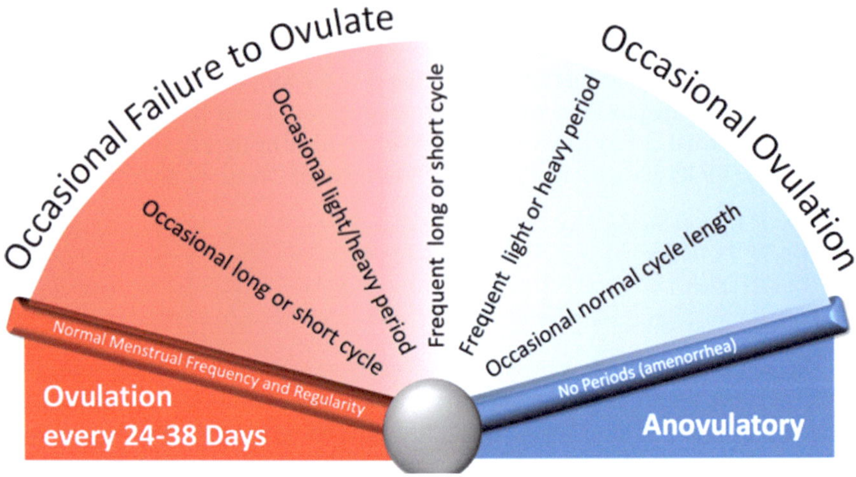

Fig. 23.3 Ovulatory disorders exist along a spectrum that ranges from occasional ovulatory failure to chronic anovulation. Taken from reference (10).

and learners, and enhances basic understanding, translational, clinical, and epidemiological research to advance our knowledge of ovulatory disorders, their diagnosis, and treatment [10] (Fig. 23.3).

In general—though not always—these disorders present with abnormalities in menstrual parameters such as frequency, regularity, duration, and volume of bleeding. In cases of chronic anovulation, amenorrhea is often present. It is evident that disorders such as luteinized unruptured follicle (LUF) and luteal phase deficiency exist along a similar spectrum with variable frequency [10]

In this chapter, we will focus primarily on the COEIN acronym from the FIGO classification, which represents a specific type of AUB in which hormonal contraceptives [11] play a more relevant role in treatment.

23.7 Diagnosis of Abnormal Uterine Bleeding

To establish a diagnosis, FIGO's two-system classification (Systems 1 and 2) can be applied by following a five-step clinical approach:

Step 1: Detailed Clinical History

Obtain a comprehensive history focusing on the menstrual pattern and perform a thorough physical exam, particularly of the reproductive system and genital area [2].

Step 2: Assess Impact on Quality of Life

The *SAMANTA questionnaire* consists of six user-friendly questions that evaluate the impact of heavy bleeding on quality of life. It has shown a sensitivity of 86.7% and specificity of 89.5% [12].

Questions

1. Do you bleed for more than 7 days each month?
2. Do you experience 3 or more days of heavy bleeding per cycle?
3. Does your menstrual flow bother you due to its heaviness?
4. During your heaviest days, do you stain your clothes at night or would you if you didn't use double protection/change clothes?
5. Are you worried about staining chairs or furniture during these days?
6. Do you avoid activities, travel, or leisure plans during heavy days because you need to change pads or tampons frequently?

- Yes to questions 1 or 3 = 3 points each
- Yes to questions 2, 4, 5, or 6 = 1 point each
- No = 0 points
- A score of 3 or more indicates HMB [12]

Step 3: Estimate Blood Loss

There are direct, indirect, or subjective methods to calculate blood loss volume during menstruation. While history-taking can help, patients often over- or underestimate blood loss. Direct methods are more accurate but not practical for routine use. Patients can be advised to track bleeding using a calendar and count of menstrual products used in order to identify AUB [6].

Step 4: Laboratory Tests

A complete blood count (CBC) is recommended, along with tests for coagulation disorders in women who have experienced heavy menstruation since menarche, or who have a personal or family history suggestive of bleeding disorders. Although the hematin/alkaline method is a direct technique with high capacity for quantifying blood loss, it should not be used routinely in all suspected cases of uterine hemorrhage. An immunological pregnancy test should be performed in all sexually active women presenting with abnormal uterine bleeding. Thyroid function tests should only be ordered when there are clinical findings suggestive of thyroid disease.

An androgen profile (total testosterone, free testosterone, androstenedione, DHEA, and DHEA-S) should be requested when there is clinical suspicion of an androgen-producing tumor. Additionally, levels of FSH, LH, and prolactin should be measured in patients with suspected chronic anovulation as the cause of AUB. Coagulation studies are especially recommended in patients with uterine bleeding that began at menarche and is difficult to control, or in those with a family history of bleeding disorders. Von Willebrand disease should be primarily ruled out [13].

Step 5: Imaging and Diagnostic Procedures

Ultrasound is the first-choice diagnostic method for patients with AUB to identify structural abnormalities. Imaging and histopathological studies are indicated when there is evidence or suspicion of anatomical changes. *Hysteroscopy* should be performed when ultrasound results are inconclusive or unsatisfactory. AUB due to

Table 23.2 Structured approach for assessing the patient presenting with AUB. Adapted from reference [2]

History	Examination
Menstrual Menarche Last menstrual period Frequency, regularity, duration, and volume of menstruation Irregular and postcoital bleeding *Anemia symptoms* *Reproductive/sexual history* Previous pregnancies and mode of delivery Desire of future fertility Subfertility Current contraceptive needs History of STIs History of defamation *Related symptoms* Pain Vaginal discharge Bladder/bowel symptoms *Systemic symptoms* Weight changes Signs of coagulopathy Hepatic, renal, thyroid, pituitary, or adrenal diseases Medications Anticoagulants, tamoxifen, hormones, menopause hormone therapy (MHT), dopamine agonists *Family history: Venous thromboembolism (VTE), malignancies* *Lifestyle: Smoking and occupation*	*Vital signs, BP, BMI* Pallor Signs of systemic disease Thyroid disorder Cushing's, bruising, hirsutism Palpable pelvic mass Speculum and bimanual Pap smear, Chlamydia test, endometrial biopsy if indicated *Investigation* Hemoglobin, possibly ferritin TSH, gonadotropins, prolactin, hCG, coagulation studies (as indicated) Imaging: ultrasound, MRI (if needed), hysteroscopy (if needed)

nonstructural causes is a *diagnosis of exclusion*, so the clinician must first rule out any organic or endocrine pathology [5, 14].

Table 23.2 shows the structured approach to evaluate a patient with abnormal uterine bleeding.

23.8 Treatment Options

The main objective is to reduce bleeding episodes and menstrual volume to improve quality of life. Treatment is tailored based on the underlying cause (once pregnancy, infection, structural, or thyroid issues are ruled out) and patient preferences, prior hormone use, cost, access, and medical history. Hormonal or no-hormonal treatment of acute or chronic bleeding is available. For patients who wish monthly regular predictable menstrual cycles, cyclic combined hormonal contraceptives (CHCs) are ideal. For fewer periods in general, progestin-only methods or continuous [15] CHC regimens are available.

23.9 Hormonal Contraceptive Treatment

Hormonal contraceptives are recommended for AUB because of the effects of estrogen and progestin on regulating endocrine function, modifying inflammatory mediators in the endometrium, and providing hemostatic control of bleeding. AUB often involves superficial vascular fragility due to altered local [16] angiogenic factors in the endometrium.

23.10 Combined Hormonal Contraceptives

CHCs are especially useful for AUB without focal anatomical lesions (e.g., no submucosal fibroids, polyps, or endometrial cancer). Their primary mechanisms include the following:

- *Estrogen* suppresses FSH secretion, halting follicular development, stabilizing the endometrium, and regulating the cycle.
- *Progestin* inhibits the LH surge, preventing ovulation and reducing endometrial proliferation.

Oral CHC users report a *35%–69% reduction in bleeding*. CHCs reduce menstrual volume and duration more effectively than luteal-phase progestin, NSAIDs, or tranexamic acid (Table 23.3) [16, 17] but are less effective than the levonorgestrel-releasing intrauterine system (LNG-IUS).

Extended or continuous CHC regimens are particularly beneficial, decreasing both bleeding episodes and overall menstrual blood loss. First-line options should include *monophasic pills with 30–50 μg of ethinyl estradiol and second-generation progestin*, as they more reliably stabilize the endometrium than lower-dose formulations [16, 17, 18].

Extended regimens (e.g., dienogest/estradiol valerate) are preferred over cyclic regimens for reducing VEGF and COX-2 expression in the endometrium, leading to better bleeding control. In the case of progestins, the cyclic regime is considered, it causes amenorrhea in 34–35% of users with a 25–64% bleeding reduction; it depends on the etiology [17, 18].

Table 23.3 Medical management options for abnormal uterine bleeding. Adapted from references [16, 17]

Medical management options for abnormal uterine bleeding	
Combined contraceptives: oral, transdermal—cyclic or noncyclic	
Oral combined	10–50 µg ethinyl E2 tablets combined. Daily
Combined patch	150 µg norelgestromin/35 µg ethinyl E2/d (transdermal). Weekly
Combined ring	0.12 mg etonogestrel/15 µg ethinyl E2/ d (vaginal). Monthly
Progestin-only therapies: *Without ovulatory dysfunction*, take 1 tablet daily starting on day 5 of the cycle for 21 days. *In case of ovulatory dysfunction*, take 1 tablet daily for 2 weeks every 4 weeks.	
Progestin-only contraceptive pills	35 µg norethindrone daily 5–15 mg norethindrone acetate for 21 days
Levonorgestrel-releasing intrauterine device	52-mg (20-µg-per-day) intrauterine device formulations (3 and 5 years, studies beginning to demonstrate that, for highest dose formulations, use may be effective for up to 7 years
Implant	68 mg etonorgestrel SC every 3 years
Medroxyprogesterone acetate (MPA)	Depo MPA 150 mg intramuscularly every 12 weeks Depo-Sub Q Provera 104 mg sq every 12 weeks Oral MPA 2.5–10 mg 12–14 d/mo
Megestrol acetate oral	20–40 mg 12–14 d/mo
Norethindrone acetate oral	2.5–5.0 mg 12–14 d/mo
Micronized progesterone	Oral 200–400 mg 12–14 d/mo

23.11 Progestin-Only Treatments

These are ideal for:

- Women who cannot tolerate estrogen
- Those with contraindications to estrogen (e.g., history of thrombosis or bleeding disorders) [19]

Mechanism Induces endometrial atrophy.

- *50% of women with irregular cycles* achieve menstrual regulation with progestin use for 12–14 days per cycle
- *Luteal-phase progestin alone* is not very effective for treating heavy and regular [20] bleeding

Administration Options

- *Luteal phase*: 10–14 days per cycle
- *Extended regimen*: 21 days per cycle

  Extended regimens are more effective at reducing bleeding volume, though not as effective as the 52 mg LNG-IUS [21].

23.12 Levonorgestrel-Releasing Intrauterine System

In the absence of significant structural pathology, the 52 mg LNG-IUS is highly effective. It releases 20 μg of levonorgestrel per day directly into the endometrium, causing atrophy and reducing vascular density.

- *Contraceptive effect* is approved for up to 8 years [22]
- *Bleeding control* is well documented for at least 5 years
- *Menstrual blood loss reduction*:
    - 86% at 3 months
    - 97% at 12 months [23]

23.13 Medical Management Options for AUB

23.13.1 Abnormal Uterine Bleeding at Different Life Stages

Approximately 10%–32% of women report experiencing heavy menstrual bleeding (HMB) at some point during their reproductive years; however, the prevalence varies depending on the region, population, age, parity, and study design.

23.14 Adolescence

- *Most common cause*: Ovulatory dysfunction due to the immaturity of the hypothalamic–pituitary–ovarian (HPO) [10] axis according to FIGO and PALM-COEIN.
- *Other causes*:
    - Coagulopathies (e.g., von Willebrand disease)
    - Platelet function disorders
    - Thrombocytopenia
    - Coagulation factor deficiencies

  Note: Structural causes of AUB are extremely rare in adolescents [13].

23.14.1 Treatment

- *Moderate AUB and active bleeding*: First-line treatment is *monophasic combined oral contraceptives (COCs)* with at least 30 μg ethinyl estradiol.
    - *Initial regimen*: 1 pill every 8 h until bleeding stops (usually within 48 h)
    - Then: 1 pill every 12 h for 2 days

  - Maintenance: 1 pill daily for at least 21 days
  - A 7-day break can be taken after the treatment course

- *Severe AUB* with symptomatic anemia or hemoglobin (Hb) < 7 g/dL:

  - Hospitalization required
  - COC regimen: 1 pill every 6 h until bleeding stops → 1 every 8 h for 3 days → 1 every 12 h for 3 more days → then 1 daily until Hb normalizes

- *If estrogen is contraindicated*: Progestin-only regimens can be used.
- *Iron supplements* and a high-iron diet are recommended.

  Note: Surgical intervention is reserved for life-threatening bleeding [24] only.

23.14.2 Maintenance Options

- CHCs, oral/injectable progestins, and LNG-IUS 52 mg [25]
- Etonorgestrel implants are not first-line due to frequent intermenstrual bleeding
- LNG-IUS is a good option, especially long-acting, for those who have difficulty with daily/weekly dosing

Currently, data on the use of intrauterine systems in women with bleeding disorders exist only for the 52 mg LNG-IUS, not for lower-dose devices. It has been shown to reduce heavy menstrual bleeding (HMB) in all women and is an effective treatment compared to conventional medical and surgical therapies [25].

23.15 Reproductive Age

According to *NICE* guidelines, medical management is suitable for:

- Women without identifiable pathology
- Fibroids < 3 cm not distorting the uterine cavity
- Suspected or confirmed adenomyosis [26]

23.15.1 Common Causes of Ovulatory Dysfunction in Patients Between 19 and 39 Years Old

- Polycystic ovary syndrome (PCOS)
- Obesity
- Endometrial hyperplasia or malignancy (in at-risk patients)

Table 23.4 Medications used in the treatment of AUB due to ovulatory dysfunction in this age group. Adapted from reference [17]

Condition	First-line treatments
1. Acute abnormal uterine bleeding	Parenteral estrogens Multidose of oral progestins
2. Heavy menstrual bleeding	Low-dose cyclic or continuous oral hormonal contraceptives at low dose Progestins including LNG-IUS Weight loss

23.15.2 *Treatment Summary for This Age Group*

Table 23.4 lists the medications used in the treatment of AUB due to ovulatory dysfunction in this age group.

23.16 Transition to Menopause

- AUB is common due to frequent *anovulatory cycles*
- Characterized by prolonged unopposed estrogen exposure → risk of *endometrial hyperplasia* [10]

23.16.1 *Special Note: "Luteal Out-of-Phase" (LOOP) Events*

- FSH spikes recruit a second follicle during the luteal phase → elevated estradiol levels → irregular cycles

23.16.2 *Management*

- *Transvaginal ultrasound (TVUS)*: Key tool to assess the endometrium
- *Endometrial thickness* helps predict bleeding risk
- In long cycles or amenorrhea: *10–14 day progestin course* [27] can prevent heavy bleeding

23.17 Menopause

- Any *postmenopausal bleeding must be investigated*
- *TVUS* is the first-line test:
  - *<4 mm endometrial thickness* → very low risk of endometrial disease → biopsy not recommended [28]
  - *≥5 mm thickness* → consider hysteroscopy and biopsy. Sensitivity to detect endometrial pathology is 92% and cancer sensitivity is 96%
  - Hysteroscopy is the gold standard due to visual and biopsy capability

23.17.1 Treatment Options

Appropriate medical treatment may include the 52 mg levonorgestrel-releasing intrauterine system (LNG-IUS), the use of combined hormonal contraceptives, injectable progestogens, extended-phase oral progestogens, tranexamic acid, danazol, and gonadotropin-releasing hormone (GnRH) agonists and antagonists (typically prescribed with add-back therapy). Table 23.5 provides an estimate of their efficacy and benefits [29].

23.17.2 Other Notes

- Contraindication and risks of each method should be taken into consideration. Age is an important factor that contributes to risk of venous thromboembolism since women aged 45–49 years have a four times higher baseline risk for VTE than women aged 15–19 years [29].
- Tailor treatment based on etiology: atrophy, hyperplasia, polyps, endometrial cancer, or HRT use.
- Vaginal estrogen (creams, rings, tablets) for genitourinary syndrome of menopause.
- Endometrial hyperplasia without atypia: cyclic or continuous progestin therapy for 3–6 months.
- With atypia: hysterectomy ± salpingo-oophorectomy [30] is recommended.

Table 23.5 Estimation of efficacy and benefits the medical treatment. From reference [29]

Treatment	Regimen	Bleeding reduction	Contraceptive effect
CHCs	Cyclic or continuous	20–50%	Yes
LNG-IUS 52 mg	Continuous	70–97%	Yes
Oral cyclic progestins	21-day cycles	87%	No
Injectable progestins (MPA 150 mg)	Every 12 weeks	60%	Yes

Declarations

Competing Interests The author(s) has no competing interests to declare that are relevant to the content of this manuscript.

Ethics Approval The author(s) declares that this manuscript does not include primary research with human participants.

The author(s) declares that this manuscript does not include primary studies involving animals.

References

1. Bradley LD, et al. The medical management of abnormal uterine bleeding in reproductive-aged women. Am J Obstet Gynecol. 2016;214(1):31–44. https://doi.org/10.1016/j.ajog.2015.07.044.
2. Whitaker L, Critchley HOD. Abnormal uterine bleeding. Best Pract Res Clin Obstet Gynaecol. 2016;34:54–65. https://doi.org/10.1016/j.bpobgyn.2015.11.012.
3. Ramalho I, Leite H, Águas F. Abnormal uterine bleeding in adolescents: a multidisciplinary approach. Acta Med Port. 2021;34(4):291–7. https://doi.org/10.20344/amp.12829.
4. Fraser IS, Critchley HOD, Munro MG, Broder M. A process designed to lead to international agreement on terminologies and definitions to describe abnormalities of menstrual bleeding. Fertil Steril. 2007;87:466–76.
5. Munro MG, Critchley HOD, Fraser IS. The two FIGO systems for normal and abnormal uterine bleeding symptoms and classification of causes of abnormal uterine bleeding in the reproductive years: 2018 revisions. Int J Gynecol Obstet. 2018;143(Suppl 2):393–408. https://doi.org/10.1002/ijgo.12666.
6. Vannuccini S, Jain V, Critchley H, Petraglia F. From menarche to menopause, heavy menstrual bleeding is the underrated compass in reproductive health. Fertil Steril. 2022;118(4):625–36. https://doi.org/10.1016/j.fertnstert.2022.07.021.
7. Munro MG, Critchley HO, Fraser I, I.S., for the FIGO Menstrual Disorders Working Group. The FIGO classification of causes of abnormal uterine bleeding in the reproductive years. Fertil Steril. 2011;95(7):2204–8.
8. Munro MG, Critchley HO, Broder MS, Fraser IS, FIGO Working Group on Menstrual Disorders. FIGO classification system (PALM-COEIN) for causes of abnormal uterine bleeding in nongravid women of reproductive age. Int J Gynaecol Obstet. 2011;113(1):3–13. https://doi.org/10.1016/j.ijgo.2010.11.011.
9. Jain V, Munro MG, Critchley HO. Contemporary evaluation of women and girls with abnormal uterine bleeding: FIGO systems 1 and 2. Int J Gynecol Obstet. 2023;162:29–42.
10. Munro MG, Balen AH, Cho S, Critchley HO, Díaz I, Ferriani R, et al. The FIGO ovulatory disorders classification system. Hum Reprod. 2022;37(10):2446–64.
11. MacGregor B, Munro MG, Lumsden MA. Therapeutic options for the management of abnormal uterine bleeding. Int J Gynecol Obstet. 2023;162(Suppl. 2):43–57. https://doi.org/10.1002/ijgo.14947.
12. Calaf J, Cancelo MJ, Andeyro M, Jiménez JM, Perelló J, Correa M, et al. Development and psychometric validation of a screening questionnaire to detect excessive menstrual blood loss that interferes in quality of life: the SAMANTA questionnaire. J Women's Health (Larchmt). 2020;29(7):1021–31. https://doi.org/10.1089/jwh.2018.7446.
13. Kadir RA. Inherited bleeding disorders in women. In: Kadir RA, James PD, Lee CA, editors. 2nd. ed. Wiley; 2019.
14. Connor ME, Clark TJ. Diagnostic and operative hysteroscopy Cambridge. United Kingdom/New York, NY: Cambridge University Press; 2020.

15. Hernandez A, Dietrich JE. Abnormal uterine bleeding in the adolescent. Obstet Gynecol. 2020;135(3):615–21. https://doi.org/10.1097/AOG.0000000000003693. PMID: 32028485
16. Bacon JL. Abnormal uterine bleeding: current classification and clinical management. Obstet Gynecol Clin North Am. 2017;44(2):179–93.
17. Bradley LD, Gueye NA. The medical management of abnormal uterine bleeding in reproductive-aged women. Am J Obstet Gynecol. 2016;214:31–44.
18. Edelman AB, Koontz SL, Nichols MD, et al. Continuous oral contraceptives: are bleeding patterns dependent on the hormones given? Obstet Gynecol. 2006;107(3):657–65.
19. Brull EP, Fernandes A, Monteiro I, Bahamondes L, Juliato CRT. Safety and bleeding patterns of the levonorgestrel 52-mg intrauterine system among women with thrombosis or coagulopathy. Int J Gynaecol Obstet. 2020;151(3):355–61. https://doi.org/10.1002/ijgo.13378. Epub 2020 Oct 26. PMID: 32966599
20. Singh S, Best C, Dunn S, Leyland N, Wolfman WL. No. 292-Abnormal uterine bleeding in premenopausal women. J Obstet Gynaecol Can. 2018;40(5):e391–415. https://doi.org/10.1016/j.jogc.2018.03.007. PMID: 29731212
21. Levy-Zauberman Y, Pourcelot AG, Capmas P, Fernandez H. Update on the management of abnormal uterine bleeding. J Gynecol Obstet Hum Reprod. 2017;46(8):613–22. https://doi.org/10.1016/j.jogoh.2017.07.005. Epub 2017 Jul 15. PMID: 28716637
22. Jensen JT, Lukkari-Lax E, Schulze A, et al. Contraceptive efficacy and safety of the 52-mg levonorgestrel intrauterine system for up to 8 years: findings from the Mirena Extension Trial. Am J Obstet Gynecol. 2022;227(873):e1–12.
23. Lethaby A, Cooke I, Rees MC. Progesterone or progesterone-releasing intrauterine systems for heavy menstrual bleeding. Cochrane Database Syst Rev. 2005;(4):CD002126.
24. Starkauskaite S, Bumbuliene Z. Abnormal uterine bleeding in adolescents: causes, challenges and concerns. Gynecol Reprod Endocrinol Metabol. 2022;3(2-3):99–102.
25. Screening and management of bleeding disorders in adolescents with heavy menstrual bleeding: ACOG COMMITTEE OPINION, Number 785. Obstet Gynecol. 2019;134(3):e71–83. https://doi.org/10.1097/AOG.0000000000003411. PMID: 31441825
26. National Institute for Health and Care Excellence. Heavy menstrual bleeding: assessment and management. NICE guideline [NG88]. 2018. 2021.
27. Hale GE, Hughes CL, Burger HG, Robertson DM, Fraser IS. Atypical estradiol secretion and ovulation patterns caused by luteal out-of-phase (LOOP) events underlying irregular ovulatory menstrual cycles in the menopausal transition. Menopause. 2009;16:50–9.
28. ACOG COMMITTEE OPINION: Number 734, May 2018: The role of transvaginal ultrasonography in evaluating the endometrium of women with postmenopausal bleeding. 2018;131(5):e124–9.
29. Black D. Diagnosis and medical management of abnormal premenopausal and postmenopausal bleeding. Climacteric. 2023;26(3):222–8. https://doi.org/10.1080/13697137.2023.
30. Sung S, Carlson K, Abramovitz A. Postmenopausal bleeding. In: StatPearls [Internet]. Treasure Island: StatPearls Publishing; 2024. [Updated 2023 Dec 20]. Available from: https://www.ncbi.nlm.nih.gov/books/NBK562188.

Chapter 24
Benefits of Hormonal Contraception Administration for Menstrual Cycle Disorders

Angelica Monterrosa-Blanco, Francesco Ricciardiello, Christian Battipaglia, and Alessandro D. Genazzani

24.1 Introduction

Globally, for the year 2022, the prevalence of contraceptive method use was estimated to be approximately between 58% and 65% [1]. Generally, the motivation for use comes from the contraceptive need; half of the women around the world of reproductive age access contraceptive methods in order to prevent an unplanned pregnancy. However, the usefulness and benefits of these medications transcend just the contraceptive purpose.

The choice of the ideal method depends on the preferences, needs, contraceptive components, context, and users' expectations. It is possible to individualize the selection of contraceptives from a safety point of view according to the presence of particular medical conditions and specific characteristics, considering the medical eligibility criteria for using contraceptives of the World Health Organization (WHO). The latter was published in the first edition in 1996 and has subsequently been updated. The most recent is the fifth edition, published in 2015 [2]. These criteria classify the safety of contraceptive methods according to different medical conditions in four categories (Table 24.1).

A. Monterrosa-Blanco
Department of Obstetrics and Gynecology, Fundación Universitaria de Ciencias de la Salud (FUCS), Bogotá, Colombia
e-mail: ammonterrosa@fucsalud.edu.co

F. Ricciardiello · C. Battipaglia · A. D. Genazzani (✉)
Center for Gynecological Endocrinology, Department of Obstetrics and Gynecology, University of Modena and Reggio Emilia, Modena, Italy
e-mail: algen@unimo.it

A. R. Genazzani et al. (eds.), *Ethical, Efficacy and Safety Issues in Contraception*, Reproductive Medicine for Clinicians 4,
https://doi.org/10.1007/978-3-032-07322-8_24

Table 24.1 Categories for the safety of contraceptive use according to medical eligibility criteria

I	Absence of restriction, able to use the method in any circumstance
II	The advantages of using the method generally outweigh the theoretical or demonstrated risks, the method could usually be used
III	Theoretical or demonstrated risks generally outweigh the advantages, so the method should not be recommended
IV	Advises against using it under any circumstances; its use represents an unacceptable health risk

Adapted from World Health Organization's medical eligibility criteria for contraceptive use [2]

24.1.1 Hormonal Contraception

Contraception is a broad concept that encompasses a variety of methods that, in turn, have different mechanisms of action, presentation, composition, dose, route of administration, duration of action, and effectiveness. In general terms, contraceptives can be classified as hormonal or non-hormonal. Hormonal contraceptives are semi-synthetic preparations that simulate the biological activity of the two main female sex hormones (estrogen and progesterone). There are two types of hormonal contraceptives: those composed of both hormones and those with only progestin. Progestins are classified according to their introduction (generation) and the chemical group from which they are derived (19-nortestosterone, 17α-progesterone, spironolactone or hybrids) or according to their antiandrogenic effect [3]. On the other hand, the estrogens available in contraceptives are ethinyl estradiol (EE), 17β–estradiol (E2), and estetrol (E4), the first considered semi-synthetic and the last two, natural estrogens [4].

Over the years, modifications have been introduced in the formulations in order to meet the requirements of those who use these contraceptives [5]. Some of these modifications include the reduction in the dose of estrogens from the macro dose to the low dose; preparations combined with natural estrogens such as 17β-estradiol and estetrol that allow better control of the cycle and reduce metabolic effects; the development of progestins with greater antiandrogenic and anti-mineralocorticoid activity; estrogen and progestin preparations where the suspension interval is not present; the creation of formulations other than monophasic, such as biphasic and sequential ones in which the hormone doses change throughout the cycle and better resemble endogenous physiological fluctuations [5]. These innovations reduce possible adverse events, increase their usefulness in different pathologies, and improve the percentage of use, tolerance, and adherence [6, 7].

However, despite the above, myths and false beliefs still exist regarding the use of hormonal contraceptive methods, giving them a negative connotation and contributing to the fact that a significant percentage of women still abstain from using contraception. Therefore, it is essential to highlight that the benefits of contraceptives extend beyond family planning. Benefits have been described in different women's health conditions in which contraceptives may be indicated as first-line treatment. Considering the variety of existing methods, it is essential to individualize the selection of the contraceptive with the appropriate components according to the needs of the patient and thus achieve the greatest benefit. The objective of the present narrative review is to highlight the benefits of hormonal contraceptive methods in six prevalent conditions in women at different stages of the life cycle: premenstrual syndrome—premenstrual dysphoric disorder; oligomenorrhea or amenorrhea in patients with hyperandrogenism and polycystic ovary syndrome; abnormal uterine bleeding during puberty; pelvic pain (adenomyosis, endometriosis, dysmenorrhea); hypothalamic amenorrhea; and premature ovarian failure and perimenopause.

24.2 Premenstrual Syndrome and Premenstrual Dysphoric Disorder (PMS/PMDD)

The occurrence of physical, emotional, and behavioral symptoms in the days surrounding the arrival of the menses, also called premenstrual symptoms, constitute a syndrome (PMS) that occurs up to 40% of women. When symptoms occur with greater intensity and severity, they are described as a disorder called premenstrual dysphoric disorder (PMDD), whose prevalence is 2–7% [8–11]. The latter has been widely described and criteria for its diagnosis are recorded in the *Diagnostic and Statistical Manual of Mental Disorders, 5th edition* [12], which includes a series of mood, physical, and behavioral symptoms such as marked affective lability, increased irritability, anger, depressed mood, hopelessness, feelings of worthlessness, anxiety, tension, feeling on edge, decreased interest in everyday activities, lethargy, difficulty concentrating, overeating, change in appetite, feeling overwhelmed or out of control, sleep disturbances, muscle and joint pain, breast tenderness, among others. The magnitude of these symptoms is significant, compromising quality of life, the performance of daily activities, and negatively impacting interpersonal relationships [10, 11].

PMS/PMDD occurs in the week before the onset of menses, improves in the week after the onset of menses, and becomes minimal or absent in the postmenstrual week [9]. It is driven by the hormonal changes as the main responsible factor, but also involves variation in neurotransmitters, individual neural vulnerability, and other neurochemical processes [13].

Androgens, estrogens, and progesterone have a neurochemical effect on brain function; emotional and cognitive control; and the activity of the neurotransmitters gamma-aminobutyric acid (GABA), serotonin, and dopamine [13]. Progesterone and its metabolites, especially 3α,5α-tetrahydroprogesterone, called allopregnanolone (Allo) and pregnanolone, function as positive allosteric modulators of $GABA_A$ receptors and are the most important neurosteroids. They open the chloride channel for a longer duration and frequency, thus increasing the receptor's affinity for GABA, the most abundant inhibitory neurotransmitter in the central nervous system acting as antidepressant and anxiolitic compounds [8, 10].

In patients diagnosed with PMDD, a greater susceptibility and the existence of some triggers have been described [14]. Variation in progesterone levels and allopregnanolone during the luteal phase affect the response of different brain regions, such as the amygdala, anterior cingulate cortex, and inferior frontal gyrus [13]. Also, PMS/PMDD symptoms have recently been related to inflammatory substances such as TNF-α, prostaglandins, interleukins, cytokines, and chemokines that rise in the late luteal phase when low estrogen and progesterone concentrations increase endometrial oxidative stress and synthesis of pro-inflammatory molecules [15]. Therefore, given the hormonal changes in the premenstrual phase, the decrease in estrogen to its lowest levels, and the rapid decrease in progesterone metabolites, there are changes at the level of neuronal excitability with an increase in the expression of the $GABA_A$ receptor subunits. However, with a significant reduction in the affinity to the receptor, which reduces the influx of chloride ion, the release of GABA is inhibited; the inhibition of pyramidal neurons is decreased and their excitability increases, resulting in the characteristic symptoms of PMDD (see Fig. 24.1) [16, 17].

PMDD symptoms are absent premenarche, in anovulatory cycles, pregnancy, menopause, and after surgical removal of the ovaries before menopause. Taking into account the relationship of neurosteroids to PMDD, hormonal contraceptives have been proposed as a therapy. Suppressing the hypothalamic-pituitary-ovarian (H-P-O) axis and ovulation can modulate brain effects caused by sudden hormonal fluctuations.

Since 2006, the only method approved by the US Food and Drug Administration (FDA) for the treatment of PMDD is the combined oral contraceptive (COC) containing drospirenone (DRSP) as a progestin administered in a 24+4 regimen. However, other hormonal formulations have proven to be useful for PMDD symptoms [18, 19]. The therapeutic benefit of DRSP is derived from its chemical

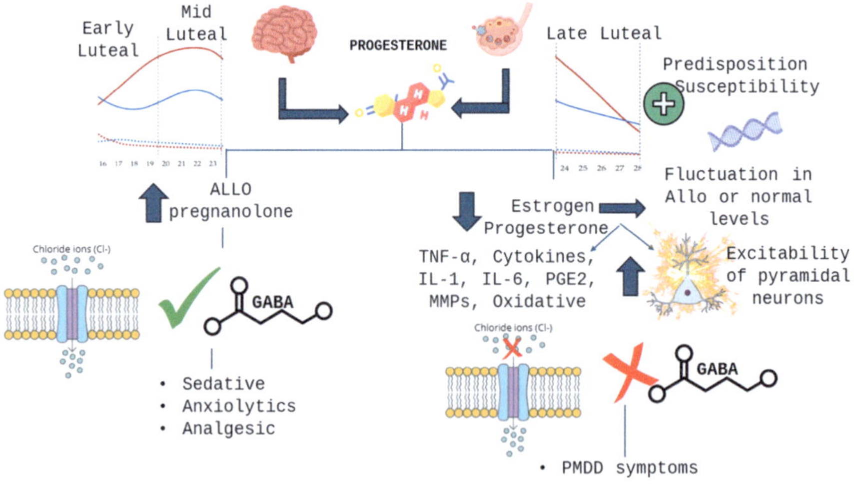

Fig. 24.1 Pathophysiology of PMDD symptoms

structure, whose similarity to progesterone allows it to exert the same sedative effects on the central nervous system, and the anti-inflammatory and anti-oxidative properties of estradiol and progesterone [14, 20, 21]. In addition, the low affinity of DRSP for sex hormone binding globulin (SHBG) results in decreased free testosterone levels, and it reduces activity of 17α-hydroxylase and hence the synthesis of testosterone [20, 21].

The 24+4 regimen, compared to the 21+7 regimen, produces greater suppression of ovarian function and reduces hormone-free days, protecting the brain from the side effects previously described [9, 14, 17, 21, 22]. In a systematic review published in 2023, Ma & Song found improvement in severity of symptoms and productivity, social activities, and relationships [23]. Significant relief of symptoms such as depressed mood, anxiety or tension, crying, anger, or irritability after 3–6 cycles of treatment with EE 20μg + DRSP has been reported [24].

The impact on PMDD symptoms depends on the profile of the progestin used; those with a more significant antiandrogenic effect are preferred due to their favorable effect on mood, with a reduction of up to 50% in more than 60% of patients [10, 21, 25]. More androgenic progestins, such as levonorgestrel (LNG), when used systemically, could worsen the symptoms of PMS and PMDD. In a network meta-analysis, combined oral contraceptives with different progestins (DRSP, LNG, desogestrel, norethindrone, nomegestrol) were compared. None of these were more efficacious than any other [26, 27]. In the same report, it was concluded that combined oral contraceptives may improve overall premenstrual symptomatology in both women with PMS and PMDD, except for depressive symptoms [26].

In conclusion, combined oral contraceptives are effective for the management of symptoms and functional impairment related to PMS and PMDD. Those that contain progestin with antiandrogenic properties are especially useful in a regimen in which the hormone-free interval is only 4 days instead of 7 [9, 21, 25, 28–30]. However, few studies support the use of progestin alone in any form (oral, injectable, IUS, implant) as a possible therapeutic alternative since progestin-only treatments would have less effectiveness due to the lack of estrogen and its regulatory effects on brain function [31, 32].

24.3 Oligomenorrhea/Amenorrhea in Hyperandrogenism/PCOS

Menstrual irregularity (oligomenorrhea or amenorrhea) caused by anovulation/oligo-ovulation is one of the most frequent reasons for medical consultation by women of reproductive age. In association with acne, hirsutism, alopecia, and polycystic ovaries, as an ultrasound finding, the most likely diagnosis is polycystic ovary syndrome (PCOS). This disorder has a prevalence of up to 15–25% in women of reproductive age [33, 34]. It is diagnosed according to the Rotterdam criteria when two out of three features are present. The diagnostic criteria point out three essential conditions: ovulatory dysfunction, hyperandrogenism, and ovarian morphology with a polycystic appearance on ultrasound (≥ 20 follicles per ovary in either ovary/≥ 10 cm^3 ovarian volume). Four patient phenotypes have been described (Table 24.2) [35].

Women with PCOS have a greater predisposition to obesity, metabolic dysfunction, insulin resistance, dyslipidemia, diabetes, infertility, thromboembolic risk, and cardiovascular disease and physiological instability [36, 37]. The presence of the above conditions will depend on factors such as age, family history, genetic predisposition, PCOS phenotype, comorbidities, and receipt of appropriate management.

There is a consensus that PCOS management must be comprehensive and holistic, where the starting point is a healthy balanced diet, incorporating physical activity, behavioral changes in habits, psychological support, and integrative medicines [37–39]. Given that the response varies, most patients require additional interventions, and COCs are the first-line option for the pharmacological management of PCOS in women who do not desire to be fertile [36, 40, 41].

COC mechanism of action in the context of PCOS is focused on three main objectives: reduction of hyperandrogenism, generation of a positive effect on metabolism, and recovery of regularity in cyclic uterine bleeding. The achievement of these objectives largely depends on the type of COC selected, considering the progestin and the dose and type of estrogen. Most contraceptives are composed of EE with different doses between 15 and 40 μg; some recent ones contain "natural" estrogens, 17β-estradiol, and only one contains estetrol [4]. In contrast, a variety of progestins are employed. These have different origins, but in practical terms, they can be categorized according to their effect on androgen receptors. Those with the greatest antiandrogenic potency are chlormadinone acetate (first generation), cyproterone acetate, dienogest (fourth generation), and DRSP (fourth generation). Progestins with little or no androgenic activity are gestodene, desogestrel, and norgestimate (all third generation). Meanwhile, levonorgestrel (LNG, second generation) has androgenic activity.

Table 24.2 PCOS phenotypes according to Rotterdam criteria

1	Hyperandrogenism + ovulatory dysfunction
2	Hyperandrogenism + polycystic ovarian morphology
3	Ovulatory dysfunction + polycystic ovarian morphology
4	Hyperandrogenism + ovulatory dysfunction + polycystic ovarian morphology

Phenotypes of PCOS according to the Rotterdam criteria [35]

Contraceptives intervene in hyperandrogenism through inhibition of pituitary gonadotropin secretion, which in turn inhibits folliculogenesis and ovarian steroidogenesis. The inhibition of the pulsatile secretion of LH prevents its action on theca cells and the subsequent production of androgens [41]. The estrogenic component of the pill stimulates hepatic production of SHBG, increasing its availability for binding with testosterone and thus contributing to the reduction of free testosterone. Hepatic protein synthesis promoted by EE increases with higher doses. However, very high doses lead to hypercoagulability, resulting in an increased risk for venous thrombotic events (VTE) [40, 42]. EE-containing COCs induce both pro- and anticoagulant factors and fibrinolytic activity, culminating in increased thrombin generation [43].

17β-estradiol, estradiol valerate (E2V)—a prodrug that is transformed into estradiol through first-pass hepatic biotransformation—and estetrol, derived from the fetal liver, have been introduced as estrogens in the recent contraceptive preparation as substitutes of ethinil estradiol (EE). In comparison to EE, all of them promote lower SBHG synthesis and have a lesser effect on angiotensin synthesis, minor effects on hemostasis markers, less impact on the coagulation and fibrinolytic systems, low bioavailability, short half-life, and lower potency, so larger doses of E2 than EE are needed for the same clinical effect. These newly used estrogens give a reduced cardiovascular and metabolic risk [5]. In a clinical trial, Haverinen et al. [43] reported that thrombin generation was lower after E2V + DNG vs. EE + DNG, thus providing evidence that natural estrogen induce less enhancement of the coagulation potential.

Antiandrogenic progestins do not change the estrogen-dependent production of SHBG, so the binding of sex hormones to SHBG is preserved. In addition, they have no affinity for SHBG, allowing their levels to be 3–4 times higher when compared to second-generation progestins, which have inhibitory effects on SHBG [5, 41, 44]. In addition, antiandrogenic progestins have a longer half-life, prolonging their effect and elimination time. They also inhibit 5α-reductase, which blocks the conversion of testosterone to the potent androgen, dihydrotestosterone, and prevents the binding of testosterone to androgen receptors [42].

Forslund et al., in a systematic review, compared second and third-generation progestins, finding greater changes in free androgen index, DHEAS, and SHBG, favoring the third-generation progestins [41]. Considering the progestins profile, in patients with significant clinical signs of hyperandrogenism, contraceptives composed of dienogest, DRSP, cyproterone acetate, and chlormadinone acetate will be preferred due to their potential to reduce total testosterone and free testosterone. However, the latter two have been associated with more adverse events and a greater risk of VTE. In some case, Desogestrel could be considered a second choice by partially blocking the increase in SHBG [40]. In patients with evident clinical hyperandrogenism, antiandrogenic progestins are preferred, and a 24+4 regimen should also be chosen, since the short hormone-free time reduces to a minimum the re-start of ovarian production of steroids [22].

Contraceptive selection should be individualized, especially in patients with PCOS and obesity. It is not advisable to manage obese + PCOS patients with the lowest doses of estrogen. Being the adipose tissue able to upload and retain steroids compounds and dismiss them with no control as a matter of time, low-dose contraceptive pill might favor a not perfect bleeding control due to the risk of eventually not having a sufficient amount of estrogen in the bloodstream. These facts might determine not to achieve the desired therapeutic effect and to expose the patient to unpredictable spotting due to the instability of the endometrium. Taking into account the requirement for a higher estrogen dose with EE, in this group of patients, counseling should be performed to emphasize weight reduction and evaluate the use of natural estrogens to avoid possible adverse cardiovascular and metabolic events [5].

The use of COCs as a treatment for PCOS has a role in the different metabolic parameters. Carbohydrate metabolism has been favored with natural estrogens and antiandrogenic progestins, especially in patients with a history of insulin resistance. Several authors have found stable or reduced insulin levels with the Homeostatic Model Assessment for Insulin Resistance (HOMA-IR) after using E2V/DNG. Dienogest, DRSP, and desogestrel may decrease HOMA-IR by improving tissue insulin sensitivity. On the contrary, a slight increase in HOMA-IR with EE/2mg chlormadinone acetate has been described [4, 40, 45]. In patients with obesity, DRSP is preferred for its diuretic effect [42]. It is also the first choice in patients with hypertension, as it is a spironolactone analog and has an anti-mineralocorticoid effect and can counteract water retention [40].

Regarding lipid metabolism, high doses of EE and androgenic progestins can increase LDL and triglycerides and decrease HDL. In patients with an impaired baseline lipid profile, such as low HDL and/or high LDL, COCs with estradiol and less androgenic progestins would be preferred; newer progestins and natural estrogens have a more beneficial effect on lipid metabolism, especially a positive effect on HDL than classic COC formulations [41]. Ågren et al. [6] compared nomegestrol acetate and 17β-estradiol (NOMAC/E2) with LNG/EE for six cycles, finding that NOMAC/E2 had minimal influence on hemostatic, lipid, and carbohydrate metabolism indices, causing less change in these parameters, while with LNG/EE, HDL decreased and LDL and triglycerides slightly increased.

Ovulatory dysfunction leading to oligomenorrhea and amenorrhea is also treated with COCs. These allow cyclic *withrawal bleeding*, ovarian, and endometrial protection from possible future neoplasias while providing contraceptive protection, since chronic anovulation and oligomenorrhea, typical of PCOS, make the endometrium subject to prolonged estrogen exposure that is unopposed by progesterone. This results in a greater risk of endometrial hyperplasia, which can lead to endometrial cancer even more if the patients have other risk factors. Thus, COCs play an essential role in protecting against endometrial cancer.

The range of options for managing PCOS with COCs is wide. Patients with strong manifestations of hyperandrogenism will benefit from progestins with a greater antiandrogenic effect; obese patients will require higher concentrations of estrogens, and those with hypertension will be able to benefit from the antimineralocorticoid and diuretic effects of the new progestins, patients with dyslipidemia and insulin resistance will be able to find a better therapeutic response with the new estrogens and the fourth-generation progestins [40, 41].

24.4 Amenorrhea and Abnormal Uterine Bleeding

Throughout life, abnormal uterine bleeding (AUB) will occur in up to 30% of women. This alteration is more prevalent at the extremes of life, in adolescents, and in the years around menopause [46]. AUB prevalence during adolescence has been reported to be 11–27%. It is defined as abnormal uterine bleeding in terms of its duration, volume, regularity, and frequency. The most common clinical presentation of AUB is through heavy menstrual bleeding, which is not caused by structural lesions of the uterus. It generates a change in the quality of life, discomfort, absences from school/work, limitations in carrying out daily life activities, associated symptoms such as pelvic pain and low blood pressure and anemia, and increase in the health care costs. The first step in offering targeted treatment is to determine the etiology, which can vary depending on the patient's age, the chronicity, and the severity of the bleeding [7].

The H-P-O axis plays a fundamental role in the proper functioning of menstrual cycles. However, it must have a maturation stage. Due to this process, anovulatory cycles are common after menarche, where ovarian stimulation by gonadotropins is just beginning to allow adequate follicular development. Therefore, during adolescence, anovulatory cycles are the most common etiology of AUB due to the immaturity of the H-P-O axis. Etiologies of other origins must be ruled out, such as insufficiency of the corpus luteum, anovulation + hyperandrogenism in patients with PCOS, hypoestrogenism, clotting pathway disorders, thyroid disorders, other endocrine disorders, pregnancy, infections, trauma, use of medications, or structural causes that, during adolescence, are usually rare [47, 48].

Cyclic uterine bleeding is the response of the endometrium to the withdrawal of progesterone and estrogen in the absence of pregnancy. Therefore, altered levels of estrogen or progesterone or their ratio along the different phases of the menstrual cycle, as well as aberrations in endometrial vasculogenesis and abnormalities in the local inflammatory response, can lead to AUB. Different therapeutic options exist for managing AUB, and hormonal pharmacological management has proven to be effective. Among the alternatives, progestin-only methods can be administered by various routes: intrauterine, intramuscular, subcutaneous, and oral, the latter cyclically or continuously. COCs are also an alternative, with different variations depending on the type of estrogen and progestin, as well as other routes: oral, transdermal, and vaginal. Its mechanism of action in the AUB context is to afford cycle control through regular withdrawal bleeds and significantly reduced blood loss. While the estrogen function is to stimulate uniform endometrial growth and promptly stop shedding, the progesterone component stabilizes the endometrium, converting it into pseudo decidua, by creating an atrophic endometrial lining by triggering apoptosis, inhibiting angiogenesis, stimulating the conversion of estradiol to the less active estrone, and thereby reducing overall blood loss at the time of withdrawal bleeding [49].

In patients with chronic AUB, with some contraindication to the use of estrogen, who cannot take pills, who desire long-term planning, or with iron deficiency anemia, the LNG-IUS generates a local effect through endometrial atrophy and reduces the mean uterine vascular density. After 3 months, the reduction in bleeding is as high as 85% and very close to 100% after 1 year. Another option for women with the conditions previously described is depot-medroxyprogesterone acetate, administered quarterly. However, among the most frequent adverse events of both methods, irregular spotting-type bleeding is described, and they are not the best option for episodes of hefty acute bleeding [48].

There is no consensus on whether to treat with COCs or progestin-only pills, even though when choosing COCs, estrogen improves hemostasis and can be even more beneficial in adolescents with active bleeding. High-dose estrogen promotes rapid growth of the epithelium and endometrial stroma, generates vasospasm of uterine arteries, induces platelet aggregation, capillary clotting, and the production of estrogen and progesterone receptors [49]. The European Consensus group and an ACOG Committee Opinion have approved, as initial management for acute bleeding in adolescents, the use of COCs in a monophasic regimen, composed of EE 30–50 μg plus any progestin every 8–12 h until the bleeding stops, then continuing with one pill per day for a total of at least 21 days. Seven days of placebo or pause should be given after the 21 days, and COC treatment should be continued for 3–6 months [7].

Bearing in mind the potential beneficial effect of contraceptives on metabolism, different COC alternatives have been proposed with novel compounds that resemble the natural estrogen and progesterone molecules [50]. 2 mg/day of E2V has an equivalent effect on the H-P-O axis, endometrium and ovarian function to 20 μg/day of EE, with a decrease in secondary events in the lipid profile, glucose metabolism, and on cardiovascular and thromboembolic risk. On the other hand, DNG has high activity on progesterone receptors; 10% circulates unbound, which is a higher percentage compared with other nortestosterone derivatives; and it has an antiandrogenic effect due to the lack of binding to SHBG. Its plasma half-life is approximately 10 h, similar to other nortestosterone derivatives. E2V/DNG in a quadriphasic dosing regimen, where DNG is increased during week 2 of the cycle while E2V is decreased on day 3 and day 25, was effective in terms of reduction of blood loss of 50% from baseline, blood loss less than 80 mL, improvements in hemoglobin, hematocrit, and ferritin after 6 months when compared with placebo, as well as an adequate safety profile. Additionally, when comparing E2V/DNG with classic COCs such as EE/LNG, the former reduced the bleeding duration, had better cycle control, and induced amenorrhea more effectively [50, 51].

During adolescence, nearly half of the peak bone mass is acquired. Endogenous circulating estrogens positively affect bone growth, development, and mineral acquisition. Estradiol inhibits bone resorption by increasing osteoclast apoptosis and reducing osteoblast apoptosis. So, estrogen deficiency during this critical period determines low bone mass density. Unfortunately, COCs during adolescence do not improve bone mineral density (BMD); they suppress insulin-like growth factor-1 secretion, a bone trophic hormone. They can compromise bone mineral acquisition in adolescence, especially in the first 3 years post-menarche [4]. Again, using natural estrogens has more benefits on bone than EE. DNG/E2V is associated with no significant change in BMD or adverse effects on bone turnover markers [52]. On the other hand, providing transdermal 100 μg of 17β-estradiol with cyclic oral progesterone was associated with more gain in spine and hip BMD; the probable reason behind this is that the transdermal route avoids the liver and the resulting inhibition of IGF-1 production. Therefore, in adolescents with AUB, alternatives with natural estrogens are preferred, but the transdermal dose is not sufficient to serve as contraception [53].

Women with high cardiovascular disease risk, especially in adulthood because it is infrequent to have this condition in adolescence, require nonestrogen-based treatment. During the acute phase, treatment with medroxyprogesterone acetate 20 mg every 8 h for 7 days or norethindrone acetate 5 mg–10 mg every 4 h may be offered. For the management of chronic AUB, oral medroxyprogesterone acetate, norethindrone, megestrol acetate, or micronized progesterone, given one tablet daily continuously or cyclically for 14–16 days prior to the anticipated start of the menstrual cycle, provides cycle control and reduction of menstrual blood loss [49].

Not all progestogens are the same; they can vary according to their classification, molecular structure, biological effects, and receptor binding. Dydrogesterone is a stereoisomer of progesterone, which differs slightly in molecular structure from natural progesterone. It has a highly selective ability to bind to the progesterone receptor and is different from others because it does not block ovulation at therapeutic doses (it is not a contraceptive) and has no estrogenic, androgenic, or glucocorticoid effects. Dydrogesterone reduces adverse events and is effective in treating menstrual disorders. During the acute episode, 20–30 mg is administered every 24 h for 10 days, and as maintenance, 10 mg is administered in the second half of the cycle, from day 14–28. This does not serve as a contraceptive [54].

In summary, during adolescence, the management of AUB should focus on reducing bleeding, regularizing menstrual cycles, protecting bone mass, and taking advantage of the risk-reducing effect on some parameters related to metabolism. Management should last at least 6 months, and in those women with an immature H-P-O axis as the etiology in the first instance, evaluate the subsequent regularization of the axis and subsequently rule out other causes of anovulation. Women who, in addition to treatment for AUB, require contraception should seek counseling since not all methods guarantee contraception.

24.5 Premature Ovarian Insufficiency, Perimenopause, and Menopause

Premature ovarian insufficiency (POI) is a pathological endocrinological condition in which there is an early interruption of ovarian function in women of fertile age. It is defined as the cessation of menses before the age of 40, affecting about 1% of women [55]. According to ESHRE guidelines, the diagnosis requires the following: oligo/amenorrhea for at least 4 months and an elevated FSH level > 25 IU/l on two occasions 4 weeks apart [56]. In some women, the etiology is uncertain, while in others, genetic predisposition, iatrogenic, and chromosomal abnormalities are the common causes. This condition will simulate perimenopause and menopause, so the clinical features are similar, predominating symptoms such as hot flashes, night sweats, mood and sleep changes, fatigue, joint pains, headaches, palpitations, and menstrual disturbance, as well as paraclinical evidence of raised gonadotrophins and low estradiol [55].

Perimenopause and menopause are physiological conditions that form part of the female life cycle. The average age of natural menopause depends on ethnicity and genetic factors but is described as around 48–53 years [55]. Perimenopause refers to the time around menopause when there is a gradual transition in which the female's ovaries slow down.

Both women with POI, as well as those in perimenopause and premenopause, should receive hormonal replacement to relieve symptoms and mitigate the consequences of hormonal loss, especially in those with POI. This substitution is carried out with preparations that contain estrogens and progesterone through the figure of combined oral contraceptive pill (COCPs) or hormone replacement therapy (HRT); the difference between the two is that HRT is generally made up of natural estrogens and a lower dose of progestins. While most COCs contain synthetic estrogens such as EE and higher doses, over the years, this gap has been reduced as COCs with natural hormones are now available.

In women diagnosed with POI, it is essential to replace the hormonal deficiency promptly, given that the negative impact on the different systems is greater because the physiological changes occur earlier than expected, and quality of life is compromised at very early ages compared to the years of life expectancy. Bone mineral density is one of the most affected; the prevalence of osteoporosis and fracture risk is double that of the general population [57]. Other consequences of hormonal shortage are genitourinary syndrome in young patients with an active sexual life and cardiovascular disease.

HRT aims to restore hormone concentrations to the premenopausal status and, as such, prevent repercussions and relieve symptoms [56]. Women with POI should be treated with hormonal therapy from the time of diagnosis until the mean age of natural menopause; it is important to consider that they require higher doses of estrogen [55, 57]. In contrast, women with average age at menopause usually require the lowest effective dose of hormonal therapy, and the optimal duration of systemic HRT in menopause is an individualized decision based on the balance between ongoing benefits, potential risks, and personal preferences [58].

17β-estradiol, because it is natural and better simulates endogenous estrogen effects, is preferred over EE or conjugated equine estrogens (CEE). Likewise, natural progesterone and dydrogesterone are preferred too because of their safety profiles in glycemic metabolism and cardiovascular and breast health [55]. In women with previous hysterectomy, estrogens can be administered as monotherapy, while in women with remaining uterus, it should be combined with progestogen to protect the endometrium against the unopposed proliferating effect of estrogens. The estrogen dose depends on whether the therapy is for POI or menopause, the control of symptoms, and their severity. The absence of response to low doses warrants its increase. Lower estrogen doses require lower progestogen doses, on the contrary, sequential regimens require higher progestogen doses than continuous regimens. The therapy can be administered orally, vaginally (cream or ring), transdermal, or through LNG-UIS [55]. Figure 24.2 shows the different therapeutic alternatives in the context of contraceptives since there are other therapies, such as tibolone or selective estrogen modulators, that exceed the scope of the review (see Fig. 24.2).

Estrogen administration is carried out continuously, and progestogen can be given cyclically 12–14 days a month, causing withdrawal bleeding; this regimen is more common in women with POI. On the contrary, a continuous estroprogestin regimen will generate endometrial atrophy with consequent amenorrhea, which is preferred in menopausal patients [55]. A recent systematic review found evidence that hormone therapy with natural estrogens and progesterone is beneficial for women with POI, not only to mitigate hypoestrogenic symptoms but also to preserve BMD, reduce plasma cholesterol concentrations, and avoid uterine atrophy [59]. Likewise, estrogen replacement in menopausal women also protects bone, decreasing circulating sclerostin levels, a potent inhibitor of bone formation [57]. Additionally, hormonal therapy indicated on time reduces the carotid atherosclerosis progression, the incidence of coronary heart disease, and lower all-cause mortality [55].

There are few contraindications for HRT in women affected by POI, as benefits tend to overcome the eventual risks, such as breast cancer, depending on the type of progestogen, stroke, or VTE. In patients who suffer from migraine with aura, transdermal delivery may be the best option for lowering its triggering. The transdermal or vaginal route can also offer the lowest risk of VTE in hypertensive or obese patients because of the avoidance of the first-pass hepatic metabolism, so there is no production of cholesterol, triglycerides, coagulation factors, and SHBG in the liver. On the other hand, estrogens administered vaginally at a very low dose have no systemic effects and do not stimulate endometrial growth [55–57].

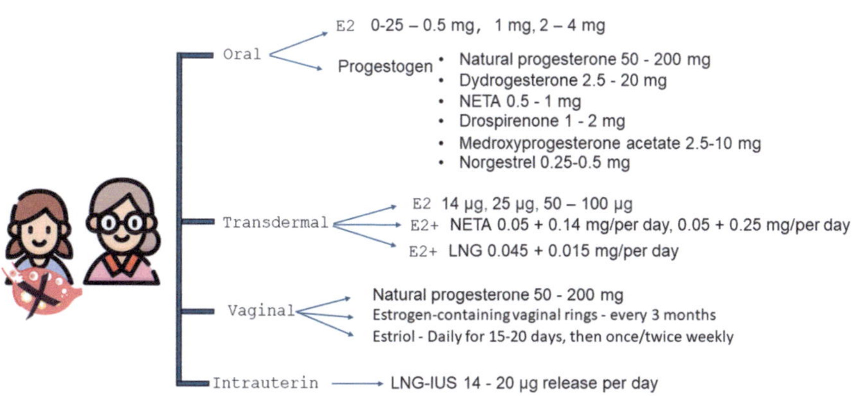

Fig. 24.2 Hormonal therapies for POI and menopause in the context of contraceptives. NETA: Norethisterone acetate

Hormonal therapy definitely benefits the three conditions mentioned previously; in summary, preparations with estrogens and progesterone that better resemble the endogenous ones will be preferred. The main objectives will be bone care, cardiovascular and breast health, and the relief of symptoms to improve quality of life.

24.6 Dysmenorrhea and Pain

Dysmenorrhea, also known as period pain, is a well-known problem affecting women in their fertile age. Its usual onset occurs around the time that menstruation begins. Its manifestation is pain, usually involving the lower abdomen or pelvis which lasts between 1 and 3 days [60]. Identifying two kinds of dysmenorrhea, primary and secondary, is possible. Primary dysmenorrhea (PD) occurs in the absence of any apparent underlying disease, whereas secondary dysmenorrhea is pain associated with underlying conditions such as endometriosis, pelvic inflammatory disease, leiomyomas, or interstitial cystitis [61].

Prostaglandins are involved in its pathogenesis, and their production also depends on hormonal control [60]. Nonsteroidal anti-inflammatory drugs (NSAIDs) are considered first-line treatment for primary dysmenorrhea. They provide adequate pain relief, but they cannot be used long-term as some patients can be allergic or may have other health conditions that present contraindicates for the use of NSAIDs. Hormonal contraception, also considered first-line treatment, has an essential role in the management of dysmenorrhea since it reduces prostaglandin and leukotriene release, which reduces uterine contractility and associated pain.

Extended and cyclic hormone regimens are available, and both are effective in treating the pain. Extended use may reduce pain in women with dysmenorrhea more effectively [60]. Differences in terms of effectiveness have not been found between different doses of EE, between newer and older formulations, or between third-, fourth-, first- and second-generation COCs [62]. Progestin-only pills (POP) or LNG-IUS are an alternative for those women who are not candidates for estrogen therapy since they have uterotrophic activity. Other combined hormonal contraceptives such as transdermal patches and vaginal rings are also acceptable for the management of dysmenorrhea [61]. The Italian Society of Gynecology and Obstetrics guidelines on contraception published in 2019 stated that oral contraceptive pills containing chlormadinone acetate are indicated when there is no response to other COCs [63].

However, dysmenorrhea/pelvic pain is frequently associated with specific organic conditions at the uterine level. Details are discussed in the following two sections.

- *Adenomyosis*

Adenomyosis is a common pathology in women of reproductive age characterized by infiltration of the myometrium by endometrial tissue. It can result in abnormal uterine bleeding, pelvic pain, and/or infertility [64]. It is challenging to establish the true prevalence of this pathology as there are some asymptomatic forms of adenomyosis. It is thought that around 20–30% of the uteri coming from women having a hysterectomy are found to have adenomyosis [65]. Until some time ago, diagnosis of adenomyosis was possible only after the anatomical examination of the uterus. Nowadays, the Morphological Uterus Sonographic Assessment (MUSA) group has established some useful ultrasound features for the diagnosis of adenomyosis. These include asymmetrical thickening of the myometrium, myometrial cysts, hyperechoic islands, fan-shaped shadowing echogenic, sub-endometrial lines and buds, translesional vascularity, irregular junctional zone, and interrupted junctional zone [66].

A variety of pharmacological and surgical therapies exist for adenomyosis. Currently, no guidelines give preference to one treatment method over another because different clinical variables have to be considered. Considering that adenomyosis, like endometriosis, is an estrogen-sensitive condition, hormonal therapy can be considered to counteract the clinical symptoms [65].

Oral contraceptives and progestins have been approved as a relevant symptomatic treatment for dysmenorrhea and heavy menstrual bleeding. Since they produce a decidualization response and subsequent atrophy of the endometrium, as well as antiproliferative and anti-inflammatory effects, helping to neutralize symptoms, reducing heavy menstrual bleeding, and for a short period, they can also cause regression of adenomyosis. Additionally, COCs containing gestodene suppress aromatase expression in the eutopic and the ectopic endometrium and the adenomyotic foci [67].

Among the available progestins, dienogest (2mg/day) has high selectivity for progesterone receptors, it causes a mild inhibition of ovarian function with slight hypoestrogenic effects, and it exerts an antiproliferative action on the endometrium. Adenomyotic cell proliferation is also inhibited by inducing apoptotic pathways [68]. Moreover, an effect of norethisterone acetate (NETA) in the management of adenomyosis has been demonstrated in women with moderate or severe pelvic pain and bleeding, obtaining a significant improvement of both dysmenorrhea and bleeding after treatment (5 mg/day) [68].

Additionally, the LNG-IUS and etonogestrel implant are both progestin alternatives, causing decidualization of the endometrium, which leads to a decrease in menstrual discharge, sometimes leading to amenorrhea, reducing uterine size, yielding pain relief. The LNG-IUS acts on the foci of adenomyosis, causing downregulation of estrogen receptors [69, 70].

- *Endometriosis*

Endometriosis is a benign illness defined by endometrial glands and stroma outside the uterine cavity. It causes chronic inflammation inside and outside of the pelvis and is linked to a variety of symptoms, including chronic pelvic pain and dysmenorrhea [71]. Its prevalence varies from 2% to 10% of females of reproductive age [72].

Treatments for endometriosis have been widely studied, and many approaches have been proposed. If ovulation and menstruation play an important role in the pathogenesis of endometriosis, hormonal contraceptives can be included as a valid therapeutic approach for controlling this disease. The goal is to reduce or suppress menstruation and/or ovulation by means of hormonal treatments [73]. In addition, contraceptive preparations significantly keep under control and/or reduce the recurrence of ovarian endometrioma.

The hormonal treatment for endometriosis-associated pain consists of COCs delivered by different routes such as oral, vaginal, or transdermal, and POPs, delivered orally, subdermally, or through an intrauterine device [72]. Women suffering from endometriosis-associated dysmenorrhea can be offered the continuous use of a combined hormonal contraceptive pill. A systematic review shows that hormonal contraceptive use (both CHCs and POCs) results in a statistically significant reduction from baseline in endometriosis-related pain, resulting in an improvement from baseline in quality of life [73]. Almost all hormonal contraceptive use in women with endometriosis who require contraception is off-label. Only two progestins, norethisterone acetate and medroxyprogesterone acetate, are approved by the US Food and Drug Administration. Another progestin, dienogest, is approved in some countries for pain relief, but it has no contraceptive properties if given alone at the usual dose of 2 mg [73]. Moreover, it is known that dienogest has a significant effect on the inflammatory microenvironment of endometriotic lesions that may contribute to its clinical efficacy. It creates a hypo-estrogenic environment that inhibits endometriotic lesion growth, reduces cell proliferation, has an immunomodulatory effect decreasing tumor necrosis factor, and an antiangiogenic effect decreasing endothelial growth factor and nerve growth factor [74]. It is also possible to consider the use of LNG-IUS or an etonogestrel-releasing subdermal implant to reduce endometriosis-associated pain, especially in women not seeking pregnancy [72].

A summary of the recommendations for hormonal treatment of pain symptoms linked to endometriosis is presented in Table 24.3. Aromatase inhibitors, GnRH agonists, and antagonists are other options that are not considered in this review.

Table 24.3 Hormonal treatment for pelvic pain symptoms

Combined hormonal contraceptives	Oral	Multiple combinations Consider continuous use
	Vaginal ring	EE 15 mcg + ETN 120 mcg/day
		EE 13 mcg + SA 150 mcg/day
	Transdermal	EE 35 mcg + norelgestromin 150 mcg/day
		EE 34 mcg + norelgestromin 203 mcg/day
		EE 30 mcg + LNG 120 mcg/day
Progestogens	POP	Dienogest 2 mg/day
		NETA 2.5 mg or 5 mg/day
	LNG-IUS	Consider side-effect profiles
	ETN-Implant	

Hormonal treatment for pelvic pain symptoms adapted from ESHRE Endometriosis Guideline Group [72]. *POP* progesterone-only pill, *SA* segesterone acetate, *LNG-IUS* levonorgestrel-releasing intrauterine system, *ETN* etonogestrel

24.7 Functional Hypothalamic Amenorrhea

There are multiple causes of primary and secondary amenorrhea during reproductive age. The etiology of amenorrhea in 20–35% of patients is of central origin. Adequate hypothalamic functioning is essential for hormonal stimulation and synthesis [75]. When release of gonadotropin-releasing hormone (GnRH) in the hypothalamus is impeded, the H-P-O axis is directly compromised, preventing secretion of FSH and LH which silences the ovaries leading to chronic anovulation and the absence of menstruation [76].

The most frequent trigger of functional hypothalamic amenorrhea (FHA) is stress. FHA is considered a rule-out diagnosis after excluding other causes of amenorrhea, such as chromosomal abnormalities, and verification of the proper functioning of different systems, such as the thyroid, the reproductive system, the adrenal gland, and the absence of pituitary tumors. Furthermore, patients with FHA share a common characteristic, which is the presence of stressors. Usually, it occurs in patients with psychosocial and metabolic imbalances, demanding work activities, eating disorders, and excessive exercise [77].

Stress activates the hypothalamic-pituitary-adrenal axis, increasing the release of corticotropin-releasing hormone (CRH) at the hypothalamic level and stimulating the pituitary synthesis of adrenocorticotropic hormone (ACTH), which will increase the production of cortisol by the adrenal glands [74]. Likewise, the elevation of CRH increases endogenous opioids, modifies the leptin secretion by adipocytes, and changes the pattern of GnRH secretion, so the frequency and amplitude of LH pulses will be low, and estrogens and progesterone will be almost absent.

The greatest repercussion of FHA is not having an absence of menstruation but what lies behind it, which is hormonal deficiency and its consequences, especially on bone metabolism during adolescence. In patients who perform excessive physical exercise before menarche, this can be delayed for 3 years. If this activity is not accompanied by adequate nutrition, the body mass index will be low. The onset and regularity of menstrual function require that weight remain above a critical threshold, with a body fat level of 17% for menarche and 22% for regular menstruation. The beneficial effects of exercise on bone are insufficient to avoid the adverse effects of estrogen deficiency, especially in adolescents. The combination of low energy availability, H-P-O axis inhibition resulting in menstrual dysfunction, and low bone density is referred to as the "female athlete triad" [77]. Similarly, in women with an eating disorder, BMD decreases by 2.5% per year in the spine and hip. The most worrying thing in these patients is osteopenia and osteoporosis, which begin at a young age and leading to the potential for pathological fractures.

OCPs do not resolve normal ovarian function; on the contrary, they suppress ovulation and as discussed in the section on amenorrhea during adolescence, semi-synthetic estrogens in OCPs do not improve bone mineral density, so in these women, preparations with natural estrogens will be preferred. The literature contains reports that yielded variable results. One study found that long-term triphasic NGM/EE administration to osteopenic women with FHA resulted in a significant increase in lumbar spine BMD and a decrease in markers of bone resorption and bone formation, with no significant changes in hip BMD [78].

Natural estrogens, in addition to being administered orally, can be delivered through transdermal patches cyclically accompanied by oral progestin, which has a positive effect on BMD. The Endocrine Society recommends the prescription of transdermal estradiol with cyclic oral progestins in high-risk patients (i.e., z-score<−2.0, prior fractures) who did not respond to 1 year of non-pharmacological therapy [76].

24.8 Conclusions

Many prevalent conditions affecting women's health benefit from hormonal contraceptive therapy. Two essential aspects must always be considered: the patient's characteristics and the components of the contraceptives, the variety of which allow for many options for selection of the optimal choice. Semi-synthetic estrogens at higher doses will generate greater liver protein synthesis and greater availability in obese patients, but in turn, greater thromboembolic risk. In contrast, lower doses and natural estrogenic preparations will have less potency but will reduce adverse effects and benefit metabolism and bone. Most androgenic progestins counteract the thromboembolic effects, but the third- and fourth-generation progestins have better performance in managing androgenic symptoms in obese patients, hypertension, and insulin resistance. The combination of dual estrogen/progestin therapy is beneficial for endometrial protection, cycle control, and pelvic pain relief, and it modulates hormonal imbalance in the brain.

Declarations

Competing Interests The author(s) has no competing interests to declare that are relevant to the content of this manuscript.

Ethics Approval The author(s) declares that this manuscript does not include primary research with human participants.

The author(s) declares that this manuscript does not include primary studies involving animals.

Bibliography

1. World Health Organization. Family planning/contraception methods 2023.
2. World Health Organization. Medical eligibility criteria for contraceptive use. 5th edn. 2015.
3. Monterrosa CÁ. Anticoncepción oral: consideraciones generales. Colombia; 2018.
4. Bastianelli C, Farris M, Rosato E, Brosens I, Benagiano G. Pharmacodynamics of combined estrogen-progestin oral contraceptives: 1. Effects on metabolism. Expert Rev Clin Pharmacol. 2017;10(3):315–26.

5. Morimont L, Haguet H, Dogné JM, Gaspard U, Douxfils J. Combined oral contraceptives and venous thromboembolism: review and perspective to mitigate the risk. Front Endocrinol (Lausanne). 2021;12:769187.
6. Ågren UM, Anttila M, Mäenpää-Liukko K, Rantala ML, Rautiainen H, Sommer WF, et al. Effects of a monophasic combined oral contraceptive containing nomegestrol acetate and 17β-oestradiol compared with one containing levonorgestrel and ethinylestradiol on haemostasis, lipids and carbohydrate metabolism. Eur J Contracept Reprod Health Care. 2011;16(6):444–57.
7. Shoupe D. The progestin revolution 2: progestins are now a dominant player in the tight interlink between contraceptive protection and bleeding control-plus more. Contracept Reprod Med. 2023;8(1):48.
8. Robertson E, Thew C, Thomas N, Karimi L, Kulkarni J. Pilot data on the feasibility and clinical outcomes of a nomegestrol acetate oral contraceptive pill in women with premenstrual dysphoric disorder. Front Endocrinol (Lausanne). 2021;12:704488.
9. Rapkin AJ, Korotkaya Y, Taylor KC. Contraception counseling for women with premenstrual dysphoric disorder (PMDD): current perspectives. Open Access J Contracept. 2019;10:27–39.
10. Rapkin AJ, Lewis EI. Treatment of premenstrual dysphoric disorder. Womens Health (Lond). 2013;9(6):537–56.
11. Reilly TJ, Patel S, Unachukwu IC, Knox C-L, Wilson CA, Craig MC, et al. The prevalence of premenstrual dysphoric disorder: Systematic review and meta-analysis. J Affect Disord. 2024;349:534–40.
12. American Psychiatric Association. Diagnostic and Statistical Manual of Mental Disorders: DSM-5. 5th edn. 2013.
13. Toffoletto S, Lanzenberger R, Gingnell M, Sundström-Poromaa I, Comasco E. Emotional and cognitive functional imaging of estrogen and progesterone effects in the female human brain: a systematic review. Psychoneuroendocrinology. 2014;50:28–52.
14. Tiranini L, Nappi RE. Recent advances in understanding/management of premenstrual dysphoric disorder/premenstrual syndrome. Fac Rev. 2022;11:11.
15. Granda D, Szmidt MK, Kaluza J. Is premenstrual syndrome associated with inflammation, oxidative stress and antioxidant status? A systematic review of case-control and cross-sectional studies. Antioxidants (Basel). 2021;10(4):604.
16. Gao Q, Sun W, Wang YR, Li ZF, Zhao F, Geng XW, et al. Role of allopregnanolone-mediated γ-aminobutyric acid a receptor sensitivity in the pathogenesis of premenstrual dysphoric disorder: Toward precise targets for translational medicine and drug development. Front Psychiatry. 2023;14:1140796.
17. Carlini SV, Lanza di Scalea T, McNally ST, Lester J, Deligiannidis KM. Management of premenstrual dysphoric disorder: a scoping review. Int J Womens Health. 2022;14:1783–801.
18. Lete I, Lapuente O. Contraceptive options for women with premenstrual dysphoric disorder: current insights and a narrative review. Open Access J Contracept. 2016;7:117–25.
19. Halbreich U, Freeman EW, Rapkin AJ, Cohen LS, Grubb GS, Bergeron R, et al. Continuous oral levonorgestrel/ethinyl estradiol for treating premenstrual dysphoric disorder. Contraception. 2012;85(1):19–27.
20. Regidor P-A, Schindler AE. Antiandrogenic and antimineralocorticoid health benefits of COC containing newer progestogens: dienogest and drospirenone. Oncotarget. 2017;8(47):83334–42.
21. Wichianpitaya J, Taneepanichskul S. A comparative efficacy of low-dose combined oral contraceptives containing desogestrel and drospirenone in premenstrual symptoms. Obstet Gynecol Int. 2013;2013:487143.
22. Genazzani AD, Sponzilli A, Mantovani M, Fusilli E, Ricciardiello F, Semprini E, et al. Modulatory effects of ethinyl estradiol plus drospirenone contraceptive pill on spontaneous and GnRH-induced LH secretion. Endocrines. 2024;5(1):36–45.
23. Ma S, Song SJ. Oral contraceptives containing drospirenone for premenstrual syndrome. Cochrane Database Syst Rev. 2023;6(6):CD006586.

24. Takeda T, Kondo A, Koga S, Hayakawa J, Hayakawa K, Hiramatsu K, et al. Effectiveness of ethinylestradiol/drospirenone for premenstrual symptoms in Japanese patients with dysmenorrhea: Open-label pilot study. J Obstet Gynaecol Res. 2015;41(10):1584–90.
25. Pearlstein TB, Bachmann GA, Zacur HA, Yonkers KA. Treatment of premenstrual dysphoric disorder with a new drospirenone-containing oral contraceptive formulation. Contraception. 2005;72(6):414–21.
26. de Wit AE, de Vries YA, de Boer MK, Scheper C, Fokkema A, Janssen CAH, et al. Efficacy of combined oral contraceptives for depressive symptoms and overall symptomatology in premenstrual syndrome: pairwise and network meta-analysis of randomized trials. Am J Obstet Gynecol. 2021;225(6):624–33.
27. Freeman EW, Halbreich U, Grubb GS, Rapkin AJ, Skouby SO, Smith L, et al. An overview of four studies of a continuous oral contraceptive (levonorgestrel 90 mcg/ethinyl estradiol 20 mcg) on premenstrual dysphoric disorder and premenstrual syndrome. Contraception. 2012;85(5):437–45.
28. Freeman EW, Kroll R, Rapkin A, Pearlstein T, Brown C, Parsey K, et al. Evaluation of a unique oral contraceptive in the treatment of premenstrual dysphoric disorder. J Womens Health Gend Based Med. 2001;10(6):561–9.
29. Marr J, Niknian M, Shulman LP, Lynen R. Premenstrual dysphoric disorder symptom cluster improvement by cycle with the combined oral contraceptive ethinylestradiol 20 mcg plus drospirenone 3 mg administered in a 24/4 regimen. Contraception. 2011;84(1):81–6.
30. Marr J, Heinemann K, Kunz M, Rapkin A. Ethinyl estradiol 20 µg/drospirenone 3 mg 24/4 oral contraceptive for the treatment of functional impairment in women with premenstrual dysphoric disorder. Int J Gynaecol Obstet. 2011;113(2):103–7.
31. Smith K, Nayyar S, Rana T, Archibong AE, Looney KR, Nayyar T. Do progestin-only contraceptives contribute to the risk of developing depression as implied by beta-Arrestin 1 levels in leukocytes? A pilot study. Int J Environ Res Public Health. 2018;15(9):1966.
32. Svendal G, Berk M, Pasco JA, Jacka FN, Lund A, Williams LJ. The use of hormonal contraceptive agents and mood disorders in women. J Affect Disord. 2012;140(1):92–6.
33. Kulkarni S, Gupta K, Ratre P, Mishra PK, Singh Y, Biharee A, et al. Polycystic ovary syndrome: current scenario and future insights. Drug Discov Today. 2023;28(12):103821.
34. Genazzani AD, Genazzani AR. Polycystic ovary syndrome as metabolic disease: new insights on insulin resistance. touchREV Endocrinol. 2023;19(1):71–7.
35. Christ JP, Cedars MI. Current guidelines for diagnosing PCOS. Diagnostics (Basel). 2023;13(6):1113.
36. Spritzer PM. Contraception for women with polycystic ovary syndrome: dealing with a complex condition. Rev Bras Ginecol Obstet. 2022;44(4):325–6.
37. Cowan S, Lim S, Alycia C, Pirotta S, Thomson R, Gibson-Helm M, et al. Lifestyle management in polycystic ovary syndrome – beyond diet and physical activity. BMC Endocr Disord. 2023;23(1):14.
38. Lim SS, Hutchison SK, Van Ryswyk E, Norman RJ, Teede HJ, Moran LJ. Lifestyle changes in women with polycystic ovary syndrome. Cochrane Database Syst Rev. 2019;3(3):CD007506.
39. Woodward A, Broom D, Harrop D, Lahart I, Carter A, Dalton C, et al. The effects of physical exercise on cardiometabolic outcomes in women with polycystic ovary syndrome not taking the oral contraceptive pill: a systematic review and meta-analysis. J Diabetes Metab Disord. 2019;18(2):597–612.
40. de Medeiros SF. Risks, benefits size and clinical implications of combined oral contraceptive use in women with polycystic ovary syndrome. Reprod Biol Endocrinol. 2017;15(1):93.
41. Forslund M, Melin J, Alesi S, Piltonen T, Romualdi D, Tay CT, et al. Different kinds of oral contraceptive pills in polycystic ovary syndrome: a systematic review and meta-analysis. Eur J Endocrinol. 2023;189(1):S1–S16.
42. Mathur R, Levin O, Azziz R. Use of ethinylestradiol/drospirenone combination in patients with the polycystic ovary syndrome. Ther Clin Risk Manag. 2008;4(2):487–92.

43. Haverinen AH, Luiro KM, Szanto T, Kangasniemi MH, Hiltunen L, Sainio S, et al. Combined oral contraceptives containing estradiol valerate vs ethinylestradiol on coagulation: a randomized clinical trial. Acta Obstet Gynecol Scand. 2022;101(10):1102–11.
44. Kovalevsky G, Ballagh SA, Stanczyk FZ, Lee J, Cooper J, Archer DF. Levonorgestrel effects on serum androgens, sex hormone-binding globulin levels, hair shaft diameter, and sexual function. Fertil Steril. 2010;93(6):1997–2003.
45. De Leo V, Fruzzetti F, Musacchio MC, Scolaro V, Di Sabatino A, Morgante G. Effect of a new oral contraceptive with estradiol valerate/dienogest on carbohydrate metabolism. Contraception. 2013;88(3):364–8.
46. Munro MG, Critchley HOD, Fraser IS, Committee FMD. The two FIGO systems for normal and abnormal uterine bleeding symptoms and classification of causes of abnormal uterine bleeding in the reproductive years: 2018 revisions. Int J Gynaecol Obstet. 2018;143(3):393–408.
47. Yaşa C, Güngör UF. Approach to abnormal uterine bleeding in adolescents. J Clin Res Pediatr Endocrinol. 2020;12(Suppl 1):1–6.
48. Elmaoğulları S, Aycan Z. Abnormal uterine bleeding in adolescents. J Clin Res Pediatr Endocrinol. 2018;10(3):191–7.
49. Bradley LD, Gueye NA. The medical management of abnormal uterine bleeding in reproductive-aged women. Am J Obstet Gynecol. 2016;214(1):31–44.
50. Nappi RE, Serrani M, Jensen JT. Noncontraceptive benefits of the estradiol valerate/dienogest combined oral contraceptive: a review of the literature. Int J Womens Health. 2014;6:711–8.
51. Rafie S, Borgelt L, Koepf ER, Temple-Cooper ME, Lehman KJ. Novel oral contraceptive for heavy menstrual bleeding: estradiol valerate and dienogest. Int J Womens Health. 2013;5:313–21.
52. Di Carlo C, Gargano V, Sparice S, Tommaselli GA, Bifulco G, Schettino D, et al. Short-term effects of an oral contraceptive containing oestradiol valerate and dienogest on bone metabolism and bone mineral density: an observational, preliminary study. Eur J Contracept Reprod Health Care. 2013;18(5):388–93.
53. Bachrach LK. Hormonal Contraception and Bone Health in Adolescents. Front Endocrinol (Lausanne). 2020;11:603.
54. Naib JM, Siddiqui MI, Ajmal W. The role of dydrogesterone in the medical management of 100 cases of Dysfunctional Uterine Bleeding (DUB) Above 35 years of age. J Postgrad Med Inst. 2011;17(2)
55. Armeni E, Paschou SA, Goulis DG, Lambrinoudaki I. Hormone therapy regimens for managing the menopause and premature ovarian insufficiency. Best Pract Res Clin Endocrinol Metab. 2021;35(6):101561.
56. Webber L, Davies M, Anderson R, Bartlett J, Braat D, Cartwright B, et al. ESHRE Guideline: management of women with premature ovarian insufficiency. Hum Reprod. 2016;31(5):926–37.
57. Meczekalski B, Niwczyk O, Bala G, Szeliga A. Managing early onset osteoporosis: the impact of premature ovarian insufficiency on bone health. J Clin Med. 2023;12(12):4042.
58. Genazzani AR, Fidecicchi T, Arduini D, Giannini A, Simoncini T. Hormonal and natural contraceptives: a review on efficacy and risks of different methods for an informed choice. Gynecol Endocrinol. 2023;39(1):2247093.
59. Gonçalves CR, Vasconcellos AS, Rodrigues TR, Comin FV, Reis FM. Hormone therapy in women with premature ovarian insufficiency: a systematic review and meta-analysis. Reprod Biomed Online. 2022;44(6):1143–57.
60. Zahradnik HP, Hanjalic-Beck A, Groth K. Nonsteroidal anti-inflammatory drugs and hormonal contraceptives for pain relief from dysmenorrhea: a review. Contraception. 2010;81(3):185–96.
61. Ferries-Rowe E, Corey E, Archer JS. Primary dysmenorrhea: diagnosis and therapy. Obstet Gynecol. 2020;136(5):1047–58.
62. Schroll JB, Black AY, Farquhar C, Chen I. Combined oral contraceptive pill for primary dysmenorrhoea. Cochrane Database Syst Rev. 2023;7(7):CD002120.

63. Hanjalic-Beck A, Schäfer WR, Deppert WR, Fischer L, Stein A, Seebacher L, et al. Chlormadinone acetate suppresses prostaglandin biosynthesis in human endometrial explants. Fertil Steril. 2012;98(4):1017–22.
64. Bourdon M, Santulli P, Marcellin L, Maignien C, Maitrot-Mantelet L, Bordonne C, et al. Adenomyosis: An update regarding its diagnosis and clinical features. J Gynecol Obstet Hum Reprod. 2021;50(10):102228.
65. Moldassarina RS. Modern view on the diagnostics and treatment of adenomyosis. Arch Gynecol Obstet. 2023;308(1):171–81.
66. Harmsen MJ, Van den Bosch T, de Leeuw RA, Dueholm M, Exacoustos C, Valentin L, et al. Consensus on revised definitions of Morphological Uterus Sonographic Assessment (MUSA) features of adenomyosis: results of modified Delphi procedure. Ultrasound Obstet Gynecol. 2022;60(1):118–31.
67. Maia H, Casoy J, Correia T, Freitas L, Pimentel K, Athayde C, et al. Effect of the menstrual cycle and oral contraceptives on aromatase and cyclooxygenase-2 expression in adenomyosis. Gynecol Endocrinol. 2006;22(10):547–51.
68. Vannuccini S, Luisi S, Tosti C, Sorbi F, Petraglia F. Role of medical therapy in the management of uterine adenomyosis. Fertil Steril. 2018;109(3):398–405.
69. Kelekci S, Kelekci KH, Yilmaz B. Effects of levonorgestrel-releasing intrauterine system and T380A intrauterine copper device on dysmenorrhea and days of bleeding in women with and without adenomyosis. Contraception. 2012;86(5):458–63.
70. Niu X, Luo Q, Wang C, Zhu L, Huang L. Effects of Etonogestrel implants on pelvic pain and menstrual flow in women suffering from adenomyosis or endometriosis: results from a prospective, observational study. Medicine (Baltimore). 2021;100(6):e24597.
71. Yu EH, Joo JK. Commentary on the new 2022 European Society of Human Reproduction and Embryology (ESHRE) endometriosis guidelines. Clin Exp Reprod Med. 2022;49(4):219–24.
72. Becker CM, Bokor A, Heikinheimo O, Horne A, Jansen F, Kiesel L, et al. ESHRE guideline: endometriosis. Hum Reprod Open. 2022;2022(2):hoac009.
73. Grandi G, Barra F, Ferrero S, Sileo FG, Bertucci E, Napolitano A, et al. Hormonal contraception in women with endometriosis: a systematic review. Eur J Contracept Reprod Health Care. 2019;24(1):61–70.
74. Grandi G, Mueller M, Bersinger NA, Cagnacci A, Volpe A, McKinnon B. Does dienogest influence the inflammatory response of endometriotic cells?A systematic review. Inflamm Res. 2016;65(3):183–92.
75. Męczekalski B, Niwczyk O, Battipaglia C, Troia L, Kostrzak A, Bala G, et al. Neuroendocrine disturbances in women with functional hypothalamic amenorrhea: an update and future directions. Endocrine. 2023;84(3):769–85.
76. Indirli R, Lanzi V, Mantovani G, Arosio M, Ferrante E. Bone health in functional hypothalamic amenorrhea: what the endocrinologist needs to know. Front Endocrinol (Lausanne). 2022;13:946695.
77. Battipaglia C, Petrillo T, Semprini E, Ricciardiello F, Rusce ML, Prampolini G, et al. Low-dose estrogens as neuroendocrine modulators in Functional Hypothalamic Amenorrhea (FHA): the putative triggering of the positive feedback mechanism(s). Biomedicines. 2023;11(6):1763.
78. Warren MP, Miller KK, Olson WH, Grinspoon SK, Friedman AJ. Effects of an oral contraceptive (norgestimate/ethinyl estradiol) on bone mineral density in women with hypothalamic amenorrhea and osteopenia: an open-label extension of a double-blind, placebo-controlled study. Contraception. 2005;72(3):206–11.

Chapter 25
Combined Hormonal Contraceptives Effects on Brain and Mood: A Focus on Migraine

Rossella E. Nappi, Lara Tiranini, Manuela Piccinino, Roberta Rossini, Ellis Martini, Chiara Placentino, Greta Monne, Giulia Martina Colombo, Giorgia Elisabetta Parrotta, and Laura Cucinella

25.1 Introduction

Combined hormonal contraceptives (CHCs) are considered one of the most important public health achievements of the last century [1]. The majority of CHCs have ethinylestradiol (EE) as the estrogenic component at different doses, whereas oral options containing natural estrogens (estradiol valerate, estradiol, and estetrol) have become available more recently with the aim of reducing the cardiometabolic impact [2]. The progestogenic component of CHCs includes several classes of molecules differing in potency, affinity for steroid receptors, interaction with estrogens, and physiological effects [3]. Alternative routes of administration have been proposed, including the vaginal, and transdermal route, to increase efficacy, compliance, and tolerance as compared to the traditional oral route [4]. "Pills" have significantly evolved also in terms of administration regimens, moving from the traditional 21/7 to the 24/4 and even 26/2,

R. E. Nappi (✉) · C. Placentino · G. Monne · G. M. Colombo · G. E. Parrotta · L. Cucinella
Department of Clinical, Surgical, Diagnostic and Pediatric Sciences, University of Pavia, Pavia, Italy

Research Center for Reproductive Medicine, Gynecological Endocrinology and Menopause, IRCCS San Matteo Foundation, Pavia, Italy

L. Tiranini
Obstetrics and Gynecology Unit, IRCCS San Matteo Foundation, Pavia, Italy

M. Piccinino · R. Rossini · E. Martini
Department of Clinical, Surgical, Diagnostic and Pediatric Sciences, University of Pavia, Pavia, Italy

A. R. Genazzani et al. (eds.), *Ethical, Efficacy and Safety Issues in Contraception*, Reproductive Medicine for Clinicians 4,
https://doi.org/10.1007/978-3-032-07322-8_25

with the goal of minimizing the impact of the HFI on women's well-being, along with improvement of ovarian suppression for contraceptive efficacy and therapeutic purposes [5]. Extended, continuous, and flexible regimens have been proposed for those women who wish to avoid monthly withdrawal bleeding to gain extra-contraceptive or lifestyle benefits [6].

Here, we briefly summarize the impact of CHCs on brain and mood with a focus on migraine.

25.2 Brain Impact of CHCs

Sex hormones modulate a number of brain functions [7], and CHCs do not have uniform effects within the central nervous system (CNS) because the variable combinations in terms of type and dose of estrogens and progestogens may have a diverse impact on the complex balance affecting neuroplasticity and individual mood vulnerabilities [8]. CHCs may contribute to the onset of negative mood by decreasing endogenous estrogen levels. On the other hand, the estrogenic component of CHCs may exert an antidepressant effect [9]. The progestogenic component seems to contribute significantly to mood and behaviour by exerting a direct effect on the CNS and an indirect effect, being converted into active neurosteroids such as allopregnanolone. Different progestogens have peculiar effects depending on their ability to modulate the neuroendocrine balance, integrating reproductive function with emotional and executive aspects [10]. Both human and rodent studies have shown that brain structure and function vary with naturally cycling ovarian hormones [11, 12], and CHCs may be considered as endocrine disruptor of mood, pain, and other brain-mediated functions in vulnerable women [13, 14]. However, the majority of women adapt quite well to the new neuroendocrine balance induced by the use of CHCs, and negative mood effects are infrequent (4–10%) [14]. It is important to remember that women who suffer adverse effects from CHC may have underlying physiological or psychological differences [14], and depressive symptoms in adolescent CHC users should be considered [15]. In fact, CHC may lead to side effects, including deterioration of mood, especially in vulnerable women (i.e., those with a previous diagnosis of mood, anxiety, or eating disorders) [16].

On the other hand, CHCs may represent an option for treatment of premenstrual disorders (premenstrual syndrome/premenstrual dysphoric disorder) given the blockade of the ovulatory surge of sex steroids [17]. Indeed, premenstrual disorders are not observed during anovulatory cycles and disappear when women undergo treatment with agonists of gonadotropin releasing hormone (GnRH) or bilateral oophorectomy [18]. Women with premenstrual symptoms are more sensitive to normal, fluctuating concentrations of gonadal steroids [18]. For this reason, extended regimens or with shorter HFI seem to offer better results [19], especially with the use of an anti-androgenic progestogen such as drospirenone [20].

25.3 CHCs and Migraine

Migraine disproportionately affects women, particularly during their reproductive years, due to the complex interplay of hormonal, neurological, and lifestyle factors [21]. It is a neurobiological disorder characterized by recurrent unilateral, pulsating headache of moderate to severe intensity, lasting up to 72 h, and associated with nausea, vomiting, photophobia, or phonophobia [22]. The most frequent subtype is migraine without aura, whereas one in four migraineurs experience an aura, which is a cluster of transient positive or negative neurological symptoms before headache onset, each lasting 20–30 min [22, 23]. Migraine is two to three times more prevalent in women than in men, with 17% of all women meeting the diagnostic criteria for migraine [23]. The prevalence of migraine varies across different life stages, with peaks during puberty, childbearing years, and around perimenopause, reflecting the influence of hormonal changes on migraine patterns [24]. Understanding the interplay between hormones and migraine is essential to optimize diagnostic and therapeutic approaches for affected women.

Estrogens influence nociceptive and inflammatory pathogenetic mechanisms of migraine by acting on brain circuitries and pelvic function in women [25]. The so-called theory of hormonal balance in the trigeminal ganglion has been proposed, taking into account the role of estrogens, oxytocin and calcitonin gene-related peptide (CGRP) in the pathogenesis of migraine [26]. The activation of trigeminal nociceptors by cortical spreading depression, which facilitates intracranial vasculature and meningeal inflammation, enhances head pain [27]. When estrogens are present, it is likely that the balance shifts toward protection from migraine; when they are absent, the balance shifts toward vulnerability [26]. The modulation of progesterone and androgenic milieu has been less investigated [25].

Hormonal fluctuations in spontaneous menstrual cycles or with administration of exogenous sex steroids by using CHCs or even hormone replacement therapy influence the clinical characteristics of migraine attacks [28–30]. Historically, CHCs have been shown to exert an aggravation of migraine in 18–50% of cases, an improvement in 3–35% and no change in 39–65% [31]. A more recent cross-sectional study on a large population found that migraine is significantly associated with CHCs, but no causal relationship between exposure and disease could be demonstrated [32]. Analysis of the different effect of the CHCs on the two forms of migraine revealed that migraine with aura worsens more (56.4%) than migraine without aura (25.3%) [33]. The cyclical decline of estrogen during the late luteal phase is a well-established trigger for menstrual migraines, which tend to be more severe and less responsive to treatment compared to nonmenstrual migraines [34]. Migraine headaches frequently occur during the HFI (so-called estrogen withdrawal), and when pharmacologically induced, they are long-lasting, very intense, and less responsive to treatment, especially in women who suffered from migraines before CHCs use [35]. Hormonal contraception can have variable effects on migraine, influenced by the type of contraception used and the individual's migraine history. CHCs, which contain both estrogen and progestin, may stabilize hormonal fluctuations and potentially reduce the frequency of menstrual migraines in some women by maintaining steady estrogen levels [25, 36]. The current availability of oral regimens with a shorter (6, 4, or 2 days) or absent HFI can prevent migraine worsening in the HFI, modulating pain threshold and leading to decreases in frequency, intensity, and duration [36, 37]. Indeed, those hormonal contraceptive regimens (continuous or extended-cycle), which eliminate or shorten the HFI, have been recommended as therapeutic strategies, potentially reducing migraine frequency and severity by maintaining stable hormone levels and preventing withdrawal effects [38]. Another potential strategy is to prevent estrogen withdrawal in natural cycles or in standard 21/7 regimens with low dose of transdermal estradiol, which has shown mixed results [39].

The main concern for CHCs use in women with migraine is vascular risk and, specifically, stroke risk [40]. CHCs are not contraindicated for women with migraines without aura and menstrual migraine [41]. However, they can induce the onset of aura in women who have not experienced this symptom in the past [41]. Women with migraine with aura are advised to exercise caution when using CHCs, as they may have an increased risk of ischemic stroke, especially if additional risk factors like smoking or hypertension are present [42]. Indeed, migraine with aura carries around a twofold increased risk of stroke [43]. Thus, it constitutes a contraindication to CHC use [39], whereas progestin-only contraceptives can be safely used [42] and may even provide some benefits to the clinical pattern of migraine with aura [44]. There is some hope that CHC containing natural estrogens can become the gold standard for women suffering from migraines, both for the possible favourable impact on the course of pain attacks [45] and for their lower cardiovascular and thromboembolic risk [2, 46]. Future research should further investigate the impact of CHC containing natural estrogens on migraines, especially on migraine with aura [47].

25.4 Conclusions

Sex hormones are potent psychoactive agents used with the aim of aligning reproduction to emotional and cognitive aspects that characterize human behavior. CHCs composition has continuously evolved over the years with the aim of improving safety, efficacy, tolerability, and noncontraceptive benefits. However, their ability to affect brain functions involved in mood and pain threshold has to be considered in clinical practice. Education and awareness are important components in the management of possible side effects of CHCs on the CNS. Knowledge of the current contraceptive options and provision of personalized, high-quality care to support each woman's decision-making process are the key elements to minimize side effects and enhance overall satisfaction.

Declarations

Competing Interests The author(s) has no competing interests to declare that are relevant to the content of this manuscript.

Ethics Approval The author(s) declares that this manuscript does not include primary research with human participants.

The author(s) declares that this manuscript does not include primary studies involving animals.

References

1. Genazzani AR, Fidecicchi T, Arduini D, Giannini A, Simoncini T. Hormonal and natural contraceptives: a review on efficacy and risks of different methods for an informed choice. Gynecol Endocrinol. 2023;39(1):2247093. https://doi.org/10.1080/09513590.2023.2247093.
2. Stanczyk FZ, Winer SA, Foidart JM, Archer DF. Comparison of estrogenic components used for hormonal contraception. Contraception. 2024;130:110310. https://doi.org/10.1016/j.contraception.2023.110310.
3. Schindler AE, Campagnoli C, Druckmann R, Huber J, Pasqualini JR, Schweppe KW, Thijssen JH. Classification and pharmacology of progestins. Maturitas. 2003;10(46 Suppl 1):S7–S16. https://doi.org/10.1016/j.maturitas.2003.09.014.
4. Bounous VE, Actis S, Rosso R, Giorgi M, Tiranini L, Nappi RE, Biglia N. No-daily hormonal contraception today: general overview and application in specific clinical settings. Gynecol Endocrinol. 2023;39(1):2214626. https://doi.org/10.1080/09513590.2023.2214626.
5. Christin-Maitre S. History of oral contraceptive drugs and their use worldwide. Best Pract Res Clin Endocrinol Metab. 2013;27(1):3–12. https://doi.org/10.1016/j.beem.2012.11.004.
6. Nappi RE, Kaunitz AM, Bitzer J. Extended regimen combined oral contraception: a review of evolving concepts and acceptance by women and clinicians. Eur J Contracept Reprod Health Care. 2016;21(2):106–15. https://doi.org/10.3109/13625187.2015.1107894.
7. Genazzani AR, Gastaldi M, Bidzinska B, Mercuri N, Genazzani AD, Nappi RE, Segre A, Petraglia F. The brain as a target organ of gonadal steroids. Psychoneuroendocrinology. 1992;17(4):385–90. https://doi.org/10.1016/0306-4530(92)90043-7.
8. Kundakovic M, Rocks D. Sex hormone fluctuation and increased female risk for depression and anxiety disorders: from clinical evidence to molecular mechanisms. Front Neuroendocrinol. 2022;66:101010. https://doi.org/10.1016/j.yfrne.2022.101010.
9. Maki PM, Kornstein SG, Joffe H, Bromberger JT, Freeman EW, Athappilly G, Bobo WV, Rubin LH, Koleva HK, Cohen LS, Soares CN, Board of Trustees for The North American Menopause Society (NAMS) and the Women and Mood Disorders Task Force of the National Network of Depression Centers. Guidelines for the evaluation and treatment of perimenopausal depression: summary and recommendations. Menopause. 2018;25(10):1069–85. https://doi.org/10.1097/GME.0000000000001174.
10. Pluchino N, Cubeddu A, Giannini A, Merlini S, Cela V, Angioni S, Genazzani AR. Progestogens and brain: an update. Maturitas. 2009;62(4):349–55. https://doi.org/10.1016/j.maturitas.2008.11.023.
11. Porcu P, Serra M, Concas A. The brain as a target of hormonal contraceptives: evidence from animal studies. Front Neuroendocrinol. 2019;55:100799. https://doi.org/10.1016/j.yfrne.2019.100799.
12. Rehbein E, Hornung J, Sundström Poromaa I, Derntl B. Shaping of the female human brain by sex hormones: a review. Neuroendocrinology. 2021;111(3):183–206. https://doi.org/10.1159/000507083.

13. Fruzzetti F, Fidecicchi T. Hormonal contraception and depression: updated evidence and implications in clinical practice. Clin Drug Investig. 2020;40(12):1097–106. https://doi.org/10.1007/s40261-020-00966-8.
14. Schaffir J, Worly BL, Gur TL. Combined hormonal contraception and its effects on mood: a critical review. Eur J Contracept Reprod Health Care. 2016;21(5):347–55. https://doi.org/10.1080/13625187.2016.1217327.
15. Kraft MZ, Rojczyk P, Weiss T, Derntl B, Kikinis Z, Croy I, Heller C. Symptoms of mental disorders and oral contraception use: a systematic review and meta-analysis. Front Neuroendocrinol. 2024;72:101111. https://doi.org/10.1016/j.yfrne.2023.101111.
16. Bengtsdotter H, Lundin C, Gemzell Danielsson K, Bixo M, Baumgart J, Marions L, Brynhildsen J, Malmborg A, Lindh I, Sundström Poromaa I. Ongoing or previous mental disorders predispose to adverse mood reporting during combined oral contraceptive use. Eur J Contracept Reprod Health Care. 2018;23(1):45–51. https://doi.org/10.1080/13625187.2017.1422239.
17. Stute P, Bodmer C, Ehlert U, Eltbogen R, Ging A, Streuli I, von Wolff M. Interdisciplinary consensus on management of premenstrual disorders in Switzerland. Gynecol Endocrinol. 2017;33(5):342–8. https://doi.org/10.1080/09513590.2017.1284788.
18. Tiranini L, Nappi RE. Recent advances in understanding/management of premenstrual dysphoric disorder/premenstrual syndrome. Fac Rev. 2022;11:11. https://doi.org/10.12703/r/11-11.
19. Sulak PJ, Cressman BE, Waldrop E, Holleman S, Kuehl TJ. Extending the duration of active oral contraceptive pills to manage hormone withdrawal symptoms. Obstet Gynecol. 1997;89(2):179–83. https://doi.org/10.1016/S0029-7844(96)00488-7.
20. Rapkin AJ, Korotkaya Y, Taylor KC. Contraception counseling for women with premenstrual dysphoric disorder (PMDD): current perspectives. Open Access J Contracept. 2019;10:27–39. https://doi.org/10.2147/OAJC.S183193.
21. Barbanti P, Nappi RE. Framing and management of migraines in women: an expert opinion on challenges, current approaches, and future multidisciplinary perspectives. Healthcare (Basel). 2025;13(2):164. https://doi.org/10.3390/healthcare13020164.
22. Headache classification Committee of the International Headache Society (IHS) the international classification of headache disorders, 3rd edition. Cephalalgia. 2018;38(1):1–211.
23. Vetvik KG, MacGregor EA. Sex differences in the epidemiology, clinical features, and pathophysiology of migraine. Lancet Neurol. 2017;16(1):76–87. https://doi.org/10.1016/S1474-4422(16)30293-9.
24. Nappi RE, Nappi G. Neuroendocrine aspects of migraine in women. Gynecol Endocrinol. 2012;28(Suppl 1):37–41. https://doi.org/10.3109/09513590.2012.651931.
25. Nappi RE, Tiranini L, Sacco S, De Matteis E, De Icco R, Tassorelli C. Role of estrogens in menstrual migraine. Cells. 2022;11(8):1355. https://doi.org/10.3390/cells11081355.
26. Krause DN, Warfvinge K, Haanes KA, Edvinsson L. Hormonal influences in migraine—interactions of oestrogen, oxytocin and CGRP. Nat Rev Neurol. 2021;17(10):621–33. https://doi.org/10.1038/s41582-021-00544-2.
27. Zhang X, Levy D, Kainz V, Noseda R, Jakubowski M, Burstein R. Activation of central trigeminovascular neurons by cortical spreading depression. Ann Neurol. 2011;69(5):855–65. https://doi.org/10.1002/ana.22329.
28. van Casteren DS, Verhagen IE, van der Arend BWH, van Zwet EW, MaassenVanDenBrink A, Terwindt GM. Comparing perimenstrual and nonperimenstrual migraine attacks using an e-diary. Neurology. 2021;97(17):e1661–71. https://doi.org/10.1212/WNL.0000000000012723.
29. Nappi RE, Sances G, Brundu B, De Taddei S, Sommacal A, Ghiotto N, Polatti F, Nappi G. Estradiol supplementation modulates neuroendocrine response to M-chlorophenylpiperazine in menstrual status migrainosus triggered by oral contraception-free interval. Hum Reprod. 2005;20(12):3423–8. https://doi.org/10.1093/humrep/dei260.

30. Facchinetti F, Nappi RE, Tirelli A, Polatti F, Nappi G, Sances G. Hormone supplementation differently affects migraine in postmenopausal women. Headache. 2002;42(9):924–9. https://doi.org/10.1046/j.1526-4610.2002.02215.x.
31. Massiou H, MacGregor EA. Evolution and treatment of migraine with oral contraceptives. Cephalalgia. 2000;20(3):170–4. https://doi.org/10.1046/j.1468-2982.2000.00038.x.
32. Aegidius K, Zwart JA, Hagen K, Schei B, Stovner LJ. Oral contraceptives and increased headache prevalence: the head-HUNT study. Neurology. 2006;66(3):349–53. https://doi.org/10.1212/01.wnl.0000196481.57994.09.
33. Granella F, Sances G, Pucci E, Nappi RE, Ghiotto N, Napp G. Migraine with aura and reproductive life events: a case control study. Cephalalgia. 2000;20(8):701–7. https://doi.org/10.1111/j.1468-2982.2000.00112.x.
34. Granella F, Sances G, Allais G, Nappi RE, Tirelli A, Benedetto C, Brundu B, Facchinetti F, Nappi G. Characteristics of menstrual and nonmenstrual attacks in women with menstrually related migraine referred to headache centres. Cephalalgia. 2004;24(9):707–16. https://doi.org/10.1111/j.1468-2982.2004.00741.x.
35. Merki-Feld GS, Sandor PS, Nappi RE, Pohl H, Schankin C. Clinical features of migraine with onset prior to or during start of combined hormonal contraception: a prospective cohort study. Acta Neurol Belg. 2022;122(2):401–9. https://doi.org/10.1007/s13760-021-01677-3.
36. Tiranini L, Cucinella L, Martella S, Bosoni D, Martini E, Nappi RE. Is now the time to reconsider risks, benefits, and limitations of estrogen preparations as a treatment for menstrually related migraine? Expert Rev Neurother. 2023;23(4):377–88. https://doi.org/10.1080/14737175.2023.2198705.
37. De Icco R, Cucinella L, De Paoli I, Martella S, Sances G, Bitetto V, Sandrini G, Nappi G, Tassorelli C, Nappi RE. Modulation of nociceptive threshold by combined hormonal contraceptives in women with oestrogen-withdrawal migraine attacks: a pilot study. J Headache Pain. 2016;17(1):70. https://doi.org/10.1186/s10194-016-0661-6.
38. Sulak PJ, Scow RD, Preece C, Riggs MW, Kuehl TJ. Hormone withdrawal symptoms in oral contraceptive users. Obstet Gynecol. 2000;95(2):261–6. https://doi.org/10.1016/s0029-7844(99)00524-4.
39. Sacco S, Merki-Feld GS, Ægidius KL, Bitzer J, Canonico M, Gantenbein AR, Kurth T, Lampl C, Lidegaard Ø, Anne MacGregor E, MaassenVanDenBrink A, Mitsikostas DD, Nappi RE, Ntaios G, Paemeleire K, Sandset PM, Terwindt GM, Vetvik KG, Martelletti P, European Headache Federation (EHF), the European Society of Contraception and Reproductive Health (ESCRH). Effect of exogenous estrogens and progestogens on the course of migraine during reproductive age: a consensus statement by the European Headache Federation (EHF) and the European Society of Contraception and Reproductive Health (ESCRH). J Headache Pain. 2018;19(1):76. https://doi.org/10.1186/s10194-018-0896-5.
40. Ornello R, Canonico M, Merki-Feld GS, Kurth T, Lidegaard Ø, MacGregor EA, Lampl C, Nappi RE, Martelletti P, Sacco S. Migraine, low-dose combined hormonal contraceptives, and ischemic stroke in young women: a systematic review and suggestions for future research. Expert Rev Neurother. 2020;20(4):313–7. https://doi.org/10.1080/14737175.2020.1730816.
41. Sacco S, Merki-Feld GS, Ægidius KL, Bitzer J, Canonico M, Kurth T, Lampl C, Lidegaard Ø, Anne MacGregor E, MaassenVanDenBrink A, Mitsikostas DD, Nappi RE, Ntaios G, Sandset PM, Martelletti P, European Headache Federation (EHF) and the European Society of Contraception and Reproductive Health (ESC). Hormonal contraceptives and risk of ischemic stroke in women with migraine: a consensus statement from the European Headache Federation (EHF) and the European Society of Contraception and Reproductive Health (ESC). J Headache Pain. 2017;18(1):108. https://doi.org/10.1186/s10194-017-0815-1.
42. Nappi RE, Merki-Feld GS, Terreno E, Pellegrinelli A, Viana M. Hormonal contraception in women with migraine: is progestogen-only contraception a better choice? J Headache Pain. 2013;14(1):66. https://doi.org/10.1186/1129-2377-14-66.

43. Chiang MC, Dumitrascu OM, Chhabra N, Chiang CC. Migraine with visual aura and the risk of stroke- a narrative review. J Stroke Cerebrovasc Dis. 2021;30(11):106067. https://doi.org/10.1016/j.jstrokecerebrovasdis.2021.106067.
44. Nappi RE, Sances G, Allais G, Terreno E, Benedetto C, Vaccaro V, Polatti F, Facchinetti F. Effects of an estrogen-free, desogestrel-containing oral contraceptive in women with migraine with aura: a prospective diary-based pilot study. Contraception. 2011;83(3):223–8. https://doi.org/10.1016/j.contraception.2010.07.024.
45. Nappi RE, Terreno E, Sances G, Martini E, Tonani S, Santamaria V, Tassorelli C, Spinillo A. Effect of a contraceptive pill containing estradiol valerate and dienogest (E2V/DNG) in women with menstrually-related migraine (MRM). Contraception. 2013;88(3):369–75. https://doi.org/10.1016/j.contraception.2013.02.001.
46. Didembourg M, Locquet M, Raskin L, Tchimchoua BT, Dogné JM, Beaudart C, Douxfils J. Lower reporting of venous thromboembolisms events with natural estrogen-based combined oral contraceptives compared to ethinylestradiol-containing pills: a disproportionality analysis of the Eudravigilance database. Contraception. 2025;142:110727. https://doi.org/10.1016/j.contraception.2024.110727.
47. Lee CD, Nappi RE, Cwiak C. Oral contraceptives for menstrual migraine with Aura. N Engl J Med. 2023;389(22):2102–4. https://doi.org/10.1056/NEJMclde2303811.

Chapter 26
The Importance of Individual Choice

Macaluso Sara, Andrea Giannini, Tiziana Fidecicchi, Stefano Luisi, Tommaso Simoncini, and Andrea R. Genazzani

26.1 Contraceptive Pill and Its Central Effect

Contraceptive pill, in combination or progestin-only pills, is the most popular contraceptive method worldwide (22.9%). According to World Contraceptive Use 2015 (UN), 56% of women aged 20–45 years who are married or in a union use contraception. The choice of contraceptive method is usually determined by patient preference, tolerability, and side effects [1]. When choosing the best contraceptive pill for their patients, clinicians should consider the impact of hormonal therapies on female brain vulnerability. The female brain is a complex dynamic system in which hormonal factors (with their ultradian, circadian, monthly, and seasonal secretions), genetic, interpersonal factors, developmental, and social factors play an important role.

26.2 Neurotransmission and Brain Function

Endogenous hormone secretion and oral administration determine changes in neurotransmission patterns. Firstly, estrogen and its receptors ERa and ERb directly modify neurotransmission by promoting memory and learning, increasing arousal, and stimulating attention and reward. Furthermore, progesterone and its metabolites act as $GABA_A$ agonists, producing an anxiolytic effect. In addition, progesterone has several other neuroendocrine effects, such as on norepinephrine and dopamine

M. Sara · A. Giannini (✉) · T. Fidecicchi · S. Luisi · T. Simoncini · A. R. Genazzani
Division of Obstetrics and Gynecology, Department of Clinical and Experimental Medicine, University of Pisa, Pisa, Italy
e-mail: andrea.giannini@unipi.it; stefano.luisi@unipi.it; tommaso.simoncini@unipi.it

A. R. Genazzani et al. (eds.), *Ethical, Efficacy and Safety Issues in Contraception*, Reproductive Medicine for Clinicians 4,
https://doi.org/10.1007/978-3-032-07322-8_26

turnover, mood disorders, mood, and pain threshold. Specifically, to be effective as a neurosteroid, progesterone (stored in neurons, oligodendrocytes and type 1 and 2 astrocytes) is converted by 5a-reductase into 5a-dihydroprogesterone and then by 3α-hydroxysteroid dehydrogenase (3a-HSD) into allopregnanolone (ALLO). Allopregnanolone, together with other neurosteroids such as dehydroepiandrosterone (DHEA) and pregnenolone, with their sulfated derivatives DHEA sulfate (DHEAS) and pregnenolone sulfate, and progesterone and deoxycorticosterone, mediate their effects through ion-gated neurotransmitter receptors rather than the classical steroid hormone nuclear receptors.

26.3 Neurosteroids and Their Variations During a Woman's Life

Neurosteroids levels are modified by neurodegenerative conditions (i.e., Alzheimer's and Parkinson's diseases, multiple sclerosis) or in other mental diseases (i.e., depression, schizophrenia) or brain trauma diseases. They may have an important role in physiological conditions, such as the reorganization of gray and white matter during intrauterine life, puberty, and adolescence or as a consequence of emotional/cognitive responses. These variations in reproductive experience imply that central neurosteroidogenesis may influence, or may be influenced by, circulating endogenous or exogenous steroids. In particular, during women's fertile life, ALLO circulating levels seem to vary according to the menstrual cycle, as they are secreted by corpus luteum, showing higher levels in the luteal than in the follicular phase, probably contributing to preserve the woman against mood changes typical of the luteal phase. Furthermore, it has been observed that women suffering from premenstrual syndrome (PMS) have both low ALLO basal levels and high DHEA levels in the luteal phase, suggesting that the onset of premenstrual anxiety may depend on the interplay of neurosteroids with different $GABA_A$ receptor activity within the central nervous system. In women with PMS, then the responses of ALLO and progesterone to gonadotropin-releasing hormone stimulation seem to be significantly blunted. This leads to the hypothesis that patients with PMS may suffer from an inadequate production of ovarian neuroactive steroids, especially in the luteal phase [2]. Thus, both pathological and physiological conditions affect the production of neurosteroids during a woman's reproductive life. Instead, when the administration of exogenous sex steroids is taken into consideration, the study of the neurosteroids response becomes more complex. Mood changes in response to changes in neurosteroids are one of the controversial effects of oral contraceptives. Retrospective studies have reported negative mood changes in 10–30% of oral contraceptive users. Mood changes, especially depression (less commonly nervousness, irritability, anxiety, and sexual complaints), are one of the main reasons given for discontinuing oral contraceptives [3].

26.4 Hormonal Contraception and Mental Health

Skovlund et al., in a nationwide prospective cohort study data from psychiatric hospitals in Denmark, analyze the association between use of hormonal contraception and use of antidepressants. The study results showed that compared with nonusers, users of combined oral contraceptives experienced a 1.8-fold higher rate (95% CI, 1.75–1.84) of first use of antidepressants; users of progestin-only pills experienced a 2.2-fold higher rate (95% CI, 1.99–2.52) of it. Nonoral products implied a threefold increased risk for first use of antidepressants. Use of hormonal contraception was associated with subsequent use of antidepressants and a first diagnosis of depression, suggesting depression as a potential adverse effect of hormonal contraceptive use. Adolescents seemed more vulnerable to this risk than women aged 20–34 years old [4].

Adolescence is a period characterized by endogenous sex hormone changes and changing external cultural and social demands, which are likely to increase the influence of any additional factor that might cause mood disturbance, such as the use of hormonal contraception. In addition to being associated with an increased risk of developing depression, the use of oral contraceptives appears to be associated with an increased suicide and suicide attempt rate. Lidegaard et al., in a nationwide prospective cohort study, demonstrated that adolescent women are more sensitive than older women to the hormonal contraceptive influence on risk of a first suicide attempt [5].

As adolescent women are particularly vulnerable to risk factors for suicide attempt, this may come from attrition of susceptible women. In particular, it is not clear whether the emotional side effects of oral contraception are due to pharmacological or psychological mechanisms.

In women with adverse mood during oral contraceptive treatment, potential mediators of the process have been identified: psychiatric history (previous depressive episode, anxiety, and PMS), socioeconomic factors, interpersonal relationships (such as "fear of pregnancy"), psychological expectations, and indirect pharmacological factors (such as somatic changes, weight gain, or acne reduction), or even particular personality traits [3, 6].

Higher scores on particular personality traits, such as somatic anxiety and stress sensitivity, are found in women with ongoing experience of adverse mood symptoms from COC. Women who discontinued COC treatment because of adverse mood effects had higher scores for mistrust and detachment that had previously occurred [7].

In terms of an OC-related effect on affect variability, Felthous and Robinson (1981) suggest that monophasic OCs may stabilize and affect across the cycle by stabilizing cycle fluctuations, although there is no clear consensus on how the neurotransmitters work [8].

26.5 Progesterone Receptor Distribution and Its Association with Suicide

Neurosteroids can trigger biological functions in the human hypothalamus in health and disease, for example, by acting on specific stress-related neuropeptide or neurotransmitter systems. Considering the recent studies that have associated peripheral progesterone levels with suicidality and mood disorders, D. Swaab et al. conducted a study in which they mapped progesterone receptor (PR) distribution in the human hypothalamus in relation to age and sex and characterized its coexpression in specific cell types. PR+ cells were identified across various hypothalamic nuclei, with the most intense expression observed in the preoptic area (POA), infundibular nucleus (INF), ventromedial nucleus (VMN), and dorsomedial nucleus (DMN). These findings indicate that PR is present from fetal development through adulthood, with notable sex differences observed in certain structures. In particular, PR expression was stronger in male subjects before puberty and increased with age in elderly individuals. PR was coexpressed in neural progenitors and peptidergic neurons, including pro-opiomelanocortin (POMC) and neuropeptide Y (NPY) neurons. Notably, increased numbers of PR/POMC+ neurons were found in the INF of suicide completers with mood disorders (MD), suggesting a link between progesterone and the opioid system in suicidality. In contrast, NPY+ neurons were significantly reduced in the INF of MD patients, but this reduction did not correlate with PR expression. Reciprocal innervation between POMC+, NPY+, corticotropin-releasing hormone (CRH)+, and thyrotropin-releasing hormone (TRH) + neurons was observed, highlighting a complex network involved in stress regulation. These findings support the hypothesis that progesterone may influence suicidality through its effect on specific peptidergic systems in the hypothalamus, with implications for understanding the molecular mechanisms underlying MD and suicide. The study also suggests that females with MD who use hormonal contraception with high progesterone levels may be particularly vulnerable to these effects [9].

26.6 The Different Role of Different Progestins

Further studies have shown how different progesterone molecules can affect negative mood changes in different ways. For example, Bäckström et al. [10] showed that the monophasic desogestrel pill produced fewer changes in mood parameters than the monophasic and triphasic levonorgestrel oral contraceptive regimens [10].

Chlormadinone acetate (CMA), an acetylated progestin structurally related to progesterone, has strong clinical evidence of mood-balancing effects.

Results from the Coss study, an observational study published in 2007, showed that depressive symptoms reported before the start of the study were reduced in more than 60% of women who started CMA/EE treatment. There are also interesting data from women who have switched from the pill to CMA; most of them had previously been using nortestosterone-type progestins. The most common reasons for switching were seborrhea/acne cycle irregularities, headache, breast tenderness, amenorrhea, spotting, and dysmenorrhea. After switching to CMA/EE treatment, many women experienced a significant reduction or disappearance of these symptoms. The results showed that 80.5% of women were satisfied or much more satisfied with CMA/EE compared to their previous contraceptive [11, 12].

A controlled, double-blind pilot study conducted by Contreras et al. investigated the efficacy of a 5-day premenstrual tapering regimen of chlormadinone acetate for premenstrual dysphoric disorder. Patients received an initial dose of 10 mg (five 2-mg tablets) on day 24 of the menstrual cycle, and one-fifth of the dose was reduced each day until a dose of 2 mg (one 2-mg tablet) was reached on day 28 of the menstrual cycle.

The study showed that the 5-day tapering regimen of chlormadinone significantly improved Daily Symptom Report scores by the third month of treatment. Chlormadinone also clinically and statistically reduced the severity of depression, anxiety, food cravings, mood swings, and cramps [13]. A study of regimens containing estrogens and drospirenone, a nonethinylated, nortestosterone-type progestin, showed that it may improve premenstrual symptoms that lead to functional impairment in women with premenstrual dysphoric disorder, particularly in terms of anxiety, depressed mood, positive well-being, self-control, general health, and vitality [14].

When considering oral contraception, it is important to remember that the different synthetic progestins used may have different clinical effects, depending on the molecules from which they are derived and the neurosteroid synthesis that results from them.

For example, an oral contraceptive regimen containing ethinyl estradiol (EE) plus levonorgestrel (LNG)—two of the most used steroids in hormonal contraceptives—decreases the concentrations of ALLO and its precursors progesterone and pregnenolone in female rat cerebral cortex, hippocampus, and plasma. It also alters $GABA_A$ receptor expression, altering social and reproductive behaviors. EE/LNG-treated rats displayed a decrease in dominant behaviors associated with a reduction in social investigation and a reduction in proceptive behaviors when mating [15]. These findings are consistent with several studies in female nonhuman primates showing that hormonal contraceptives reduce the expression of proceptive behavior, their ability to attract mates, and can abolish or significantly reduce the cyclical increase in female anogenital swelling. Similarly, hormonal contraceptive treatment can affect sexuality in women by reducing sexual desire, sexual activity, and spontaneous arousal. Instead, progesterone administration to EE/LNG-treated rats appeared to increase sexual activity and cerebrocortical allopregnanolone concentrations. The reduced secretion of allopregnanolone and its effects are thought to be mediated by its positive modulation of $GABA_A$ receptors in specific nuclei of the hypothalamus involved in the control of reproductive behavior [16, 17].

The inhibitory effect of OC progestins and EE (not in combination) on skin 5-reductase was recently evaluated in a European in vitro study. Testosterone in the skin can be metabolized to dihydrotestosterone, a potent androgen, and this process is controlled by 5-reductase. The greater the inhibitory effect of a progestin on 5-reductase is, the less androgen is converted to dihydrotestosterone, thereby reducing circulating androgens and excess androgen levels. Progestins analyzed that are available in OCs in the United States include norgestimate (NGM), 3-keto-desogestrel, norethindrone, LNG, and norgestrel. Other steroids studied included gestodene (GSD), dienogest, and cyproterone acetate. The results showed that all progestins had some inhibitory effect, but NGM was the most potent inhibitor of 5-reductase activity, followed by LNG and dienogest. Ethinyl estradiol did not show any inhibitory potential [18].

Further studies showed that CMA increased ALLO levels in the hippocampus and, when given with E(2)V, also in the hypothalamus and anterior pituitary. This result suggests that the addition of an estrogen molecule might enhance the responsiveness of selective brain areas to CMA action on ALLO synthesis and release. Clinical studies highlight a neuroactive role of CMA: compared to placebo, CMA seems to reduce the severity of depression, anxiety, food cravings, mood swings, and cramps in fertile women affected by premenstrual dysphoric disorder. Thus, improvement of mood symptoms and anxiety evaluated after CMA administration might be the clinical consequence, at least in part, of the higher brain ALLO content [19] (Table 26.1).

In addition to the production of ALLO and subsequent activation of $GABA_A$ systems, membrane actions of progesterone such as CMA and NOMac in the CNS include modulation of opioidergic tone at the hypothalamic and subhypothalamic levels. In particular, beta-endorphin is an endogenous opiate involved in the response to stress, pain mechanism, and reward system. It has also been postulated that beta-endorphin may play an important role in the mechanism of sexual arousal and pleasure in both sexes [20].

More studies showed that beta-END content is increased in the neurointermediate lobe and anterior pituitary after CMA administration, and it did not affect the positive response of brain opioid level to the estrogen administration and the subsequent increase of beta-END levels.

Analyzing other oral progestins, nomegestrol acetate (NOMac) was also shown to increase ALLO production in the hippocampus and also in the hypothalamus and

Table 26.1 Central and peripheral expression of allopregnanolone after different progestins administration in rats model

	MP 2–4–8	CMA 0.1–0.5–1	DRSP 0.1–0.5–1	NOM Ac 0.05–0.1–0.2–0.5-1
Frontal cortex	4–8 mg/kg/d	=	=	=
Parietal cortex	2–4–8 mg/kg/d	=	=	=
Hippocampus	8 mg/kg/d	1 mg/kg/d	=	0.5–1 mg/kg/d
Hypothalamus	4–8 mg/kg/d	=	=	=
Anterior pituitary	8 mg/kg/d	=	=	=
Adrenal cortex	=	=	=	8 mg/kg/d
Serum	2–4–8 mg/kg/d	=	=	=

anterior pituitary when combined with E2V, demonstrating a synergistic effect with estrogens only in selective brain areas. Drospirenone (DRSP), instead, seemed to have a neutral effect toward the production of ALLO [19].

26.7 Conclusions

In conclusion, the use of hormonal contraceptives, particularly oral contraceptives, represents a complex interplay between reproductive health and mental well-being. While these methods remain the most popular form of contraception worldwide, their effects on mood and neurotransmission patterns underscore the need for careful consideration when prescribing. The variable effects of different progestins suggest that individual responses to oral contraceptives may vary significantly depending on the specific hormonal composition and how these hormones interact with neurosteroidogenesis in the female brain.

Research suggests that while some formulations may exacerbate mood disorders, others, such as chlormadinone acetate, have shown promise in alleviating symptoms such as depression and anxiety. In addition, the increased susceptibility of adolescents to mood changes associated with hormonal contraceptives requires a tailored approach to treatment, taking into account both psychological and pharmacological factors.

Overall, increased awareness and understanding of the neurotransmitter dynamics affected by hormonal contraceptives could lead to more personalized contraceptive counseling and better health outcomes for women. As ongoing research continues to shed light on the relationship between hormonal contraceptive use and mental health, it is vital that healthcare providers remain vigilant in ensuring that their patients are fully informed to make informed decisions about their reproductive health.

Declarations

Competing Interests The author(s) has no competing interests to declare that are relevant to the content of this manuscript.

Ethics Approval The author(s) declares that this manuscript does not include primary research with human participants.

The author(s) declares that this manuscript does not include primary studies involving animals.

Bibliography

1. undesa_pd_report_2015_trends_contraceptive_use.pdf. Accessed 15 Jan 2025. https://www.un.org/development/desa/pd/sites/www.un.org.development.desa.pd/files/undesa_pd_report_2015_trends_contraceptive_use.pdf.

2. Pluchino N, Santoro A, Casarosa E, et al. Advances in neurosteroids: role in clinical practice. Climacteric J Int Menopause Soc. 2013;16(Suppl 1):8–17. https://doi.org/10.3109/13697137.2013.809647.
3. Oinonen KA, Mazmanian D. To what extent do oral contraceptives influence mood and affect? J Affect Disord. 2002;70(3):229–40. https://doi.org/10.1016/s0165-0327(01)00356-1.
4. Skovlund CW, Mørch LS, Kessing LV, Lidegaard Ø. Association of hormonal contraception with depression. JAMA Psychiatry. 2016;73(11):1154–62. https://doi.org/10.1001/jamapsychiatry.2016.2387.
5. Skovlund CW, Mørch LS, Kessing LV, Lange T, Lidegaard Ø. Association of hormonal contraception with suicide attempts and suicides. Am J Psychiatry. 2018;175(4):336–42. https://doi.org/10.1176/appi.ajp.2017.17060616.
6. Segebladh B, Borgström A, Odlind V, Bixo M, Sundström-Poromaa I. Prevalence of psychiatric disorders and premenstrual dysphoric symptoms in patients with experience of adverse mood during treatment with combined oral contraceptives. Contraception. 2009;79(1):50–5. https://doi.org/10.1016/j.contraception.2008.08.001.
7. Borgström A, Odlind V, Ekselius L, Sundström-Poromaa I. Adverse mood effects of combined oral contraceptives in relation to personality traits. Eur J Obstet Gynecol Reprod Biol. 2008;141(2):127–30. https://doi.org/10.1016/j.ejogrb.2008.07.018.
8. Felthous AR, Robinson DB. Oral contraceptive medication in prevention of psychotic exacerbations associated with phases of the menstrual cycle. J Prev Psychiatry. 1981;1(1):5–14.
9. Zhang L, Verwer RWH, van Heerikhuize J, et al. Progesterone receptor distribution in the human hypothalamus and its association with suicide. Acta Neuropathol Commun. 2024;12(1):16. https://doi.org/10.1186/s40478-024-01733-y.
10. Bäckström T, Hansson-Malmström Y, Lindhe BA, Cavalli-Björkman B, Nordenström S. Oral contraceptives in premenstrual syndrome: a randomized comparison of triphasic and monophasic preparations. Contraception. 1992;46(3):253–68. https://doi.org/10.1016/0010-7824(92)90006-f.
11. Heskamp MLS, Schramm GAK. Efficacy of the low-dose combined oral contraceptive chlormadinone acetate/ethinylestradiol: physical and emotional benefits. Contraception. 2010;81(1):49–56. https://doi.org/10.1016/j.contraception.2009.06.011.
12. Huber JC, Heskamp MLS, Schramm GAK. Effect of an oral contraceptive with chlormadinone acetate on depressive mood: analysis of data from four observational studies. Clin Drug Investig. 2008;28(12):783–91. https://doi.org/10.2165/00044011-200828120-00006.
13. Contreras CM, Azamar-Arizmendi G, Saavedra M, Hernández-Lozano M. A five-day gradual reduction regimen of chlormadinone reduces premenstrual anxiety and depression: a pilot study. Arch Med Res. 2006;37(7):907–13. https://doi.org/10.1016/j.arcmed.2006.05.001.
14. Apter D, Borsos A, Baumgärtner W, et al. Effect of an oral contraceptive containing drospirenone and ethinylestradiol on general well-being and fluid-related symptoms. Eur J Contracept Reprod Health Care. 2003;8(1):37–51.
15. Follesa P, Porcu P, Sogliano C, et al. Changes in GABAA receptor gamma 2 subunit gene expression induced by long-term administration of oral contraceptives in rats. Neuropharmacology. 2002;42(3):325–36. https://doi.org/10.1016/s0028-3908(01)00187-3.
16. Porcu P, Mostallino MC, Sogliano C, Santoru F, Berretti R, Concas A. Long-term administration with levonorgestrel decreases allopregnanolone levels and alters GABA(A) receptor subunit expression and anxiety-like behavior. Pharmacol Biochem Behav. 2012;102(2):366–72. https://doi.org/10.1016/j.pbb.2012.05.011.
17. Santoru F, Berretti R, Locci A, Porcu P, Concas A. Decreased allopregnanolone induced by hormonal contraceptives is associated with a reduction in social behavior and sexual motivation in female rats. Psychopharmacology. 2014;231(17):3351–64. https://doi.org/10.1007/s00213-014-3539-9.
18. Rabe T, Kowald A, Ortmann J, Rehberger-Schneider S. Inhibition of skin 5 alpha-reductase by oral contraceptive progestins in vitro. Gynecol Endocrinol. 2000;14(4):223–30. https://doi.org/10.3109/09513590009167685.

19. Pluchino N, Lenzi E, Merlini S, et al. Selective effect of chlormadinone acetate on brain allopregnanolone and opioids content. Contraception. 2009;80(1):53–62. https://doi.org/10.1016/j.contraception.2009.01.005.
20. Straneva PA, Maixner W, Light KC, Pedersen CA, Costello NL, Girdler SS. Menstrual cycle, beta-endorphins, and pain sensitivity in premenstrual dysphoric disorder. Health Psychol. 2002;21(4):358–67.

Part IX
Barrier Methods: A Useful Tool in the Prevention of Sexually Transmitted Diseases

Chapter 27
Barrier Methods: A Useful Tool in the Prevention of Sexually Transmitted Diseases

Giovanna Esposito and Fabio Parazzini

The barrier methods of contraception include male and female condoms, as well as diaphragms, cervical caps, contraceptive gels, spermicides (foams, creams, and suppositories), and vaginal sponges. According to the World Health Organization (WHO) [1], in 2020, male condom is used by about 210 million couples worldwide. Barrier methods represent the most commonly used contraceptive methods (Table 27.1).

Traditionally, barrier methods of contraception have been proposed as a tool in the prevention of pregnancy and sexually transmitted diseases (STDs). However, while we have a good understanding of the effectiveness of these methods, there is little data on the real-life role of barrier methods in preventing sexually transmitted infections. This chapter briefly summarizes the available evidence.

27.1 Male Condoms

Condoms protect the wearer and his partner from infection by covering the penile glans and shaft, which are the major portals of entry and exit of sexually transmitted pathogens.

Laboratory studies observe that latex condoms are effective mechanical barriers to prevent the passage of several infectious agents, including the smallest sexually transmitted viruses, such as cytomegalovirus (CMV), human immunodeficiency virus (HIV), hepatitis B virus (HBV), herpes simplex virus type II (HSV-II) [2, 3].

G. Esposito · F. Parazzini (✉)
Department of Clinical Sciences and Community Health, University of Milan, Milan, Italy
e-mail: Fabio.parazzini@unimi.it

A. R. Genazzani et al. (eds.), *Ethical, Efficacy and Safety Issues in Contraception*, Reproductive Medicine for Clinicians 4,
https://doi.org/10.1007/978-3-032-07322-8_27

Table 27.1 Number of women of reproductive age (15–49 years) using various contraceptive methods (WHO, 2020) [1]

	Million women 15–49 years	%
Permanent and long acting		
Female sterilization	219	22.9
IUD	161	16.8
Implant	25	2.6
Male sterilization	17	1.8
Traditional		
Withdrawal	53	5.5
Rhythm	33	3.5
Short acting		
Male condom	208	21.8
Pill	150	15.7
Injectable	72	7.5
Other[a]	17	1.8

[a]Other methods include female condoms, vaginal barrier methods (including diaphragms, cervical caps, and spermicidal foams, jellies, creams, and sponges), lactational amenorrhea method (LAM), emergency contraception, and other modern or traditional methods not presented separately

27.1.1 What Do We Know About the Effectiveness of Male Condoms in Reducing the Risk of STD Transmission?

It has been suggested that consistent use of male condom decreases the risk of transmission of gonorrhea, chlamydia, trichomoniasis, syphilis, and viral infections, including HIV, HSV2, HPV, HBV, HCV [4].

However, condoms can be expected to provide protection depending on the type of STD. Because condoms do not cover and protect all exposed areas, they are likely to be more effective at preventing infections transmitted by genital fluids from mucosal surfaces (e.g., gonorrhea, chlamydia, trichomoniasis, and HIV) than those transmitted by skin-to-skin contact (e.g., HSV, HPV, syphilis, and chancroid).

The majority of published studies on the protective effect of condoms against the transmission of STD have evaluated HIV infection.

A cochrane database systematic review has included that 13 cohorts of "always" users showed an homogenous HIV incidence estimate of 1.14 (95% CI:0.56, 2.04) per 100 person-years. In comparison, 10 cohorts of "never" users (consisting mainly of studies of partners of hemophiliac and transfusion patients) showed an HIV incidence estimate of 5.75 (95% CI: 3.16, 9.66) per 100 person-years. Thus, the proportionate reduction in HIV seroconversion with condom use is approximately 80%. In particular, in heterosexual relationships, HIV-negative partners were 80% less likely to become infected with HIV than nonusers [5]. Considering MSM relationships, always-use was 60–70% effective [6]. The effect was not observed in occasional users (Table 27.2).

Table 27.2 Efficacy of condom use in heterosexual and MSM relationship

Heterosexual relationship	MSM relationship
Regular use: HIV-negative partners were 80% less likely to become HIV infected than nonusers *Cochrane Database Syst Rev. 2002;1:CD003255.*	*Bottom*: Always use: 72% effective Sometimes use: 8% effective *Top*: Always use: 63% effective Sometimes use: not more effective than never using a condom *J Acquir Immune Defic Syndr. 2015 Mar 1;68(3):337–44.*

There is epidemiological evidence that condoms markedly reduce the risk of gonorrhea [7] and less so that of chlamydia [8].

Condoms also reduce the risk of getting genital herpes if used the right way every times. In heterosexual monogamous relationships, condom use during more than 25% of sex acts was associated with protection against HSV-II acquisition for women (adjusted HR, 0.085; 95% CI, 0.01–0.67) but not for men (adjusted HR, 2.02; 95% CI, 0.32–12.50) [9]. In another pooled analysis, consistent condom users (100% use) had a 30% lower risk of HSV-2 infection than those who never used condoms, and the risk increased steadily and significantly with each unprotected sexual act (HR: 1.16, 95% CI: 1.08–1.25) [10]. A reduction of about 80% has been reported in MSM relationships [11].

For monogamous couples, the Centers for Disease Control and Prevention (CDC) does not recommend routine condom use to prevent HBV and HCV transmission. However, the CDC recommends routine condom use in HIV positive and in case of multiple short-term sexual relationships with partners who have HCV [12].

Finally, the role of condom use in the transmission of HPV is controversial [13–15]. A review, including longitudinal studies, reports that, although many aspects of this protection remain to be elucidated, consistent condom use appears to provide relatively good, albeit partial, protection against HPV infection.

27.1.2 Role of Different Male Condoms

The basic concept of the male condom has not evolved over the past 30 years, except for the use of different materials.

Natural condoms were made from animal intestines, bladders, and skins. While they were an effective barrier against sperm and bacterial STDs, they were not as effective against viral organisms such as HIV, which are smaller than bacteria.

Rubber condoms are less porous than natural condoms and, hence, form a more effective barrier that can block smaller organisms, such as HIV.

Plastic condoms provide an effective barrier against HIV as well as bacterial STDs, while at the same time allowing better transfer of heat.

However, latex condoms—which are the most widely used and offer protection against all common STDs—reduce heat transfer, which can contribute to reduced sexual pleasure.

Nonlatex condoms have not shown any advantages over latex condoms, except for people with latex allergies, and condom failure rates have been higher than latex condoms [16].

Recent innovations include polyurethane strips to assist with correct and rapid application (http://www.sensicondoms.com/) and a folded silicone condom (http://www.origami.com/) currently awaiting regulatory approval.

27.2 Female Condoms

Female condom is a flexible barrier device made of latex, comprising an outer retention ring that prevents invagination, a sheath that lines and covers the vagina, an internal retention ring to ensure the condom stays in place, and an insertion mechanism to facilitate proper placement. Laboratory studies indicate that the female condom may be as effective mechanical barrier to viruses, including HIV. However, few real-life data are available on the efficacy of female condoms in providing protection against STDs, including HIV [14]. The female condom has been approved for use by several regulatory agencies and is being marketed in Europe as Femidom and in North America as both Femidom and Reality.

27.3 Spermicides

Spermicides consist of two components, a spermicidal chemical and a delivery base for the chemical. The base can be a cream, jelly, foam, film, suppository, or tablet. The spermicidal chemicals most often used today are nonoxynol-9 (N-9), menfegol, and benzalkonium chloride (BZK). Most research has been done using N-9 since it is the most common spermicide in the world.

The spermicidal agent kills sperm and STD microorganisms. Most spermicides are surfactants, which means they act on the membrane of the sperm or microorganism. In addition, some of the delivery bases physically block the cervix to prevent sperm and microorganisms from moving into the woman's uterus, providing a secondary mode of action.

Spermicides can be used alone or with another contraceptive method. They are available without prescription in most countries, but may be expensive.

The effect of vaginal spermicides containing N-9 in preventing cervical gonorrhea, chlamydia, or HIV infection is unclear. Thus, spermicides alone are not recommended for STD/HIV prevention. Frequent use of spermicides containing N-9 has been associated with genital lesions, which may be associated with an increased risk of HIV transmission [17, 18].

The role of spermicides, sponges, and diaphragms for preventing transmission of HIV to men has not been evaluated.

27.4 Conclusions

Male latex condom is the only barrier method that has been shown in human studies to prevent the transmission of all types of STDs, including HIV. The protection is mainly observed in always users. The female condom may prove to be as effective as the male condom, but clinical studies are limited. Spermicides containing N-9 protect against common bacterial STDs and have been found to inactivate HIV in the laboratory, but their effect on HIV transmission in humans is under study. Based on available data, male condoms are currently the only contraceptive methods recommended for STD prevention.

In consideration of the role of condom use in reducing the risk of HIV infection and potentially other STD, an important public health objective is to increase its use, particularly in the case of occasional relationships or in stable couples in where one of the two partners is HIV positive.

But how can we increase the frequency of condom users? Users of barrier methods are more likely to be successful when they receive effective counseling. Thus, intensive counseling, which may involve teaching new skills, is needed to facilitate consistent use. Partner communication and cooperation are also required for effective use of barrier methods.

Clear and practical information on how to use the method correctly, how to avoid common mistakes in use, and how to get more supplies is also essential.

However, when promoting the use of condoms, doctor must avoid giving a sense of security. Condoms are an effective tool against STD transmission, but they do not eliminate the risk of infection.

In fact, one concern is the fact that condom promotion may lead to risk compensation: men who use condoms may feel safer and consequently engage in more frequent sex or sex with more partners, thus increasing the risk of transmission. However, a systematic review has shown that sexual risk reduction interventions do not increase unsafe sexual behavior [17]. Further, adding condom promotion to interventions focusing on abstinence seems to not undermine the abstinence message [18].

The use of condoms must be part of the ABC strategy where A stands for Abstinence, B for Be faithful to one partner, and C for use Condoms.

Clinicians who counsel patients about sexual health should firstly underline that people who abstain from intercourse or who are uninfected and mutually monogamous eliminate the risk of infection entirely.

Secondly, they should inform that people who choose to be sexually active can be reassured that condom use reduces the risk of most infections, but that condoms, like any other prevention tool, work only when used properly; consistent and correct use is essential for optimal risk reduction.

In any case, condom may be a useful tool for a safer sex but not for a safe sex.

Declarations

Competing Interests The author(s) has no competing interests to declare that are relevant to the content of this manuscript.

Ethics Approval The author(s) declares that this manuscript does not include primary research with human participants.

The author(s) declares that this manuscript does not include primary studies involving animals.

References

1. United Nations Department of Economic and Social Affairs, Population Division. 2022. World family planning 2022: meeting the changing needs for family planning: contraceptive use by age and method. UN DESA/POP/2022/TR/NO. 4.
2. Centers for Disease Control and Prevention (CDC). Update: barrier protection against HIV infection and other sexually transmitted diseases. MMWR Morb Mortal Wkly Rep. 1993;42(30):589–91. 597.
3. https://www.cdc.gov/condom-use/index.html#:~:text=Condom%20effectiveness%20for%20STD%20and,preventing%20the%20spread%20of%20HIV. Accessed Nov 2024.
4. Holmes KK, Levine R, Weaver M. Effectiveness of condoms in preventing sexually transmitted infections. Bull World Health Organ. 2004;82(6):454–61.
5. Weller S, Davis K. Condom effectiveness in reducing heterosexual HIV transmission. Cochrane Database Syst Rev. 2002;1:CD003255.
6. Smith DK, Herbst JH, Zhang X, Rose CE. Condom effectiveness for HIV prevention by consistency of use among men who have sex with men in the United States. J Acquir Immune Defic Syndr. 2015;68(3):337–44.
7. Niccolai LM, Rowhani-Rahbar A, Jenkins H, Green S, Dunne DW. Condom effectiveness for prevention of Chlamydia trachomatis infection. Sex Transm Infect. 2005;81(4):323–5.
8. Warner L, Stone KM, Macaluso M, Buehler JW, Austin HD. Condom use and risk of gonorrhea and Chlamydia: a systematic review of design and measurement factors assessed in epidemiologic studies. Sex Transm Dis. 2006;33(1):36–51. https://doi.org/10.1097/01.olq.0000187908.42622.fd.
9. Wald A, Langenberg AG, Link K, Izu AE, Ashley R, Warren T, Tyring S, Douglas JM Jr, Corey L. Effect of condoms on reducing the transmission of herpes simplex virus type 2 from men to women. JAMA. 2001;285(24):3100–6.
10. Martin ET, Krantz E, Gottlieb SL, Magaret AS, Langenberg A, Stanberry L, Kamb M, Wald A. A pooled analysis of the effect of condoms in preventing HSV-2 acquisition. Arch Intern Med. 2009;169(13):1233–40. https://doi.org/10.1001/archinternmed.2009.177.
11. Lin KW. Condom use lowers genital herpes risk. Am Fam Physician. 2006;73(10):1832–7.
12. https://www.cdc.gov/std/treatment-guidelines/hcv.htm. Accessed Nov 2024.
13. Liang W. Condom use and the risk of HPV infection. N Engl J Med. 2006;355(13):1388. author reply 1389. https://doi.org/10.1056/NEJMc061933.
14. Steiner MJ, Dominik R, Rountree RW, Nanda K, Dorflinger LJ. Contraceptive effectiveness of a polyurethane condom and a latex condom: a randomized controlled trial. Obstet Gynecol. 2003;101(3):539–47. https://doi.org/10.1016/s0029-7844(02)02732-1. Erratum in: Obstet Gynecol. 2003 May;101(5 Pt 1):1026.
15. Lam JU, Rebolj M, Dugué PA, Bonde J, von Euler-Chelpin M, Lynge E. Condom use in prevention of human papillomavirus infections and cervical neoplasia: systematic review of longitudinal studies. J Med Screen. 2014;21(1):38–50. https://doi.org/10.1177/0969141314522454.
16. Wiyeh AB, Mome RKB, Mahasha PW, Kongnyuy EJ, Wiysonge CS. Effectiveness of the female condom in preventing HIV and sexually transmitted infections: a systematic

review and meta-analysis. BMC Public Health. 2020;20(1):319. https://doi.org/10.1186/s12889-020-8384-7. PMID: 32164652; PMCID: PMC7068875.
17. Wilkinson D, Ramjee G, Tholandi M, Rutherford G. Nonoxynol-9 for preventing vaginal acquisition of HIV infection by women from men. Cochrane Database Syst Rev. 2002;2002(4):CD003936. https://doi.org/10.1002/14651858.CD003936. PMID: 12519622; PMCID: PMC8407148.
18. Wilkinson D, Ramjee G, Tholandi M, Rutherford G. Nonoxynol-9 for preventing vaginal acquisition of sexually transmitted infections by women from men. Cochrane Database Syst Rev. 2002;4:CD003939. https://doi.org/10.1002/14651858.CD003939.
19. Smoak ND, Scott-Sheldon LA, Johnson BT, Carey MP. Sexual risk reduction interventions do not inadvertently increase the overall frequency of sexual behavior: a meta-analysis of 174 studies with 116,735 participants. J Acquir Immune Defic Syndr. 2006;41(3):374–84.
20. Underhill K, Operario D, Montgomery P. Systematic review of abstinence-plus HIV prevention programs in high-income countries. PLoS Med. 2007;4(9):e275.

Part X
Contraception at Different Stages of Life

Chapter 28
Postpartum Contraception

Edson Santos Ferreira-Filho, Luciano de Melo Pompei, and Nilson Roberto de Melo

28.1 Introduction

Contraception is a matter of public health. Increasing contraceptive use reduces substantially the number of maternal deaths, mainly by reducing the number of unintended pregnancies [1]. The postpartum period is the perfect time to discuss family planning [2], since the woman is no longer pregnant, she is highly motivated to protect against pregnancy, and she is under specialized healthcare. Contraception improves obstetric and perinatal outcomes, once that short interpregnancy intervals are associated with multiple complications: maternal death, preterm birth, low birthweight, fetal death, and early neonatal death [1].

E. S. Ferreira-Filho
Gynecology Division at Hospital das Clínicas HCFMUSP, Faculdade de Medicina, Universidade de São Paulo, São Paulo, Brazil

University of São Paulo, São Paulo, Brazil
e-mail: edson.f@fm.usp.br

L. de Melo Pompei
Disciplina de Ginecologia da Faculdade de Medicina do ABC, Faculdade de Medicina da Universidade de São Paulo, São Paulo, Brazil

N. R. de Melo (✉)
Faculdade de Medicina da Universidade de São Paulo, São Paulo, Brazil

A. R. Genazzani et al. (eds.), *Ethical, Efficacy and Safety Issues in Contraception*, Reproductive Medicine for Clinicians 4,
https://doi.org/10.1007/978-3-032-07322-8_28

28.2 Contraceptive Options in the Postpartum Period

The choice of the contraceptive method depends on several factors: desire for a next pregnancy, attributes of contraceptive methods (effectiveness, safety), date and type of delivery, comorbidities, breastfeeding. Therefore, this decision must be made after proper counseling. It is important that professionals discuss this issue since prenatal care, during labor, and before hospital discharge. This conversation should not be postponed, once that mean day of first ovulation after delivery ranges from 45 to 94 days postpartum; the earliest ovulation occurs on day 25–27 postpartum; 20%–71% of first menses are preceded by ovulation, and up to 60% of these ovulations are potentially fertile [3].

Since the postpartum is a period with higher risk of venous thromboembolism (VTE), combined hormonal contraception (CHC)–including pill, patch, ring, and monthly injectables—is not the first choice. The incidence proportion of postpartum VTE is highest during the first 3 weeks after delivery, dropping from 9 per 10,000 during the first week to 1 per 10,000 at 4 weeks after delivery [4]. Other VTE risk factors given in Table 28.1 should also be assessed.

Considering that an ideal interpregnancy interval would be at least 6–24 months, long-acting reversible contraception (LARC) is highly indicated [1] and safe. For instance, the etonogestrel-releasing contraceptive subdermal implant inserted immediately postpartum has no negative effects on the hemostatic system [6]. As short-acting methods depend on the user's action, there is a greater abandonment rate, which implies a greater recurrence of pregnancy [7].

Table 28.1 Venous thromboembolism (VTE) risk factors

	Strong risk factors	Weak risk factors
Persistent	Active cancer Antiphospholipid syndrome	Chronic inflammatory disorders Nursing home confinement Obesity Personal or family history of venous thromboembolism Pacemaker placement
Transient	Antiphospholipid syndrome Caesarean section Heparin-induced thrombocytopenia Hospitalization for acute illness Major trauma or fracture Prolonged immobility (e.g., bedridden >3 days) Surgery >30 min	Nursing home confinement Obesity Brief immobility (e.g., travel >4 h) Oestrogen therapy Infection Minor trauma or fracture Pacemaker placement Pregnancy or puerperium Surgery <30 min Venous catheterization

Source: Khan et al. [5]

It is important to say that this contraindication does not apply to emergency contraception: if Yuzpe method [8] is the only one available, it can be administered. If levonorgestrel method is available, it should be preferred, due to a higher efficacy and less side effects [9]. However, the copper IUD has lower rates of pregnancy in the next year compared to oral levonorgestrel [10].

28.3 Timing of Contraceptive Initiation

Ideally, the discussion concerning contraception should be held during the prenatal appointments, to choose the method wisely and with enough time. If this is not possible, the subject must be approached when the patient is admitted to the hospital for delivery, whether vaginal or cesarean. Ultimately, the debate about the contraceptive method takes place in the ward, before hospital discharge.

The best situation is to take advantage of the opportunity when the patient is in front of the obstetrician-gynecologist to receive the contraceptive method. Delaying this offer may reduce access to the methods. For example, among people interested in an IUD who went through a protocol of two consultations, only 54.4% had their IUD inserted [11, 12]. An IUD can be inserted any time after delivery, but some contraindications must be respected: puerperal sepsis, uncontrolled puerperal hemorrhage, chorioamnionitis, prolonged ruptured membranes.

Insertion of an IUD in the immediate postpartum period is safe and appropriate for most women. Despite the higher risk of expulsion as compared with interval insertion, the benefits of insertion in the immediate postpartum period are significant and include improved rates of contraception continuance and reduced instances of short interval birth [13]. The risk of expulsion is 10.2% when the IUD is inserted in the first 10 min after delivery, 13.2% if inserted between 10 min and 48 h after delivery, and 1.8% if inserted 4 weeks after delivery [14]. WHO Medical Eligibility Criteria [15] for contraceptive use are presented in Table 28.2.

Table 28.2 Medical Eligibility Criteria for intrauterine device (IUD) use

Postpartum	Cu-IUD	LNG-IUD
<48 h	1	1/2 (if breastfeeding)
Between 48 h and 4 weeks	3	3
≥4 weeks	1	1
Puerperal sepsis	4	4

Caption: *Cu-IUD* copper intrauterine device, *LNG-IUD* levonorgestrel-releasing intrauterine device

28.4 Breastfeeding

Considering the importance of breastfeeding for both mother and child, it is crucial that contraception does not impact negatively on one's ability to breastfeed. Since combined pills may have a negative effect on breast milk volume or content [16], WHO Medical Eligibility Criteria recommend against the use of CHC in the first 6 months after childbirth [17]. Most recently, the Centers for Disease Control and Prevention (CDC) published their Medical Eligibility Criteria, restricting the use of CHC to the first 6 weeks postpartum [18].

Professionals must be aware of the absence of impact of progestogen-only methods. For instance, etonogestrel-containing subdermal implant does not alter the volume of breast milk intake by newborns [19]. Similarly, the total amount of drospirenone that passes into breast milk of postpartum women in a 24-h period is tiny [20].

WHO Medical Eligibility Criteria [15] for contraceptive use are presented in Table 28.3.

Table 28.3 WHO Medical Eligibility Criteria for contraceptive use

Breastfeeding	CHC	POP	DMPA	ENG and LNG implants
<6 weeks postpartum	4	2	3	2
Between 6 weeks and 6 months postpartum	3	1	1	1
≥6 months postpartum	2	1	1	1
Postpartum (not breastfeeding)	**CHC**	**POP**	**DMPA**	**ENG and LNG implants**
<21 days without other risk factors for VTE	3	1	1	1
<21 days with other risk factors for VTE	4	1	1	1
Between 21 and 42 days without other risk factors for VTE	2	1	1	1
Between 21 and 42 days with other risk factors for VTE	3	1	1	1
>42 days	1	1	1	1

Caption: *CHC* combined hormonal contraception, *POP* progestin-only pills, *DMPA* depot medroxyprogesterone acetate, *ENG* etonogestrel, *LNG* levonorgestrel

28.5 Counseling and Shared Decision-Making

Avoiding unintended pregnancies is the utmost goal of good contraceptive counseling. The contraceptive choice in the postpartum period must respect the Medical Eligibility Criteria [17, 18]. Thus, if the woman presents any comorbidity, this also should be considered. Since women with chronic medical conditions have even higher rates of unintended pregnancies, there is an urgent need to offer adequate options especially in the high-risk prenatal setting. Besides, we must take into account what the woman wants: a method that she can control or that does not require any action, noncontraceptive benefits, availability, cost, etc. The best method is the one whose choice comes from an honest dialog between patient and healthcare provider.

Declarations

Competing Interests The author(s) has no competing interests to declare that are relevant to the content of this manuscript.

Ethics Approval The author(s) declares that this manuscript does not include primary research with human participants.

The author(s) declares that this manuscript does not include primary studies involving animals.

References

1. Cleland J, Conde-Agudelo A, Peterson H, Ross J, Tsui A. Contraception and health. Lancet. 2012;380(9837):149–56.
2. Grandi G, Del Savio MC, Tassi A, Facchinetti F. Postpartum contraception: a matter of guidelines. Int J Gynaecol Obstet. 2024;164(1):56–65.
3. Jackson E, Glasier A. Return of ovulation and menses in postpartum nonlactating women: a systematic review. Obstet Gynecol. 2011;117(3):657–62.
4. Tepper NK, Boulet SL, Whiteman MK, Monsour M, Marchbanks PA, Hooper WC, et al. Postpartum venous thromboembolism: incidence and risk factors. Obstet Gynecol. 2014;123(5):987–96.
5. Khan F, Tritschler T, Kahn SR, Rodger MA. Venous thromboembolism. Lancet. 2021;398(10294):64–77.
6. Brito MB, Ferriani RA, Meijers JCM, Garcia AA, Quintana SM, Silva de Sá MF, et al. Effects of the etonogestrel-releasing contraceptive implant inserted immediately postpartum on maternal hemostasis: a randomized controlled trial. Thromb Res. 2012;130(3):355–60.
7. Brunson MR, Klein DA, Olsen CH, Weir LF, Roberts TA. Postpartum contraception: initiation and effectiveness in a large universal healthcare system. Am J Obstet Gynecol. 2017 Jul;217(1):55.e1–9.
8. World Health Organization. Emergency contraception [Internet] 2021. Available from: https://www.who.int/news-room/fact-sheets/detail/emergency-contraception.

9. Task Force on Postovulatory Methods of Fertility Regulation. Randomised controlled trial of levonorgestrel versus the Yuzpe regimen of combined oral contraceptives for emergency contraception. Lancet. 1998;352(9126):428–33.
10. Turok DK, Jacobson JC, Dermish AI, Simonsen SE, Gurtcheff S, McFadden M, et al. Emergency contraception with a copper IUD or oral levonorgestrel: an observational study of 1-year pregnancy rates. Contraception. 2014;89(3):222–8.
11. Whitaker AK, Chen BA. Society of family planning guidelines: postplacental insertion of intrauterine devices. Contraception. 2018;97(1):2–13.
12. Bergin A, Tristan S, Terplan M, Gilliam ML, Whitaker AK. A missed opportunity for care: two-visit IUD insertion protocols inhibit placement. Contraception. 2012;86(6):694–7.
13. Lopez LM, Bernholc A, Hubacher D, Stuart G, Van Vliet HAAM. Immediate postpartum insertion of intrauterine device for contraception. Cochrane Database Syst Rev. 2015;2015(6):CD003036.
14. Averbach SH, Ermias Y, Jeng G, Curtis KM, Whiteman MK, Berry-Bibee E, et al. Expulsion of intrauterine devices after postpartum placement by timing of placement, delivery type, and intrauterine device type: a systematic review and meta-analysis. Am J Obstet Gynecol. 2020;223(2):177–88.
15. World Health Organization. Medical eligibility criteria for contraceptive use. Geneva: World Health Organization; 2015.
16. Lopez LM, Grey TW, Stuebe AM, Chen M, Truitt ST, Gallo MF. Combined hormonal versus nonhormonal versus progestin-only contraception in lactation. Cochrane Database Syst Rev. 2015;2015(3):CD003988.
17. World Health Organization. Medical eligibility criteria for contraceptive use. 5th ed. World Health Organization; 2015.
18. Nguyen AT, Curtis KM, Tepper NK, Kortsmit K, Brittain AW, Snyder EM, et al. U.S. medical eligibility criteria for contraceptive use, 2024. MMWR Morb Mortal Wkly Rep. 2024;73(4):1–126.
19. Braga GC, Ferriolli E, Quintana SM, Ferriani RA, Pfrimer K, Vieira CS. Immediate postpartum initiation of etonogestrel-releasing implant: a randomized controlled trial on breastfeeding impact. Contraception. 2015;92(6):536–42.
20. Archer DF, Ahrendt H-J, Drouin D. Drospirenone-only oral contraceptive: results from a multicenter noncomparative trial of efficacy, safety and tolerability. Contraception. 2015;92(5):439–44.

Chapter 29
Contraception at Different Stages of Life: Early Ovarian Failure and Perimenopause

Marisa Ardito, Matilde Giudetti, Tiziana Fidecicchi, Stefano Luisi, and Tommaso Simoncini

29.1 Contraception in Perimenopause

The function of the hypothalamus–pituitary axis varies throughout a woman's lifetime. The gradual decline in the function of the hypothalamic–pituitary–gonadal axis at last brings to irregularities in menstrual cycles and increasing of anovulatory cycles, and it is responsible for the onset of menopause. All the neurotransmitter systems undergo to a progressive decline during life, especially cholinergic, serotoninergic, and dopaminergic systems that produce a disruption of the hypothalamus–pituitary–gonad axis due to the influence of the neurotransmitters on the activity of the neurons producing GnRh. All these events could explain the occurrence of many typical menopausal transitions and of the menopausal period symptoms. According to the World Health Organization (WHO) definition, menopause occurs with the permanent cessation of menses due to the loss of ovarian follicular activity and typically occurs around 51 years of age, with an age range varying between 40 and 60 years. Perimenopouse starts 5–10 years before the menopause, at approximately 40 years of age. The 2001 Stages of Reproductive Ageing Workshop (STRAW) proposed a staging system for ovarian aging. Based on that, we can identify different stages of the menopausal transition: early menopausal (early perimenopause), characterized by an irregular cycle; late menopausal (late perimenopause), characterized by an interval of amenorrhea ≥60 days in the prior 12 months; early postmenopause, which is the first year following the final menstrual period (FMP) [1]. Perimenopause is characterized by the worst menopausal symptom burden, like sleep disorders, depression, vasomotor symptoms like hot

M. Ardito · M. Giudetti · T. Fidecicchi · S. Luisi · T. Simoncini (✉)
Division of Obstetrics and Gynecology, Department of Clinical ad Experimental medicine, University of Pisa, Pisa, Italy
e-mail: stefano.luisi@unipi.it; tommaso.simoncini@unipi.it

A. R. Genazzani et al. (eds.), *Ethical, Efficacy and Safety Issues in Contraception*, Reproductive Medicine for Clinicians 4,
https://doi.org/10.1007/978-3-032-07322-8_29

flushes and sweating (occurring in up to 80% of women). Approximately half of women [2, 3] women suffer from these symptoms usually 2 years before the FMP and for 4 years after the FMP. Sleep problems, particularly nocturnal awakenings, concern 40–60% of menopausal women [4, 5]. Long-term manifestations of definite estrogen decline are urogenital atrophy, aging of the skin, osteoporosis, and sarcopenia that might develop during the postmenopausal period. Some perimenopausal symptoms might be predictive of future health complications, especially disorders such as vasomotor symptoms or sleep disturbance and mood disorders. MHT (menopausal hormone therapy) is an effective treatment for bothersome perimenopausal and menopausal disturbances. Clinician's challenge is creating a benefit–risk profile and tailoring hormonal therapy to each woman. In addition to investigating the woman's health status, it is crucial to make patient understand the importance of contraception also in perimenopause. The fertility of a woman during the perimenopause is lower but, at the same time, there are higher rates of unintended pregnancies among these women [6]. The definition of "advanced pregnancy" is now used for pregnant women over 40 years of age. Pregnancies carried at an advanced age can run into several complications and adverse outcome: increased miscarriages, ectopic pregnancies, twinning, fetal and chromosomal abnormalities, low birth weight, and prematurity. Pregnancy may be considered "at risk" for or the increased risk of including diabetes, preeclampsia, haemorrhage, preterm ruptured membranes, prolonged and dysfunctional labor, and caesarean delivery [7–9]. In order to avoid unwanted pregnancies and these possible adverse effects, it is critical to make the patient aware with the aim of increased compliance with therapy. The first step approaching a perimenopausal woman, to choose the best treatment option, is to create a benefit–risk profile and to assess the patient's comorbidities and risk factors, considering the signs and symptoms. First among them are cardiovascular risk, thromboembolic risk, cardiovascular events in patient's history, cigarette smoking, diabetes, and high BMI. The incidence of CVD in women increases substantially with aging, probably because with menopause, decreased estrogen concentration results in reduced protection contributing to an adverse impact on cardiovascular risk variables. Estrogens regulate vascular reactivity, blood pressure, endothelial function, and cardiac remodeling. After menopause, traditional cardiovascular risk factors are adversely affected, particularly hypertension [10–13]. Additionally menopause is associated with central adiposity, insulin resistance, and a pro-atherogenic lipid profile, increasing the CV risk. Investigating regarding the cancer history of the patient and their family is also important, especially regarding breast cancer, whose risk increases with advancing age as the cardiovascular risk. All these factors should be considered during the therapy's choice in perimenopausal women with symptoms in order to reach a risk–benefit balance. For example, MHT in the young woman with vasomotor symptoms approaching menopause is useful to prevent VRS, at the same time MHT is absolutely contraindicated in patients with high cardiovascular risk.

Different types and formulations of therapies have been developed over the years: estroprogestin pills or exclusively with progesterone, formulation with etinil-estradiol or with natural estrogen, local therapies or those with systemic effects, long-acting reversible contraception (LARC) or short acting. In case the woman suffers from symptoms mainly due to estrogen decline, e.g., hot flashes, night sweats, mood alterations, etc. the best option is a hormone therapy made by estroprogestin and contraceptive in the perimenopausal woman. If, on the other hand, the symptoms involve more menstrual flow alterations, oligomenorrhea, abnormal flow, spotting, a medicated IUD or POP with progestin only will be better chosen. Combination therapy is preferred if the goal is contraception, menstrual cycle control, metrorrhagic cycles, dysmenorrhea, vasomotor symptoms, body mass density protection, and endometrial hyperplasia prevention. The progestin-only pill is not effective against bone mass decay, nor in relieving vasomotor symptoms, and it has poor control over the menstrual cycle, often causing amenorrhea or spotting [14]. Regarding the choice of estrogen, natural estrogen has numerous benefits. Estrogen E4, estetrol, has been introduced as contraceptive and experimented in the treatment of perimenopausal symptoms. Preclinical studies have largely demonstrated that the combination of E4 with drospirenone (DSP) is optimal [15]. It has been showed that the E4/DSP combination (15 mg/3 mg) has minimal impact on hemostasis, coagulation factors, fibrinolysis, angiotensinogen, cholesterol, and triglycerides [16] with optimal endometrial control also compared with the E4/Levonorgestrel combination [17]. Safety profile of estrogen E4 has been proven in multiple areas. Its effect is mammary neutral, excellent for endometrium and bone. As far as currently known, E4 is also effective in treating vasomotor symptoms with doses that are neutral on breast cancer cells [18]. In addition to being used as a therapy for premenopausal symptoms and for contraception, hormonal therapy with estrogen–progestin has many other extra-contraceptive benefits and real possibilities for therapeutic use in particular diseases and clinical conditions, particularly of protection from several malignancies. Officially recognized data have shown how hormonal contraception has an overall effect in reducing cancer occurrence [19]. Specifically, the cancers that appear most positively affected by long-term hormonal contraceptive use appear to be colorectal, endometrial, and ovarian cancers. Moreover, the reduction in the incidence of these cancer persists for at least 30 years after cessation of use. Combined OC has a significant protective effect on the risk of ovarian cancer, and the protection increases with duration of use. The largest meta-analysis of studies on the subject [20] demonstrates a significantly reduced risk of ovarian cancer by about 27% in oral contraceptive users The significant risk reduction has been confirmed for BRCA 1 and 2 mutation carriers [21]. The exact mechanism of protection has not been fully clarified: ovulation's inhibition, suppression of gonadotropin levels, direct effect of progestin, and reduction of retrograde menstruation might play a role. This effect occurs for all histologic types of malignant and borderline ovarian epithelial carcinoma, except for mucinous histotype. There is strong evidence showing that hormonal contraceptive use reduces the risk of endometrial cancer by about 50%. The protective effect increases with longer use and persists for more than 20 years after discontinuation and during postmenopause, the period of the highest incidence of this neoplasy [22].

Positive effects have been proven also on body mass density (BMD). Estrogen and estrogen–progestogen combinations can prevent all fractures [23–27] and increase BMD [28, 29]. MHT is the only therapy with proven effects on fracture reduction in patients without osteoporosis in early postmenopausal years [30]. The use of oral contraceptives in perimenopausal oligomenorrheic women appears to have beneficial effects on bone, restoring a normal bone turnover and maintaining or even increasing BMD. Treatment must be started upon the onset of anovulatory cycles to affect BMD in both perimenopausal and young women. However, in healthy women with normal ovarian function, oral contraceptives have no benefits on bone [31–33].

Menopause is confirmed after 12 consecutive months without menstruation in women aged 40 and older. It is recommended to continue contraception until menopause is confirmed. For women using progestin-only pills (POP), FSH levels can be monitored once. If FSH is above 30 IU/L, the contraceptive method can be continued for an additional year before stopping. If FSH is below 30 IU/L, the method should be used for another year before rechecking FSH levels. Alternatively, these methods may be discontinued at age 55 without further hormonal evaluation. For users of CHCs, the situation is more complex because CHCs can suppress FSH levels. For women aged 50 and older, one approach is to stop CHCs and switch to a nonhormonal contraceptive method temporarily. If menstruation does not resume after 6 weeks, FSH levels should be measured twice, 1–2 months apart. If both readings are above 30 IU/L, contraception can be stopped [14].

29.2 Contraception in Premature Ovarian Failure

Premature ovarian failure (POF), also known as primary ovarian insufficiency (POI), affects women under 40 who experience amenorrhea, elevated gonadotropins, and infertility. This condition has a major effect on women of reproductive age and manifests through a range of symptoms, which may be due to various underlying causes. POF has serious health consequences, including psychological distress, infertility, osteoporosis, autoimmune disorders, ischemic heart disease, and increased risk of mortality [34, 35]. Research has demonstrated that the age at which a woman experiences menopause significantly influences her cardiovascular health. Specifically, women who undergo early menopause (before age 45) or premature menopause (before age 40) have an increased risk of experiencing a nonfatal cardiovascular disease (CVD) event before the age of 60, compared to women who enter menopause after the age of 50. However, this elevated risk does not extend beyond the age of 70. Numerous studies have shown that premature ovarian insufficiency (POI) and early menopause adversely affect several physiological factors, such as lipid levels, body composition, systolic blood pressure, insulin sensitivity, risk of metabolic syndrome, endothelial function, and inflammatory markers. Additionally, women who experience early menopause face a 12% increased risk of developing diabetes compared to those who go through menopause at a later age. The lack of natural hormones after menopause, combined with a genetic predisposition for faulty DNA repair, may lead to accelerated aging and a higher risk of cardiovascular disease [36]. Earlier age at menopause has been linked to shorter leukocyte telomere length. This telomere length has been identified as a mediator in the association between earlier age at natural menopause and incident coronary artery disease. The highest risks have been observed in women with premature menopause and below-average telomere length [35].

The initial symptoms of estrogen deficiency are characterized by the onset of hot flushes, excessive sweating, nervousness, diminished libido, weakness, and urogenital atrophy which can manifest as vaginal dryness and infections.

Furthermore, premature estrogen deficiency is associated with a reduction in bone mineral density, which can lead to the development of conditions such as osteopenia and osteoporosis. It is essential for young women with POF to have densitometry testing due to the high risk of significant bone mineral density loss. Patients with POF have been demonstrated to have an elevated risk of fractures relative to women who have developed osteoporosis for reasons other than POF, including hyperthyroidism, steroid treatment, and hyperparathyroidism. It is also recommended that patients undergo measurement of vitamin D levels. Autoimmune hypothyroidism is the disease most commonly associated with POF; thus, screening by measurement of TSH, free T4, anti-thyroid peroxidase, and antithyroglobulin antibody levels is recommended. The most common disease associated with POF is celiac disease. However, the most distressing consequence of POF for young women is the reduction in fertility or even the inability to conceive [34].

Primary ovarian insufficiency and early menopause have significant health implications, and managing these conditions effectively is crucial to mitigate their adverse effects. Hormone replacement therapy (HRT) is the primary treatment for POI, designed to relieve symptoms and normalize sex steroid levels. It is essential for managing POI, alleviating symptoms, and preventing long-term health problems due to estrogen deficiency. Early diagnosis and a personalized, integrated treatment approach are key to achieving the best outcomes and enhancing the quality of life for women with POI. In the treatment of POI, it is essential not to forget the importance of healthy habits, supplementation with folic acid, calcium, and vitamin D, as well as psychological and emotional support to help patients manage the psychological aspects characteristic of POI.

Another aspect to consider is that a woman with POI may still desire pregnancy. Therefore, we must first try to understand the cause. This may include genetic testing, autoimmune screening, and assessment of ovarian reserve.

Identify any potentially reversible causes of POI, such as autoimmune conditions or infections, and lead them appropriately. If the cause of POI is iatrogenic, egg donation remains a valid option for achieving pregnancy. In some cases, ovarian stimulation might be tried to collect any remaining usable eggs. This approach is less commonly successful but may be considered. If the cause of POI is autoimmune, specific considerations and interventions are necessary. Conduct tests to identify specific autoimmune conditions that might be causing POI, such as thyroid disease, adrenal insufficiency, or autoimmune oophoritis. In some cases, immunosuppressive medications may help manage the autoimmune condition, potentially preserving some ovarian function. It's also important to monitor and treat the others autoimmune conditions, such as Hashimoto's thyroiditis or Addison's disease, that may coexist with POI. If a woman with POI does not desire pregnancy and there is no risk of spontaneous conception, HRT can be an effective treatment option to manage symptoms and prevent long-term health complications associated with estrogen deficiency. If there is a risk of spontaneous pregnancy and does not desire to conceive, contraceptive therapy is an effective option. Contraceptive therapy can serve dual purposes: managing symptoms of estrogen deficiency and offering effective contraception.

HRT for POI must be personalized based on age and individual needs. Unlike contraceptive therapy with fixed estrogen levels, HRT dosage can be adjusted. For inducing puberty, estrogen should be increased gradually with regular monitoring. After puberty, effectiveness should be evaluated through symptom relief and assessments of bone and cardiovascular health.

For prepubertal girls with POI, HT should begin around ages 10–11 years. Oral contraceptive pills are generally not recommended. Systemic low-dose estradiol is preferred, with doses gradually increased over 4 years or more, depending on puberty development. Progesterone should be introduced when ultrasound shows a sufficient endometrium, vaginal bleeding starts, or after 2 years of estrogen treatment. This strategy is key for achieving proper pubertal development, a fully mature uterus, and optimal bone growth. For postpubertal women with POI, adequate menopausal hormone therapy (MHT), combined with regular exercise, sufficient dietary calcium, and vitamin D, is essential for maintaining bone health and supporting cardiovascular health [37].

In conclusion, if we compare CHCs (combined hormonal contraceptives) with HRT, we can say that contraceptive therapy is useful to treat symptoms and is more accepted by women rather than HRT, prevents pregnancy, but may be less effective for long-term prevention of menopause-related consequences. The estrogen dosage is not modifiable with a very narrow range. Additionally, long-term use can increase the risk of VTE.

On the other hand, hormone replacement therapy is highly effective for symptom management, has very low risks for young girls, and is more effective in preventing long-term complications of POI. It is also used to induce puberty, as dosages can be adjusted and increased. However, it is less psychologically accepted by young women, and it does not have a contraceptive function. There are no specific guidelines regarding the duration of contraceptive therapy in POF, theoretically until the age of likely menopause. However, it is important to consider the woman's risk factors and symptoms for a personalized decision [37].

Declarations

Competing Interests The author(s) has no competing interests to declare that are relevant to the content of this manuscript.

Ethics Approval The author(s) declares that this manuscript does not include primary research with human participants.

The author(s) declares that this manuscript does not include primary studies involving animals.

Conflict of Interest None.

Financial Support None.

References

1. Harlow SD, Gass M, Hall JE, et al. Executive summary of the stages of reproductive aging workshop + 10: addressing the unfinished agenda of staging reproductive aging. J Clin Endocrinol Metab. 2012;97:1159–68.
2. Politi MC, Schleinitz MD, Col NF. Revisiting the duration of vasomotor symptoms of menopause: a meta-analysis. J Gen Intern Med. 2008;23:1507–13.
3. Woods NF, Mitchell ES. Symptoms during the perimenopause: prevalence, severity, trajectory, and significance in women's lives. Am J Med. 2005;118:14–24.
4. Joffe H, Massler A, Sharkey K. Evaluation and management of sleep disturbance during the menopause transition. Semin Reprod Med. 2010;28:404–21.
5. Polo-Kantola P. Sleep problems in midlife and beyond. Maturitas. 2011;68:224–32.
6. FSRH clinical guideline: contraception for women aged over 40 years (August 2017, amended September 2019). Faculty of sexual and reproductive healthcare; 2018. Available from: https://www.fsrh.org/standards-and-guidance/documents/fsrh-guidance-contraception-for-women-aged-over-40-years-2017/. Accessed 7 July 2022.en.
7. Kim DS, Dorchester W, Freeman RC. Advanced maternal age: the mature gravida. Am J Obstet Gynecol. 1985;152:7–12.
8. Gilbert WM, Nesbitt TS, Danielsen B. Childbearing beyond age 40: pregnancy outcome in 24,032 cases. Obstet Gynecol. 1999;93:9–14.
9. Bianco A, Stone J, Lynch L, et al. Pregnancy outcome at age 40 and older. Obstet Gynecol. 1996;87:917–22.
10. Schunkert H, Danser AHJ, Hense H-W, Derkx FHM, Ku¨Rzinger S, Riegger G€NAJ. Effects of estrogen replacement therapy on the renin-angiotensin system in postmenopausal women. Circulation. 1997;95:39–45.
11. Yanes LL, Romero DG, Iliescu R, Zhang H, Davis D, Reckelhoff JF. Postmenopausal hypertension: role of the renin-angiotensin system. Hypertension. 2010;56:359–63.
12. Hart EC, Charkoudian N. Sympathetic neural regulation of blood pressure: influences of sex and aging. Physiology (Bethesda). 2014;29:8–15.
13. GBD 2019 Risk Factors Collaborators. Global burden of 87 risk factors in 204 countries and territories, 1990–2019: a systematic analysis for the Global Burden of Disease Study 2019. Lancet. 2020;396:1223–49.
14. Grandi G, Di Vinci P, Sgandurra A, Feliciello L, Monari F, Facchinetti F. Contraception during perimenopause: practical guidance. Int J Womens Health. 2022;14:913–29.
15. Mawet M, et al. Unique effects on hepatic function, lipid metabolism, bone and growth endocrine parameters of estetrol in combined oral contraceptives. Eur J Contracept Reprod Health Care. 2015;20:463–75.
16. Kluft C, et al. Reduced hemostatic effects with drospirenone-based oral contraceptives containing estetrol vs. ethinyl estradiol. Contraception. 2017;95:140–7.
17. Duijkers IJM, et al. Inhibition of ovulation by administration of estetrol in combination with drospirenone or levonorgestrel: results of a phase II dose-finding pilot study. Eur J Contracept Reprod Health Care. 2015;20:476–89.

18. Gallez A, Dias Da Silva I, Wuidar V, Foidart J-M, Péqueux C. Estetrol and mammary gland: friends or foes? J Mammary Gland Biol Neoplasia. 2021;26:297–308.
19. Gierisch JM, et al. Oral contraceptive use and risk of breast, cervical, colorectal, and endometrial cancers: a systematic review. Cancer Epidemiol Biomarkers Prev. 2013;22:1931–43.
20. Beral V, Doll R, Hermon C, Peto R, Reeves G. Ovarian cancer and oral contraceptives: collaborative reanalysis of data from 45 epidemiological studies including 23,257 women with ovarian cancer and 87,303 controls. Lancet. 2008;371:303–14.
21. Cibula D, Gompel A, Mueck AO, La Vecchia C, Hannaford PC, Skouby SO, Zikan M, Dusek L. Hormonal contraception and risk of cancer. Hum Reprod Update. 2010;16(6):631–50.
22. The ESHRE Capri Workshop Group. Noncontraceptive health benefits of combined oral contraception. Hum Reprod Update. 2005;11:513–25.
23. Zhu L, Jiang X, Sun Y, et al. Effect of hormone therapy on the risk of bone fractures. Menopause. 2016;23:461–70.
24. Marjoribanks J, Farquhar C, Roberts H, et al. Long-term hormone therapy for perimenopausal and postmenopausal women. Cochrane Database Syst Rev. 2017;2017:CD004143.
25. Cauley JA. Effects of estrogen plus progestin on risk of fracture and bone mineral density. The women's health initiative randomized trial. JAMA. 2003;290:1729.
26. Jackson RD, LaCroix AZ, Gass M, et al. Calcium plus vitamin D supplementation and the risk of fractures. N Engl J Med. 2006;354:669–83.
27. Writing Group for the Women's Health Initiative Investigators. Risks and benefits of estrogen plus progestin in healthy postmenopausal women: principal results from the women's health initiative randomized controlled trial. JAMA J Am Med Assoc. 2002;288:321–33.
28. Manson JE, Chlebowski RT, Stefanick ML, et al. Menopausal hormone therapy and health outcomes during the intervention and extended Poststopping phases of the women's health initiative randomized trials. JAMA. 2013;310:1353.
29. Miller VT. Effects of estrogen or estrogen/progestin regimens on heart disease risk factors in postmenopausal women. JAMA. 1995;273:199.
30. Bagger YZ, Tankó LB, Alexandersen P, et al. Two to three years of hormone replacement treatment in healthy women have long-term preventive effects on bone mass and osteoporotic fractures: the PERF study. Bone. 2004;34:728–35.
31. Biller BMK, Coughlin JF, Saxe V, et al. Osteopenia in women with hypothalamic amenorrhea: a prospective study. Obstet Gynecol. 1991;78:996–1001.
32. Slemenda C, Longcope C, Peacock M, et al. Sex steroids, bone mass and bone loss: a prospective study of pre-, peri-, postmenopausal women. J Clin Invest. 1996;97:14–21.
33. Steinberg KK, Freni-Titulaer LW, De Puey EG, et al. Sex steroids and bone density in premenopausal and postmenopausal women. J Clin Endocrinol Metab. 1988;69:533–9.
34. Jankowska K. Premature ovarian failure. Prz Menopauzalny. 2017;16(2):51–6.
35. Schuermans A, Nakao T, Uddin MM, Hornsby W, Ganesh S, Shadyab AH, Liu S, Haring B, Shufelt CL, Taub MA, Mathias RA, Kooperberg C, Reiner AP, Bick AG, Manson JE, Natarajan P, Honigberg MC. Age at menopause, leukocyte telomere length, and coronary artery disease in postmenopausal women. Circ Res. 2023;133(5):376–86.
36. Maas AHEM, Rosano G, Cifkova R, Chieffo A, van Dijken D, Hamoda H, Kunadian V, Laan E, Lambrinoudaki I, Maclaran K, Panay N, Stevenson JC, van Trotsenburg M, Collins P. Cardiovascular health after menopause transition, pregnancy disorders, and other gynaecologic conditions: a consensus document from European cardiologists, gynaecologists, and endocrinologists. Eur Heart J. 2021;42(10):967–84.
37. Fruzzetti F, Palla G, Gambacciani M, Simoncini T. Tailored hormonal approach in women with premature ovarian insufficiency. Climacteric. 2020;23(1):3–8.

Part XI
Violence Against Women and Contraceptive Rights

Chapter 30
Violence Against Women and Contraceptive Rights

S. Shantha Kumari

30.1 Introduction

Violence against women is a global crisis with devastating consequences for their physical, mental, sexual, and reproductive health. It increases the risk of injuries, depression, anxiety, unplanned pregnancies, and sexually transmitted infections, including HIV. Beyond individual harm, it impacts children, families, communities, and national economies. Addressing violence is crucial for safeguarding women's health and ensuring their contraceptive rights [1].

Violence against women, including sexual and domestic abuse, is deeply linked to reproductive health in three primary ways [2]:

I. The ability to control one's body is essential to breaking the cycle of violence.
II. Violence can lead to reproductive rights violations.
III. Laws, policies, and practices that restrict access to reproductive rights constitute violence against women.

Women when restricted from their rights to access contraception for safe reproductive health are exposed to risks of increased morbidity and mortality due to unsafe abortions resorted to for the unwanted pregnancies. We need to address this if we want to achieve the SDG 2030.

Over the past decade, Indian courts have increasingly recognized women's reproductive rights as fundamental to the right to life. Landmark rulings have affirmed reproductive rights as essential for women's equality, emphasizing autonomy in pregnancy-related decisions. Cases on maternal health, contraception, abortion, and child marriage have aligned with human rights standards, with some

S. S. Kumari (✉)
Yashoda Hospitals, Hyderabad, India

A. R. Genazzani et al. (eds.), *Ethical, Efficacy and Safety Issues in Contraception*, Reproductive Medicine for Clinicians 4,
https://doi.org/10.1007/978-3-032-07322-8_30

judgments setting global precedents, such as recognizing maternal health as a right. While not uniform, these decisions have strengthened legal protections and reinforced the judiciary's role in addressing violations of reproductive rights [3].

30.2 Understanding Contraceptive Rights

A woman's right to decide if and when to have children depends on access to a full range of contraceptive methods and the ability to make informed choices. Governments have a duty under international human rights law to ensure contraceptives are available and accessible. Failure to do so—whether by restricting certain methods or neglecting to provide essential reproductive healthcare—violates women's rights.

Coercive practices such as forced sterilization further undermine bodily autonomy and dignity. In low- and middle-income countries, over 200 million women lack access to effective contraception, leading to 76 million unplanned pregnancies annually. Addressing this unmet need could significantly reduce unintended pregnancies and prevent 142,000 pregnancy-related deaths each year, including 53,000 from unsafe abortions. Ensuring contraceptive rights is essential for women's health, autonomy, and overall well-being [4].

- *To Quote a Country as an Example is India Role of Government; Judicial Recognition of Reproductive Rights as Fundamental and Human Rights in India* [3]

Indian courts, including the Supreme Court and various High Courts, have recognized reproductive rights as fundamental and human rights, holding the government accountable for providing reproductive healthcare. Key areas of recognition include maternal health, contraceptive access, abortion rights, and child marriage.

- Maternal health

  Courts have ruled that denial of maternal healthcare violates Article 21 (Right to Life).

  - Landmark cases:

    - Laxmi Mandal v. Deen Dayal Harinagar Hospital (2011): Established maternal healthcare as an inalienable survival right.
    - Sandesh Bansal v. Union of India (2012): Government financial constraints are not an excuse for poor maternal care; mandated proper healthcare infrastructure.
- Contraceptive access
  - Devika Biswas v. Union of India (2016): Recognized reproductive autonomy and gender equality.
  - Coercive sterilization policies were declared unconstitutional.
  - Governments must ensure noncoercive access to contraceptive options.

- Abortion and forced pregnancy
  - Courts have progressively upheld women's autonomy over abortion.
  - Hallo Bi v. State of Madhya Pradesh (2013): Allowed rape survivors access to abortion without judicial authorization.
  - Recent Supreme Court cases (2015–2017) have permitted abortions beyond the 20-week limit in cases of fetal impairment or risk to the mother's health.
  - High Court on its Own Motion v. State of Maharashtra (2016): Established that abortion rights are part of a woman's bodily autonomy and dignity.
- Child marriage
  - Courts recognize child marriage as a violation of human rights.
  - Delhi High Court rulings (2010, 2012) highlighted the impact on girls, linking it to domestic violence, sexual abuse, and lack of reproductive autonomy.
- *Human Rights and Access to Contraception*

International and regional human rights treaties, along with national laws, guarantee access to contraceptive information and services. Over the years, human rights bodies have reinforced the need for timely, affordable, and high-quality reproductive healthcare. They emphasize that contraception must be provided with full respect for dignity, autonomy, privacy, and informed decision-making, ensuring services are tailored to individuals' needs and rights [5].

- *ICPD and the Recognition of Reproductive Rights*

The 1994 International Conference on Population and Development (ICPD) marked a pivotal moment in global reproductive rights. With 179 countries adopting the Programme of Action, it established that reproductive rights are human rights recognized in domestic and international law. The agreement emphasized empowering individuals, especially women, to make informed family planning decisions and ensuring access to reproductive health services. The ICPD defined reproductive health as a state of complete physical, mental, and social well-being in all matters related to the reproductive system [6].

30.3 Impact of Violence on Contraceptive Access

- *The Impact of Domestic Violence on Contraceptive Use and Unwanted Pregnancies: Evidence from India*

  Stephenson R et al. reported a significant link between male-to-female domestic violence and unwanted pregnancies across different regions of India. Analyzing data from the 1998–1999 National Family Health Survey and a 2002–2003 follow-up survey, they found that women who experienced physical violence from their husbands were less likely to adopt contraception and more likely to have unwanted pregnancies. The study also highlighted that prospective measures of pregnancy unwantedness revealed a higher prevalence of unwanted pregnancies compared to traditional retrospective methods. These findings underscore the profound impact of domestic violence on women's reproductive autonomy and the need for improved methods to measure pregnancy intendedness [7].

- Other barriers include the following [8]:
  - *Forced early marriage* and social pressure for early childbearing
  - *Limited access* to contraceptive information and services
  - *Restricted decision-making power* within households
  - *Limited physical mobility* and restricted access to healthcare providers
  - *Physical violence and coercion* in sexual and family relations

- *Intimate Partner Violence and Reproductive Coercion* [9]

Research on the relationship between intimate partner violence (IPV) and contraceptive use discontinuation in low- and middle-income countries (LMICs) has remained limited. A study by Upadhyay et al. aimed to address this gap using data from the 2015–2016 National Family Health Survey (NFHS) in India, analyzing the contraceptive behaviors of women aged 15–49 years.

Findings have revealed that experiences of IPV were significantly associated with discontinuation of contraceptive methods while still in need (DWSIN). Women who had experienced physical violence were more likely to discontinue long-acting reversible contraceptives (LARC) or intrauterine devices (IUDs) (RRR: 3.73, 95% CI [1.55–8.95]). Similarly, condom discontinuation was found to be higher among women who had endured emotional violence (RRR: 4.16, 95% CI [1.59–10.90]). While no association was identified between IPV and overall contraceptive discontinuation, the strong link between IPV and discontinuation of specific contraceptive methods was observed in India.

These findings have highlighted the role of IPV in reproductive coercion, influencing women's contraceptive choices and autonomy. Addressing IPV has been recognized as a critical component of high-quality family planning services, ensuring that women are supported in making uninterrupted contraceptive decisions that align with their individual circumstances and reproductive goals.

- *Sexual Violence and Barriers to Emergency Contraception*

Sexual violence remains a significant public health concern, with nearly one in five women experiencing completed or attempted rape. Despite professional guidelines recommending emergency contraception (EC) for sexual assault survivors, access in emergency departments (EDs) remains inconsistent. A scoping review of US hospital EDs found that only 60% had EC policies, 75% provided EC counseling, 44% offered EC, and 62% dispensed it onsite. Barriers such as hospital policies, provider training gaps, and state laws contribute to this variability, potentially limiting survivors' access to essential post assault reproductive care. Addressing these disparities is crucial to ensuring comprehensive support for survivors [10].

- *Societal and Cultural Stigmas*

Religious and cultural beliefs significantly influence contraceptive acceptance and use, shaping reproductive choices differently across faiths and communities. While religious teachings may guide perspectives on contraception, interpretations vary across sects, and individuals may choose to disregard them. Cultural expectations regarding family size and fertility also play a crucial role, particularly among immigrant populations adapting to new societal norms. These influences, combined with societal stigmas, can create barriers to contraceptive access, particularly for women in restrictive environments [11].

30.4 Legal and Policy Challenges

Since the US Department of Health and Human Services (HHS) regulation on preventive services for women, over 80 corporations have filed lawsuits challenging contraceptive coverage. For-profit corporations argue it violates their First Amendment rights and burdens them under the Religious Freedom Restoration Act (RFRA). Nonprofit organizations also claim exemptions under religious grounds, particularly opposing emergency contraception, despite its FDA classification as a contraceptive [12].

In India, legal and policy challenges around contraception include ensuring access to a full range of methods, addressing social and cultural barriers, and promoting male involvement in family planning, while also navigating the complexities of the legal framework and public health policies [3].

30.5 DHEERA: Advocating Against Violence and for Reproductive Rights [13]

DHEERA—meaning Courage and Conviction—is an initiative launched in 2016 in Hyderabad India by Prof S. Shantha kumari as a member of FIGO Working group on NO TO Violence Against Women with the International Federation of Gynecology and Obstetrics (FIGO), the Federation of Obstetric and Gynaecological Societies of India (FOGSI), and the Obstetric and Gynaecological Society of Hyderabad (OGSH). It advocates for gender equality and reproductive rights by partnering with key stakeholders, including the following:

- Sensitization—Educating communities on reproductive rights and gender-based violence
- Advocacy—Engaging policymakers, media, and legal bodies to drive systemic change

- Action-oriented impact—Implementing programs to ensure women's safety, autonomy, and quality of life
- *DHEERA initiative is to give women the courage to access the healthcare for sexual and reproductive health rights and for contraception.*

30.6 Conclusion

Violence against women, including reproductive coercion, remains a significant barrier to achieving gender equality. Governments, international organizations, and civil society must collaborate to protect and advance reproductive rights. The denial of contraceptive access, restrictive abortion laws, and coercive family planning policies must be recognized as violations of fundamental human rights. Ending violence against women requires a comprehensive approach—one that guarantees autonomy, informed choice, and access to quality reproductive healthcare for all.

Declarations

Competing Interests The author(s) has no competing interests to declare that are relevant to the content of this manuscript.

Ethics Approval The author(s) declares that this manuscript does not include primary research with human participants.

The author(s) declares that this manuscript does not include primary studies involving animals.

References

1. Violence against women. Impact. Available at: https://www.who.int/health-topics/violence-against-women#tab=tab_2. Accessed 29 Mar 2025.
2. Violence against women and reproductive rights in the Americas. Available at: https://www.reproductiverights.org/sites/crr.civicactions.net/files/documents/(EN)%20Advocacy%20Doc%20for%20OAS%20Convening.pdf. Accessed 29 Mar 2025.
3. Reproductive rights in Indian courts. Available at: https://reproductiverights.org/sites/default/files/documents/Reproductive-Rights-In-Indian-Courts.pdf. Accessed 29 Mar 2025.
4. Chapter III: Contraception. Available at: https://reproductiverights.org/wp-content/uploads/2018/08/pub_bo_GG_contraception.pdf. Accessed 29 Mar 2025.
5. Ensuring human rights in the provision of contraceptive information and services. Guidance and recommendations. Available at: https://iris.who.int/bitstream/handle/10665/102539/9789241506748_eng.pdf. Accessed 29 Mar 2025.
6. ICPD and human rights: 20 years of advancing reproductive rights through UN treaty bodies and legal reform. Available at: https://www.unfpa.org/sites/default/files/pub-pdf/icpd_and_human_rights_20_years.pdf. Accessed 29 Mar 2025.
7. Stephenson R, Koenig MA, Acharya R, et al. Domestic violence, contraceptive use, and unwanted pregnancy in rural India. Stud Fam Plan. 2008;39(3):177–86.
8. Sanneving L, Trygg N, Saxena D, Mavalankar D, Thomsen S. Inequity in India: the case of maternal and reproductive health. Glob Health Action. 2013;6:19145.

9. Association between intimate partner violence and contraceptive use discontinuation in India. Available at: https://iipsindia.ac.in/sites/default/files/Association_Between_Intimate_Partner_Violence.pdf. Accessed 29 Mar 2025.
10. Wang MJ, Khodadadi AB, Turan JM, et al. Scoping review of access to emergency contraception for sexual assault victims in emergency departments in the United States. Trauma Violence Abuse. 2021;22(2):413–21.
11. Srikanthan A, Reid RL. Religious and cultural influences on contraception. J Obstet Gynaecol Can. 2008;30(2):129–37.
12. A guide to the Supreme Court's review of the contraceptive coverage requirement. Available at: https://www.kff.org/report-section/8523-contraceptive-coverage-requirement-legal-challenges/. Accessed 29 Mar 2025.
13. Shantha KS. DHEERA: no to violence against women. J Obstet Gynaecol India. 2021;71(Suppl 2):59–63.

Chapter 31
Sexual Violence, Dignity, and Contraception

Rubina Sohail and Mariam Iqbal

Sexual violence is a human rights violation and a global issue. It is defined as physical, sexual, or psychological violence directed towards an individual based on gender, but mostly affecting women and girls. It occurs mostly by intimate partners but can happen by strangers or sometimes authoritarian figures. It includes sexual harassment, sexual exploitation, sexual assault, rape, and trafficking. The survivors of sexual violence may experience physical injuries, psychological trauma, and long-term health consequences, including sexually transmitted infections and unintended pregnancies, which can have lasting consequences on the lives of survivors. Survivors of GBV may experience depression, anxiety, posttraumatic stress disorder, and other mental health issues [1].

Sexual violence has impact on the self-esteem and dignity of survivors, often resulting in feelings of shame, guilt, worthlessness, and self-blame [2]. This can result in inability to pursue educational goals and profession. It is essential to ensure the dignity of individuals who have experienced sexual violence.

The aftermath of sexual violence includes concerns about unwanted pregnancy, and the emotional, financial, and social implications under the circumstances. Therefore, providing access to emergency contraception and long-term contraceptives must be an essential part of support and care for survivors. Contraception empowers women and allows them to make informed choices about their reproductive health and enables them to plan their future without the added burden of an unintended pregnancy. Contraception also allows women to participate fully in society, pursue education, and use available career opportunities.

R. Sohail (✉)
FIGO, SOGP - Hameed Latif Hospital, Lahore, Pakistan

M. Iqbal
Integrated Medical Center, Lahore, Pakistan

A. R. Genazzani et al. (eds.), *Ethical, Efficacy and Safety Issues in Contraception*, Reproductive Medicine for Clinicians 4,
https://doi.org/10.1007/978-3-032-07322-8_31

Sometimes in low-resource countries, access to contraception may be limited due to lack of resources. Perpetrators may deny access to contraception to maintain control over the victim. Fear of recurring violence can prevent the survivors from seeking contraception [3].

31.1 Gender-Based Sexual Violence

Violence against women is mostly underreported due to social, cultural, and legal barriers. According to the World Health Organization (WHO), one in three women around the world has experienced physical or sexual violence. In developed countries, the prevalence of gender-based violence is around 20–25% [4]. In developing countries, the situation is scary. The United Nations Population Fund (UNFPA) reports that one-third of women worldwide experience violence. In sub-Saharan Africa, the figure rises to 45%, with 36% of women reported experiencing intimate partner violence in South-East Asia [5]. Child marriage is also a form of GBV. One in five girls in developing countries is married before 18, putting them at risk of violence and abuse.

Prevalence of GBV is influenced by gender inequality, cultural norms that condone violence against women, and weak legal systems that fail to protect women rights. Poverty and conflict also contribute to the high rates of GBV, while armed conflicts lead to an increase in sexual violence.

31.2 Consequences of Gender-Based Violence

Gender-based violence reinforces gender inequalities and create a barrier for achieving sustainable development goals. It has multifaceted consequences, impacting the physical, mental, social, and economic well-being.

Sexual violence can have *physical consequences* for the victim, ranging from bruises and cuts to permanent disabilities or even death. In both developed and developing countries, women and girls are the primary victims of sexual violence and endure long-lasting effects on their health and personal well-being leading to a decline in their overall quality of life. Studies demonstrate that physical violence is associated with chronic health conditions, such as chronic pain, hypertension, and GI disorders [6]. There is increased risk of sexually transmitted infections, including HIV. Vaginismus maybe associated with a history of violence and abuse.

Mental health problems, such as depression, anxiety, posttraumatic stress disorder (PTSD), and suicidal thoughts, are common in survivors [7]. It is associated with a feeling of shame, guilt, and fear of judgment, making it difficult for them to seek help, further exacerbating the mental health issues.

Social consequences of GBV affect relationships of the victim with family, friends, and community. Survivors may face social isolation and marginalization due to associated stigma resulting in loss of identity and abandonment from families, making it challenging for them to reintegrate into society.

There are significant *economic consequences* of sexual violence such as difficulty in obtaining and maintaining employment. According to an estimate, sexual violence costs the global economy about 5.2 trillion USD annually [8].

31.2.1 Factors Contributing to Sexual Violence (Fig. 31.1)

In developing countries, the reasons of sexual violence are deep-rooted into social and cultural norms. One of the main triggers is gender inequality, where women are considered inferior to men. This leads to a perceived normalization of sexual violence against women [9]. The gender inequality as determined by the gender gap is dependent upon four factors—economic participation, educational attainment, political empowerment, and health and survival. At the current pace, it will take more than 100 years to achieve gender equality in the world.

Gender inequality drives violence against women and girls in four keyways.

1. Condoning of violence against women
2. Men's control of decision making and limits to independence in public and private place [10]
3. Male colleagues and peer relations that emphasize aggression and disrespect towards women
4. Rigid gender roles and stereotyped constructs of masculinity and femineity [11]

These factors produce an underlying social milieu in which violence against women occurs. In patriarchal societies, all the four keyways exist and create a recipe that promotes sexual violence. Similarly, poverty and economic disparity are also significant drivers of sexual violence, as women and girls may be forced into exploitative relationships to provide for themselves and their families [12].

Women and girls from disadvantaged communities are more vulnerable to sexual exploitation and trafficking. Conflict and displacement increase the risk of sexual violence. During times of war, women and girls are frequently targeted as tools of degradation and are dominated and controlled [9]. In refugee camps, women and children are particularly vulnerable to sexual violence, as perpetrators take advantage of their vulnerability and lack of protection.

Inadequate education and lack of awareness about consent and healthy relationships can also contribute to sexual violence. Many educational institutions do not have comprehensive sex education programs that address consent and healthy relationships, leaving individuals vulnerable to manipulation and coercion. Laws to protect citizens from sexual violence exist in developed countries. However, the objectification of women in media and advertising can reinforce the idea that women's bodies are solely for men's pleasure, leading to a culture that normalizes sexual violence and makes it easier for perpetrators to justify their actions [12]. The expectation for men to be dominant, aggressive, and in control can lead to a sense of

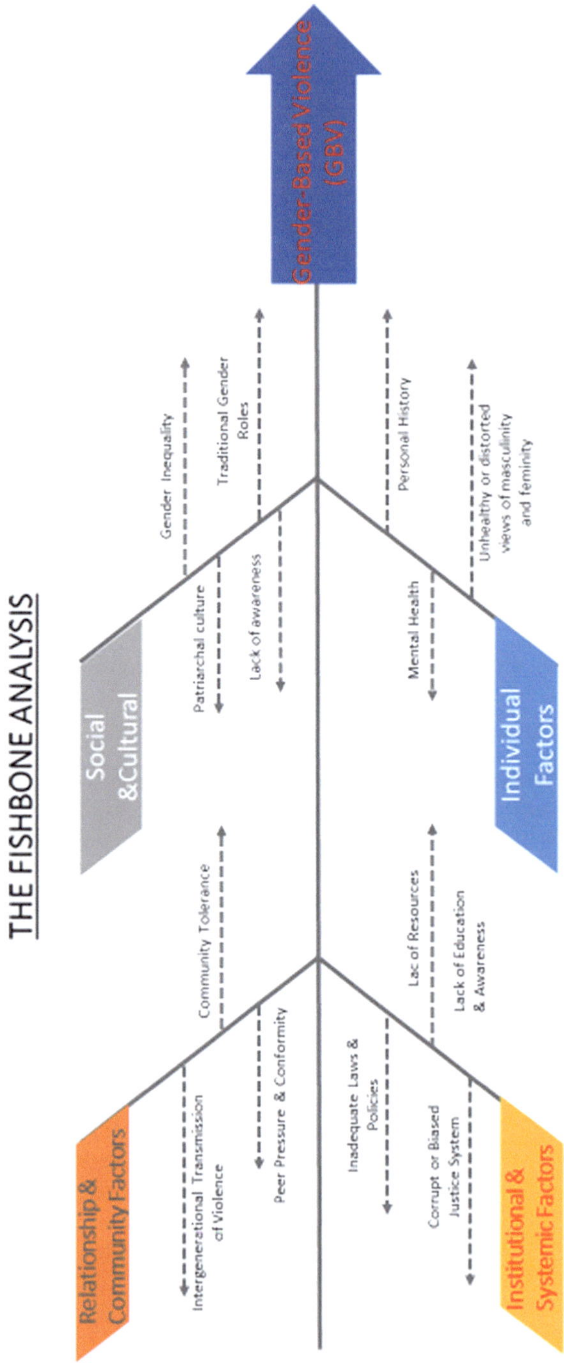

Fig. 31.1 Factors contributing to sexual violence

entitlement and normalization of sexual violence towards women. This pressure and expectation placed on men can also lead to the stigmatization of male victims of sexual violence and discourage them from seeking help [13].

31.3 Addressing Gender-Based Violence

The Convention on the Elimination of All Forms of Discrimination Against Women (CEDAW) and the Beijing Declaration are important international instruments that provide a framework for promoting gender equality.

In developed countries, legal and policy measures have been successful in preventing and responding to violence against women. In developing countries, the situation needs efforts to raise awareness, rethinking gender roles, and improving access to justice.

31.4 The Interplay of Sexual Violence, Dignity, and Contraception

The interplay between sexual violence, dignity, and access to contraception create opportunities for discrimination and emphasize the fact that comprehensive and rights-based solutions are needed to address this issue (Fig. 31.2).

The term *intersectionality* was coined by legal scholar Kimberlé Crenshaw in 1989 [14] and refers to the interconnected nature of social categories, such as gender, race, class, and sexuality, and how they intersect to create unique forms of discrimination and oppression [15]. Girls from marginalized groups, such as migrants and low-income populations, face a higher risk of sexual violence due to their intersectional identities [16]. Intersectionality accepts that sexual violence can manifest differently based on individual identities. For example, LGBTQ+ individuals may experience sexual violence that is shaped by their sexuality and gender identity [17].

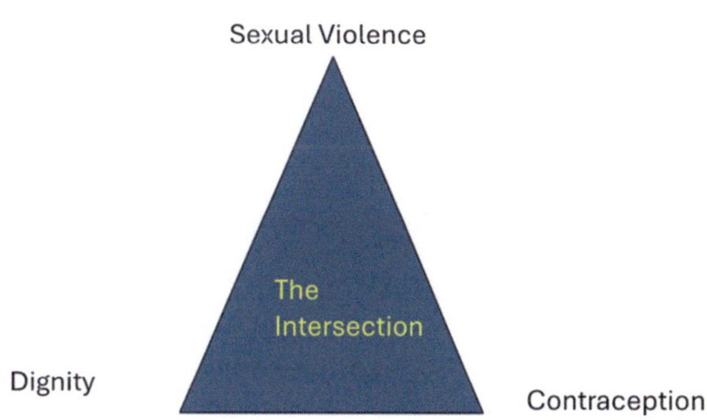

Fig. 31.2 The triad of sexual violence, contraception, and dignity highlighting the intersection of the three and how these themes interplay for women in crises

One of the most important areas is the concept of dignity, which is central to human rights principles and refers to an individual's inherent worth [18]. Sexual violence results in loss of dignity, undermining their sense of self-worth and autonomy. The mental health issues occurring because of GBV can further erode the sense of dignity [19]. In conservative societies, there is emphasis on preserving a woman's chastity and honor, which can result in a feeling of shame and worsen the situation. Power dynamics can make the situation more complex and is commonly seen in conflict-affected areas, where sexual violence is used as a weapon of war to assert power and control over communities [20].

Access to contraception is another significant intersection of sexual violence. The right to access contraception is a human right and is necessary for the health, well-being, and autonomy of individuals [21]. However, their exist many barriers for accessing contraception including lack of information and resources, social stigma, cultural barriers, opposition from family members, and ignorance of the healthcare providers. A study from Africa suggests that successful contraceptive initiatives should also work towards reducing GBV as it is the most common cause of high unmet need for contraception [22]. The intersection of sexual violence and contraception can have implications for marginalized communities. Indigenous women in Canada faced forced sterilization as a form of reproductive violence which violates the right to autonomy and bodily integrity [23].

The risk of sexually transmitted infections is increased in women who experience GBV and may lead to issues such as infertility [24, 25]. Contraception is an essential tool in preventing unintended pregnancies, but access can be limited for survivors and the perpetrators may deliberately target women and girls for reproductive control through forced pregnancies and coerced pregnancies [26–28] A study conducted by the United Nations Population Fund (UNFPA) in 2013 concluded that women who experienced intimate partner violence were 50% more likely to have an unintended pregnancy and were less likely to use modern methods of contraception [29, 30].

Women who experience economic abuse in the form of control of their income or finances may have limited resources to pay for contraceptives, leading to reduced contraceptive use [31]. In developing countries, poverty, lack of education and healthcare, and harmful cultural and traditional practices exacerbate the impact of sexual violence on dignity and contraception. In such situations, sexual violence is often normalized, and survivors may be blamed for the violence they experienced.

The impact of sexual violence on contraception is not limited to the survivors, the perpetrators are likely to indulge in risky sexual behaviors, like multiple sexual partners and not using condoms [32]. This increases the risk of sexually transmitted infections (STIs), which can have a significant impact on their reproductive health. Men who experience sexual violence may also have limited control over their reproductive choices, as their partners may pressure them to have unprotected sex [33].

Interventions are needed to address these issues. Community-based education programs, targeted interventions for men, and economic empowerment programs for women have shown promising results in promoting gender equality and reducing sexual violence [34]. These result in more women making decisions and increasing their autonomy, leading to improved contraceptive use and better reproductive health outcomes.

31.5 Contraceptive Provision and Barriers to Contraceptive Access

Barriers to contraceptive access can be related to distance from facility, lack of uniformity in availability of contraceptive commodities, availability and lack of long-acting reversible contraception. Structural and institutional barriers, including cost, lack of information, and stigma, can make it challenging for survivors to obtain and use contraception. Furthermore, survivors may face additional barriers, such as power imbalances and lack of agency, in negotiating contraceptive use with their partners [40]. Lack of government policies facilitating contraceptive distribution can lead to this situation. Undesirable attitudes of healthcare providers can contribute to worsening the situation. One needs to consider the community level barriers which include perceived side effects, myths and misconceptions, stigma associated with use from peers and friends, and negative traditional and religious beliefs. Women in crises, especially the ones affected by war or who are internally displaced, are particularly vulnerable, as availability and affordability of counseling and commodities is a challenge in these situations. Political will can play a significant enabling role in these situations by improving the availability, access, couple counseling, and provision of trained personnel services to women in need.

31.6 Women in Crisis and Impact on Sexual Violence

Women in crisis include those in conflict zones, displacement camps, and suffering from natural and man-made disasters. They constitute a significant proportion of displaced populations and face challenges such as lack of shelter, sanitation, and protection. Displacement camps and informal settlements can expose women to increased risk of sexual violence, exploitation, and trafficking.

Crises disproportionately affect women leading to loss of livelihoods, hunger, malnutrition, and poverty. Hence, disasters can increase a woman's vulnerability and susceptibility to violence and exploitation [35]. This was exhibited after the Loma Prieta earthquake when reports of sexual violence increased by 300-fold [36]. Similarly, during Hurricane Katrina, sexual violence increased from a baseline of 4.6 to 16.3 reported cases per 100,000 per day. This reflects failure of disaster response to protect these women [37]. According to the United Nations Population Fund (UNFPA), about 75% of all women and girls aged 15–49 who are living in areas affected by armed conflict are at risk of being sexually abused. The United Nations Office for the Coordination of Humanitarian Affairs (OCHA) states that in armed conflicts, sexual violence is often used as a weapon of war to intimidate, humiliate, and control communities [38]. Though providing comprehensive sexual and reproductive health services in crisis settings is a daunting task, provision of these services is an integral part of disaster response, which is somehow often missing from the humanitarian agenda [39].

31.6.1 Needs and Rights of Women in Crises

1. Protection from gender-based violence including prevention, response, and access to support services. This includes ensuring safe spaces, psychosocial support, legal assistance, and economic empowerment initiatives.
2. Access to sexual and reproductive health services, including contraceptives, treatment for STIs, and maternal healthcare.
3. Support for maternal and child health such as good quality antenatal care, presence of skilled birth attendants, neonatal care, and postnatal support.
4. Empowering women to engage in advocacy initiatives, community leadership, and job support to improve livelihood, resulting in greater social cohesion, agency, and resilience. Empowerment and participation of women in humanitarian response planning, and peacebuilding efforts is also necessary.

31.7 SWOT Analysis

The following is a SWOT analysis of gender-based violence (GBV) in both developed and developing countries.

Strengths

Increased awareness and recognition: One of the strengths in addressing GBV is the growing awareness and recognition of its existence. More individuals and organizations are acknowledging GBV as a serious human rights issue, and efforts are being made to eliminate it.

Increasingly stringent laws and policies: Many countries have developed and implemented laws and policies to address GBV. For example, the United Nations has adopted the Convention on the Elimination of All Forms of Discrimination Against Women (CEDAW), which requires member states to implement measures to protect women from violence.

Availability of support services: In both developed and developing countries, there are increasing numbers of support services for victims of GBV. These include hotlines, shelters, legal aid, and counseling services.

International co-operation: There has been a growing recognition that GBV is a global issue, and there are initiatives to address it at the international level. For example, the United Nations has designated 25th November as the International Day for the Elimination of Violence Against Women.

Weaknesses

Under-reporting: GBV is vastly underreported due to various factors such as lack of trust in the justice system, fear of retaliation, and shame and stigma associated with being a victim of violence. This makes it difficult to understand the full extent of the problem.

Lack of enforcement: Despite the existence of laws and policies, there is often a lack of enforcement, especially in developing countries. This can be due to corruption, inadequate resources, and deep-rooted cultural norms that perpetuate GBV.

Limited access to support services: In many developing countries, support services for victims of GBV are limited or non-existent. This leaves victims with few options for seeking help and addressing their situation.

Insufficient funding: The resources allocated to address GBV are often insufficient, particularly in developing countries. This limits the ability to implement effective prevention and intervention programs.

Opportunities

Integration of GBV into broader development policies: There is an opportunity to incorporate efforts to address GBV into broader development policies and strategies. This can help increase resources and attention towards this issue.

Strengthening partnerships: Increased collaboration and partnership between governments, civil society organizations, and individuals can help address GBV more comprehensively. This can bring together different perspectives, knowledge, and skills to develop more effective strategies.

Use of technology: Technological advancements can be utilized to raise awareness, provide support services, and collect data on GBV. For example, mobile apps and online platforms can be used to reach out to victims and provide them with resources and support.

Threats

Patriarchal attitudes and norms: Deeply ingrained societal attitudes that reinforce gender inequality and perpetuate patriarchal power structures can hinder efforts to address GBV.

Limited resources: As mentioned earlier, limited resources can hinder the implementation of effective programs and initiatives to address GBV.

Political instability and conflict: Political instability and conflict can create a chaotic and dangerous environment where GBV thrives. This makes it difficult to implement long-term solutions and sustain progress in addressing GBV.

Discrimination and marginalization: Certain groups, such as women from marginalized communities, may face even greater barriers in accessing support services and seeking justice for GBV (Fig. 31.3).

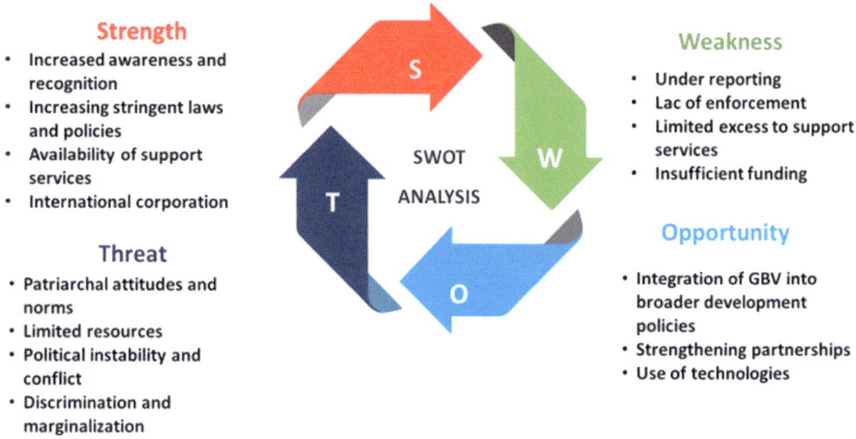

Fig. 31.3 The SWOT analysis

31.8 Role of Healthcare Providers

Healthcare professionals should be able to work in a multidisciplinary team environment and spearhead the campaign to identify, support, treat victims of sexual violence and refer if needed. However, in many countries, they need to be sensitized to the issue first and provided proper training to build their capacity for the next steps. The physicians should be advocates of women and girls and become a part of the change, working with women to empower them, and working in collaboration with the government and policy makers to develop and implement policies to protect and strengthen women.

With several standards and guidelines in place to direct their practice, healthcare practitioners in developed nations have a well-established role in managing gender-based violence. The Center for Disease Control and Prevention (CDC) has developed a National Intimate Partner and Sexual Violence Survey (NISVS) that gathers information on the frequency, pattern, and prevalence of sexual violence in the country [41]. This information has been instrumental in informing healthcare professionals on the diverse types of sexual violence, the influence on victims and their families, as well as the risk factors that contribute to the execution of sexual violence. In Europe, the Council of Europe has also established the Istanbul Convention, which is a legally binding instrument that sets minimum standards for the protection of women against all types of sexual violence [42]. The convention expects member states to have developed measures to prevent sexual violence, protect victims, and ensure accountability for perpetrators, in which healthcare professionals play a crucial role. These protocols and guidelines have equipped healthcare professionals

Table 31.1 The role of healthcare provider

	Role of healthcare provider
1	Sensitize
2	Train
3	Identify
4	Counsel
5	Treat
6	Support
7	Refer
8	Advocate
9	Empower
10	Collaborate

with the knowledge and skills to identify signs of gender-based violence, provide suitable care to victims, and refer them to relevant services, such as counseling and legal support.

In developing countries, healthcare professionals face several obstacles in management of sexual violence victims due to lack of resources, inadequate training, and cultural barriers. They often work in resource-limited settings, which requires their involvement in community-based interventions to address sexual violence. In rural areas of India, community health workers have been trained to identify cases and offer basic counseling, as well as refer victims to legal and support services [44]. This approach has proven to be effective in raising awareness and decreasing the prevalence of sexual violence.

In countries like South Africa, which has one of the highest statistics for sexual violence, the government has developed the National Strategic Plan on Gender-Based Violence and Femicide (GBVF) to address this matter [43]. As part of the plan, healthcare professionals are required to undergo training to recognize and treat sexual violence victims, provide post-exposure prophylaxis (PEP) for victims, and refer them to appropriate services (Table 31.1).

31.9 Policy Implications

- Need policy initiatives aimed at addressing sexual violence, promoting dignity, and increasing access to contraception
- Advocacy for legislative reforms, funding allocations, and community-based interventions to support survivors and prevent sexual violence
- Multi-sectoral collaboration and advocacy efforts to enhance the rights and well-being of survivors

31.10 Current Work for Survivors of Sexual Violence: The Red Line Initiative

The Red Line Initiative, led by the Mukwege Foundation, has the mission to put an end to conflict-related sexual violence in all its forms, including when used as a weapon of war. The use of sexual violence in conflict can be prevented and must be prioritized as absolutely unacceptable [45]. The initiative works in close collaboration with SEMA, the Global Network of Victims and Survivors to End Wartime Sexual Violence. The Mukwege Foundation works at national and international levels and with states to:

1. *Ask for a strong response*, clearly rejecting conflict-related sexual violence in all its forms, including as a method of warfare
2. *Clarify and strengthen legal obligations* of States, to actively prevent and punish conflict-related sexual violence
3. *Advocate and educate* to build political will to push for a more robust and timely response by States in line with their international obligations

31.11 Recommendations for Addressing Sexual Violence, Dignity, and Contraception

Addressing sexual violence requires a comprehensive approach that recognizes and addresses the underlying factors that perpetuate this issue. This includes promoting gender equality and challenging societal norms and systems that uphold power imbalances and discrimination. Additionally, facilitating access to comprehensive sexual and reproductive health services, including contraception, is crucial in supporting survivors of sexual violence and preventing future incidents. There is a need for a holistic approach to addressing sexual violence, which considers the intersecting identities of individuals and promotes their rights and dignity. As global efforts to combat sexual violence continue, it is essential to recognize and address these intersections to ensure the protection and well-being of all individuals. A multifaceted approach involves education, awareness, policy changes, and community support.

31.11.1 Raise Awareness

Increase public awareness about sexual violence and its impact on individuals and communities. Use media campaigns [46], workshops, and community events to educate people about the signs of sexual violence, how to prevent it, and where to seek help. Raising awareness can also contribute to changing societal attitudes and norms that condone violence against women.

31.11.2 Comprehensive Sex Education

Age-appropriate and culturally sensitive comprehensive sex education programs teach about consent, healthy relationships, and reproductive health.

31.11.3 Community Engagement

Engage communities in efforts to prevent sexual violence and promote dignity and respect for all individuals. Work with community leaders, religious organizations, and other stakeholders to challenge attitudes and norms that condone violence and discrimination.

31.11.4 Promote Consent

Promote a culture of consent by emphasizing the importance of obtaining explicit and enthusiastic consent in all sexual encounters. This will include teaching people how to recognize and respect boundaries, as well as challenging harmful attitudes and beliefs about gender and sexuality.

31.11.5 Empowerment

Empower individuals, especially women and marginalized communities, to assert their rights and make informed decisions about their bodies and reproductive health. Provide access to contraception and family planning services, including a range of contraceptive options to suit different needs and preferences.

31.11.6 Address Root Cause

Address the root causes of sexual violence, including gender inequality, poverty, and social norms that perpetuate harmful attitudes and behaviors. Promote gender equity and challenge harmful stereotypes that contribute to violence and discrimination.

31.11.7 Governments Support Survivors

They are creating safe spaces where survivors can share their experiences without fear of judgment or retaliation. Survivors of sexual violence should have access to confidential support services for counseling, medical care, and legal assistance. Survivors of GBV often face physical, psychological, and economic challenges, which require a range of support services to aid their recovery and empowerment and help them rebuild their lives. Governments, NGOs, and civil society organizations should provide various support services such as counseling, legal aid, and shelters for survivors. These services include medical care, legal assistance, psychosocial support, and economic empowerment programs. It is essential to ensure that these services are accessible, culturally appropriate, and free of charge for survivors, especially in developing countries where resources may be limited. These services should be tailored to the unique needs of survivors and be readily available in both urban and rural areas [47].

31.11.8 Policy Changes

Advocate for policy changes at the local, national, and international levels to strengthen laws and regulations related to sexual violence prevention, prosecution, and support for survivors.

31.11.9 Training and Capacity Building

Provide training for healthcare providers, law enforcement officers, and other professionals who work with survivors of sexual violence. This includes training on trauma-informed care, cultural competence, and how to respond effectively to disclosures of violence.

31.11.10 Research and Evaluation

Invest in research and evaluation to better understand the causes and consequences of sexual violence, as well as what interventions are most effective in preventing and responding to it. Use evidence-based practices to inform policy and programming decisions. Data and research are essential for understanding the scope and nature of GBV, identifying the underlying causes, and developing evidence-based interventions. Therefore, it is crucial to strengthen data collection systems, including disaggregated data that captures the experiences of marginalized groups such as refugees, indigenous communities, and LGBTQ+ individuals. Additionally, investing in research on GBV can help generate evidence to inform policies and programs to address the issue effectively.

31.11.10.1 Implement Strong Laws and Policies

Governments play a crucial role in eliminating gender-based violence. Strong laws and policies are needed to protect victims and hold perpetrators accountable. These laws should cover all forms of gender-based violence, including physical, sexual, emotional, and economic abuse [48]. In addition, governments must ensure that these laws are effectively enforced and accessible to all, regardless of their socioeconomic status. In many countries, rules and policies related to GBV may be inadequate or not effectively enforced. Therefore, reviewing and strengthening existing legal frameworks to ensure they address all forms of GBV and provide adequate protection and support for survivors is crucial. This includes criminalizing all forms of GBV, establishing specialized courts and legal mechanisms, and providing training for law enforcement and judicial personnel to address GBV cases effectively.

31.11.10.2 Promote Gender Equality

Gender inequality is a root cause of gender-based violence. Therefore, promoting gender equality is crucial in eliminating this issue. This can be achieved by addressing underlying factors such as patriarchal attitudes, social and cultural norms, and economic disparities between men and women. Governments must ensure that women have equal access to education, employment, and leadership opportunities [49].

31.11.10.3 Address Economic Inequality and Empower Women

Gender inequality, including economic inequality, is a significant driver of GBV. Therefore, it is essential to address gender disparities in education, employment, and economic opportunities. This can be achieved by promoting women's education and skills training, promoting women's entrepreneurship, and eliminating discriminatory laws and practices that limit women's economic participation.

31.11.10.4 Engage Males

GBV is a result of harmful gender norms and stereotypes, which can also negatively impact males. Engaging men and boys in efforts to challenge and transform these norms is crucial in the elimination of GBV [50]. Males can be powerful advocates for change by challenging traditional gender roles and promoting healthy

Table 31.2 Solutions—the ten steps

1	Strategies to empower survivors of GBV to make decisions about their RH
2	Survivor centered care to promote resilience
3	Provision of comprehensive sexual and RH services integrating trauma informed care
4	Free access to contraception empowering women to make informed choice about their SRH
5	Ensure autonomy, dignity, confidentiality, safety of survivors and access to justice
6	Providing counseling, compassionate support, and respecting survivors choices
7	Addressing the root cause of violence and using intersectional approaches to deal with sexual violence, dignity, and contraception
8	Recognize the special needs of diverse individuals and address underlying inequalities and discrimination
9	Legal and policy reforms to protect survivors and to hold the perpetrators accountable
10	Implement measures to prevent and respond to GBV and ensure the rights of survivors are protected in the legal process

masculinity. This can be achieved through targeted campaigns and programs that challenge toxic masculinity, foster healthy relationships and positive masculinities, and involve men and boys as allies in creating gender-equal societies. Governments, together with NGOs, can engage men and boys through education and awareness programs that highlight their role in ending gender-based violence.

In developing countries and conservative societies, particularly in the South Asian regions, men are the decision-makers; having them on board would not only help in eliminating GBV but also would help in increasing the contraception uptake rate if they are convinced (Table 31.2).

31.12 Conclusions

In conclusion, sexual violence has a profound impact on the dignity and reproductive health of individuals, particularly women and girls, in both developed and developing countries. It is imperative that efforts are made to prevent and respond to sexual violence, not only to protect the physical and mental well-being of survivors but also to uphold their fundamental human rights and promote their dignity. This includes addressing gender inequality, promoting gender-sensitive education and interventions, and providing comprehensive support services to survivors. Only by addressing the root causes of sexual violence can we create a world where individuals are free from violence and can exercise their sexual and reproductive rights with dignity and autonomy.

Call to action for coordinated efforts to address sexual violence, protect women's dignity, and promote access to contraception for women in crises.

Declarations

Competing Interests The author(s) has no competing interests to declare that are relevant to the content of this manuscript.

Ethics Approval The author(s) declares that this manuscript does not include primary research with human participants.

The author(s) declares that this manuscript does not include primary studies involving animals.

References

1. World Health Organization. Violence against women: key facts. 2020. Retrieved from https://www.who.int/news-room/fact-sheets/detail/violence-against-women.
2. Knaul FM, Gomez-Dantes O, Rozental R, García-Junco D, Arreola-Ornelas H, Mujica OJ, Sarukhán J. Sexual violence against women: understanding the responses in Mexico and Latin America. Lancet Glob Health. 2017;5(3):e276–7.
3. Miller E, Decker MR, McCauley HL, Tancredi DJ, Levenson RR, Waldman J. Pregnancy coercion, intimate partner violence and unintended pregnancy. Contraception. 2010;81(4):316–22.
4. World Health Organization. Violence against women: key facts. 2017. Retrieved from https://www.who.int/news-room/fact-sheets/detail/violence-against-women.
5. United Nations Population Fund. Ending gender-based violence is crucial to achieving the sustainable development goals. 2020. Retrieved from https://www.unfpa.org/ending-gender-based-violence-crucial-achieving-sustainable-development-goals.
6. Mahapatra B, Gupta RN, Mahapatra S. Consequences of domestic violence on women's mental and physical health. Int J Res Med Sci. 2018;6(5):1548–52.
7. World Health Organization. Global and regional estimates of violence against women: prevalence and health effects of intimate partner violence and non-partner sexual violence. Geneva: World Health Organization; 2013.
8. World Bank. Gender-based violence: issues and approaches in the Pacific. Washington: World Bank; 2018.
9. Sarkar NN, Dasgupta A. Chapter 28 – Women's health in developing countries. In: Comprehensive gynecology. 7th ed. Elsevier; 2018. p. 412–26.
10. Edström J, Hassink A, Shahrokh T, Stern E. Engendering men: A collaborative review of evidence on men and boys in social change and gender equality; 2015.
11. Heimer K, Coster SD. The gendering of violent delinquency. Criminology. 1999;37(2):277–318.
12. Brownmiller S. Against our will: men, women and rape. Penguin UK; 2018. Chabbra D, Jackson SR, Patel R. Sexual violence against women and girls in India. J Glob Health. 2017;7(1):1–11.
13. Kilmartin C, Kampf R. Male privilege and toxic masculinity. In: Handbook of masculinity and toxicent- ulinity in contemporary society. Routledge; 2019. p. 1–16.
14. Crenshaw K. Demarginalizing the intersection of race and sex: a black feminist critique of antidiscrimination doctrine, feminist theory, and antiracist politics. Univ Chic Leg Forum. 1989;1989:139–67.
15. Collins PH. Intersectionality's definitional dilemmas. Annu Rev Sociol. 2015;52:299–319. https://doi.org/10.1146/annurev-soc-073014-112142.
16. United Nations Human Rights Office of the High Commissioner. Violence against women: about gender and inequality. 2018. Retrieved from https://www.ohchr.org/EN/Issues/Women/WRGS/Pages/AboutGender.aspx.
17. Logie CH, Earnshaw V. Sexuality, stigma, and intersectionality: non-normative sexualities and sexual- and gender-minority status. In: Johnson ML, Tebes ME, editors. Handbook of

multicultural mental health: assessment and treatment of diverse populations. Amsterdam: Elsevier; 2018. p. 363–81.
18. International Society of Human Rights. Human dignity. 2020. Retrieved from https://www.ishr.org/wp-content/uploads/2020/05/SHR-HumanDignityFactSheet2020.pdf.
19. World Health Organization. Responding to intimate partner violence and sexual violence against women: clinical and policy guidelines. 2009. Retrieved from https://www.who.int/reproductivehealth/publications/violence/9789241599379/en/.
20. United Nations Security Council. Resolution 2467 (2019). 2019. Retrieved from https://undocs.org/S/RES/2467(2019).
21. United Nations Population Fund. Human rights based contraceptive information and services: a final training resource for family planning. 2012. Retrieved from https://www.unfpa.org/publications/human-rights-based-contraceptive-information-and-services-final-training-resource.
22. Ahinkorah BO, Ameyaw EK, Seidu AA, Agbaglo E, Budu E, Mensah F, Adu C, Yaya S. Sexual violence and unmet need for contraception among married and cohabiting women in sub-Saharan Africa: evidence from demographic and health surveys. PLoS One. 2020;15(11):e0240556.
23. Truth and Reconciliation Commission of Canada. Honouring the truth, reconciling for the future: summary of the final report of the truth and Reconciliation Commission of Canada. 2015. Retrieved from http://www.trc.ca/assets/pdf/Hon.
24. Decker MR, Miller E, McCauley HL, Tancredi DJ, Anderson H, Levenson R, et al. Recent partner violence and sexual and drug related STI/HIV risk among adolescent and young adult women attending family planning clinics. Sex Transm Infect. 2014;90(2):145–9.
25. Tumlinson K, Speizer I, Davis JT, Fotso JC, Kuria P, Archer LH. Partner violence and fertility: a longitudinal study in urban Kenya. BMC Public Health. 2013;13:11.
26. United Nations Population Fund. Marital rape: registered legal submissions in developing and developed countries. 2013. Retrieved from http://www.unfpa.org/sites/default/files/pub-pdf/MaritalRape.pdf. United Nations Population Fund. (2013).
27. Devries KM, Mak JY, Bacchus LJ, et al. Intimate partner violence and incident depressive symptoms and suicide attempts: a systematic review of longitudinal studies. PLoS Med. 2013;10(5):e1001439.
28. García-Moreno C, Jansen HA, Ellsberg M, Heise L, Watts CH. WHO multi-country study on women's health and domestic violence against women: initial results on prevalence, health outcomes and women's responses. Geneva: WHO; 2005.
29. Intimate partner and sexual violence against women: common health consequences. Retrieved from https://www.unfpa.org/sites/default/files/pub-pdf/EN-SWOP14-ESTIMATES-EN-v17.pdf.
30. Kaye D, Mirembe F, Bantebya G, Johansson A, Ekstrom AM. Implications of women's fertility desires for uptake of modern contraceptive methods in Busia District, Uganda. Reprod Health. 2010;7:27.
31. Lian OS, Linhares MB, Körners TM, et al. Physical and emotional intimate partner violence and contraceptive behaviour among young women in Brazil. BMJ Open. 2018;8(12):e021130.
32. Simbayi LC, Kalichman SC, Jooste S, et al. Intimate partner violence and condom use among south African men who have sex with men. J Acquir Immune Defic Syndr. 2007;46(2):216–21.
33. Lichtenstein B, Reisner SL, Bianchi FT, Mimiaga MJ. Sexual violence, sexual risk, and sexual protective behaviors among a nationally representative sample of transgender adults. J Acquir Immune Defic Syndr. 2018;79(1):123–9.
34. World Health Organization. Preventing intimate partner and sexual violence against women: taking action and generating evidence. Geneva: World Health Organization; 2010.
35. Kilpatrick DG. Rape in America: a report to the nation. Technical report 1992.
36. Enarson E. Commission for the prevention of violence against women. violence against women in the aftermath of the October 17, 1989, earthquake: a report to the mayor and City Council of the City of Santa Cruz. Santa Cruz 1989.

37. Schumacher JA, Coffey SF, Norris FH, Tracy M, Clements K, Galea S. Intimate partner violence and hurricane Katrina: predictors and associated mental health outcomes. Violence Vict. 2010;25(5):588–603.
38. United Nations Office for the Coordination of Humanitarian Affairs. Preventing and responding to sexual violence in humanitarian emergencies. 2018. https://www.unocha.org/sites/unocha/files/Sexual violence in humanitarian emergencies infographic.pdf.
39. Foster AM, Evans DP, Garcia M, Knaster S, Krause S, McGinn T, Rich S, Shah M, Tappis H, Wheeler E. The 2018 inter-agency field manual on reproductive health in humanitarian settings: revising the global standards. Reprod Health Matters. 2017;25(51):18–24.
40. Silumbwe A, Nkole T, Munakampe MN, Milford C, Cordero JP, Kriel Y, Zulu JM, Steyn PS. Community and health systems barriers and enablers to family planning and contraceptive services provision and use in Kabwe District, Zambia. BMC Health Serv Res. 2018;18:1–1.
41. Centers for Disease Control and Prevention. National intimate partner and sexual violence survey. 2020. Retrieved from https://www.cdc.gov/violenceprevention/sexualviolence/overview.html. Council of Europe. (2011).
42. The Istanbul Convention: preventing and combating violence against women and domestic violence. Retrieved from https://www.coe.int/en/web/istanbul-convention/the-convention.
43. Government of South Africa. National strategic plan on gender-based violence and femicide. 2020. Retrieved from https://www.gov.za/documents/national-strategic-plan-gender-based-violence-and-femicide.
44. Ganju D, Saggurti N. Community health worker-delivered counselling for women survivors of intimate partner violence in India: a case study of intervention adaptation and feasibility. Glob Health Action. 2017;10(1):1355052. https://doi.org/10.1080/16549716.2017.1355052.
45. Dolan C, Hovil L, Pasquero L. Translating survivor-centredness into pedagogical approaches to training on sexual violence in conflict and emergency settings: a case study. Int Rev Red Cross. 2024;106:1–24.
46. Sherlock N, Turner J. The role of media in raising awareness about gender-based violence. 2018. Retrieved from https://doi.org/10.1080/13552074.2018.1488477.
47. International Rescue Committee. Key services for survivors of gender-based violence. 2019. Retrieved from https://www.rescue.org/article/key-services-survivors-gender-based-violence.
48. United Nations Entity for Gender Equality and the Empowerment of Women. Strengthening laws and policies to eliminate gender-based violence. n.d. Retrieved from http://www.endvawnow.org/en/articles/382-strengthening-laws-and-policies-to-eliminate-gender-based-violence.html.
49. World Health Organization. Gender equality: a key factor in preventing violence against women. 2019. Retrieved from http://www.who.int/reproductivehealth/topics/violence/preventing_violence/en/.
50. Silberschmidt M. Engaging men and boys against gender-based violence. 2006. Retrieved from https://www.unfpa.org/sites/default/files/pub-pdf/ogvrw_engaging.pdf.

MIX
Papier aus verantwortungsvollen Quellen
Paper from responsible sources
FSC® C105338

If you have any concerns about our products,
you can contact us on
ProductSafety@springernature.com

In case Publisher is established outside the EU,
the EU authorized representative is:
Springer Nature Customer Service Center GmbH
Europaplatz 3, 69115 Heidelberg, Germany

Printed by Libri Plureos GmbH
in Hamburg, Germany